Clinical Hypertension

Clinical Hypertension

Edited by Jayden Miller

hayle medical

New York

Hayle Medical,
750 Third Avenue, 9th Floor,
New York, NY 10017, USA

Visit us on the World Wide Web at:
www.haylemedical.com

ISBN: 978-1-63241-552-3

Printed in China.

Cataloging-in-Publication Data

Clinical hypertension / edited by Jayden Miller.
p. cm.
Includes bibliographical references and index.
ISBN 978-1-63241-552-3
1. Hypertension. 2. Hypertension--Treatment. 3. Blood circulation disorders.
4. Cardiology. I. Miller, Jayden.
RC685.H8 C55 2019
616.132--dc23

Table of Contents

Preface

Every book is a source of knowledge and this one is no exception. The idea that led to the conceptualization of this book was the fact that the world is advancing rapidly; which makes it crucial to document the progress in every field. I am aware that a lot of data is already available, yet, there is a lot more to learn. Hence, I accepted the responsibility of editing this book and contributing my knowledge to the community.

Hypertension, also termed as high blood pressure, is a medical condition characterized by persistent elevation of blood pressure in the arteries. Hypertension that persists for a long-time is considered a major risk factor for heart failure, stroke, peripheral vascular disease, chronic kidney disease, dementia and coronary artery disease, among others. Hypertensive crisis may also occur due to severely elevated blood pressure, which can cause damage to kidney, brain, heart and lungs. Making the right lifestyle choices such as maintaining a steady and healthy weight, regular exercising, adopting a healthy diet and decreased salt intake can reduce blood pressure and prevent health complications. Hypertension usually does not cause clear identifiable symptoms and hence its identification usually occurs through screening. Physical examination involves screening for changes in the optic fundus using ophthalmoscopy. This book aims to shed light on some of the unexplored aspects of clinical hypertension and the recent researches in this field. The topics included herein are of utmost significance and bound to provide incredible insights to readers. It attempts to assist those with a goal of delving into this field.

While editing this book, I had multiple visions for it. Then I finally narrowed down to make every chapter a sole standing text explaining a particular topic, so that they can be used independently. However, the umbrella subject sinews them into a common theme. This makes the book a unique platform of knowledge.

I would like to give the major credit of this book to the experts from every corner of the world, who took the time to share their expertise with us. Also, I owe the completion of this book to the never-ending support of my family, who supported me throughout the project.

Editor

1

Modulation of miRNAs in Pulmonary Hypertension

Sudhiranjan Gupta[1,2,3] and Li Li[1,4]

[1]*Division of Molecular Cardiology, Department of Medicine, Texas A&M Health Science Center College of Medicine, Temple, TX 76504, USA*
[2]*Baylor Scott & White Health, Temple, TX 76508, USA*
[3]*Central Texas Veterans Health Care System, Temple, TX 76504, USA*
[4]*Department of Physiology and Pathophysiology, Peking University Health Science Center, Beijing 100191, China*

Correspondence should be addressed to Sudhiranjan Gupta; sgupta@medicine.tamhsc.edu

Academic Editor: Nitish R. Mahapatra

MicroRNAs (miRNAs) have emerged as a new class of posttranscriptional regulators of many cardiac and vascular diseases. They are a class of small, noncoding RNAs that contributes crucial roles typically through binding of the 3′-untranslated region of mRNA. A single miRNA may influence several signaling pathways associated with cardiac remodeling by targeting multiple genes. Pulmonary hypertension (PH) is a rare disorder characterized by progressive obliteration of pulmonary (micro) vasculature that results in elevated vascular resistance, leading to right ventricular hypertrophy (RVH) and RV failure. The pathology of PH involves vascular cell remodeling including pulmonary arterial endothelial cell (PAEC) dysfunction and pulmonary arterial smooth muscle cell (PASMC) proliferation. There is no cure for this disease. Thus, novel intervention pathways that govern PH induced RVH may result in new treatment modalities. Current therapies are limited to reverse the vascular remodeling. Recent studies have demonstrated the roles of various miRNAs in the pathogenesis of PH and pulmonary disorders. This review provides an overview of recent discoveries on the role of miRNAs in the pathogenesis of PH and discusses the potential for miRNAs as therapeutic targets and biomarkers of PH at clinical setting.

1. Introduction

Pulmonary hypertension (PH) is predominantly defined by a mean pulmonary artery pressure at rest greater than or equal to 25 mm Hg. It is an enigmatic vascular disease and the pathogenesis of PH is multifactorial of origin and, hence, is categorized as idiopathic type [1–4]. As PH develops in a wide variety of clinical circumstances and is associated with diverse histological manifestations, a classification system is developed [5, 6]. The Dana Point expert group has published a consensus of PH classification based on pathology, survival, natural history/epidemiology, etiology, and response to the treatment [5]. Among them, one of the most classical types is pulmonary arterial hypertension (PAH). PAH specifies that the disease primarily restricted to the pulmonary arterioles, a typical characteristic which shows an elevated pulmonary arterial pressure [2, 3]. The pathological consequence of PAH is the structural remodeling of pulmonary arteries (PA), where increased proliferation of pulmonary artery smooth muscle cells (PASMC) and dysfunction of pulmonary artery endothelial cells (PAEC) occur in the vascular bed [7–9]. The morphological changes consist of hypertrophy of the tunica media, multicellular vascular lesions which obstruct and obliterate pulmonary arterioles leading to intimal thickening. The obstructed vessels limit the blood flow *via* PA and increase right ventricular afterload leading to right ventricular hypertrophy (RVH) and RV dysfunction [10–12]. At molecular level, it is believed that the remodeling events in PH demand the participation of all cell-types present in the pulmonary arteries and that influence the pathological manifestation in the pulmonary vessel wall. The contributing factors that influence the remodeling process are hypoxic state, inflammation, vessel injury, and oxidative stress in the pulmonary vessels. As all forms of PH have in common

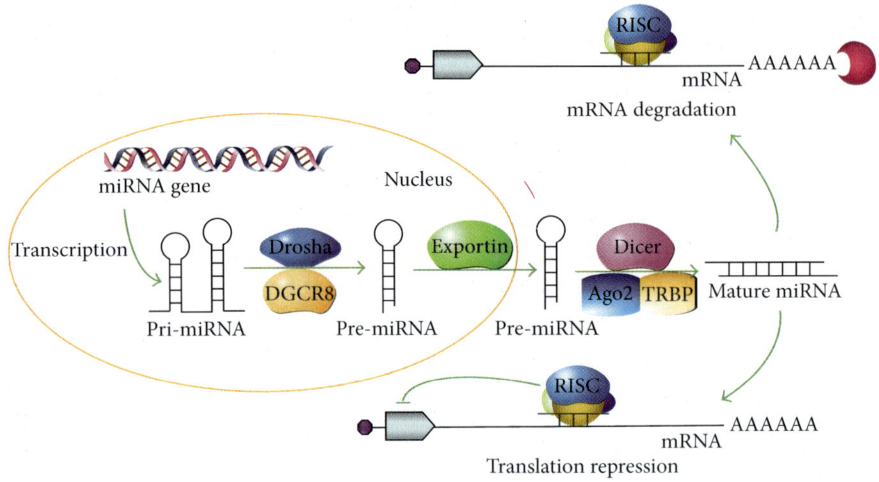

Figure 1: miRNA biogenesis. The miRNAs are transcribed by RNA polymerase II as primary transcript of miRNA (pri-miRNA). The pri-miRNA is the cleaved by RNase III enzyme, Drosha, along with several cofactors including DGCR8 and produces the stem-loop precursor miRNA (pre-miRNA). The pre-miRNA is then exported out of the nucleus by Exportin-5 to the cytoplasm. In the cytoplasm, the pre-miRNA is diced-up by Dicer resulting miRNA duplex, ~22 nucleotides long. The mature miRNA is incorporated into the RNA-induced silencing complex (RISC) which contains Argonaute (Ago) and is guided to the 3′-UTR of target mRNAs. The gene silencing is achieved by either mRNA degradation or translational repression.

an altered production of various endothelial vasoactive mediators, such as nitric oxide, prostacyclin, or endothelin- (ET-) 1, to establish the correct balance between vasoconstriction and vasodilatation [13–16]. Currently, the management for PH is aimed at optimizing cardiopulmonary interactions by targeting prostacyclin, endothelin, and nitric oxide signaling pathways [17]. The most commonly used treatment regimen of PH is the use of prostacyclin analogues (Alprostadil, Epoprostenol, Treprostinil, and Iloprost), endothelin receptor antagonists (Bosentan, Ambrisentan), and inhaled NO. In addition, phosphodiesterases (PDEs) inhibitors; PDE-3 inhibitors (e.g., Milrinone and Enoximone), and PDE-5 inhibitors (e.g., Sildenafil and Tadalafil) are used to treat PH. They were used as an alternative therapeutic strategy which targets downstream components of the NO signaling pathway by inhibiting PDE-5, the enzyme that catalyzes the conversion of cGMP to GMP. Despite the advancement of modern surgery or PH-specific therapy, the mortality of PH patients still remains high, ranging between 22.2% and 54.5% [18].

Although PH (or PAH) is well-studied encompassing both cardiac and vascular boundaries, the precise cellular and molecular mechanism of initiation and progression of PH are not completely understood and are still being explored. There is no cure of this disease and current therapies are limited to reverse the vascular remodeling. Evolving evidence indicates that dysregulation of microRNAs (miRNA or miR) contributes to PH pathogenesis [19–24]. Indeed, an emerging body of evidence demonstrates that a fine balance in miRNA levels seems to be a fundamental to maintaining homeostasis in the pulmonary vasculature and an imbalance with miRNA level playing a critical role in the pathogenesis of PH by regulating a set of targeted genes [25]. This review will collate vascular remodeling during PH, miRNA biogenesis, recent advances on miRNA modulation in PH, therapeutic opportunity, and conclusion.

2. miRNA Biogenesis

The miRNA(s) are composed of a vast family of short, noncoding RNAs (~22 nucleotide long). miRNAs are found from a single cell organism to plant and higher animals and even viruses [37–39]. In humans, more than 2,500 miRNAs have been reported in miRBase 20.0 database [40]. The biogenesis (canonical) pathway of mammalian miRNAs is a two-step enzymatic process initiated in the nucleus and then transported to cytoplasm (Figure 1). The transcription of miRNAs generally processed by RNA polymerase II (less frequently by RNA polymerase III) and are typically capped and polyadenylated [41, 42]. As a result, a long primary miRNA transcripts (pri-miRNA) containing a stem-loop structure is developed which is recognized by a large protein complex, called the Microprocessor, the main components of which are the RNase III Drosha and DiGeorge Syndrome Critical Region 8 (DGCR8) [43–48] (Figure 1). For most pri-miRNA, Drosha is contributing the cleavage process called "cropping" with the assistance of its binding partner protein, DGCR8 [41, 48, 49]. The resultant product is a ~60 nucleotides long, hairpin-structured, called precursor miRNA (pre-miRNA). DGCR8 directly interacts with the pri-miRNA stem and flanking segments, a crucial measurement for one end of the mature miRNA [45]. In addition to the canonical pathway of miRNA biogenesis described above, an alternative pathway also exists that are independent of Drosha. In alternative pathways, the miRNA can be released as mitrons (pre-miRNA like introns) [50] from pri-miRNA and proceed for miRNA processing unit without assistance of Microprocessor [50, 51].

The pre-miRNAs are actively transported from the nucleus into the cytoplasm by Exportin-5 (Exp-5) [52] (Figure 1). In the cytoplasm, another RNase III enzyme, called Dicer, catalyzing the process with the assistance of partner molecules Argonaute (Ago2), HIV-1 transactivation response RNA-binding protein (TRBP) and/or Protein activator of PKR kinase (PACT), producing a short dsRNA duplex, miRNA/miRNA* of approximately 22-nucleotide length [44, 53–56]. The miRNA/miRNA* duplexes are then incorporated into a ribonucleoprotein (RNP) complex—called miRISC (RNA-induced silencing complex)—that plays a critical role in the miRNA-mediated mechanism of gene regulation. During assembly process of the miRISC, the miRNA/miRNA* duplex is loaded into the Ago, and the strands (called the "passenger strand") are released and degraded [57]. Eventually, the bound miRNA strand (called the "guide strand") dictates miRISC to interact with partially complementary sequences in target transcripts (localized within the $3'$UTR) and primarily triggers mRNA deadenylation and degradation [58].

3. Key miRNA in the Pathogenesis of PH

MicroRNAs (miRNAs) are small, endogenously expressed noncoding RNAs that regulate gene expression at posttranscriptional level, via degradation or translational inhibition of their target mRNAs [37, 59]. miRNAs are ~22 nucleotides in length which bind to the $3'$ untranslated region of specific target genes and thereby suppress/inhibit the translation of target genes [60, 61]. miRNAs are key regulators of a wide range of cellular processes and play a pivotal role in vascular inflammation and cardiovascular pathologies inclusive of PH. From extensive studies from the past few years, it has become apparent that miRNAs are expressed in a cell- and tissue-specific manner and are critically involved in various biological processes. The degree of imbalances in their expression may lead to various diseases. Emerging evidence indicates that miRNAs contribute an important role in the maintenance of pulmonary vascular homeostasis and in the pathogenesis of PH [62]. In the following part, a discussion of the roles of miRNAs in PH-related signaling pathways is provided.

3.1. miR-21. miR-21 is a ubiquitously expressed miRNA that is traditionally considered to be an oncogenic miRNA (oncomiR). The two-channel microarray was performed to quantify miRNA expression in whole lung extracts during the development of PH or PAH caused by chronic hypoxia or monocrotaline in rats. It was suggested that miR-21 expression was downregulated in MCT-induced PH model, but not in chronic hypoxia rats. The similar change of miR-21 was observed in cultured PASMCs and PAF. miR-21 showed a similar expression level in both normoxic hypoxic cells, whereas TGF-β1, an important regulator of pulmonary vascular remodeling in PH, reduced expression of miR-21. This suggests that although hypoxia- and monocrotaline-induced PH shares some common cellular processes driving the characteristic vascular remodeling, the different pathobiology induced by hypoxia and monocrotaline may lead to the different regulation of miR-21 expression. Furthermore, the downregulation of miR-21 was confirmed in human lung tissue and serum from patients with idiopathic PH [20]. Since BMPs induce smooth muscle cell differentiation through upregulating the expression of miR-21, the downregulation of miR-21 in this setting may relate to the reduced BMP signaling and contribute to the alteration of smooth muscle cell phenotype in PH [63].

However, Yang and colleagues reported that miR-21 expression was increased in distal small pulmonary arteries of hypoxia-exposed PAH mice and levels of BMPR2, WWP1, SATB1, and YOD1, the putative miR-21 targets, were decreased in the same tissue. Transfection of miR-21 mimics also led to the reduced expression of BMPR2, SATB1, and YOD1 in PASMCs [23]. The crucial role of miR-21 in vascular pathology has been evidenced by the results that the blockade of miR-21 impeded the development of intimal hyperplasia after acute vascular injury and bleomycin-induced pulmonary fibrosis [28, 64]. Yang et al. also found that inhibition of miR-21 alleviated chronic hypoxia-induced PH and attenuated pulmonary vascular remodeling. In human PASMCs, overexpression of miR-21 promoted, whereas sequestration of miR-21 abrogated cell proliferation and the expression of cell proliferation-associated proteins. The miR-21 null mice showed an exaggerated PH response to hypoxia, suggesting a major role of miR-21 in the pathogenesis of chronic hypoxia-induced pulmonary vascular remodeling and PH [23]. Although an association between miR-21 and PH (PAH) is identified, the function of miR-21 in the development of PH is inconsistent in many experimental models. Therefore, further investigations are required to clarify the role of miR-21 in the pathogenesis of PH.

3.2. miR-204. The miR-204 appears to be the first miRNA that showed a mechanistic link between pulmonary arterial remodeling and cellular function. miR-204 was reported to be decreased in rodent lungs with hypoxia- and MCT-induced PAH and lung specimens from patients with PAH [65]. The reports suggested that STAT3 activation contributed a crucial role in regulating miR-204 in PASMC. It was further demonstrated that miR-204 inhibition increased expression of SHP2, triggered the activation of Src kinase, STAT3, and nuclear factor of activated T cells (NFAT), and thereby reduced apoptosis and was promoted proliferation of PASMCs. Finally, delivery of synthetic miR-204 mimic to the lungs lowered pulmonary artery pressure, reduced medial wall thickness, normalized levels of miR-204, SHP2, and STAT3, and alleviated the disease severity [65]. This study may indicate the safe and effective use of mimic delivery to the pulmonary vasculature for future therapeutic purpose. Interestingly, Wei et al. have identified reduced level of miR-204 in the buffy coat of human subjects may correlate with PAH severity and might serve as a circulatory biomarker for PH [66].

3.3. miR-143/145 Cluster. The miR-143/145 cluster was considered to be expressed specifically in vascular smooth muscle cells [67]. Expression of miR-143/145 was driven by TGF-β and BMP4 and induced contractile gene expression through downregulating KLF4 and myocardin [31, 68, 69]. The elevated levels of miR-145 were observed in primary PASMCs cultured from patients with BMPR2 mutations and also in the lungs of BMPR2-deficient mice, suggesting a role of BMPR2 signaling in modulating miR-145 expression [24]. Caruso and colleagues also found that miR-145 was downregulated in patient samples obtained from idiopathic and congenital PH but upregulated in plexiform lesions. The role of miR-145 in PAH was further explored and elevated expression of miR-145 was shown in the wild type mice exposed to hypoxia. miR-145 deficiency and a locked nucleic acid anti-miR-145 resulting in significant protection from hypoxia-induced PH may represent a potential therapeutic target [24].

3.4. miR-17-92 Cluster. The miR-17-92 cluster encodes seven related miRNAs, which result from the transcription of a single pre-miRNA and is further processed and cleaved to the mature miRNAs [70]. miR-17-92 cluster was retrieved as potential modulators of BMPR2 signaling by performing a computational algorithm on the BMPR2 gene. Overexpression of miR-17-92 resulted in a marked reduction of BMPR2 protein level, and BMPR2 was proved to be directly targeted by miR-17 and miR-20a by using a BMPR2 reporter in HEK293 cells. STAT3 was found to be involved in IL-6 signaling-mediated upregulation of miR-17-92 cluster and the subsequent downregulation of BMPR2, since a highly conserved STAT3-binding site exists in the promoter region of miR-17-92 gene [71].

The role of a cholesterol-modified antagomir to miR-20a in hypoxia-induced PH was explored by Brock et al. miR-20a restored functional BMPR2 signaling in human PASMCs and intraperitoneal administration of anti-miR-20a increased BMPR2 levels and alleviated vascular remodeling in lung tissue of hypoxic mice [72]. Antagomirs to miR-17 and miR-92a reduced muscularization of pulmonary arteries in the hypoxic mouse and monocrotaline rat models of PH, but only anti-miR-17 decreased RVSP and parameters of right heart dysfunction [22].

3.5. miR-130/301. Bertero and colleagues identified miR-130/301 family as a master regulator of cellular proliferation in PH by constructing *in silico* a network of genes and interactions based on curated seed genes with known importance in PH. miR-130/301 expression was found to be increased in lungs of mice suffering from PH induced by SU5416 administration with chronic hypoxia, in lungs of rats with MCT-induced PH and in lungs of juvenile sheep with shunt-induced PH. In both human PAECs and PASMCs, multiple PH inducers, including hypoxia, IL-1β, and IL-6, increased miR-130/301 expression and hypoxia was found to upregulate miR-130/301 *via* a dependence on HIF-2α and POU5F1/OCT4. It was further validated that miR-130/301 modulated apelin-miR-424/503-FGF2 signaling in PAECs and miR-130/301-PPAR-γ axis controlled proliferation of PASMCs by increasing STAT3 expression and activity and repressing miR-204 expression. In hypoxia-induced PH mouse model, induction of miR-130/301 was promoted while miR-130/301 inhibition prevented PH pathogenesis [73].

4. miRNA in PASMCs Plasticity in PH

PH is broadly considered to be a vascular disease as vasoconstriction in the pulmonary artery is a prime cause for the development of PH. The hyperproliferation of pulmonary vascular cells (mainly VSMC) and subsequent neointima formation in the small PAs are hallmark in PH. On the other hand, pulmonary arterial endothelial cells (PAECs) further contribute a critical role in vascular homeostatic balance in the pulmonary vascular bed by orchestrating the vessel tone, leucocytes trafficking, and so forth [74, 75]. Another cell type called adventitial fibroblasts also participate a critical role in PH [76]. Proliferation of fibroblasts is reported in hypoxia-induced PH that plays a role in adventitial thickening [77, 78]. Under pathological situation like PH (PAH), the endothelium becomes dysfunctional which allows the penetration of infiltrating molecules, increased leucocytes adhesion, getting resistant to apoptosis that result in severe remodeling in the pulmonary vessels. These infiltrating molecules invade the barrier of neighboring cells like smooth muscle cells and activating the resident of adventitious fibroblasts. The remodeling process is basically an interaction between these cell-types present in the pulmonary arterial layers that resulting in a marked histological change in the pulmonary vasculature [75]. An emerging body of evidences suggests that the miRNAs play a pivotal role in the vascular cell integrity and plasticity during the progression of PH. Here, we assemble those miRNAs that participate in vascular remodeling in PH.

Although identification of miRNAs in vascular diseases like PH is relatively new, but the earliest association connecting VSMC remodeling with miRNAs was reported in 2007. Ji et al. described the miRNA signature in the vascular wall of balloon-injured carotid artery rat model [64]. They showed that miR-21 was upregulated and the cellular effects were targeted by PTEN and Bcl_2 for neointimal lesion formation [64]. The initial studies of miR-21 in vascular remodeling were followed by series of milestone works that include miR-143/145 cluster [24, 31, 79–83]. Two of the key miRNAs involved in regulation of the phenotype of SMCs are miR-143 and miR-145. miR-145 is transcribed bicistronically along with miR-143 from human chromosome 5 [24]. With relevance to PAH, downregulation of miR-145 is associated with increased proliferation of neointimal cells [31]. Downregulation of target genes klf4 and klf5 by activation of miR-143/miR-145 upregulates SMC-specific genes such as SMA, calponin, and SM22-α, triggering differentiation and lowering the proliferation rates in vascular SMCs [31, 82]. Another miRNA, miR-221/222 that triggers PDGF signaling in VSMC is thought to contribute in neointimal proliferation [35, 84, 85]. It is demonstrated that inhibition of miR-221 prevented PDGF induced proliferation, while forced expression of miR-221 increased proliferation and reduced the expression of VSMC marker [35, 84].

Table 1: Vascular smooth muscle cells and miRNA modulation.

miRNA	Function	Target gene(s)	Reference
miR-1	Promote VSMC differentiation	Myocardin, KLF4	[26, 27]
miR-21	Promote VSMC differentiation	PDCD4	[28]
miR-24	VSMC proliferation and repression of contractile gene expression	Tribbles-like protein 3, SMURF1	[29]
miR-26a	Promote VSMC dedifferentiation	Smad1 and Smad4	[30]
miR-143/145	Promote VSMC differentiation	KLF4, KLF5, ELK1, versican, BMP4, MRTF	[31–33]
miR-146	Promote VSMC dedifferentiation and proliferation	KLF4	[34]
miR-221/222	Promote VSMC dedifferentiation and proliferation	p27Kip, c-kit	[35, 36]

In addition to the above miRNAs, other miRNAs are reported to regulate SMC gene expression in hypoxia-induced PH. They included miR-210, miR-124, miR-204, and miR-138. It is demonstrated that miR-210 that acts as a hypoxia-inducible miRNA both *in vitro* and *in vivo*, inhibits PASMC apoptosis in hypoxia by specifically repressing E2F3 [86]. A cell-based high throughput screening of a human miRNA library with the NFAT luciferase reporter system identified miR-124 as a new candidate in PH. It showed decreased NFAT reporter activity and, decreased dephosphorylation and the nuclear translocation of NFAT [87]. An elegant study by Courboulin et al. demonstrated that miR-204 downregulation correlates with PH severity and responsible for proliferative and antiapoptotic phenotypes of PH-PASMCs targeting STAT3 and NFATc [65]. Interestingly, a recent study showed that a serine/threonine kinase Mst1, a modulator of cell death, appears to be a target of miR-138 [88]. The authors suggest that miR-138 may be a negative regulator of PASMC apoptosis in hypoxic mediated PAH. A panel of miRNAs which are shown to modulate SMC fate and modulation are listed in Table 1 [26–36].

5. miRNA as Therapeutic Target for PH

Therapeutic target which defines the treatment of a disease by means of a well-defined biological molecule. In this regard, miRNAs, a "tiny" RNA molecule, have become an important gene modulator of various biochemical, physiological, and cellular functions. As we observed that either deficiency or abundance of a specific miRNA or cluster of miRNAs contributed a pathological state of many cardiovascular diseases including PH, it is reasonable to accept those miRNAs as therapeutic target for diagnosis and therapeutic intervention. This is because we can utilize ability of a single miRNA to control the expression of multiple (hundreds) proteins suggest that changes of a single miRNA may influence several signaling pathways associated with pathological disease state. While each target is regulated subtly, the additive effect of coordinated regulation of a large suite of transcripts is believed to result in strong phenotypic outputs. Several animal models in diverse disease pathology showed usefulness of miRNAs as target molecules for therapeutic benefit; this review will focus on vascular remodeling associated with PH. At therapeutic strategic stand-point, the aberrant miRNA expression can be modulated or restored to normal by two main approaches: an anti-miRNA (anti-miR) and miRNA mimic. The former can be applicable to those miRNAs whose expressions were increased in disease pathology and, therefore, silencing or inhibiting will be beneficial. To modulate miRNA expression, the current strategy utilized chemically modified, cholesterol-conjugated single-stranded RNA analogues complementary to the mature miRNAs for antagomir or mimics, respectively [89]. Synthetic modified oligonucleotides are currently used as potential "antagomirs" for miRNA silencing [90]. An elegant work demonstrated by Liu et al. in a balloon-injury model represents a successful knocking down of miR-221/222 that suppressed VSMC proliferation and neointimal lesion formation [35]. Recently, Brock et al. have shown that treatment with antagomiR-20a restores the levels of BMPR2 in pulmonary arteries and prevents vascular remodeling in hypoxia-induced PAH [72]. For downregulated miRNAs, a mimic approach is generally undertaken which basically rescued the underexpressed miRNA in the tissue under pathological situation [89]. This strategy is sometimes referred to as miRNA replacement as it reintroduced the similar depleted miRNA those were downregulated during diseases progression. Therefore, by introducing the miRNA "mimic," the cells can restore the function as the miRNA "mimic" is expected to target the same set of mRNAs that is also regulated by the endogenous miRNA. In a very comprehensive study by Courboulin et al., they demonstrated that reestablishing of miR-204 level by delivery of synthetic miR-204 into the lungs of experimentally-induced PAH animals significantly reduced the disease pathology [65].

Although the miRNA-based intervention is attractive and seems to be feasible, however, several challenges are noted. First, the critical miRNAs responsible for PH must be confirmed definitively in well-accepted animal models along with explanted human PAH samples, biopsies, and so forth, second, the cellular, molecular and physiological function of these miRNAs should be performed in diseases progression and prevention; third, the delivery route should be precisely targeted or restricted to lung vascular cells, for example, PAEC, PASMC, or fibroblasts. This will minimize the off-target effects on the neighboring cells. Finally, the dose of antagomir or mimic delivery to the vascular bed should be carefully monitored further to avoid off-target effects. Therefore, our future direction should be focus of vascular cell-specific delivery of miRNA mimic or inhibitors. Additionally, a regulated release of miRNAs by conjugating nanoparticle will be considered for long-term use.

Finally, miRNA-mediated therapeutics can be achieved by inhalation which may reduce the potential off-target issues to the other organs.

6. Can Circulatory miRNA Be Used as a Biomarker in PH?

Biomarker generally refers to measurable substance in biological state. At clinical stand-point, it is extremely important as it predicts the "medical" outcome of a disease and its progression. Over the past few years, it has been demonstrated that miRNAs are found in the blood, plasma, urine, platelets, and saliva in a surprisingly stable form [91–97]. The stability of miRNA in the extracellular environment offers a great opportunity to consider as "biomarker" at clinical settings. Using miRNA as a "biomarker" offers many advantages like early prediction of diseases, differential expression during disease progression/pathologies, high degree of specificity, and sensitivity and importantly having longer half-life in the system. Accumulating evidence suggested that the stability of miRNA in extracellular environment illustrated by packed with lipid vesicles, wrapped in protein or lipoprotein complexes [98–100]. In the context of cardiac diseases that include myocardial infarction, hypertrophy and heart failure; several miRNAs are identified and predicted to be considered as "biomarker" [101–104].

The miRNAs are circulating freely in the mammalian blood and can be predicted as "biomarker" for early diagnosis of cardiovascular diseases in humans [102, 105–108]. Several evidences indicate that miRNAs are secreted as micro vesicles or exosome and apoptotic bodies that may be responsible for release the miRNAs into the circulation [109–112] and are extremely stable in the blood or serum [91]. Rhodes and colleagues measured plasma levels of miRNAs in eight patients newly diagnosed with PAH and eight healthy controls by use of microarray analysis. Fifty-eight miRNAs showed differences in plasma concentration between the two groups and miR-150 was largest downregulated in PAH. Reduced expression of miR-150 predicted 2-year survival and correlated with disease severity. The miR-150 level was also found to be significantly reduced in circulating microvesicles and lymphocytes from patients with PAH [113]. Courboulin et al. reported that downregulation of miR-204 in buffy-coat cells correlated with PAH severity and might serve as a circulatory biomarker of PAH [65]. On the contrary, increasing higher plasma levels of miR-130/301 family members were observed in patients with increasing hemodynamic severity of PH [73].

Our previous study detected the pattern of miRNAs in buffy-coat samples from mild-to-severe human PH subjects compared with the control subjects by miRNA array. Our study revealed that moderate to severe PH in human subjects are associated with significant downregulation of plasma levels of circulatory miR-1, miR-26a, and miR-29c. The kinetics of the changes differed from moderate to severe PH human subjects as we observed further downregulation of the above miRNAs in severe PH. We also found a set of upregulated miRNA in the circulation of PH subjects. miR-21, miR-23b, miR-130a, miR-491, and miR-1246 were moderately upregulated in moderate PH subjects and were more pronounced in severe PH. Another set of miRNAs that include miR-133b, miR-204, and miR-208b were significantly upregulated in all moderate PH subjects and showed further increment in severe PH subjects [66]. Our study provided the evidence for the first time that circulating miRNAs in the setting of PH may be used as early detection parameters for PH. Nevertheless, the data presented were based on limited study population and the results need to be confirmed in a larger cohort study. Furthermore, the dysregulation miRNA in PH remains to be tested whether these circulatory miRNAs have any influence in the target genes.

Circulatory miRNAs are considered to be novel promising biomarkers for detection of PH. However, at current stage, using circulatory miRNA as diagnostic tool for detecting PH is still in its infancy. The key advantage of circulating miRNAs is a noninvasive testing procedure and relies on the stability of miRNAs in the circulation and their storage condition. We give credit to the concept of quick determination of secretory molecules (miRNAs) in the blood; but the importance of miRNA must be reevaluated at the clinical setting or model at multiple laboratories. Another limitation is the small number of cohort study which appears to be heterogeneous clinical sample-type. These points may consider as preliminary-type of observation and need further confirmatory studies for considering miRNAs as biomarkers for clinical use.

7. Conclusion

Understanding of miRNAs role and function in the pulmonary circulation will offer and contribute a great potential to the pathogenesis of PH or PAH. The miRNA signature can be used as a diagnostic tool for the development of therapeutic strategy. The characterization of these miRNAs under various experimental settings (*in vitro* and *in vivo*) should be performed along with the human subjects. The outcome will validate both physiological and pathological roles of these miRNAs during the development and progression of PH prior to consider them for therapeutic intervention or future clinical trials. Furthermore, use of disease specific mouse models, conditional transgenic, and knockouts are necessary to elucidate the functional role *in vivo* and verify its therapeutic potential, both of which remain largely unexplored. More novel approaches such as combination of Argonaute protein immunoprecipitation, deep sequencing, or proteomic profiling approaches are required to identify its potential *bona fide* targets responsible for its functional impact.

Acknowledgments

The authors acknowledge the Central Texas Veterans Affairs Health Care System for providing the research facility to complete this work. This study was partly supported by start-up funds from the Texas A&M Health Science Center College of Medicine and by the American Heart Association-Grant-in-Aid (14 GRNT 20490320) to S. Gupta (SG).

References

[1] M. Humbert, D. Montani, O. V. Evgenov, and G. Simonneau, "Definition and classification of pulmonary hypertension," *Handbook of Experimental Pharmacology*, vol. 218, pp. 3–29, 2013.

[2] C. Guignabert and P. Dorfmuller, "Pathology and pathobiology of pulmonary hypertension," *Seminars in Respiratory and Critical Care Medicine*, vol. 34, no. 5, pp. 551–559, 2013.

[3] R. M. Tuder, E. Stacher, J. Robinson, R. Kumar, and B. B. Graham, "Pathology of pulmonary hypertension," *Clinics in Chest Medicine*, vol. 34, no. 4, pp. 639–650, 2013.

[4] B. A. Maron and J. Loscalzo, "Pulmonary hypertension: pathophysiology and signaling pathways," *Handbook of Experimental Pharmacology*, vol. 218, pp. 31–58, 2013.

[5] "New developments in pulmonary hypertension/pulmonary arterial hypertension. Proceedings of Pulmonary Hypertension UP2DATE 2008—post Dana Point. March 14-15, 2008. Munich, Germany," *Deutsche Medizinische Wochenschrift*, vol. 133, supplement 6, pp. S165–S218, 2008.

[6] G. Simonneau, I. M. Robbins, M. Beghetti et al., "Updated clinical classification of pulmonary hypertension," *Journal of the American College of Cardiology*, vol. 54, no. 1, supplement, pp. S43–S54, 2009.

[7] M. Humbert, N. W. Morrell, S. L. Archer et al., "Cellular and molecular pathobiology of pulmonary arterial hypertension," *Journal of the American College of Cardiology*, vol. 43, no. 12, supplement S, pp. 13S–24S, 2004.

[8] A. Shifren, A. G. Durmowicz, R. H. Knutsen, G. Faury, and R. P. Mecham, "Elastin insufficiency predisposes to elevated pulmonary circulatory pressures through changes in elastic artery structure," *Journal of Applied Physiology*, vol. 105, no. 5, pp. 1610–1619, 2008.

[9] L. A. Shimoda and S. S. Laurie, "Vascular remodeling in pulmonary hypertension," *Journal of Molecular Medicine*, vol. 91, no. 3, pp. 297–309, 2013.

[10] A. Vonk-Noordegraaf, F. Haddad, K. M. Chin et al., "Right heart adaptation to pulmonary arterial hypertension: physiology and pathobiology," *Journal of the American College of Cardiology*, vol. 62, no. 25, supplement, pp. D22–D33, 2013.

[11] V. Franco, "Right ventricular remodeling in pulmonary hypertension," *Heart Failure Clinics*, vol. 8, no. 3, pp. 403–412, 2012.

[12] T. G. di Salvo, "Pulmonary hypertension and right ventricular failure in left ventricular systolic dysfunction," *Current Opinion in Cardiology*, vol. 27, no. 3, pp. 262–272, 2012.

[13] L. R. Frumkin, "The pharmacological treatment of pulmonary arterial hypertension," *Pharmacological Reviews*, vol. 64, no. 3, pp. 583–620, 2012.

[14] R. Nogueira-Ferreira and T. Henriques-Coelho, "Cellular interplay in pulmonary arterial hypertension: implications for new therapies," *Biochimica et Biophysica Acta—Molecular Cell Research*, vol. 1843, no. 5, pp. 885–893, 2014.

[15] S. S. Pullamsetti, R. Schermuly, A. Ghofrani, N. Weissmann, F. Grimminger, and W. Seeger, "Novel and emerging therapies for pulmonary hypertension," *The American Journal of Respiratory and Critical Care Medicine*, vol. 189, no. 4, pp. 394–400, 2014.

[16] A. Seferian and G. Simonneau, "Therapies for pulmonary arterial hypertension: where are we today, where do we go tomorrow?" *European Respiratory Review*, vol. 22, no. 129, pp. 217–226, 2013.

[17] N. Brunner, V. A. de Jesus Perez, A. Richter et al., "Perioperative pharmacological management of pulmonary hypertensive crisis during congenital heart surgery," *Pulmonary Circulation*, vol. 4, no. 1, pp. 10–24, 2014.

[18] L. Lindberg, A. K. Olsson, P. Jögi, and C. Jonmarker, "How common is severe pulmonary hypertension after pediatric cardiac surgery?" *Journal of Thoracic and Cardiovascular Surgery*, vol. 123, no. 6, pp. 1155–1163, 2002.

[19] Y. Wang, X.-Y. Xue, Y.-X. Liu et al., "Pulmonary arterial hypertension and MicroRNAs-an ever-growing partnership," *Archives of Medical Research*, vol. 44, no. 7, pp. 483–487, 2013.

[20] P. Caruso, M. R. MacLean, R. Khanin et al., "Dynamic changes in lung microRNA profiles during the development of pulmonary hypertension due to chronic hypoxia and monocrotaline," *Arteriosclerosis, Thrombosis, and Vascular Biology*, vol. 30, no. 4, pp. 716–723, 2010.

[21] K. M. Drake, D. Zygmunt, L. Mavrakis et al., "Altered MicroRNA processing in heritable pulmonary arterial hypertension: an important role for Smad-8," *The American Journal of Respiratory and Critical Care Medicine*, vol. 184, no. 12, pp. 1400–1408, 2011.

[22] S. S. Pullamsetti, C. Doebele, A. Fischer et al., "Inhibition of microRNA-17 improves lung and heart function in experimental pulmonary hypertension," *American Journal of Respiratory and Critical Care Medicine*, vol. 185, no. 4, pp. 409–419, 2012.

[23] S. Yang, S. Banerjee, A. de Freitas et al., "miR-21 regulates chronic hypoxia-induced pulmonary vascular remodeling," *The American Journal of Physiology—Lung Cellular and Molecular Physiology*, vol. 302, no. 6, pp. L521–L529, 2012.

[24] P. Caruso, Y. Dempsie, H. C. Stevens et al., "A role for miR-145 in pulmonary arterial hypertension: evidence from mouse models and patient samples," *Circulation Research*, vol. 111, no. 3, pp. 290–300, 2012.

[25] A. Lee, D. McLean, J. Choi, H. Kang, W. Chang, and J. Kim, "Therapeutic implications of microRNAs in pulmonary arterial hypertension," *BMB Reports*, vol. 47, no. 6, pp. 311–317, 2014.

[26] D. Z. Wang and X. L. Zheng, "Induction of microRNA-1 by myocardin in smooth muscle cells inhibits cell proliferation," *Arteriosclerosis, Thrombosis, and Vascular Biology*, vol. 31, no. 2, pp. 368–375, 2011.

[27] C. Xie, H. Huang, X. Sun et al., "MicroRNA-1 regulates smooth muscle cell differentiation by repressing kruppel-like factor 4," *Stem Cells and Development*, vol. 20, no. 2, pp. 205–210, 2011.

[28] G. Liu, A. Friggeri, Y. Yang et al., "miR-21 mediates fibrogenic activation of pulmonary fibroblasts and lung fibrosis," *The Journal of Experimental Medicine*, vol. 207, no. 8, pp. 1589–1597, 2010.

[29] M. C. Chan, A. C. Hilyard, C. Wu et al., "Molecular basis for antagonism between PDGF and the TGFβ family of signalling pathways by control of miR-24 expression," *The EMBO Journal*, vol. 29, no. 3, pp. 559–573, 2010.

[30] N. J. Leeper, A. Raiesdana, Y. Kojima et al., "MicroRNA-26a is a novel regulator of vascular smooth muscle cell function," *Journal of Cellular Physiology*, vol. 226, no. 4, pp. 1035–1043, 2011.

[31] Y. Cheng, X. Liu, J. Yang et al., "MicroRNA-145, a novel smooth muscle cell phenotypic marker and modulator, controls

vascular neointimal lesion formation," *Circulation Research*, vol. 105, no. 2, pp. 158–166, 2009.

[32] K. R. Cordes, N. T. Sheehy, M. P. White et al., "MiR-145 and miR-143 regulate smooth muscle cell fate and plasticity," *Nature*, vol. 460, no. 7256, pp. 705–710, 2009.

[33] T. Boettger, N. Beetz, S. Kostin et al., "Acquisition of the contractile phenotype by murine arterial smooth muscle cells depends on the *Mir143/145* gene cluster," *The Journal of Clinical Investigation*, vol. 119, no. 9, pp. 2634–2647, 2009.

[34] S. G. Sun, B. Zheng, M. Han et al., "MiR-146a and Krüppel-like factor 4 form a feedback loop to participate in vascular smooth muscle cell proliferation," *EMBO Reports*, vol. 12, no. 1, pp. 56–62, 2011.

[35] X. Liu, Y. Cheng, S. Zhang, Y. Lin, J. Yang, and C. Zhang, "A Necessary role of miR-221 and miR-222 in vascular smooth muscle cell proliferation and neointimal hyperplasia," *Circulation Research*, vol. 104, no. 4, pp. 476–486, 2009.

[36] C. Le Sage, R. Nagel, D. A. Egan et al., "Regulation of the p27Kip1 tumor suppressor by miR-221 and miR-222 promotes cancer cell proliferation," *EMBO Journal*, vol. 26, no. 15, pp. 3699–3708, 2007.

[37] D. P. Bartel, "MicroRNAs: genomics, biogenesis, mechanism, and functio," *Cell*, vol. 116, no. 2, pp. 281–297, 2004.

[38] R. W. Carthew and E. J. Sontheimer, "Origins and Mechanisms of miRNAs and siRNAs," *Cell*, vol. 136, no. 4, pp. 642–655, 2009.

[39] M. K. Meshesha, I. Veksler-Lublinsky, O. Isakov et al., "The microRNA transcriptome of human cytomegalovirus (HCMV)," *The Open Virology Journal*, vol. 6, pp. 38–48, 2012.

[40] A. Kozomara and S. Griffiths-Jones, "MiRBase: integrating microRNA annotation and deep-sequencing data," *Nucleic Acids Research*, vol. 39, no. 1, pp. D152–D157, 2011.

[41] V. N. Kim, "MicroRNA biogenesis: coordinated cropping and dicing," *Nature Reviews Molecular Cell Biology*, vol. 6, no. 5, pp. 376–385, 2005.

[42] X. Cai, C. H. Hagedorn, and B. R. Cullen, "Human microRNAs are processed from capped, polyadenylated transcripts that can also function as mRNAs," *RNA*, vol. 10, no. 12, pp. 1957–1966, 2004.

[43] R. I. Gregory, K.-P. Yan, G. Amuthan et al., "The Microprocessor complex mediates the genesis of microRNAs," *Nature*, vol. 432, no. 7014, pp. 235–240, 2004.

[44] A. Stroynowska-Czerwinska, A. Fiszer, and W. J. Krzyzosiak, "The panorama of miRNA-mediated mechanisms in mammalian cells," *Cellular and Molecular Life Sciences*, vol. 71, no. 12, pp. 2253–2270, 2014.

[45] J. Han, Y. Lee, K.-H. Yeom, Y.-K. Kim, H. Jin, and V. N. Kim, "The Drosha-DGCR8 complex in primary microRNA processing," *Genes and Development*, vol. 18, no. 24, pp. 3016–3027, 2004.

[46] M. Morlando, M. Ballarino, N. Gromak, F. Pagano, I. Bozzoni, and N. J. Proudfoot, "Primary microRNA transcripts are processed co-transcriptionally," *Nature Structural and Molecular Biology*, vol. 15, no. 9, pp. 902–909, 2008.

[47] J. Bauersachs and T. Thum, "Biogenesis and regulation of cardiovascular MicroRNAs," *Circulation Research*, vol. 109, no. 3, pp. 334–347, 2011.

[48] Y. K. Kim and V. N. Kim, "Processing of intronic microRNAs," *The EMBO Journal*, vol. 26, no. 3, pp. 775–783, 2007.

[49] Y. Lee, C. Ahn, J. Han et al., "The nuclear RNase III Drosha initiates microRNA processing," *Nature*, vol. 425, no. 6956, pp. 415–419, 2003.

[50] E. Berezikov, W.-J. Chung, J. Willis, E. Cuppen, and E. C. Lai, "Mammalian mirtron genes," *Molecular Cell*, vol. 28, no. 2, pp. 328–336, 2007.

[51] S. Cheloufi, C. O. Dos Santos, M. M. W. Chong, and G. J. Hannon, "A dicer-independent miRNA biogenesis pathway that requires Ago catalysis," *Nature*, vol. 465, no. 7298, pp. 584–589, 2010.

[52] R. Yi, Y. Qin, I. G. Macara, and B. R. Cullen, "Exportin-5 mediates the nuclear export of pre-microRNAs and short hairpin RNAs," *Genes and Development*, vol. 17, no. 24, pp. 3011–3016, 2003.

[53] T. P. Chendrimada, R. I. Gregory, E. Kumaraswamy et al., "TRBP recruits the Dicer complex to Ago2 for microRNA processing and gene silencing," *Nature*, vol. 436, no. 7051, pp. 740–744, 2005.

[54] K. H. Kok, M.-H. J. Ng, Y.-P. Ching, and D.-Y. Jin, "Human TRBP and PACT directly interact with each other and associate with dicer to facilitate the production of small interfering RNA," *The Journal of Biological Chemistry*, vol. 282, no. 24, pp. 17649–17657, 2007.

[55] E. Koscianska, J. Starega-Roslan, and W. J. Krzyzosiak, "The role of dicer protein partners in the processing of microRNA precursors," *PLoS ONE*, vol. 6, no. 12, Article ID e28548, 2011.

[56] E. Bernstein, A. A. Caudy, S. M. Hammond, and G. J. Hannon, "Role for a bidentate ribonuclease in the initiation step of RNA interference," *Nature*, vol. 409, no. 6818, pp. 363–366, 2001.

[57] G. Meister, "Argonaute proteins: Functional insights and emerging roles," *Nature Reviews Genetics*, vol. 14, no. 7, pp. 447–459, 2013.

[58] A. Lingel, B. Simon, E. Izaurralde, and M. Sattler, "Nucleic acid 3′-end recognition by the Argonaute2 PAZ domain," *Nature Structural and Molecular Biology*, vol. 11, no. 6, pp. 576–577, 2004.

[59] D. S. Schwarz, G. Hutvágner, T. Du, Z. Xu, N. Aronin, and P. D. Zamore, "Asymmetry in the assembly of the RNAi enzyme complex," *Cell*, vol. 115, no. 2, pp. 199–208, 2003.

[60] D. Baek, J. Villén, C. Shin, F. D. Camargo, S. P. Gygi, and D. P. Bartel, "The impact of microRNAs on protein output," *Nature*, vol. 455, no. 7209, pp. 64–71, 2008.

[61] M. Selbach, B. Schwanhäusser, N. Thierfelder, Z. Fang, R. Khanin, and N. Rajewsky, "Widespread changes in protein synthesis induced by microRNAs," *Nature*, vol. 455, no. 7209, pp. 58–63, 2008.

[62] J. Kim, Y. Kang, Y. Kojima et al., "An endothelial apelin-FGF link mediated by miR-424 and miR-503 is disrupted in pulmonary arterial hypertension," *Nature Medicine*, vol. 19, no. 1, pp. 74–82, 2013.

[63] B. N. Davis, A. C. Hilyard, G. Lagna, and A. Hata, "SMAD proteins control DROSHA-mediated microRNA maturation," *Nature*, vol. 454, no. 7200, pp. 56–61, 2008.

[64] R. Ji, Y. Cheng, J. Yue et al., "MicroRNA expression signature and antisense-mediated depletion reveal an essential role of MicroRNA in vascular neointimal lesion formation," *Circulation Research*, vol. 100, no. 11, pp. 1579–1588, 2007.

[65] A. Courboulin, R. Paulin, N. J. Giguère et al., "Role for miR-204 in human pulmonary arterial hypertension," *The Journal of Experimental Medicine*, vol. 208, no. 3, pp. 535–548, 2011.

[66] C. Wei, H. Henderson, C. Spradley et al., "Circulating miRNAs as potential marker for pulmonary hypertension," *PLoS ONE*, vol. 8, no. 5, Article ID e64396, 2013.

[67] C. L. Bockmeyer, L. Maegel, S. Janciauskiene et al., "Plexiform vasculopathy of severe pulmonary arterial hypertension and microRNA expression," *Journal of Heart and Lung Transplantation*, vol. 31, no. 7, pp. 764–772, 2012.

[68] B. N. Davis-Dusenbery, M. C. Chan, K. E. Reno et al., "Down-regulation of Krüppel-like Factor-4 (KLF4) by microRNA-143/145 is critical for modulation of vascular smooth muscle cell phenotype by transforming growth factor-β and bone morphogenetic protein 4," *Journal of Biological Chemistry*, vol. 286, no. 32, pp. 28097–28110, 2011.

[69] X. Long and J. M. Miano, "Transforming growth factor-β1 (TGF-β1) utilizes distinct pathways for the transcriptional activation of microRNA 143/145 in human coronary artery smooth muscle cells," *Journal of Biological Chemistry*, vol. 286, no. 34, pp. 30119–30129, 2011.

[70] V. Pospisil, K. Vargova, J. Kokavec et al., "Epigenetic silencing of the oncogenic miR-17-92 cluster during PU.1-directed macrophage differentiation," *The EMBO Journal*, vol. 30, no. 21, pp. 4450–4464, 2011.

[71] M. Brock, M. Trenkmann, R. E. Gay et al., "Interleukin-6 modulates the expression of the bone morphogenic protein receptor type ii through a novel STAT3-microRNA cluster 17/92 pathway," *Circulation Research*, vol. 104, no. 10, pp. 1184–1191, 2009.

[72] M. Brock, V. J. Samillan, M. Trenkmann et al., "AntagomiR directed against miR-20a restores functional BMPR2 signalling and prevents vascular remodelling in hypoxia-induced pulmonary hypertension," *European Heart Journal*, vol. 35, no. 45, pp. 3203–3211, 2014.

[73] T. Bertero, Y. Lu, and S. Annis, "Systems-level regulation of microRNA networks by miR-130/301 promotes pulmonary hypertension," *Journal of Clinical Investigation*, vol. 124, no. 8, pp. 3514–3528, 2014.

[74] G. G. Pietra, F. Capron, S. Stewart et al., "Pathologic assessment of vasculopathies in pulmonary hypertension," *Journal of the American College of Cardiology*, vol. 43, no. 12, supplement S, pp. 25S–32S, 2004.

[75] K. Abe, M. Toba, A. Alzoubi et al., "Formation of plexiform lesions in experimental severe pulmonary arterial hypertension," *Circulation*, vol. 121, no. 25, pp. 2747–2754, 2010.

[76] K. R. Stenmark, N. Davie, M. Frid, E. Gerasimovskaya, and M. Das, "Role of the adventitia in pulmonary vascular remodeling," *Physiology*, vol. 21, no. 2, pp. 134–145, 2006.

[77] M. Das, E. C. Dempsey, J. T. Reeves, and K. R. Stenmark, "Selective expansion of fibroblast subpopulations from pulmonary artery adventitia in response to hypoxia," *The American Journal of Physiology—Lung Cellular and Molecular Physiology*, vol. 282, no. 5, pp. L976–L986, 2002.

[78] K. R. Stenmark, D. Bouchey, R. Nemenoff, E. C. Dempsey, and M. Das, "Hypoxia-induced pulmonary vascular remodeling: contribution of the adventitial fibroblasts," *Physiological Research*, vol. 49, no. 5, pp. 503–517, 2000.

[79] G. Lagna, M. M. Ku, P. H. Nguyen, N. A. Neuman, B. N. Davis, and A. Hata, "Control of phenotypic plasticity of smooth muscle cells by bone morphogenetic protein signaling through the myocardin-related transcription factors," *The Journal of Biological Chemistry*, vol. 282, no. 51, pp. 37244–37255, 2007.

[80] A. Y. Rangrez, Z. A. Massy, V. M.-L. Meuth, and L. Metzinger, "MiR-143 and miR-145 molecular keys to switch the phenotype of vascular smooth muscle cells," *Circulation: Cardiovascular Genetics*, vol. 4, no. 2, pp. 197–205, 2011.

[81] M. Xin, E. M. Small, L. B. Sutherland et al., "MicroRNAs miR-143 and miR-145 modulate cytoskeletal dynamics and responsiveness of smooth muscle cells to injury," *Genes and Development*, vol. 23, no. 18, pp. 2166–2178, 2009.

[82] K. R. Cordes, N. T. Sheehy, M. P. White et al., "miR-145 and miR-143 regulate smooth muscle cell fate and plasticity," *Nature*, vol. 460, no. 7256, pp. 705–710, 2009.

[83] L. Elia, M. Quintavalle, J. Zhang et al., "The knockout of miR-143 and -145 alters smooth muscle cell maintenance and vascular homeostasis in mice: correlates with human disease," *Cell Death and Differentiation*, vol. 16, no. 12, pp. 1590–1598, 2009.

[84] B. N. Davis, A. C. Hilyard, P. H. Nguyen, G. Lagna, and A. Hata, "Induction of MicroRNA-221 by platelet-derived growth factor signaling is critical for modulation of vascular smooth muscle phenotype," *Journal of Biological Chemistry*, vol. 284, no. 6, pp. 3728–3738, 2009.

[85] S. Albinsson and W. C. Sessa, "Can microRNAs control vascular smooth muscle phenotypic modulation and the response to injury?" *Physiological Genomics*, vol. 43, no. 10, pp. 529–533, 2011.

[86] D. Gou, R. Ramchandran, X. Peng et al., "Mir-210 has an antiapoptotic effect in pulmonary artery smooth muscle cells during hypoxia," *The American Journal of Physiology—Lung Cellular and Molecular Physiology*, vol. 303, no. 8, pp. L682–L691, 2012.

[87] K. Kang, X. Peng, X. Zhang et al., "MicroRNA-124 suppresses the transactivation of nuclear factor of activated T cells by targeting multiple genes and inhibits the proliferation of pulmonary artery smooth muscle cells," *Journal of Biological Chemistry*, vol. 288, no. 35, pp. 25414–25427, 2013.

[88] S. Li, Y. Ran, D. Zhang, J. Chen, and D. Zhu, "MicroRNA-138 plays a role in hypoxic pulmonary vascular remodeling by targeting Mst1," *Biochemical Journal*, vol. 452, no. 2, pp. 281–291, 2013.

[89] J. Weiler, J. Hunziker, and J. Hall, "Anti-miRNA oligonucleotides (AMOs): ammunition to target miRNAs implicated in human disease?" *Gene Therapy*, vol. 13, no. 6, pp. 496–502, 2006.

[90] J. Krützfeldt, N. Rajewsky, R. Braich et al., "Silencing of microRNAs in vivo with 'antagomirs'," *Nature*, vol. 438, no. 7068, pp. 685–689, 2005.

[91] P. S. Mitchell, R. K. Parkin, E. M. Kroh et al., "Circulating microRNAs as stable blood-based markers for cancer detection," *Proceedings of the National Academy of Sciences of the United States of America*, vol. 105, no. 30, pp. 10513–10518, 2008.

[92] R. Recchioni, F. Marcheselli, F. Olivieri, S. Ricci, A. D. Procopio, and R. Antonicelli, "Conventional and novel diagnostic biomarkers of acute myocardial infarction: a promising role for circulating microRNAs," *Biomarkers*, vol. 18, no. 7, pp. 547–558, 2013.

[93] D.-Z. Zhang, K.-M. Lau, E. S. Y. Chan et al., "Cell-free urinary microRNA-99a and microRNA-125b are diagnostic markers for the non-invasive screening of bladder cancer," *PLoS ONE*, vol. 9, no. 7, Article ID e100793, 2014.

[94] R. Nassirpour, S. Mathur, M. M. Gosink et al., "Identification of tubular injury microRNA biomarkers in urine: comparison of next-generation sequencing and qPCR-based profiling platforms," *BMC Genomics*, vol. 15, article 485, 2014.

[95] N. J. Park, H. Zhou, D. Elashoff et al., "Salivary microRNA: discovery, characterization, and clinical utility for oral cancer detection," *Clinical Cancer Research*, vol. 15, no. 17, pp. 5473–5477, 2009.

[96] J. Saikumar, D. Hoffmann, T.-M. Kim et al., "Expression, circulation, and excretion profile of microRNA-21, -155, and -18a following acute kidney injury," *Toxicological Sciences*, vol. 129, no. 2, pp. 256–267, 2012.

[97] Z. Xie, G. Chen, X. Zhang et al., "Salivary microRNAs as promising biomarkers for detection of esophageal cancer," *PLoS ONE*, vol. 8, no. 4, Article ID e57502, 2013.

[98] K. C. Vickers, B. T. Palmisano, B. M. Shoucri, R. D. Shamburek, and A. T. Remaley, "MicroRNAs are transported in plasma and delivered to recipient cells by high-density lipoproteins," *Nature Cell Biology*, vol. 13, no. 4, pp. 423–435, 2011.

[99] J. D. Arroyo, J. R. Chevillet, E. M. Kroh et al., "Argonaute2 complexes carry a population of circulating microRNAs independent of vesicles in human plasma," *Proceedings of the National Academy of Sciences of the United States of America*, vol. 108, no. 12, pp. 5003–5008, 2011.

[100] K. Wang, S. Zhang, J. Weber, D. Baxter, and D. J. Galas, "Export of microRNAs and microRNA-protective protein by mammalian cells," *Nucleic Acids Research*, vol. 38, no. 20, pp. 7248–7259, 2010.

[101] Y. D'Alessandra, P. Devanna, F. Limana et al., "Circulating microRNAs are new and sensitive biomarkers of myocardial infarction," *European Heart Journal*, vol. 31, no. 22, pp. 2765–2773, 2010.

[102] X. Ji, R. Takahashi, Y. Hiura, G. Hirokawa, Y. Fukushima, and N. Iwai, "Plasma miR-208 as a biomarker of myocardial injury," *Clinical Chemistry*, vol. 55, no. 11, pp. 1944–1949, 2009.

[103] A. J. Tijsen, E. E. Creemers, P. D. Moerland et al., "MiR423-5p as a circulating biomarker for heart failure," *Circulation Research*, vol. 106, no. 6, pp. 1035–1039, 2010.

[104] E. E. Creemers, A. J. Tijsen, and Y. M. Pinto, "Circulating MicroRNAs: novel biomarkers and extracellular communicators in cardiovascular disease?" *Circulation Research*, vol. 110, no. 3, pp. 483–495, 2012.

[105] V. di Stefano, G. Zaccagnini, M. C. Capogrossi, and F. Martelli, "microRNAs as peripheral blood biomarkers of cardiovascular disease," *Vascular Pharmacology*, vol. 55, no. 4, pp. 111–118, 2011.

[106] M. Tanaka, K. Oikawa, M. Takanashi et al., "Down-regulation of miR-92 in human plasma is a novel marker for acute leukemia patients," *PLoS ONE*, vol. 4, no. 5, Article ID e5532, 2009.

[107] G.-K. Wang, J.-Q. Zhu, J.-T. Zhang et al., "Circulating microRNA: a novel potential biomarker for early diagnosis of acute myocardial infarction in humans," *European Heart Journal*, vol. 31, no. 6, pp. 659–666, 2010.

[108] O. Gidlöf, P. Andersson, J. van der Pals, M. Götberg, and D. Erlinge, "Cardiospecific microRNA plasma levels correlate with troponin and cardiac function in patients with ST elevation myocardial infarction, are selectively dependent on renal elimination, and can be detected in urine samples," *Cardiology*, vol. 118, no. 4, pp. 217–226, 2011.

[109] Y. Akao, A. Iio, T. Itoh et al., "microvesicle-mediated RNA molecule delivery system using monocytes/macrophages," *Molecular Therapy*, vol. 19, no. 2, pp. 395–399, 2011.

[110] X. Chen, H. Liang, J. Zhang, K. Zen, and C.-Y. Zhang, "Secreted microRNAs: a new form of intercellular communication," *Trends in Cell Biology*, vol. 22, no. 3, pp. 125–132, 2012.

[111] M. P. Hunter, N. Ismail, X. Zhang et al., "Detection of microRNA expression in human peripheral blood microvesicles," *PLoS ONE*, vol. 3, no. 11, Article ID e3694, 2008.

[112] A. Zernecke, K. Bidzhekov, H. Noels et al., "Delivery of microRNA-126 by apoptotic bodies induces CXCL12-dependent vascular protection," *Science Signaling*, vol. 2, no. 100, p. ra81, 2009.

[113] C. J. Rhodes, J. Wharton, R. A. Boon et al., "Reduced microRNA-150 is associated with poor survival in pulmonary arterial hypertension," *American Journal of Respiratory and Critical Care Medicine*, vol. 187, no. 3, pp. 294–302, 2013.

2

The Association between ESR and CRP and Systemic Hypertension in Sarcoidosis

Mehdi Mirsaeidi,[1] Hesham R. Omar,[2] Golnaz Ebrahimi,[1] and Micheal Campos[1]

[1] *Division of Pulmonary, Critical Care, Sleep and Allergy, Department of Medicine, University of Miami, FL, USA*
[2] *Internal Medicine Department, Mercy Medical Center, Clinton, IA, USA*

Correspondence should be addressed to Mehdi Mirsaeidi; msm249@med.miami.edu

Academic Editor: Markus P. Schlaich

Introduction. The association between the level of systemic inflammation and systemic hypertension (sHTN) among subjects with sarcoidosis has not been previously explored. *Methods.* A retrospective study was conducted to investigate the relation between the level of systemic inflammation in sarcoidosis, measured by various serum inflammatory markers, and sHTN. *Results.* Among a total of 108 cases with sarcoidosis (mean age: 53.4 years, 76.9% females), 55 (50.9%) had sHTN and 53 (49.1%) were normotensive. ESR was highly associated with sHTN. The patients with sHTN had higher mean ESR levels compared with normotensives (48.8 ± 35 versus 23.2 ± 27 mm/hr, resp.; $P = 0.001$). ROC curve analysis for ESR revealed an AUC value of 0.795 (95% CI: 0.692–0.897; $P = 0.0001$). With regard to CRP, there was a trend towards higher mean values in sHTN group (3.4 versus 1.7 mg/L; $P = 0.067$) and significantly higher prevalence of sHTN in the highest CRP quartile compared to the lowest one (69.6% versus 30%; OR 4.95; $P = 0.017$). ROC curve analysis for CRP revealed an AUC value of 0.644 (95% CI: 0.518–0.769; $P = 0.03$). On multivariate analysis, ESR and the CRP remained independent predictors for sHTN among subjects with sarcoidosis. *Conclusion.* Systemic inflammation is associated with the presence of sHTN in sarcoidosis.

1. Introduction

Inflammation is recognized as a main pathogenic element in the development of pulmonary arterial hypertension (PH) [1, 2] with several studies showing a significant association between systemic inflammatory markers and PH [3, 4]. Inflammation is also a precursor for the development and progression of atherosclerosis and systemic hypertension (sHTN). The association between C-reactive protein (CRP) and sHTN has been established in multiple cross-sectional studies [5–9], in particular after the advent of high sensitivity CRP (hs-CRP) assays capable of detecting levels that were earlier considered to be normal. Higher levels of CRP may contribute to the development of sHTN through the reduction of endothelium-dependant relaxation by reducing nitric oxide production in endothelial cells [10, 11], resulting in vasoconstriction and increased production of endothelin 1 [12]. CRP may also promote atherosclerosis through upregulating angiotensin type 1 receptor expression [13]. Another marker of systemic inflammation is albumin which is an acute phase reactant that is influenced by multiple factors mainly including malnutrition and inflammation which may reduce albumin levels irrespective of the patient's nutritional status [14, 15]. Other inflammatory markers include erythrocyte sedimentation rate (ESR), ferritin, angiotensin-converting enzyme (ACE), and 25 OH vitamin D.

Sarcoidosis is a systemic inflammatory disease that is associated with higher incidence of PH not only in cases with evidence of advanced parenchymal fibrosis, but also in cases without significant interstitial lung disease. In fact, anti-inflammatory therapies can have an impact on the progression of sarcoidosis-associated PH [16]. The relationship between chronic granulomatous inflammatory disease and systemic hypertension had not been previously explored.

The aim of this study was to investigate the relation between the degree of systemic inflammation measured by various inflammatory markers and sHTN in sarcoidosis patients.

2. Materials and Methods

This is a retrospective observational study of consecutive adult subjects >18 years who were diagnosed with sarcoidosis at the University of Illinois at Chicago between January 2010 and January 2015. The diagnosis of sarcoidosis was made according to the European Respiratory Society (ERS), American Thoracic Society (ATS), and World Association of Sarcoidosis and other Granulomatous Disorders (WASOG) criteria [17]. The Institutional Review Board of the University of Illinois at Chicago approved the study and waived the need for patient consent (approval number of 20130195001). Cases were divided into two groups based on the presence or absence of an underlying diagnosis of sHTN. The diagnosis of sHTN was made according to the seventh report of the joint national committee guidelines (JNC 7) if the blood pressure was ≥140/90 mmHg [18] in at least two separate visits or if the patient has been taking antihypertensive medication(s).

The inflammatory markers evaluated in this study were serum ESR, CRP, albumin, ferritin, ACE, and 25 OH vitamin D. Patients had been routinely tested for these inflammatory biomarkers to track the treatment response in several visits during a year. We used the mean recorded values for ESR, CRP albumin, ferritin, and 25 OH vitamin D. Data on patient demographic characteristics, medical comorbidities, clinical and laboratory variables, pulmonary function test (PFT), treatment, and outcome were collected. Blood sampling for biomarkers was performed by venipuncture. ESR was read after 30 minutes of bed rest and the reference range for it is 0–20 mm/hr. The blood levels of CRP were measured by immunonephelometry and the reference range for CRP was 0.5–2 mg/L. Albumin is measured by protein electrophoresis and reported in gm/dL. Serum 25 (OH) vitamin D was assayed using a competitive protein binding assay employing automated chemiluminescence and expressed in ng/mL. Serum ferritin concentration is determined by enzyme immunoassay and expressed in μg/L.

2.1. Statistical Analysis. Primary analysis was to compare biomarker values between sarcoidosis cases with and without sHTN. Continuous variables are expressed as mean ± standard deviation or median and interquartile range (IQR) and compared using Student t-test. Categorical variables are described as counts and percentages and compared using the Chi-square test. In order to study the effect of increase ESR, CRP, and albumin level on the prevalence of sHTN, we have divided the cohort into 4 groups according to the 4 quartiles of the ESR, CRP, and albumin, and the Cochran-Mantel-Haenszel common odds ratio test was used to evaluate the odds ratio (OR) and P value for the prevalence of hypertension in the 2nd, 3rd, and 4th ESR and CRP quartiles using the first quartile as the comparator, or the 1st, 2nd, and 3rd quartile using the fourth quartile as a comparator in the case of albumin. Chi-square test was utilized to detect whether the trend in sHTN prevalence across the four ESR and CRP quartiles was significant or not. A ROC (receiver operating characteristics) curve analysis was implemented to detect the ideal cutoff value of ESR, CRP, and albumin that yields the highest sensitivity and specificity for predicting sHTN and to calculate the area under the curve (AUC). In order to examine independent predictors for sHTN in sarcoidosis patients and avoid confounding factors, we used a multivariate logistic regression model with backward stepwise elimination. The variables used in the model were either those that achieved statistical significance at $P < 0.01$ upon univariate analysis or variables considered to be clinically relevant. A P value less than 0.05 is considered statistically significant. All statistical analyses were 2-sided. Data were analyzed using IBM SPSS 21.0 statistical software (IBM SPSS Version 21.0, Armonk, NY).

3. Results

3.1. Patient Characteristics. A total of 108 cases diagnosed with sarcoidosis were included in the study, among which 55 patients (50.9%) had sHTN and 53 (49.1%) were normotensive. The mean age of the study population was 53.4 ± 9.4 years, 76.9% were females, 70% were African Americans, and the average duration of sarcoidosis was 12 years. The results of univariate comparison of baseline demographics, clinical and laboratory characteristics, PFT, echocardiographic data, and treatment in sarcoidosis subjects with and without sHTN are summarized in Table 1. Compared with normotensive patients, those with sHTN were older (56 versus 50.6 years, $P = 0.002$), had a higher body mass index (33.5 versus 30.2 Kg/m^2, $P = 0.037$), had a higher proportion of African American race (89.1% versus 50.9%, $P = 0.0001$), and had a longer mean duration of sarcoidosis (14.3 versus 10 days, $P = 0.014$). Pulmonary-wise, subjects with sHTN have a higher proportion of PH (37% versus 15.1%, $P = 0.012$), were more likely to complain of dyspnea (62.7% versus 43.1%, $P = 0.049$), and had significantly lower lung function values (FVC%, FEV1%, TLC%, and DLCO). Most of the study cohort (83%) was receiving oral steroids, 43.9% were on disease modifying antirheumatic drugs, 29.6% were on methotrexate, and 4.7% were on azathioprine. At 5 years, 84 cases were still available for follow-up information while the rest were lost to follow-up.

3.2. Association between ESR and Systemic Hypertension. Subjects with sHTN had significantly higher mean and median ESR levels (Table 2). Furthermore, the prevalence of sHTN significantly increased from the 1st to the 4th ESR quartile, with crude prevalence rates of sHTN being 10%, 40.9%, 63.2%, and 75%, respectively (P value for the trend = 0.0001). A total of 23 subjects (67.6%) in the sHTN group had ESR levels in the 3rd or 4th higher quartiles, compared with only 11 (32.4%) of the subjects without sHTN ($P = 0.002$). Using the Cochran-Mantel-Haenszel method, compared to the lowest ESR quartile, the OR to have sHTN were 6.2 ($P = 0.034$), 15.4 ($P = 0.002$), and 33.8 ($P = 0.0001$) for the 2nd, 3rd, and 4th ESR quartiles, respectively. ROC curve

Table 1: Demographic and clinical characteristics of the sarcoidosis cohort.

	All subjects (n = 108)	Sarcoidosis with HTN (n = 55)	Sarcoidosis without HTN (n = 53)	P value
	Baseline demographics and comorbidities			
Age (years, mean ± SD)	53.4 ± 9.4	56 ± 9.2	50.6 ± 8.9	0.002
Female sex% (n)	76.9% (83)	76.4% (42)	77.4% (41)	0.902
BMI (Kg/m^2, mean ± SD)	31.9 ± 8	33.5 ± 8.2	30.2 ± 7.4	0.037
Duration of sarcoidosis (y, mean ± SD)	12.2 ± 9.1	14.3 ± 9.8	10 ± 7.9	0.014
African American% (n)	70.4% (76)	89.1% (49)	50.9% (27)	0.0001
Diabetes% (n)	31.1% (33)	38.2% (21)	23.5% (12)	0.106
Dyslipidemia% (n)	24.3% (26)	33.3% (18)	15.1% (8)	0.031
CKD% (n)	3.7% (4)	5.5% (3)	1.9% (1)	0.348
PCI or CABG% (n)	1.9% (2)	1.8% (1)	1.9% (1)	0.979
Atrial fibrillation% (n)	5.6% (6)	7.3% (4)	3.8% (2)	0.435
CHF% (n)	6.6% (7)	9.3% (5)	3.8% (2)	0.276
Pulmonary hypertension% (n)	26.2% (28)	37% (20)	15.1% (8)	0.012
Rheumatoid arthritis% (n)	3.7% (4)	5.5% (3)	1.9% (1)	0.348
Asthma% (n)	26.2% (28)	27.8% (15)	24.5% (13)	0.702
OSA% (n)	24.3% (28)	30.9% (17)	17.3% (9)	0.105
Dyspnea% (n)	52.9% (54)	62.7% (32)	43.1% (22)	0.049
	Pulmonary function tests and echocardiography			
FVC% (mean ± SD)	93.2 ± 20.9	87.7 ± 19.9	99.4 ± 20.4	0.008
FEV1% (mean ± SD)	88 ± 24.9	80.5 ± 23.9	96.7 ± 23.4	0.002
TLC% (mean ± SD)	89.1 ± 15.6	84.7 ± 15	94.1 ± 15.1	0.005
RV% (mean ± SD)	99.4 ± 26.7	98.4 ± 29.4	100.9 ± 22.7	0.711
DLCO% (mean ± SD)	67 ± 20.3	58.8 ± 18.4	76.4 ± 18.4	0.000
EF (mean ± SD)	57.8 ± 4.8	57.1 ± 4.8	58.6 ± 4.7	0.108
	Treatment			
Oral steroid% (n)	83.5% (86)	88% (44)	79.2% (42)	0.237
DMARD% (n)	43.9% (47)	43.6% (24)	44.2% (23)	0.951
Methotrexate% (n)	29.6% (32)	25.5% (14)	34% (18)	0.334
Azathioprine% (n)	4.7% (5)	3.6% (2)	5.6% (3)	0.620
Lasix% (n)	17.6% (19)	23.6% (13)	11.3% (6)	0.099
Warfarin% (n)	2.8% (3)	5.5% (3)	0% (0)	0.129
Statin% (n)	28.7% (31)	38.2% (21)	18.9% (10)	0.029
ACE or ARB% (n)	46.7% (50)	74.1% (40)	18.9% (10)	0.0001
Aspirin	26.9% (29)	34.5% (19)	18.9% (10)	0.069

PHTN: pulmonary hypertension, BMI: body mass index, CKD: chronic kidney disease, PCI: percutaneous coronary intervention, CABG: coronary artery bypass graft, OSA: obstructive sleep apnea, PASP: pulmonary artery systolic pressure, EF: ejection fraction, ESR: erythrocyte sedimentation rate, CRP: C-reactive protein, DMARD: disease modifying antirheumatic drug, ACE: angiotensin converting enzyme, y: year, m: mean, and SD: standard deviation.

analysis performed to detect the best cutoff value for ESR in predicting sHTN in sarcoidosis patients revealed an AUC value of 0.795 (95% CI 0.692–0.897, P = 0.0001) (Figure 1). A cutoff value for ESR of 30 mm/hr yielded a 62% sensitivity and 80% specificity for predicting the presence of sHTN in this sarcoidosis patient cohort.

3.3. Association between CRP and Systemic Hypertension. Subjects with sHTN had a trend towards higher median and interquartile range of CRP levels [1.1 (0.65, 3.65) versus 0.9 (0.5, 1.8), resp., P = 0.067] compared with normotensive subjects as shown in Table 2. On dichotomizing CRP values, sarcoidosis patients with sHTN had a significantly higher frequency of CRP >2 mg/L (P = 0.003), CRP >2.5 mg/L (P = 0.004), CRP >3 mg/L (P = 0.001), and CRP >3.5 mg/L (P = 0.01). When we dichotomized the cohort according to CRP levels, the prevalence of sHTN was 88.9% when CRP >3 mg/L versus 45% when CRP <1 mg/dL (univariate OR for the prevalence of sHTN when CRP >3 mg/dL versus CRP <1 mg/dL 9.778, 95% CI 1.981–48.261, P = 0.005). The crude

TABLE 2: Associations between various inflammatory markers with prevalence of systemic hypertension in sarcoidosis patients.

	Inflammatory markers			
	All subjects (n = 108)	Sarcoidosis with HTN (n = 55)	Sarcoidosis without HTN (n = 53)	P value
	Erythrocyte sedimentation rate			
ESR (mm/hr, mean ± SD)	35.2 ± 33.4	48.8 ± 35	23.2 ± 27	0.001
ESR (mm/hr, median, IQR)	25 (12.5–44)	34.5 (23.8–81)	13 (10–28)	—
ESR quartile 1 (ESR < 12.5 mm/hr), % (n)	24.7% (20)	10% (2)	90% (18)	0.001
ESR quartile 2 (ESR 12.5–24 mm/hr), % (n)	27.2% (22)	40.9% (9)	59.1% (13)	0.509
ESR quartile 3 (ESR 25–44 mm/hr), % (n)	23.5% (19)	63.2% (12)	36.8% (7)	0.11
ESR quartile 4 (ESR > 44 mm/hr), % (n)	24.7% (20)	75% (15)	25% (5)	0.006
	C-reactive protein			
CRP (mg/L, mean ± SD)	2.5 ± 4.2	3.4 ± 4.5	1.7 ± 3.7	0.067
CRP (mg/L, median, IQR)	1 (0.6, 2.37)	1.1 (0.65, 3.65)	0.9 (0.5, 1.8)	—
CRP > 2% (n)	28.9% (24)	45% (18)	14% (6)	0.003
CRP > 2.5% (n)	22.9% (19)	37.5% (15)	9.3% (4)	0.004
CRP > 3% (n)	20.7% (17)	38.5% (15)	4.7% (2)	0.001
CRP > 3.5% (n)	14.5% (12)	27.5% (11)	2.3% (1)	0.01
CRP quartile 1 (CRP < 0.6 mg/dL), % (n)	23.8% (20)	30% (6)	70% (14)	0.059
CRP quartile 2 (CRP 0.6–0.99 mg/dL), % (n)	28.6% (24)	58.3% (14)	41.7% (10)	0.272
CRP quartile 3 (CRP 1.0–2.37 mg/dL), % (n)	22.6% (19)	26.3% (5)	73.7% (14)	0.031
CRP quartile 4 (CRP > 2.37 mg/dL), % (n)	25% (21)	76.2% (16)	23.8% (5)	0.006
	Albumin			
Albumin (gm/dL, mean ± SD)	3.6 ± 0.58	3.44 ± 0.63	3.77 ± 0.49	0.004
Albumin (gm/dL, median, IQR)	3.7 (3.4–4)	3.6 (3.2–3.8)	3.8 (3.6–4.1)	—
Albumin quartile 1 (albumin < 3.4 gm/dL), % (n)	24% (24)	70.8% (17)	29.2% (7)	0.017
Albumin quartile 2 (albumin 3.4–3.69 gm/dL), % (n)	19% (19)	52.6% (10)	47.4% (9)	0.725
Albumin quartile 3 (albumin 3.7–4.1 gm/dL), % (n)	29% (29)	48.3% (14)	51.7% (15)	0.926
Albumin quartile 4 (albumin > 4.1 gm/dL), % (n)	28% (28)	28.6% (8)	71.4% (20)	0.013
	Other inflammatory markers			
Ferritin (ng/mL, mean ± SD)	161.4 ± 602	245 ± 857	83 ± 91	0.262
ACE level (U/L, mean ± SD)	63.2 ± 49.5	52.9 ± 55	71.4 ± 43.8	0.121
25 OH vitamin D (μg/L, mean ± SD)	16.1 ± 8.5	15.7 ± 8.7	16.5 ± 8.3	0.657

HTN: systemic hypertension, ESR: erythrocyte sedimentation rate, CRP: C-reactive protein, ACE: angiotensin converting enzyme, m: mean, SD: standard deviation, and IQR: interquartile range.

prevalence of sHTN increased from 30% in the first CRP quartile to 76.2% in the 4th quartile (OR 6.933, P = 0.006). P value for the trend in sHTN prevalence across the 4 CRP quartiles was 0.003. ROC curve analysis for CRP revealed an AUC value of 0.644 (95% CI 0.518–0.769, P = 0.03) (Figure 1) and a cutoff value of 3 mg/L yielded a 37% sensitivity and 95% specificity for predicting the presence of sHTN in this cohort of sarcoidosis subjects.

3.4. Association between Hypoalbuminemia and Systemic Hypertension. The median and interquartile range (IQR) of albumin for the entire cohort was 3.7 g/dL (IQR 3.4–4 gm/dL). Sarcoidosis patients with sHTN had a significantly lower mean albumin level compared with normotensives (3.44 versus 3.77 gm/dL, resp., P = 0.004). Opposite to what was observed with ESR and CRP, the prevalence of hypertension significantly decreased along albumin quartiles (1st quartile < 3.4, 2nd quartile 3.4–3.69, 3rd quartile 3.7–4, and 4th quartile > 4 gm/dL), with the crude prevalence rates of sHTN being 70.8%, 52.6%, 48.3%, and 28.6% for the 1st, 2nd, 3rd, and 4th quartile, respectively (P value for the trend = 0.025). Using the Cochran-Mantel-Haenszel method, the OR to have sHTN in the first albumin quartile compared with the 4th albumin quartile was 5.77 (95% CI 1.725–19.287, P = 0.004). ROC curve analysis revealed an AUC value of 0.670 (95% CI 0.564–0.776, P = 0.003) (Figure 2). An albumin level < 3.3 gm/dL yielded a 35% sensitivity and 87% specificity for predicting systemic hypertension in this sarcoidosis cohort.

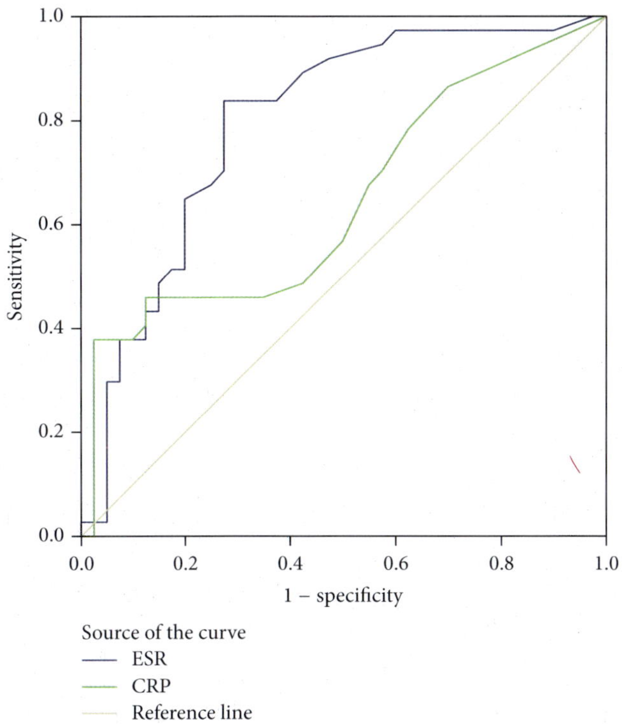

FIGURE 1: Receiver operating characteristic (ROC) curve to detect the best cutoff value for ESR and CRP in the prediction of systemic hypertension in sarcoidosis patients. ESR had an AUC value of 0.795 (95% CI 0.692–0.897, $P = 0.0001$). A cutoff value for ESR of 30 mm/hr yielded a 62% sensitivity and 80% specificity for predicting systemic hypertension in sarcoidosis patients. With regard to CRP, the AUC value is 0.644 (95% CI 0.518–0.769, $P = 0.03$). A cutoff value for CRP of 3 mg/L yielded a 37% sensitivity and 95% specificity for predicting systemic hypertension in sarcoidosis patients.

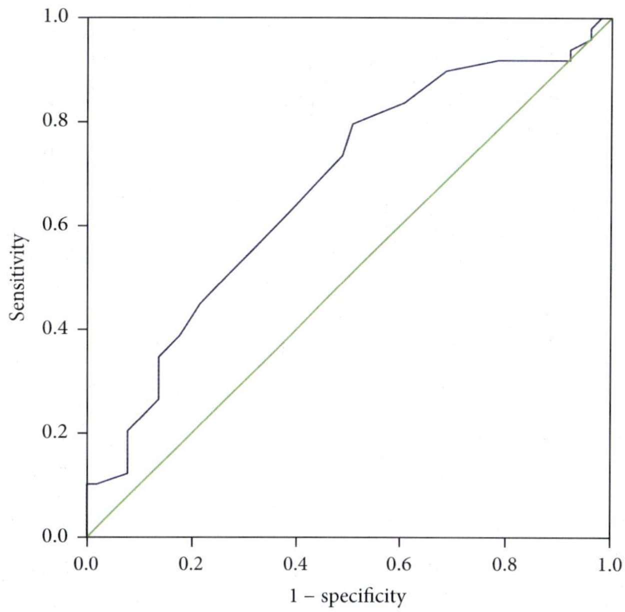

FIGURE 2: Receiver operating characteristic (ROC) curve to detect the best cutoff value for albumin in the prediction of systemic hypertension in sarcoidosis patients. AUC value of 0.670 (95% CI 0.564–0.776, $P = 0.003$). An albumin level < 3.3 gm/dL yielded a 35% sensitivity and 87% specificity for predicting systemic hypertension in sarcoidosis patients.

3.5. Relationship between Other Inflammatory Markers and Systemic Hypertension. We have also evaluated the relationship between sHTN and other nontraditional markers of inflammation including ferritin, ACE, and 25-hydroxy vitamin D. On univariate analysis, there was no significant difference between those with sHTN and normotensive subjects with regard to the mean ferritin level (245 versus 83 μg/L, $P = 0.262$), mean ACE level (52.9 versus 71.4 U/L, $P = 0.121$), and mean 25 OH vitamin D (15.7 versus 16.5 ng/mL, $P = 0.657$).

3.6. Multivariable Logistic Regression Analysis. Multivariate logistic regression analysis with backward stepwise elimination did not change the positive dose-response relationship between the ESR and CRP levels and the prevalence of sHTN. In the multivariate logistic regression model ($N = 70$, Nagelkerke $R^2 = 0.332$, and P from Hosmer and Lemeshow = 0.775), we found that having ESR levels in the 3rd and 4th quartiles combined (OR 3.165, 95% confidence interval 1.044–9.593, $P = 0.042$) and CRP levels in the 4th quartile (OR 6.057, 95% confidence interval 1.567–23.415, $P = 0.009$) remained independent predictors for a subject with sarcoidosis to have sHTN after adjustment for age, sex, body mass index, dyslipidemia, sarcoidosis duration, the use of oral steroids, and hypoalbuminemia. We have not found a relationship between other inflammatory markers such as ferritin, 25 OH vitamin D level, and neutrophil-to-lymphocyte ratio and sHTN on univariate or multivariable analysis. The variables used in the multivariate model are shown as a Forest plot (Figure 3).

4. Discussion

We were able to show in this retrospective analysis that an independent relationship exists between the degree of systemic inflammation and sHTN in sarcoidosis patients. Previous work showed that ESR [19, 20] and CRP [20] levels are higher in sarcoidosis patients compared to controls. We observed that, among sarcoidosis subjects, ESR and CRP levels are almost twice as high in hypertensive subjects compared with normotensive patients (48.8 versus 23.2 mm/hr, $P = 0.001$ for ESR, and 3.4 versus 1.7, $P = 0.067$ for CRP). Furthermore, the link between sHTN and inflammation is supported by the stepwise increase in sHTN prevalence across quartiles of both ESR and CRP. These results imply that a more intense inflammatory response may have an important pathophysiologic contribution for the development of sHTN in sarcoidosis. Patients with pulmonary sarcoidosis and systemic hypertension also had significantly higher frequency of pulmonary hypertension ($P = 0.012$) where inflammation is a recognized factor in its pathogenesis.

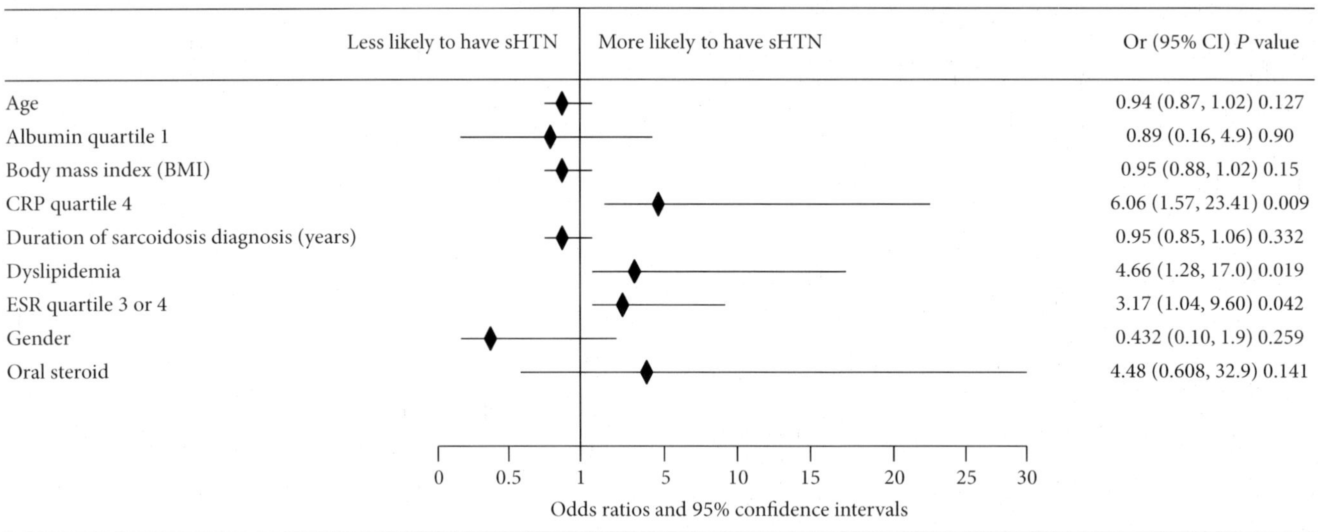

FIGURE 3: Forest plot of multivariate logistic regression analysis demonstrating independent factors associated with systemic hypertension in sarcoidosis patients. Hosmer and Lemeshow $P = 0.775$.

The association between CRP and sHTN has been previously demonstrated in other studies not related to sarcoidosis. For example, in a cross-sectional study of 300 subjects ≥30 years old, Bautista and colleagues found that the prevalence of sHTN was 1.56 times (95% CI 1.14–2.13, $P = 0.005$) higher in subjects in the fourth quartile of CRP as compared to subjects in the first quartile [21]. In a later cross-sectional survey of 8347 apparently healthy Koreans, Sung and colleagues found a significant positive association between the blood pressure and CRP level ($P < 0.0001$) and after adjustment for confounding variables, the prevalence of hypertension by CRP was significantly higher in subjects in the second, third, and fourth quartiles of CRP compared to subjects in the first quartile [22]. Furthermore CRP was found to be a predictor of future development of hypertension. In an analysis of the Women's Health Study [23], 20,525 females with initially normal blood pressure were followed up for 7.8 years and CRP was found to be significantly associated with an increased risk of developing sHTN over time [24]. Furthermore, Magen and colleagues found a significant positive correlation between systolic blood pressure and CRP levels, with significantly higher levels in the resistant hypertension group compared with the controlled hypertension group (6.9 ± 5.8 versus 4.2 ± 4.8, $P = 0.021$) [25]. These studies utilized the hypothesis that inflammation is important in the pathogenesis of sHTN. In our study, we are trying to show whether systemic inflammation caused by other diseases such as sarcoidosis would predispose to the development of systemic hypertension just like it predisposes these patients to pulmonary hypertension irrespective of lung involvement.

In the above mentioned studies, the association of sHTN with elevated ESR was either insignificant [25], not studied, or not reported. However, we found that ESR gives the highest AUC value in predicting sHTN compared with any of the inflammatory markers studies. Hypoalbuminemia has been studied in multiple respiratory and cardiac diseases and was found to be poor prognostic indicator and an independent predictor of mortality [26]. A large prospective study on emergency department patients showed that the short-term mortality of patients with hypoalbuminemia was three times higher compared with patients with normal albumin after adjusting for several confounders [15]. Albumin is a negative acute phase reactant that is influenced by mainly two factors: patient's nutritional status and inflammation; however, prior studies showed that inflammation reduces albumin levels irrespective of the patient's nutritional state [27]. Serum albumin level is reduced in acute and chronic inflammatory states due to increased degradation from the high catabolic rate in addition to its transudation to extravascular space from increased capillary permeability [15].

The current study is subject to all limitations inherent to nonrandomized observational studies. Our experience is from a single center, the design is retrospective, and the cohort is relatively small due to rarity of the disease. The main study limitation is that we have not taken into account whether the diagnosis of sHTN was made before or after the diagnosis of sarcoidosis and therefore a proportion of these hypertensive patients may have had sHTN prior to and independent of sarcoidosis. However, this is very difficult to control for as both diseases (hypertension and sarcoidosis) are chronic diseases and to know the exact onset of either pathology is not possible. There may have been confounding variables that were not accounted in our analysis. For example, it is known that sarcoidosis patients with active disease have very high levels of ESR and CRP [28]. These inflammatory markers are also significantly elevated in sarcoidosis-associated arthritis [29], erythema nodosum [30], concomitant connective tissue disease, or simultaneous acute infections and these factors have not been accounted for. We have only used sHTN as a diagnosis without staging its severity and therefore we were unable to study the correlation between the level of these inflammatory markers and the severity of sHTN. The OR for the prevalence of sHTN across the quartiles is notably elevated because it is known that, in diseases with high prevalence, the OR may overestimate the effect of exposure (the prevalence of sHTN in this cohort is 50.9%).

We conclude that the level of systemic inflammation in sarcoidosis patients—reflected by a higher ESR, CRP—may be associated with the presence of sHTN. This study provides insight of the role of systemic inflammation in the development of sHTN as an additional complication of the disease, suggesting the importance of a closer follow-up of blood pressure in normotensive sarcoidosis patients with elevated inflammatory markers. The study may also stimulate the conduction of further trials to assess the role of anti-inflammatory drugs in the control and/or regression of sHTN in sarcoidosis subjects who had developed sHTN after the diagnosis of sarcoidosis.

Competing Interests

The authors declare that they have no competing interests.

Authors' Contributions

Conception, hypotheses delineation, and design of the study were by Mehdi Mirsaeidi and Hesham R. Omar, data analysis and interpretation was by Mehdi Mirsaeidi and Hesham R. Omar, and writing the paper or substantial involvement in its revision before submission was by Mehdi Mirsaeidi, Hesham R. Omar, Golnaz Ebrahimi, and Micheal Campos.

References

[1] R. T. Schermuly, H. A. Ghofrani, M. R. Wilkins, and F. Grimminger, "Mechanisms of disease: pulmonary arterial hypertension," *Nature Reviews Cardiology*, vol. 8, no. 8, pp. 443–455, 2011.

[2] L. C. Price, S. J. Wort, F. Perros et al., "Inflammation in pulmonary arterial hypertension," *Chest*, vol. 141, no. 1, pp. 210–221, 2012.

[3] A. Yildiz, H. Kaya, F. Ertas et al., "Association between neutrophil to lymphocyte ratio and pulmonary arterial hypertension," *Turk Kardiyoloji Dernegi Arsivi's*, vol. 41, no. 7, pp. 604–609, 2013.

[4] E. Özpelit, B. Akdeniz, M. E. Özpelit et al., "Prognostic value of neutrophil-to-lymphocyte ratio in pulmonary arterial hypertension," *Journal of International Medical Research*, vol. 43, no. 5, pp. 661–671, 2015.

[5] E. S. Ford and W. H. Giles, "Serum C-reactive protein and fibrinogen concentrations and self-reported angina pectoris and myocardial infarction: findings from National Health and Nutrition Examination Survey III," *Journal of Clinical Epidemiology*, vol. 53, no. 1, pp. 95–102, 2000.

[6] L. E. P. Rohde, C. H. Hennekens, and P. M. Ridker, "Survey of C-reactive protein and cardiovascular risk factors in apparently healthy men," *American Journal of Cardiology*, vol. 84, no. 9, pp. 1018–1022, 1999.

[7] E. A. Bermudez, N. Rifai, J. Buring, J. E. Manson, and P. M. Ridker, "Interrelationships among circulating interleukin-6, C-reactive protein, and traditional cardiovascular risk factors in women," *Arteriosclerosis, Thrombosis, and Vascular Biology*, vol. 22, no. 10, pp. 1668–1673, 2002.

[8] C. U. Chae, R. T. Lee, N. Rifai, and P. M. Ridker, "Blood pressure and inflammation in apparently healthy men," *Hypertension*, vol. 38, no. 3, pp. 399–403, 2001.

[9] S. Yamada, T. Gotoh, Y. Nakashima et al., "Distribution of serum C-reactive protein and its association with atherosclerotic risk factors in a Japanese population: Jichi Medical School Cohort study," *American Journal of Epidemiology*, vol. 153, no. 12, pp. 1183–1190, 2001.

[10] S. Verma, C.-H. Wang, S.-H. Li et al., "A self-fulfilling prophecy: c-reactive protein attenuates nitric oxide production and inhibits angiogenesis," *Circulation*, vol. 106, no. 8, pp. 913–919, 2002.

[11] S. K. Venugopal, S. Devaraj, I. Yuhanna, P. Shaul, and I. Jialal, "Demonstration that C-reactive protein decreases eNOS expression and bioactivity in human aortic endothelial cells," *Circulation*, vol. 106, no. 12, pp. 1439–1441, 2002.

[12] S. Verma, S.-H. Li, M. V. Badiwala et al., "Endothelin antagonism and interleukin-6 inhibition attenuate the proatherogenic effects of C-reactive protein," *Circulation*, vol. 105, no. 16, pp. 1890–1896, 2002.

[13] C.-H. Wang, S.-H. Li, R. D. Weisel et al., "C-reactive protein upregulates angiotensin type 1 receptors in vascular smooth muscle," *Circulation*, vol. 107, no. 13, pp. 1783–1790, 2003.

[14] S. Ishida, I. Hashimoto, T. Seike, Y. Abe, Y. Nakaya, and H. Nakanishi, "Serum albumin levels correlate with inflammation rather than nutrition supply in burns patients: a retrospective study," *Journal of Medical Investigation*, vol. 61, no. 3-4, pp. 361–368, 2014.

[15] O. Lyons, B. Whelan, K. Bennett, D. O'Riordan, and B. Silke, "Serum albumin as an outcome predictor in hospital emergency medical admissions," *European Journal of Internal Medicine*, vol. 21, no. 1, pp. 17–20, 2010.

[16] D. M. Rodman and J. Lindenfeld, "Successful treatment of sarcoidosis-associated pulmonary hypertension with corticosteroids," *Chest*, vol. 97, no. 2, pp. 500–502, 1990.

[17] Joint Statement of the American Thoracic Society (ATS), The European Respiratory Society (ERS), and The World Association of Sarcoidosis and Other Granulomatous Disorders (WASOG), "Statement on sarcoidosis," *American Journal of Respiratory and Critical Care Medicine*, vol. 160, no. 2, pp. 736–755, 1999.

[18] A. V. Chobanian, G. L. Bakris, H. R. Black et al., "Seventh report of the Joint National Committee on Prevention, Detection, Evaluation, and Treatment of High Blood Pressure," *Hypertension*, vol. 42, no. 6, pp. 1206–1252, 2003.

[19] D. Gupta, V. M. Rao, A. N. Aggarwal, G. Garewal, and S. K. Jindal, "Haematological abnormalities in patients of sarcoidosis," *The Indian Journal of Chest Diseases & Allied Sciences*, vol. 44, no. 4, pp. 233–236, 2002.

[20] R. Su, M.-L. T. Nguyen, M. R. Agarwal et al., "Interferon-inducible chemokines reflect severity and progression in sarcoidosis," *Respiratory Research*, vol. 14, article 121, 2013.

[21] L. E. Bautista, P. López-Jaramillo, L. M. Vera, J. P. Casas, A. P. Otero, and A. I. Guaracao, "Is C-reactive protein an independent risk factor for essential hypertension?" *Journal of Hypertension*, vol. 19, no. 5, pp. 857–861, 2001.

[22] K. C. Sung, J. Y. Suh, B. S. Kim et al., "High sensitivity C-reactive protein as an independent risk factor for essential hypertension," *American Journal of Hypertension*, vol. 16, no. 6, pp. 429–433, 2003.

[23] K. M. Rexrode, I.-M. Lee, N. R. Cook, C. H. Hennekens, and J. E. Buring, "Baseline characteristics of participants in the

Women's Health Study," *Journal of Women's Health & Gender-Based Medicine*, vol. 9, no. 1, pp. 19–27, 2004.

[24] H. D. Sesso, J. E. Buring, N. Rifai, G. J. Blake, J. M. Gaziano, and P. M. Ridker, "C-reactive protein and the risk of developing hypertension," *The Journal of the American Medical Association*, vol. 290, no. 22, pp. 2945–2951, 2003.

[25] E. Magen, J. Mishal, J. Paskin et al., "Resistant arterial hypertension is associated with higher blood levels of complement C3 and C-reactive protein," *Journal of Clinical Hypertension*, vol. 10, no. 9, pp. 677–683, 2008.

[26] M. E. Jellinge, D. P. Henriksen, P. Hallas, and M. Brabrand, "Hypoalbuminemia is a strong predictor of 30-day all-cause mortality in acutely admitted medical patients: a prospective, observational, cohort study," *PLoS ONE*, vol. 9, no. 8, Article ID e105983, 2014.

[27] S. Ishida, I. Hashimoto, T. Seike, Y. Abe, Y. Nakaya, and H. Nakanishi, "Serum albumin levels correlate with inflammation rather than nutrition supply in burns patients: A Retrospective Study," *Journal of Medical Investigation*, vol. 61, no. 3-4, pp. 361–368, 2014.

[28] S. Rothkrantz-Kos, M. P. van Dieijen-Visser, P. G. H. Mulder, and M. Drent, "Potential usefulness of inflammatory markers to monitor respiratory functional impairment in sarcoidosis," *Clinical Chemistry*, vol. 49, no. 9, pp. 1510–1517, 2003.

[29] A. F. Shorr, F. T. Murphy, W. R. Gilliland, and O. W. Hnatiuk, "Osseous disease in patients with pulmonary sarcoidosis and musculoskeletal symptoms," *Respiratory Medicine*, vol. 94, no. 3, pp. 228–232, 2000.

[30] G. Greenberg, D. G. James, T. Feizi, and R. Bird, "Serum-proteins in sarcoidosis," *The Lancet*, vol. 284, no. 7373, pp. 1313–1315, 1964.

3

Hypertension Management in Brazil: Usual Practice in Primary Care—A Meta-Analysis

Rafael V. Picon,[1] Juvenal S. Dias-da-Costa,[2] Flavio D. Fuchs,[3] Maria Teresa A. Olinto,[2] Niteesh K. Choudhry,[4] and Sandra C. Fuchs[1,5]

[1] *Postgraduate Studies Program in Cardiology, School of Medicine, Universidade Federal do Rio Grande do Sul, R. Ramiro Barcelos 2600, 90035-003 Porto Alegre, RS, Brazil*
[2] *Postgraduate Program of Collective Health, Universidade do Vale do Rio dos Sinos, São Leopoldo, RS, Brazil*
[3] *Division of Cardiology, Hospital de Clinicas de Porto Alegre, Universidade Federal do Rio Grande do Sul, Porto Alegre, RS, Brazil*
[4] *Division of Pharmacoepidemiology and Pharmacoeconomics, Brigham and Women's Hospital, Harvard School of Medicine, Harvard University, Boston, MA, USA*
[5] *Postgraduate Studies Program in Epidemiology, School of Medicine, Universidade Federal do Rio Grande do Sul, R. Ramiro Barcelos 2600, 90035-003 Porto Alegre, RS, Brazil*

Correspondence should be addressed to Sandra C. Fuchs; scfuchs@terra.com.br

Academic Editor: Tomohiro Katsuya

Knowing the usual clinical practice is relevant for evaluations in health care and economic policies of management of hypertension. This study aimed to describe the usual management of hypertension in the Brazilian primary healthcare system through a systematic review and meta-analysis. The search of population-based studies conducted in Brazil was undertaken using PubMed, EMBASE, and Brazilian databases. Eligible studies were those conducted in adults with hypertension (blood pressure (BP) ≥ 140/90 mmHg or using BP lowering drugs). Three datasets' data were analyzed: SESI study (in Brazilian workers); HIPERDIA (Brazilian Registration and Monitoring of Hypertensive and Diabetic Patients Program); and a population-based study. Meta-analysis has been performed using the fixed and random effect models. A total of 11 studies or data sets were included in the systematic review. Hypertensive individuals had, on average, 2.6 medical visits annually and 18.2% were on diuretics ($n = 811$ hypertensive patients) and 16.2% on ACE inhibitors ($n = 1768$ hypertensive patients). BP control rate ranged from 43.7 to 67.5%; 35.5% had measured total cholesterol and 36.5% determined fasting plasma glucose in the previous 12 months. Thiazide diuretics and ACE inhibitors were the most used BP lowering medications as single drugs, but the control rate of hypertension is insufficient.

1. Introduction

Assessment of costs and health outcomes can generate estimates to compare and choose among screening, diagnostic, or therapeutic strategies, which should be incorporated into the healthcare system. The endpoint is to achieve maximum health gains with the available resources, respecting the expectations of the population covered by the healthcare system and considering the limited resources [1]. Health economic evaluations (HEES) are useful tools for managers and policy makers to choose the best allocation of available resources, or even about the assimilation of a new health technology. HEES are particularly useful to decide on incorporation of new strategies for prevention or control of noncommunicable diseases. In Brazil, the public health system, *Sistema Único de Saúde* (SUS), is based on universal free access to healthcare to the whole population, with decentralization provided at all levels, from prevention to high complexity level, shared by federal, state, and municipal government [2]. Blood pressure lowering medication are available at the SUS, freely distributed, and a list of drugs include thiazide diuretic, beta-blocker, ACE inhibitor, and an angiotensin receptor blocker (ARB). Health plan physicians are an alternative placed between the public and private systems, ranging from partial to full coverage, and usually with no refund for costs with blood pressure lowering agents.

HEE is necessary to decide whether new drugs will be made available by the SUS.

It is estimated that hypertension (HT) affects 28.7% (95% CI: 26.2–31.4%) of the Brazilian adult population, with decreasing temporal trend in the rate of hypertension control [9]. In a meta-analysis of population-based studies, the control rate was 25% [9]. HT is responsible for significant global morbidity and mortality [10]. However, there is no systematic analysis of economic costs for diagnosis, risk stratification, and treatment of HT in Brazil [11].

A suitable HEE should include the comparison between the strategy of the Brazilian Guidelines of Hypertension [12] and the usual practice (status-quo), aiming at the primary prevention of CVD in patients of primary care. The status-quo can serve as a baseline for comparisons whenever a new health strategy is being considered for implementation [13]. Hence, our study aimed to describe the usual practice, in the context of primary care of the SUS in Brazil, regarding the diagnosis, risk stratification, and pharmacological treatment of HT.

2. Methods

2.1. Design and Data Sources. Studies conducted at population-based or outpatient, cross-sectional, or cohort studies, carried out since 2000, were searched in the databases of PubMed, EMBASE, and population-based databases of the Brazilian Virtual Health Library (VHL; http://brasil.bvs.br/en/). The following search strategies were used: VHL using Descriptors in Health Sciences: "Hipertensão" AND "Atenção Primária à Saúde" AND "Brasil"; on EMBASE using entrees: "brazil"/exp AND "hypertension"/exp AND "primary health care"/exp; and on PubMed using MeSH Terms: (("Hypertension"[Mesh]) AND "Primary Health Care"[Mesh]) AND "Brazil"[Mesh]. We also evaluated articles, which were included in a meta-analysis of the prevalence of hypertension [9], conducted by the authors. Articles that met the eligibility criteria were included: population-based cross-sectional or cohort studies performed in participants with 18 years or more, between 1980 and 2010. We also incorporated in meta-analysis four sets of data available to us, regardless of the systematic review searches [14–16].

2.2. Eligibility Criteria for the Review and Screening Process. Studies conducted in Brazil including patients with HT treated in any primary care facility affiliated to the SUS or population-based studies, which reported data in adults with HT were considered eligible for data extraction. Hospitalized patients were outside of the scope of this analysis and were excluded. The search results were handled in a double-screening process: their titles and abstracts were scrutinized and those eligible had their full-texts examined. Duplicated results were excluded. Studies conducted in pregnant women were excluded.

2.3. Target Population and Variables of Interest. The target population consisted of Brazilian adults (≥18 years) who either had blood pressure (BP) ≥ 140/90 mmHg or were on treatment with BP lowering agents (BPLM), enrolled from the general population or among those who were undertaking treatment in primary care settings. In order to collect information on management of patients and ensure comparability with the Brazilian Guidelines of Arterial Hypertension [12] and among guidelines [17], the following variables have been extracted: frequency of medical consultations and type of health insurance (e.g., SUS, private health plan) used most of the time, number and frequency of diagnostic tests suggested by this guideline (e.g., ECG, fasting glucose, and chest X-ray), antihypertensive classes, clinical characteristics, such as systolic BP (SBP), total and high-density lipoprotein cholesterol (HDL), and prevalence of other relevant comorbidities (diabetes mellitus (DM) and smoking) [18]. The rates of smoking and prevalence of DM among hypertensive individuals enrolled in the HIPERDIA (Brazilian Registration and Monitoring of Hypertensive and Diabetic Patients Program), from May 2002 to April 2012, were also evaluated [5].

2.4. Data Analysis. Continuous variables with normal distribution were presented as means and standard deviations (SD). Binary data were presented as proportions using point estimates and 95% confidence interval (95% CI). Meta-analyses were performed with the pooling of means or proportions: when the same variable of interest was measured using the same method across studies (e.g., self-reported diabetes versus fasting plasma glucose) and the same, or interchangeable, metric (e.g., one laboratory test per month equals 12 tests per year). Random effects model was mostly used; however, fixed effect model was employed when non-significant heterogeneity (p value ≥ 0.05) was observed, as measured by Cochran's Q. The I^2 statistic was employed as a continuous measure of heterogeneity. Statistical analysis was performed in the Statistical Package for the Social Science (SPSS; version 17.0, IL, USA) and meta-analysis using Comprehensive Meta-Analysis (software version 2.0; Biostat, Englewood, NJ). Since this study is entirely descriptive, we did not formulate nor test any hypothesis.

3. Results

Figure 1 depicts the flow of search results in this review. The VHL search retrieved 31 results, PubMed 18 results, and EMBASE another 31 results. EMBASE and VHL retrieved identical results, which encompassed all the 18 articles found in PubMed. After the first screening and removal of overlapping result across databases, 19 articles were deemed eligible. Four studies reported data on at least one of the studied variables and were included in the meta-analysis. There were three available datasets: (i) two datasets from population-based cross-sectional studies conducted in large representative samples of two cities from Southern Brazil, Porto Alegre (capital of the state; SOFT study; $n = 1858$) [6, 7]; (ii) a third dataset was originated from a nationwide cross-sectional study conducted among 1148 industry workers (SESI study previously carried out by one of the authors) [3, 4]; (iii) a nationwide registry of hypertensive and diabetic patients treated in primary care of SUS (with of 7.3 million individuals on treatment for hypertension) collected from the

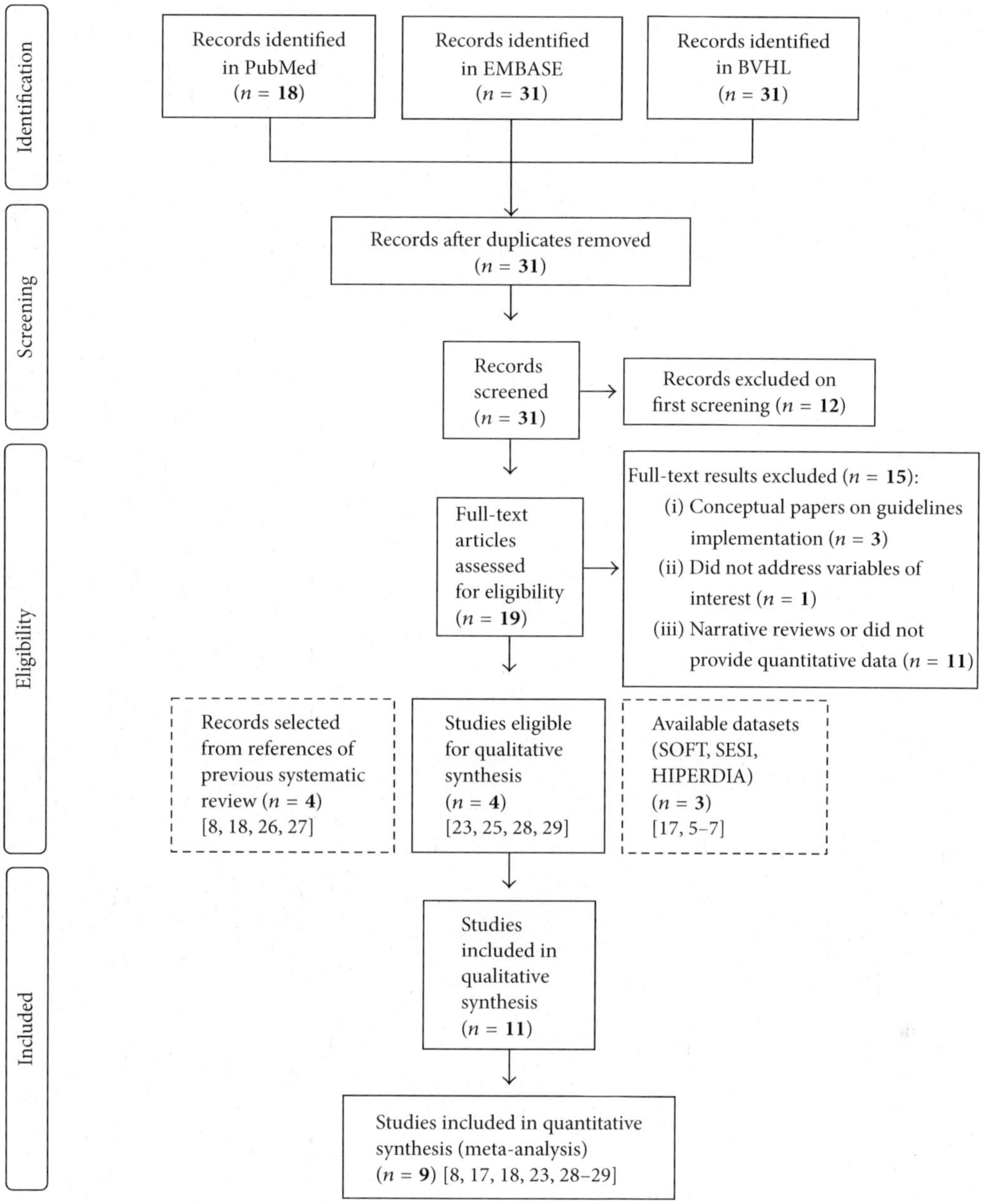

FIGURE 1: Flow chart of records retrieved, screened, and included in the systematic review.

HIPERDIA [5]. Another four studies included in a previous systematic review were considered eligible and, hence, were added to this meta-analysis along with the three aforementioned datasets, rendering a total of 11 studies [8, 19–21].

Table 1 shows characteristics of the studies and HIPERDIA registry that provided data on clinical characteristics of individuals with HT according to sex. Studies that have data on mean systolic blood pressure and blood pressure control are presented in Table 1 as well. In the SESI study, men and women had similar SBP, but women had higher rate of hypertension control than men. In the population-based studies men and women had similar mean systolic blood pressure and rates of hypertension control. Higher prevalence of DM was observed among patients registered in HIPERDIA, especially in comparison to the participants of the SESI study. Smoking prevalence rates were more evenly distributed across the SESI study, HIPERDIA registry, and population-based studies, with higher prevalence of current smokers in men in comparison to women.

Table 2 presents information from seven studies that provided data on pharmacotherapy, diagnostic tests, and medical appointments. Less than half of the hypertensive subjects were using a single BPLM, and the most common class of BPLM was thiazide diuretics, followed by angiotensin-converting enzyme (ACE) inhibitors. Thiazide diuretics combined with ACE inhibitors were the most frequent 2-drug combination in use (14.9%), followed by thiazides and beta-blockers (9.4%).

TABLE 1: Clinical characteristics of individuals with hypertension from the SESI study, the HIPERDIA registry, and from meta-analyses of four population-based studies.

Studies and clinical characteristics	Mean (±SD)/prevalence (95% CI)	
	Men	Women
SESI study [3, 4]: participants (n)	1034	114
Age (years)	40.6 (11.8)	41.5 (9.2)
Systolic blood pressure (mmHg)	152.5 (15.9)	150.4 (21.7)
Controlled blood pressure	31.8 (26.3–37.7)	56.9 (45.5–67.7)
Total cholesterol (mg/dL)	188.8 (40.0)	196.0 (39.2)
HDL cholesterol (mg/dL)	49.3 (20.9)	56.8 (12.7)
Current smokers	18.3 (15.9–20.7)	15.5 (8.9–22.1)
Diabetes mellitus (DM)	5.6 (4.2–7.0)	3.5 (0.1–6.9)
HIPERDIA registry [5]: participants (n)	2.5 million	4.8 million
Current smokers	21.42 (20.4–22.5)	15.6 (14.7–16.5)
Diabetes mellitus	21.9 (19.8–24.0)	24.9 (22.9–27.0)
Current smokers with DM	6.3 (5.8–6.8)	5.6 (5.2–6.0)
Population-based studies: participants (n)	5064	8126
Systolic blood pressure (mm Hg)		
Trevisol et al. [6]	146.8 (20.7)	138.9 (22.6)
Dias da Costa et al. [7]	144.5 (8.3)	146.1 (20.7)
Controlled blood pressure		
Trevisol et al. [6]	47.8 (39.7–56.1)	43.7 (38.5–49.2)
Dias da Costa et al. [7]	65.7 (53.7–75.9)	67.5 (60.7–73.7)
Moreira et al. [8]	53.0 (46.9–58.4)	52.7 (45.6–58.9)
Current smokers	21.7 (17.2–27.0)‡	14.8 (10.1–21.0)*
Diabetes mellitus**	13.5 (12.5–14.4)†	13.2 (8.3–20.7)††

‡Q $p < 0.01$; $I^2 = 90.0\%$. *Data from 7867 women. Q $p < 0.01$; $I^2 = 94.1\%$. †Fixed effect model analysis. Q $p = 0.24$; $I^2 = 27.4\%$. **Data from 4912 men and 7867 women; ††Q $p < 0.01$; $I^2 = 87.3\%$.

Data on diagnostic tests came from one study, and estimates on most used type of medical services came from another study. Approximately a third of individuals with known HT had fasting plasma glucose, serum triglycerides, total cholesterol, and creatinine level measured in the previous 12 months. On average, an adult with HT had 2.6 medical appointments per year, and more than half of subjects who sought medical appointments used mostly those provided by the SUS. Figures 2, 3, and 4 are forest plots illustrating contents from Table 2. Figure 2 shows considerable heterogeneity among studies, mostly due to the study of Lima et al. [19], carried out in Rio de Janeiro.

4. Discussion

This systematic review examined all available databases that provide information on the management of HT among the Brazilian adult population. Some of them described the compliance with treatment guidelines of the State Health Department or provided an opinion on this matter [22, 23]. One article assessed physicians' compliance with HT treatment according to a Municipal Health Department guideline and detected noncompliance rates of 56.8%, 63.8%, and 54.0% regarding HT staging, cardiovascular risk classification, and choice of treatment, respectively [20].

Official data estimate that about 75% of the country's population depends exclusively on SUS for health care [24], but it has not been confirmed by the information from a population-based study carried out in the city of Pelotas [7]. The divergence may be explained by at least two biases from both sources of information: (i) the use of SUS services probably does not reach the 75% rate for all health conditions; (ii) recall bias of the medical appointments made in the previous month by participants of the population-based study. Nonetheless, the systematic review data derives from a single city; therefore it is hardly representative of the entire country.

Medical treatment by use of blood pressure lowering agents, conversely, was more often reported, so HT treatment data might be more representative of nationwide clinical practice within the SUS. Blood pressure control rates among individuals with HT could not be summarized through the results of all included studies, but it was reported for three population-based studies. The rates of controlled hypertension were higher than that reported in a previously systematic review, which identified a pooled control estimate of 24.1%

TABLE 2: Frequency of blood pressure lowering medication use, diagnostic tests, and medical appointments among hypertensive subjects.

	Prevalence (95% CI)/mean (±SD)	Heterogeneity	
	Status quo	Q *p* value	I^2
Blood pressure lowering medication (%)			
In use of one BPLM	42.7 (28.6–58.1)	<0.01	99.0
In use of two BPLM	33.0 (23.7–43.9)	<0.01	92.4
Type of BPLM			
Thiazide diuretics			
Single-drug therapy or combined with another drug	41.1 (26.4–57.6)	<0.01	98.3
Single-drug therapy	18.2 (7.4–38.4)	<0.01	96.6
Combined with ACEI	14.9 (11.1–19.8)	<0.01	84.6
Combined with BB	9.4 (5.7–15.2)	<0.01	86.5
Combined with CCB‡	5.0 (2.4–7.6)	NA	NA
Angiotensin-converting enzyme inhibitors (ACEI)			
Single-drug therapy or combined with another drug	41.1 (20.2–65.7)	<0.01	97.7
Single-drug therapy	16.2 (11.6–22.1)	<0.01	85.0
Combined with BB†	3.4 (2.5–4.7)	0.07	62.1
Combined with CCB‡	4.0 (2.1–5.9)	NA	NA
Beta-blockers (BB)			
Single-drug therapy or combined with other BPLM	21.2 (17.3–25.8)	<0.01	84.3
Single-drug therapy†	10.0 (8.1–12.3)	0.17	46.2
Combined with CCB‡	2.3 (0.5–4.1)	NA	NA
Calcium channel blockers (CCB)			
Single-drug therapy or combined with other BPLM	10.0 (7.5–13.3)	<0.01	72.4
Single-drug therapy‡	3.9 (1.6–6.2)	NA	NA
Angiotensin receptor blockers (ARB)			
Single-drug therapy or combined with other BPLM†	2.3 (1.4–3.6)	0.06	71.2
Diagnostic tests and procedures (%) among hypertensive subjects			
Previous month testing			
Electrocardiography‡	6.3 (3.9–8.8)	NA	NA
Any radiography‡	9.7 (6.8–12.7)	NA	NA
Any urine test‡	8.4 (5.6–11.2)	NA	NA
Any blood test‡	12.6 (9.3–16.0)	NA	NA
Direct ophthalmoscopy‡*	35.0 (30.2–39.8)	NA	NA
Previous 12-month testing			
Serum potassium‡	19.5 (13.9–25.2)	NA	NA
Serum creatinine‡	31.0 (24.4–29.6)	NA	NA
Total serum cholesterol‡	35.5 (28.7–42.3)	NA	NA
Serum LDL or HDL cholesterol‡	25.0 (18.3–31.2)	NA	NA
Serum triglycerides‡	34.0 (27.3–40.8)	NA	NA
Fasting plasma glucose‡	36.5 (29.6–43.4)	NA	NA
Urine analysis‡	25.0 (18.8–31.2)	NA	NA
Medical appointments (%) among hypertensive subjects			
Annual mean of medical appointments	2.62 (2.37)	0.5	0
Mostly using Brazilian Health Care System‡	51.2 (46.1–56.2)	NA	NA
Mostly using private physicians‡	20.9 (16.8–25.1)	NA	NA
Mostly using health plan physician‡	13.0 (9.6–16.4)	NA	NA
Mostly using emergency services‡	1.9 (0.5–3.2)	NA	NA
Others‡	13.0 (9.6–16.4)	NA	NA

†Fixed effect analysis. ‡Based on one study. *Since the diagnosis of hypertension; LDL: low-density lipoprotein; HDL: high-density lipoprotein; Q *p* value and I^2–: nonapplicable; that is, only one study provided data; NA: not applicable.

First author	Year	City	Sample size	%	95% CI
Dias da Costa [7]	2002	Pelotas	262	53.0	46.9–59.0
de Souza [21]	2003	São Paulo	392	46.7	41.8–51.6
Moreira [8]	2009	São José do Rio Preto	549	44.6	40.5–48.8
Lima [19]	2009	Rio de Janeiro	3133	18.4	17.1–19.8
Maluf [20]	2010	Curitiba	189	57.0	49.8–63.9
Summary			*4525*	*42.7*	*28.6–58.1*

Summary $T^2 = 0.82$, $Q < 0.01$, $I^2 = 99.0\%$

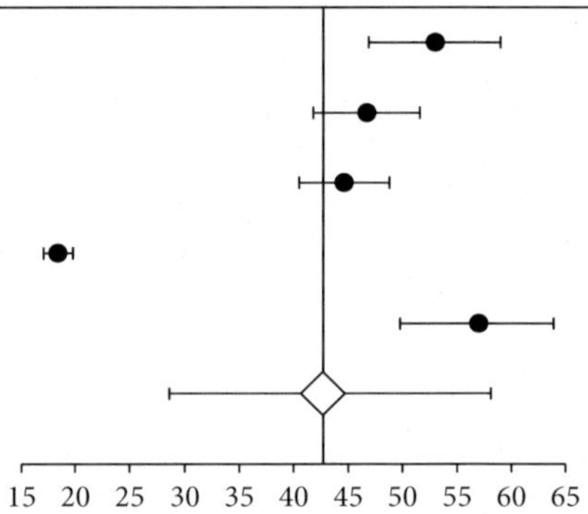

BPLM: blood pressure lowering medication; 95% CI: 95% confidence interval.

FIGURE 2: Meta-analysis of proportion of use of one BPLM (in chronological order according to the data collection year).

First author	Year	City	Sample size	%	95% CI
de Souza [21]	2003	São Paulo	392	22.4	18.5–26.8
Moreira [8]	2009	S. José do Rio Preto	549	41.2	37.2–45.4
Lima [19]	2009	Rio de Janeiro	3133	37.2	35.5–38.9
Maluf [20]	2010	Curitiba	189	32.5	26.2–39.5
Summary			*4263*	*33.0*	*23.7–43.9*

Summary $T^2 = 0.09$, $Q < 0.01$, $I^2 = 92.4\%$

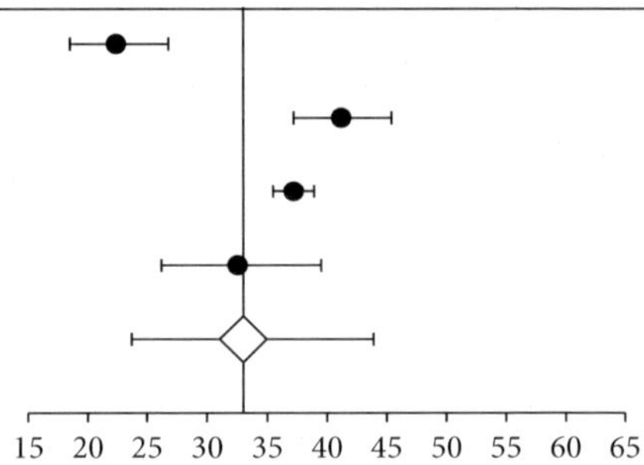

BPLM: blood pressure lowering medication; 95% CI: 95% confidence interval.

FIGURE 3: Meta-analysis of proportion of use of two blood pressure lowering medication.

(10.1–47.3%) [9]. The use of thiazide-type diuretics (as single or combined-drug therapy) was widespread in our analysis. This is in concordance with the best available evidence of effectiveness and current guidelines that advocate for the use of these drugs as first line treatment [12]. However, considering that there are few absolute contraindications for the use of diuretics, one may argue that the 41% usage rate should have been higher. On the other side, thiazide diuretics are more often used in Brazil than in Denmark, Finland, Germany, Norway, Sweden, Netherlands [25], Portugal [26], Spain [27], Mexico [28], and the United States [29]. Among other antihypertensive drugs, the use of beta-blockers was similar to that reported in other countries, but the prevalence of calcium channel blockers (CCB), ACE inhibitors, and ARBs use was much lower. CCB and ARB were rarely used to treat HT, since these drugs were not available in the SUS by the time that most of the studies were conducted. An ARB agent, by the opposite, was recently incorporated in the SUS.

Although there are several population-based studies that evaluated the prevalence of HT all over the country, only four studies provided information on how participants with hypertension were treated. The vast majority of these field studies restricted their assessment to measuring the prevalence of HT and other diseases among the general population, reporting little or no information with regard to individuals with HT (mean age of participants with HT, blood pressure control rates, etc.). Five studies reported the prevalence of hypertensive patients using one BPLM. The summary estimate of prevalence was reduced due to the weight of a study performed at a primary care center in Rio de Janeiro [19]. This study introduced heterogeneity due to the variability in the number of follow-up visits, ranging from 1 to 27, and to participants who did not use any medication (7.8%) and used two or more BPLMs (73.8%) and 18.4% who used only one drug to decrease BP. This study had a major contribution to the overall results.

Another limitation of the present study is the overall paucity of publications. This scarcity contrasts with a huge amount of data on patient management generated every day inside the SUS [2], with more than 40.4 million medical appointments recorded in the HIPERDIA registry from August 2011 to July 2012 [5].

Finally, our data did not cover the years since the new public program, Farmácia popular (popular pharmacy), for delivery of drugs and devices was launched, including the

Type of therapy	First author	Year	Sample size	%	95% CI
Single-drug or combined					
	Dias da Costa	2002	262	57.9	51.8–63.7
	de Souza	2003	392	32.6	28.2–37.4
	Moreira	2009	549	39.9	35.8–44.0
	Maluf	2010	189	51.5	44.4–58.5
	Santa Helena	2006	565	26.0	22.5–29.8
	Hoepfner	2007	415	72.4	67.9–76.5
	Trevisol	2012	426	44.4	39.7–49.1
	Summary		*2798*	*46.1*	*33.2–59.6*
		Summary $\tau^2 = 0.44$, $Q < 0.01$, $I^2 = 97.5\%$			
Single-drug					
	Dias da Costa	2002	262	27.4	22.3–33.1
	Moreira	2009	549	11.6	9.2–14.6
	Summary		*811*	*18.2*	*7.4–38.4*
		Summary $\tau^2 = 0.53$, $Q < 0.01$, $I^2 = 96.6\%$			
Combined with ACEI					
	Dias da Costa	2002	262	11.0	7.7–15.4
	de Souza	2003	392	11.0	8.3–14.5
	Moreira	2009	549	19.5	16.4–23.0
	Santa Helena	2006	565	18.6	15.6–22.0
	Summary		*1768*	*14.9*	*11.07–19.7*
		Summary $\tau^2 = 0.10$, $Q < 0.01$, $I^2 = 84.6\%$			
Combined with BB					
	Dias da Costa	2002	262	15.0	11.2–19.9
	de Souza	2003	392	6.0	4.0–8.8
	Moreira	2009	549	8.7	6.7–11.4
	Summary		*1203*	*9.4*	*5.7–15.2*
		Summary $\tau^2 = 0.20$, $Q < 0.01$, $I^2 = 86.5\%$			

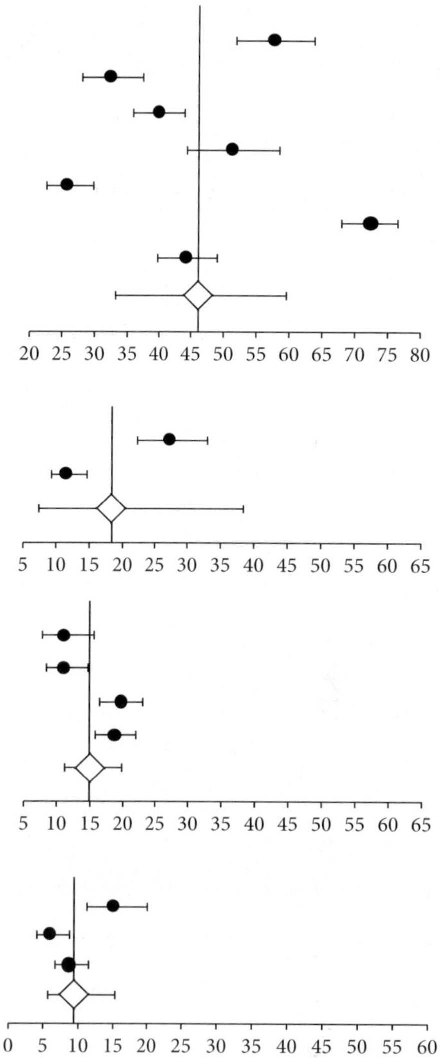

ACEI: angiotensin-converting enzyme inhibitors; BB: beta-blockers; 95% CI: 95% confidence interval.

FIGURE 4: Meta-analysis of proportion of use of thiazide-based therapy.

subsidized offering of losartan (90% of rebate). Twenty percent of the population is presently covered (http://www.brasil.gov.br/saude/2016/03/aqui-tem-farmacia-popular-atende-38-milhoes-de-brasileiros-em-10-anos, accessed in December, 22, 2016). The impact of this program in the use of BP lowering drugs was not captured in the surveys available for this systematic review.

5. Conclusions

Despite these limitations, the estimates presented by this review are the best available evidence about the pattern of use of BP lowering drugs and rate of BP control in Brazil. Further studies should prospectively collect data to better describe the impact of new BP lowering agents. Thiazide diuretics and ACE inhibitors were the most frequently used as a single drug, and ACE inhibitors were the BP lowering medications more frequently prescribed, but the rate of hypertension control is insufficient.

Disclosure

The funding agencies had no participation in the planning or execution of the study or the analyses of the study data. An earlier version of this work was presented as an abstract at International Symposium on Cardiovascular Epidemiology.

Authors' Contributions

The authors contributed equally to the conceptual development of the study and subsequent draft of the manuscript. All authors read and approved the final manuscript.

Acknowledgments

This work was supported by the Coordination for the Improvement of Higher Education Personnel (CAPES; MD/PhD Program), the National Council of Technological and Scientific Development (CNPq), and the Fundo de Incentivo à Pesquisa (FIPE) of the Hospital de Clínicas de Porto Alegre, RS, Brazil.

References

[1] M. Velasco-Garrido and R. Busse, "Health technology assessment: an introduction to objectives, role of evidence, and structure in Europe," World Health Organization 2005, on behalf of the European Observatory on Health Systems and Policies, http://www.euro.who.int/Document/E87866.pdf.

[2] J. Paim, C. Travassos, C. Almeida, L. Bahia, and J. MacInko, "The Brazilian health system: history, advances, and challenges," *The Lancet*, vol. 377, no. 9779, pp. 1778–1797, 2011.

[3] Serviço Social da Indústria, "Departamento Nacional. Unidade de Saúde e Segurança do Trabalho. Estudo SESI: perfil epidemiológico de fatores de risco para doenças não-transmissíveis em trabalhadores da indústria do Brasil. Brasília: CNI/SESI," 2007.

[4] D. B. Vinholes, I. M. F. Melo, C. A. MacHado, H. De Castro Chaves, F. D. Fuchs, and S. C. Fuchs, "The association between socioeconomic characteristics and consumption of food items among Brazilian industry workers," *The Scientific World Journal*, vol. 2012, Article ID 808245, 14 pages, 2012.

[5] Departamento de Informática do SUS, "Informações de Saúde: Epidemiológicas e Morbidade," April 2012, http://www2.datasus.gov.br/DATASUS/index.php?area=0203&VObj=http://tabnet.datasus.gov.br/cgi/deftohtm.exe?hiperdia/cnv/hd.

[6] D. J. Trevisol, L. B. Moreira, F. D. Fuchs, and S. C. Fuchs, "Health-related quality of life is worse in individuals with hypertension under drug treatment: results of population-based study," *Journal of Human Hypertension*, vol. 26, no. 6, pp. 374–380, 2012.

[7] J. S. Dias Da Costa, S. C. Fuchs, M. T. Anselmo Olinto et al., "Cost-effectiveness of hypertension treatment: a population-based study," *Sao Paulo Medical Journal*, vol. 120, no. 4, pp. 100–104, 2002.

[8] G. C. Moreira, J. P. Cipullo, J. F. Vilela Martin et al., "Evaluation of the awareness, control and cost-effectiveness of hypertension treatment in a Brazilian city: populational study," *Journal of Hypertension*, vol. 27, no. 9, pp. 1900–1907, 2009.

[9] R. V. Picon, F. D. Fuchs, L. B. Moreira, G. Riegel, and S. C. Fuchs, "Trends in prevalence of hypertension in Brazil: a systematic review with meta-analysis," *PLoS ONE*, vol. 7, no. 10, Article ID e48255, 2012.

[10] S. Lewington, R. Clarke, N. Qizilbash, R. Peto, and R. Collins, "Age-specific relevance of usual blood pressure to vascular mortality: a meta-analysis of individual data for one million adults in 61 prospective studies," *The Lancet*, vol. 360, no. 9349, pp. 1903–1913, 2002.

[11] M. I. Schmidt, B. B. Duncan, G. A. E Silva et al., "Chronic non-communicable diseases in Brazil: burden and current challenges," *The Lancet*, vol. 377, no. 9781, pp. 1949–1961, 2011.

[12] M. V. B. Malachias, W. K. S. B. Souza, F. L. Plavnik et al., "7th Brazilian Guideline of Arterial Hypertension," *Arquivos Brasileiros de Cardiologia*, vol. 107, pp. 1–83, 2016.

[13] M. F. Drummond, M. J. Sculpher, K. Claxton, G. L. Stoddart, and G. W. Torrance, Eds., *Methods for the economic evaluation of health care programmes*, chapters 8 and 9, Oxford University Press, Oxford, UK, 4th edition, 2015.

[14] M. Egger, G. D. Smith, and D. G. Altman, *Systematic Review in Health Care: Meta-Analysis in Context*, BMJ Publishing Group, London, UK, 2nd edition, 2003.

[15] M. Pai, M. McCulloch, J. D. Gorman et al., "Systematic reviews and meta-analyses: an illustrated, step-by-step guide," *National Medical Journal of India*, vol. 17, no. 2, pp. 86–95, 2004.

[16] M. J. Sculpher, F. S. Pang, A. Manca et al., "Generalisability in economic evaluation studies in healthcare: a review and case studies," *Health Technology Assessment*, vol. 8, no. 49, pp. 1–192, 2004.

[17] A. V. Chobanian, G. L. Bakris, H. R. Black et al., "Joint National Committee on Prevention, Detection, Evaluation, and Treatment of High Blood Pressure. National Heart, Lung, and Blood Institute; National High Blood Pressure Education Program Coordinating Committee. Seventh Report of the Joint National Committee on Prevention, Detection, Evaluation, and Treatment of High Blood Pressure," *Hypertension*, vol. 42, no. 6, pp. 1206–1252, 2003.

[18] R. B. D'Agostino Sr., R. S. Vasan, M. J. Pencina et al., "General cardiovascular risk profile for use in primary care: the Framingham heart study," *Circulation*, vol. 117, no. 6, pp. 743–753, 2008.

[19] S. M. L. Lima, M. C. Portela, I. Koster et al., "Use of clinical guidelines and the results in primary healthcare for hypertension," *Cadernos de Saúde Pública*, vol. 25, pp. 2001–2011, 2009.

[20] I. Maluf Jr., M. R. Zahdi, N. Unterstell, E. M. C. P. Maluf, A. B. D. Sousa, and F. D. Loures, "Evaluation of physicians' compliance with the hypertension protocol of the Municipal Health Department of the city of Curitiba," *Arquivos Brasileiros de Cardiologia*, vol. 94, no. 1, pp. 86–91, 2010.

[21] J. J. G. de Souza, *Hipertensão arterial referida e uso de anti-hipertensivos em adultos na cidade de São Paulo, 2003: um estudo de base populacional [M.S. thesis]*, Universidade de São Paulo, Faculdade de Saúde Pública, São Paulo, Brazil, 2006.

[22] J. M. B. D. S. Costa, M. R. F. da Silva, and E. F. de Carvalho, "The implementation analysis of the arterial hypertension care by the Family Health teams in Recife city (Pernambuco, Brazil)," *Ciencia e Saude Coletiva*, vol. 16, no. 2, pp. 623–633, 2011.

[23] V. M. V. Paniz, A. G. Fassa, L. A. Facchini et al., "Free access to hypertension and diabetes medicines among the elderly: a reality yet to be constructed," *Cadernos de Saude Publica*, vol. 26, no. 6, pp. 1163–1174, 2010.

[24] Brasil. Ministério da Saúde. Organização Pan-Americana da Saúde, *Avaliação do plano de reorganização da atenção à hipertensão arterial e ao diabetes mellitus no Brasil*, Ministério da Saúde, Brasilia, Brazil, 2004.

[25] P. Stolk, B. L. G. Van Wijk, H. G. M. Leufkens, and E. R. Heerdink, "Between-country variation in the utilization of antihypertensive agents: guidelines and clinical practice," *Journal of Human Hypertension*, vol. 20, no. 12, pp. 917–922, 2006.

[26] C. Furtado and M. Pinto, "Antihypertensive drug utilization in Continental Portugal (1999-2004)," *Revista Portuguesa de Cardiologia*, vol. 25, article 27392, 2006.

4

Adherence to Antihypertensive Medications in Iranian Patients

Azin Behnood-Rod,[1] Omid Rabbanifar,[2] Pirouz Pourzargar,[3] Alireza Rai,[4] Zahra Saadat,[3] Habibollah Saadat,[3] Yashar Moharamzad,[3,4] and Donald E. Morisky[5]

[1] *Islamic Azad University, Tehran Medical Branch, Tehran, Iran*
[2] *Zanjan University of Medical Sciences, Zanjan, Iran*
[3] *Cardiovascular Research Center, Shahid Beheshti University of Medical Sciences, Tehran, Iran*
[4] *School of Medicine, Kermanshah University of Medical Sciences, Kermanshah, Iran*
[5] *Department of Community Health Sciences, UCLA Fielding School of Public Health, Los Angeles, CA, USA*

Correspondence should be addressed to Alireza Rai; alireza.rai2014@yahoo.com

Academic Editor: Tomohiro Katsuya

Introduction. Appropriate adherence to medication is still a challenging issue for hypertensive patients. We determined adherence to antihypertensive(s) and its associated factors among 280 Iranian patients. *Methods.* They were recruited consecutively from private and university health centers and pharmacies in four cities. The validated Persian version of the 8-item Morisky Medication Adherence Scale (MMAS-8) was administered to measure adherence. *Results.* Mean (±SD) overall MMAS-8 score was 5.75 (±1.88). About half of the sample (139 cases, 49.6%) showed low adherence (MMAS-8 score < 6). There was a negative linear association between the MMAS-8 score and systolic BP ($r = -0.231$, $P < 0.001$) as well as diastolic BP ($r = -0.280$, $P < 0.001$). In linear regression model, overweight/obesity ($B = -0.52$, $P = 0.02$), previous history of admission to emergency services due to hypertensive crisis ($B = -0.79$, $P = 0.001$), and getting medication directly from drugstore without refill prescription in hand ($B = -0.51$, $P = 0.04$) were factors recognized to have statistically significant association with the MMAS-8 score. *Conclusion.* Antihypertensive adherence was unsatisfactory. We suggest that health care providers pay special attention and make use of the aforementioned findings in their routine visits of hypertensive patients to recognize those who are vulnerable to poor adherence.

1. Introduction

Hypertension (HTN) is a major public health challenge in many parts of the world [1]. Left uncontrolled, HTN poses serious health problems on sufferers including heart attack, heart failure, and stroke [2]. Health care providers should make use of all armamentariums available for better control of HTN. Beside regular checkups, medication intensification, health surveillance, and patient education, a factor that health care providers should be more aware about in facing this population is assessing the extent to which hypertensive patients comply with medications as prescribed for them (i.e., adherence to medication) [3].

Considering the fact that there are effective medications available to control HTN and the aggressive stance required with hypertensive patients, we think that assessing the issue of medication adherence could be an integral part of management of such patients. In other words, medication adherence, although a complex issue with various associated factors, is a very critical component in controlling blood pressure (BP) of patients within the recommended normal ranges and consequently achieving good health outcome in long term and holding up the cardiovascular complications [4]. Nonadherence has been noted as one of the contributing factors in uncontrolled BP [5].

The pertinent literature review from different countries revealed that adherence to medications prescribed for patients with high BP may not be satisfactory. Good/acceptable adherence, determined via various tools, has been reported as 15.8% [6], 20.3% [7], 43.1% [8], 43.7% [9], 46% [10], 53% [11], 58% [12], and 77% [13]. As seen, most studies reported that good adherence to antihypertensives was documented in half of the patients studied. Most of the aforementioned studies also conceded that poor medication adherence was significantly associated with uncontrolled BP.

Hitherto, studies regarding medication adherence among hypertensive patients from Iran are insufficient. There are reports that a substantial proportion of patients have uncontrolled BP, reportedly 56.3% [14], 62% [15], and 65% [16]. In a comparative analysis carried out on data from national surveys of 20 countries, Iran was recognized as one of the countries with poor diagnosis and control of HTN [17]. With respect to lack of enough information about this issue in Iran, we intended to determine the antihypertensive adherence status of a sample of Iranian patients with HTN and find out any allied significant factor contributing to low medication adherence.

2. Materials and Methods

This cross-sectional study lasted from August to December 2014. This was a multicenter study including tertiary referral center of university-affiliated hospital, private cardiology office, pharmacy, and private general practitioner office in the cities of Tehran, Karaj, Kermanshah, and Bafgh. Inclusion criteria were adult patients of either gender who had documented HTN and were taking antihypertensive medications. The patients were interviewed directly at health centers or offices upon their presentation for checking their BP or to refill their prescriptions. A coordination session was held before the study initiation and the participating doctors and pharmacists were instructed by the principal investigator to interview any patient meeting the inclusion criteria consecutively during their daily visit of the patients in predetermined research locations. The pharmacists were asked to refer the eligible subjects to one of the nearest physicians involved in this research. For known patients for whom a medical record existed, in addition to the interview, other pertinent data were extrapolated from their records and were documented in the forms.

To determine the adherence to antihypertensives, the Persian version of the MMAS-8 which was validated by our team in a previous study was administered to the patients. The MMAS-8 was developed as a simple and reliable tool which can be used by clinicians to determine the adherence of patients to prescribed medications [18]. The 8-item scale was originally studied in hypertensive patients and the results revealed that it was a reliable ($\alpha = 0.83$) tool and showed significant correlation with BP control ($P < 0.05$). It showed a sensitivity of 93% in detecting patients with poor BP control [19]. In our previous study on 200 Iranian patients who were suffering from HTN, we determined the Persian version of the MMAS-8 to be valid and reliable tool with an overall Cronbach's α coefficient of 0.697 and test-retest reliability showed good reproducibility ($r = 0.940$) [20].

In addition to the MMAS-8, a checklist was designed by the authors to gather demographic as well as variables about other diseases or medications the patients were taking. First, the MMAS was completed by the patients. If the patient was illiterate, the researcher read the questions for the patient and asked him/her to answer the questions orally. Then the correspondent answer was marked by the researcher on the MMAS and checklist. After completing the MMAS, the checklist data was completed. The data included in the checklist were demographic data (age, gender, weight, height, occupation, and educational level), duration of HTN, medications prescribed for HTN, other comorbidities, other medications other than antihypertensives, and control of HTN during the last 6 months by a health care provider. One of the variables included in the checklist was history of HTN crisis, in the form of emergency or urgency, leading to emergency admission. This variable was investigated using the medical records available at the research location or those from other medical centers in the past. Only documented reports/discharge notes signed by medical professionals containing detailed information were used to decide the previous history of HTN crisis. At the end, BP of the patients was measured by the researchers using a sphygmomanometer on the left arm when the patient was in seated position. The patients were asked to seat relaxed and not smoke for half an hour before BP recording. Korotkoff sounds were the basis to define systolic and diastolic BP. For the purpose of this study, brand new sphygmomanometers were provided to the doctors and an educational video was displayed and reviewed to ensure the lowest level of variation between BP readings by the research team members.

2.1. Statistical Analyses. All gathered data were entered into the SPSS software for Windows (ver. 18.0) (SPSS Inc., Chicago, IL). To express the results, we used descriptive indices including mean and its standard deviation (SD), frequency and percentage. Regarding the MMAS-8 score, we divided the patients into two groups of low adherence (i.e., MMAS-8 score of less than 6) versus moderate/high adherence (i.e., MMAS-8 scores of 6–8). The Chi-squared and Mann-Whitney U tests were applied to compare, respectively, the gathered categorical and continuous data between these two groups of MMAS-8 scores. To find any relationship between controlled BP (i.e., systolic BP < 140 and diastolic BP < 90 mmHg in nondiabetics and $< 130/80$ mmHg in diabetics) and MMAS score, the Pearson correlation test was used. Significance level was set at 0.05. To find correlation between systolic and diastolic BP values and the MMAS-8 score, Spearman's rho test was used. A multiple logistic regression analysis was done to predict effective variables that can affect poor drug adherence. In this analysis, all variables were indicated as independent and poor drug adherence (i.e., MMAS score < 6) was indicated as the dependent variable.

2.2. Ethics. Firstly, the objective of the study was explained to the patients. If the patient was interested in contributing to the study and gave his/her oral consent, then instructions about how to complete the MMAS-8 and the demographic form were provided to them. They were assured that the information will be used only for scientific purposes. The protocol of the study was in conformity with the Helsinki Declaration.

Table 1: Comparison of demographic characteristics between low and moderate/high adherence groups among 280 Iranian hypertensive patients.

	Total (N = 280)	Low adherence (N = 139)	Moderate/high adherence (N = 141)	Sig.
Gender				
Male	118 (42.1%)	59 (50%)	59 (50%)	0.919
Female	162 (57.9%)	80 (49.4%)	82 (50.6%)	
Age, years				
≤50	51 (18.2%)	25 (49%)	26 (51%)	0.922
>50	229 (81.8%)	114 (49.8%)	115 (50.2%)	
BMI, kg/m^2				
<25	76 (27.1%)	28 (36.8%)	48 (63.2%)	0.011
≥25	204 (72.9%)	111 (54.4%)	93 (45.6%)	
Education				
Lower than high school diploma/illiterate	164 (58.5%)	86 (52.4%)	78 (47.6%)	
High school diploma	71 (25.4%)	40 (56.3%)	31 (43.7%)	0.008
Academic degree	45 (16.1%)	13 (28.9%)	32 (71.7%)	
Occupation				
Market/self-employed	73 (26.1%)	43 (58.9%)	30 (41.4%)	
Clerk/military	41 (14.6%)	9 (22.0%)	32 (78.0%)	0.001
Housewife	119 (42.5%)	65 (54.6%)	54 (45.4%)	
Retired/unemployed	47 (16.8%)	22 (46.8%)	25 (53.2%)	
Current smoker	49 (17.5%)	29 (59.2%)	20 (40.8%)	0.141
Insurance coverage	246 (87.8%)	119 (48.4%)	127 (51.6%)	0.253
Residence place				
Urban	273 (97.5%)	133 (48.7%)	140 (51.3%)	0.053
Rural	7 (2.5%)	6 (85.7%)	1 (14.3%)	

Sig. = significance level.

3. Results

In total, 280 patients were included. Mean (±SD) age of the participants was 60.3 (±10.0) years, 118 cases (42.1%) were male, 204 (72.9%) were overweight/obese (BMI values of ≥25 kg/m^2), 164 (58.5%) had education level below high school diploma or were illiterate, and 49 (17.5%) were current smokers. Mean (±SD) overall MMAS-8 score was 5.75 (±1.88). About half of the sample (139 cases, 49.6%) showed low adherence to antihypertensives. Ninety-five cases (33.9%) had moderate adherence and 46 cases (16.4%) showed high adherence.

Table 1 presents demographic characteristics of the sample and comparison of these data between low and medium/high adherence groups. As depicted, there was higher percentage of patients with BMI values of less than 25 kg/m^2 in moderate/high adherence group compared to low adherence group. Also, those who had received academic training and had occupations as clerk or in military personnel represented better adherence. However, considering other demographic information including gender, age, having an insurance coverage, residential place (urban areas versus rural ones), and being a smoker did not reveal significant difference between low and moderate/high adherers.

Mean (±SD) duration of HTN was 7.2 (±5.9) years (range, 6 months to 40 years). General practitioner (67 cases, 23.9%) and cardiologist (65 cases, 23.2%) were the most common presented physicians whose patients reported that they visit to control their high BP. Others reported visiting internist (24 cases, 8.6%), nephrologist (9 cases, 3.2%), or more than one physician to check their BP (115 patients, 41.0%). According to the criteria, 122 patients out of 280 cases (43.6%) had controlled BP. Among diabetics (i.e., 55 hypertensive diabetics with/without other concomitant conditions), only 2 cases (3.6%) had controlled BP. Table 2 shows comparison of BP-related variables between low and moderate/high adherers. As seen, those who were low adherers had higher percentage of hypertensive crisis (hypertensive emergency or urgency) which required admission to hospital emergency services, lower rate of visiting their doctors to get their BP checked during the preceding 6 months from the study, and higher systolic and diastolic BP measurements when compared to moderate/high adherers. Controlled BP was also significantly higher in moderate/high nondiabetic adherers compared to those who had low MMAS-8 score. About diabetics, since the sample size was not enough, statistical significance was not seen.

Table 2: Comparison of blood pressure variables between low and moderate/high adherence groups among 280 Iranian hypertensive patients.

	Total ($N = 280$)	Low adherers ($N = 139$)	Moderate/high adherers ($N = 141$)	Sig.
HTN duration, mean (±SD), year	7.23 (±5.97)	7.06 (±5.71)	7.40 (±6.23)	0.966
History of HTN crisis	99 (35.3%)	62 (62.5%)	37 (37.4%)	0.001
BP measurement by a health care provider in the last 6 months	230 (82.1%)	107 (46.5%)	123 (53.5%)	0.025
Self-awareness of BP	161 (57.5%)	81 (50.3%)	80 (49.7%)	0.795
Mean systolic BP, mmHg	136.7 (±16.2)	139.6 (±15.2)	133.8 (±16.8)	0.003
Mean diastolic BP, mmHg	83.9 (±9.0)	85.7 (±8.3)	82.1 (±9.2)	<0.001
Controlled BP in nondiabetics	120	49 (40.8%)	71 (59.2%)	<0.001
Controlled BP in diabetics	2	0	2 (100%)	0.504

Table 3: Comparison of number of antihypertensives and comorbidities between low and moderate/high adherence groups among 280 Iranian hypertensive patients.

	Total ($N = 280$)	Low adherers ($N = 139$)	Moderate/high adherers ($N = 141$)	Sig.
Antihypertensive therapy				
Monotherapy	127 (45.3%)	68 (53.5%)	59 (46.5%)	0.234
Combination therapy	153 (54.6%)	71 (46.4%)	82 (53.6%)	
Number of antihypertensive(s) classes taken				
1	127 (45.3%)	68 (53.5%)	59 (46.5%)	0.079
2	95 (34%)	37 (38.9%)	58 (61.1%)	
3–5	58 (20.7%)	34 (58.6%)	24 (41.4%)	
Presence of comorbidity	160 (57.1%)	77 (48.1%)	83 (51.9%)	0.629
Mean (±SD) number of comorbidities, $N = 160$ patients with at least one comorbidity	1.54 (±0.76)	1.53 (±0.75)	1.54 (±0.77)	0.984
Taking anti-hypertensive from pharmacy without doctor visit	212 (75.7%)	113 (53.3%)	99 (46.7%)	0.031

Nearly half of the cases (127 patients, 45.3%) were taking one class of antihypertensive for their condition. Among these, angiotensin-receptor blocker (74 cases, 26.4%) was the most prevalent medication used, followed by selective beta-blockers (22 cases, 7.9%), hydrochlorothiazide (13 cases, 4.6%), angiotensin-converting enzyme inhibitor (10 cases, 3.6%), calcium-channel blocker (7 patients, 2.5%), and finally alpha-blocker (one patient, 0.4%). Others (153 cases, 54.6%) were taking more than one class of antihypertensive to control their high BP. One-hundred sixty patients (57.1%) had a concomitant condition other than HTN. The most common comorbidity was ischemic heart disease (with or without having undergone coronary artery bypass grafting (CABG) or minimally invasive percutaneous interventions; PCI) which was documented in 28 patients (10.0%). Then, diabetes mellitus (23 cases, 8.2%) and dyslipidemia (12 cases, 4.3%) were, respectively, most common comorbidities. Most patients (212 patients, 75.7%) reported that they had presented to pharmacies during the last 6 months to take their medication without controlling their BP by their doctor. In Table 3, comparison of antihypertensives taken and comorbidities between low and moderate/high adherers is presented. As observed, no association was detected between number of antihypertensives or number of comorbidities and medication adherence categories. The only statistically significant association was observed regarding those who reported that they personally without visiting their doctors requested the pharmacist to refill their prescription or in some cases, even without prescription in hand, purchased their medication directly from the drugstore.

There was a negative linear association between the MMAS-8 score and systolic BP ($r = -0.231$, $P < 0.001$) as well as diastolic BP ($r = -0.280$, $P < 0.001$). Table 4 shows linear regression model results. Being overweight or obese, previous history of admission to emergency services due to hypertensive crisis, and getting medication directly from drugstore without refill prescription in hand were factors recognized to have statistically significant association with the MMAS-8 score.

4. Discussion

Good adherence to antihypertensives is a key factor in achieving appropriate BP control in hypertensive patients.

Table 4: Linear regression analysis of variables associated with the MMAS-8 score.

	B	Standard error of B	Significance
History of HTN crisis	−0.796	0.228	0.001
Taking antihypertensive from pharmacy without doctor visit	−0.515	0.251	0.041
BMI ≥ 25 kg/m^2	−0.523	0.237	0.028
Constant	9.764	0.913	0.001

BMI = body mass index; HTN = hypertension.

The results obtained here show that compliance with antihypertensive(s) is not satisfactory among Iranian hypertensive patients. The rate of controlled BP and the significant association detected between systolic and diastolic BP measurements with adherence level support this finding. In other words, poor adherence affected negatively BP control. Adherence studies from Iran are not sufficient in terms of quantity and quality. The limited literature has noted diverse designs and tools to define adherence and subsequently direct comparison with the current results may not be feasible. According to a review article, though there has been good effort to determine adherence to diabetes medicines, no high quality study has been done so far in Iran on hypertensive patients. In particular, the tools used to define adherence included pill counting and self-reported questionnaire [21]. It has been noted that methods such as 24-hour recall and refill history do not accurately measure medication adherence [22]. We administered the MMAS-8 to define medication adherence. This scale has been established in several studies across different cultures and languages and various populations to be a reliable tool in determining adherence [6, 7, 23–25]. As mentioned above, we observed a good reliability and validity of this scale in Persian speaking patients in a previous study [20].

In a former study on 250 patients with high BP in Shiraz city, Iran, using a self-report questionnaire and ratio of taken pills to prescribed pills in one-month period, it was found that having a positive attitude toward antihypertensives and the interval between visits to physician of less than 3 months were two independent predictors of good adherence [26]. We did not study attitude or knowledge of the patients here, but about 40% of the patients reported that they had visited more than one doctor to control their BP. Adding this to the figure of one-fifth of the cases who had never scheduled an appointment to visit their doctors during the preceding 6 months of the study may reflect faults in health care system. Reviewing the literature, it seems that there is no general consensus among experts and scientific organizations about visit frequency in hypertensive patients, but studies confirm the fact that shorter intervals yield better BP control and earlier normalization [27, 28].

In a study on older adults with HTN and using the Morisky 4-Item Self-Report Measure of Medication-Taking Behavior (MMAS-4), the authors found that older people with a comorbidity and longer history of HTN had better adherence. These are in contrast to our finding as age, presence of comorbidity or its number and duration of HTN were not different between poor and moderate/good adherers. This may be due to different scales to define adherence (MMAS-4 in Chinese study versus MMAS-8 in our study) and the nature of patients studied in the mentioned article which included only those who aged more than 55 years. The only similar finding was higher educational level in both studies which was associated with better adherence. The finding that the number of antihypertensives did not associate with adherence is compatible with an Indian study performed in a tertiary care center [29]. They, similar to what we found here, reported that those who had experienced symptoms of HTN were significantly more likely to have low adherence to antihypertensives. In our opinion, this is a mutual relationship that patients who do not take their medicines regularly are more likely to experience hypertensive crisis and need for admission to get inpatient treatment. The same patients who were interviewed at a later date were still found to be nonadherent. It could be inferred that, despite experiencing hypertensive crisis, the patients' attitude and practice regarding taking his/her antihypertensive is not changed and they are still considered poor adherers. Likewise, the Indian article did not find any association between number of antihypertensives taken daily and adherence. This is contradictory to what was reported by a Pakistani study where it was found that higher number of patients who were taking two drugs (82% versus 18%) or more than 3 drugs (87% versus 12%) were adherent when compared to low adherers. They used the 4-item MMAS to define adherence level [13]. Self-medication and self-prescription are two quite widespread practices in Iranian patients. Although governmental authorities have consistently warned publicly about self-medication health hazards and despite advice from experts to pass legislations to limit easy access to prescription-only medications [30], unfortunately this problem still remains a health problem in Iran. Former studies on this topic focused mainly on antibiotic and analgesic self-medication which reported high prevalence of this public health concern [31]. In a similar fashion, we observed a high number of the cases who reported self-prescription and that this sample had lower adherence level. It is important to note that adherence to medication is one of the factors that contribute to acceptable BP control. There are other factors such as patient education, correct intensification of medication, and economic issues that determine good BP control [5].

We suggest that future studies focus on antihypertensive self-medication and related behavioral, economic, and social factors. It is also prudent to compare various methods to find the most effective to raise medication adherence in Iranian hypertensive patients.

Regarding strengths and limitations we faced here, in our opinion, the fact that the data were gathered from several health centers as well as pharmacies in different cities would enable us to generalize the data in a better form to the Iranian community. Particularly, the city of Karaj which is located about 30 km from the capital, Tehran, has faced an increasing growth in its population during the last 2 decades, mainly as a result of immigration from other cities.

The limitation here to be considered is that adherence is a complex phenomenon and various factors can affect that. For instance, patient awareness and knowledge about HTN and medicines prescribed, the role of the physicians in providing information and patient education, behavioral and psychological factors, doctor-patient relationship, and the like are potential factors that can be investigated in more detail in the future studies. Another limitation is related to BP recording. Since this study was done in different centers and BP recording was based on measurement by sphygmomanometer and taken by different physicians, it is likely that there might be variations in devices and maybe some variations, though we think not very significant, differences in BP readings. Our resources and limited time did not allow us to implement more accurate devices for BP monitoring such as Holter monitor.

5. Conclusion

Adherence to antihypertensive(s) among Iranian patients is not satisfactory and more than half of the patients had uncontrolled BP which was in direct relationship with poor adherence to medications. The patients who were overweight/obese, who had been admitted to hospital or clinic emergency services because of HTN crisis, housewives or those who were unemployed or retired, those with lower educational level, and those getting their medication directly from pharmacies without visiting their doctors to control their BP and refill prescription in hand were more likely to be low adherers. We recommend that health care professionals who manage hypertensive patients consider these factors during their routine visit of such patients in an attempt to alert the patients for better adherence.

Additional Points

The use of the ©MMAS is protected by US copyright laws. Permission for use is required. A license agreement is available from Professor Donald E. Morisky, Sc.D., Sc.M., MSPH, Department of Community Health Sciences, UCLA Fielding School of Public Health, 650 Charles E. Young Drive South, Los Angeles, CA 90095-1772; dmorisky@ucla.edu.

Competing Interests

The authors declare that there are no competing interests regarding the publication of this paper.

References

[1] P. Kaur, S. R. Rao, E. Radhakrishnan, D. Rajasekar, and M. D. Gupte, "Prevalence, awareness, treatment, control and risk factors for hypertension in a rural population in South India," *International Journal of Public Health*, vol. 57, no. 1, pp. 87–94, 2012.

[2] M. A. Krousel-Wood, P. Muntner, T. Islam, D. E. Morisky, and L. S. Webber, "Barriers to and determinants of medication adherence in hypertension management: perspective of the cohort study of medication adherence among older adults," *The Medical Clinics of North America*, vol. 93, no. 3, pp. 753–769, 2009.

[3] L. Osterberg and T. Blaschke, "Adherence to medication," *The New England Journal of Medicine*, vol. 353, no. 5, pp. 487–497, 2005.

[4] M. Krousel-Wood, S. Thomas, P. Muntner, and D. Morisky, "Medication adherence: a key factor in achieving blood pressure control and good clinical outcomes in hypertensive patients," *Current Opinion in Cardiology*, vol. 19, no. 4, pp. 357–362, 2004.

[5] M. Heisler, M. M. Hogan, T. P. Hofer, J. A. Schmittdiel, M. Pladevall, and E. A. Kerr, "When more is not better: treatment intensification among hypertensive patients with poor medication adherence," *Circulation*, vol. 117, no. 22, pp. 2884–2892, 2008.

[6] R. H. Aşılar, S. Gözüm, C. Çapık, and D. E. Morisky, "Reliability and validity of the Turkish form of the eight-item morisky medication adherence scale in hypertensive patients," *Anadolu Kardiyoloji Dergisi*, vol. 14, no. 8, pp. 692–700, 2014.

[7] A. D. de Oliveira-Filho, D. E. Morisky, S. J. F. Neves, F. A. Costa, and D. P. De Lyra Jr., "The 8-item morisky medication adherence scale: validation of a brazilian-portuguese version in hypertensive adults," *Research in Social & Administrative Pharmacy*, vol. 10, no. 3, pp. 554–561, 2014.

[8] A. AlHewiti, "Adherence to long-term therapies and beliefs about medications," *International Journal of Family Medicine*, vol. 2014, Article ID 479596, 8 pages, 2014.

[9] V. Korb-Savoldelli, F. Gillaizeau, J. Pouchot et al., "Validation of a french version of the 8-item morisky medication adherence scale in hypertensive adults," *Journal of Clinical Hypertension*, vol. 14, no. 7, pp. 429–434, 2012.

[10] M. Fernandez-Arias, A. Acuna-Villaorduna, J. J. Miranda, F. Diez-Canseco, and G. Malaga, "Adherence to pharmacotherapy and medication-related beliefs in patients with hypertension in Lima, Peru," *PLoS ONE*, vol. 9, no. 12, Article ID e0112875, 2014.

[11] A. Ramli, N. S. Ahmad, and T. Paraidathathu, "Medication adherence among hypertensive patients of primary health clinics in Malaysia," *Patient Preference and Adherence*, vol. 6, pp. 613–622, 2012.

[12] M. Krousel-Wood, T. Islam, L. S. Webber, R. N. Re, D. E. Morisky, and P. Muntner, "New medication adherence scale versus pharmacy fill rates in seniors with hypertension," *The American Journal of Managed Care*, vol. 15, no. 1, pp. 59–66, 2009.

[13] S. K. Hashmi, M. B. Afridi, K. Abbas et al., "Factors associated with adherence to anti-hypertensive treatment in Pakistan," *PLoS ONE*, vol. 2, no. 3, article e280, 2007.

[14] H. Najafipour, H. R. Nasri, M. Afshari et al., "Hypertension: diagnosis, control status and its predictors in general population aged between 15 and 75 years: a community-based study in southeastern Iran," *International Journal of Public Health*, vol. 59, no. 6, pp. 999–1009, 2014.

[15] S. Arabzadeh, M. Sadeghi, K. Rabiei, N. Sarrafzadegan, L. Taheri, and A. Golshahi, "Determinants of uncontrolled hypertension in an Iranian population," *ARYA Atherosclerosis*, vol. 10, no. 1, pp. 25–31, 2014.

[16] M. Ebrahimi, M. A. Mansournia, A. A. Haghdoost et al., "Social disparities in prevalence, treatment and control of hypertension in iran: second national surveillance of risk factors of noncommunicable diseases, 2006," *Journal of Hypertension*, vol. 28, no. 8, pp. 1620–1629, 2010.

[17] N. Ikeda, D. Sapienz, R. Guerrero et al., "Control of hypertension with medication: a comparative analysis of national surveys in 20 countries," *Bulletin of the World Health Organization*, vol. 92, no. 1, pp. 10–19, 2014.

[18] D. E. Morisky and M. R. DiMatteo, "Improving the measurement of self-reported medication nonadherence: response to authors," *Journal of Clinical Epidemiology*, vol. 64, no. 3, pp. 255–263, 2011.

[19] D. E. Morisky, A. Ang, M. Krousel-Wood, and H. J. Ward, "Predictive validity of a medication adherence measure in an outpatient setting," *Journal of Clinical Hypertension*, vol. 10, no. 5, pp. 348–354, 2008.

[20] Y. Moharamzad, H. Saadat, B. Nakhjavan Shahraki et al., "Validation of the persian version of the 8-item morisky medication adherence scale (MMAS-8) in Iranian hypertensive patients," *Global Journal of Health Science*, vol. 7, no. 4, pp. 173–183, 2014.

[21] A. Sarayani, Z. Jahangard-Rafsanjani, M. Hadjibabaie, A. Ahmadvand, M. Javadi, and K. Gholami, "A comprehensive review of adherence to diabetes and cardiovascular medications in Iran; implications for practice and research," *Journal of Diabetes and Metabolic Disorders*, vol. 12, article 57, 2013.

[22] J. K. Lee, K. A. Grace, T. G. Foster et al., "How should we measure medication adherence in clinical trials and practice?" *Therapeutics and Clinical Risk Management*, vol. 3, no. 4, pp. 685–690, 2007.

[23] J. Yan, L.-M. You, Q. Yang et al., "Translation and validation of a Chinese version of the 8-item morisky medication adherence scale in myocardial infarction patients," *Journal of Evaluation in Clinical Practice*, vol. 20, no. 4, pp. 311–317, 2014.

[24] H. K. Al-Qazaz, M. A. Hassali, A. A. Shafie, S. A. Sulaiman, S. Sundram, and D. E. Morisky, "The eight-item Morisky Medication Adherence Scale MMAS: translation and validation of the Malaysian version," *Diabetes Research and Clinical Practice*, vol. 90, no. 2, pp. 216–221, 2010.

[25] Y.-S. Lin, Y. Ho, C.-J. Hu et al., "Development of a Taiwan version of the eight-item morisky medication adherence scale and factors influencing patients' comprehension," *Journal of Experimental & Clinical Medicine*, vol. 5, no. 2, pp. 77–80, 2013.

[26] N. Hadi and N. Rostami-Gooran, "Determinant factors of medication compliance in hypertensive patients of Shiraz, Iran," *Archives of Iranian Medicine*, vol. 7, no. 4, pp. 292–296, 2004.

[27] A. Turchin, S. I. Goldberg, M. Shubina, J. S. Einbinder, and P. R. Conlin, "Encounter frequency and blood pressure in hypertensive patients with diabetes mellitus," *Hypertension*, vol. 56, no. 1, pp. 68–74, 2010.

[28] R. Guthmann, N. Davis, M. Brown, and J. Elizondo, "Visit frequency and hypertension," *Journal of Clinical Hypertension*, vol. 7, no. 6, pp. 327–332, 2005.

[29] A. M. Nagarkar, S. A. Gadhave, I. Sharma, A. Choure, and D. Morisky, "Factors influencing medication adherence among hypertensive patients in a tertiary care hospital, pune, maharashtra," *National Journal of Community Medicine*, vol. 4, no. 4, pp. 559–563, 2013.

[30] A. H. Zargarzadeh, M. Minaeiyan, and A. Torabi, "Prescription and nonprescription drug use in isfahan, Iran: an observational, cross-sectional study," *Current Therapeutic Research, Clinical and Experimental*, vol. 69, no. 1, pp. 76–87, 2008.

[31] S. Sarahroodi, A. Maleki-Jamshid, A. F. Sawalha, P. Mikaili, and L. Safaeian, "Pattern of self-medication with analgesics among iranian university students in central Iran," *Journal of Family & Community Medicine*, vol. 19, no. 2, pp. 125–129, 2012.

5

Association between CD4 Cell Count and Blood Pressure and Its Variation with Body Mass Index Categories in HIV-Infected Patients

Christian Akem Dimala,[1,2,3] Benjamin Momo Kadia,[4,5] Ben-Lawrence Kemah,[3,6] Maxime Tindong,[3,7] and Simeon-Pierre Choukem[3,8,9]

[1] *Faculty of Epidemiology and Population Health, London School of Hygiene and Tropical Medicine, London, UK*
[2] *Department of Orthopaedics, Southend University Hospital, Essex, UK*
[3] *Health and Human Development (2HD) Research Network, Douala, Cameroon*
[4] *Presbyterian General Hospital Acha-Tugi, Acha-Tugi, Cameroon*
[5] *Grace Community Health and Development Association (GRACHADA), Kumba, Cameroon*
[6] *Department of Vascular Surgery, Ashford and St Peter's Hospitals NHS, Surrey, UK*
[7] *Department of Public Health, Université libre de Bruxelles, Brussels, Belgium*
[8] *Diabetes and Endocrinology Unit, Department of Internal Medicine, Douala General Hospital, Douala, Cameroon*
[9] *Department of Internal Medicine and Paediatrics, Faculty of Health Sciences, University of Buea, Buea, Cameroon*

Correspondence should be addressed to Christian Akem Dimala; christian.akem.dimala1@alumni.lshtm.ac.uk

Academic Editor: Daniel Duprez

The aim of this study was to establish whether an independent relationship exists between CD4 count and hypertension and if this relationship is modified or confounded by the body mass index (BMI). *Methods.* A secondary data analysis of a cross-sectional study on 200 HIV/AIDS patients at a referral hospital in Cameroon was conducted. Linear and logistic regression models were used as appropriate to explore the association between the variables of interest. *Results.* There was no linear association between log CD4 count and both systolic ($p = 0.200$; $r = 0.12$) and diastolic blood pressures ($p = 0.123$; $r = 0.14$), respectively. After adjusting for BMI, patients with CD4 count ≥ 350 cells/μl were more likely to have hypertension than those with CD4 count $<$ 350 cells/μl (AOR: 2.50, 95% CI: 1.05–5.93, and $p = 0.032$). There was no effect modification from BMI (test of homogeneity, $p = 0.721$). There was no independent relationship between CD4 count and hypertension after controlling for age, sex, family history of hypertension, BMI-defined overweight, HAART use, and duration of HIV infection (AOR: 1.66, 95% CI: 0.48–5.71, and $p = 0.419$). *Conclusion.* This study did not identify any independent relationship between CD4 count and hypertension. Large prospective studies are recommended to better explore this relationship between hypertension and CD4 count.

1. Introduction

The introduction of highly active antiretroviral therapy (HAART) has greatly reduced the morbidity and mortality due to Human Immunodeficiency Virus/Acquired Immunodeficiency Syndrome (HIV/AIDS), with patients experiencing longer and healthier lives [1, 2]. These increases in life expectancy and quality have, however, coincided with an epidemiological transition characterized by an increase in rates of noncommunicable diseases including cardiovascular diseases (CVD) among HIV-infected persons.

Nadir CD4 cell count in HIV-infected patients has been shown to be associated with hypertension [3, 4], through processes of persistent immune activation, chronic inflammation, endothelial dysfunction, and microbial translocation that occurs with inadequate immune recovery [5–9]. The lipid metabolism derangements and accelerated atherosclerosis associated with HAART have also been reported to affect the blood pressure in these patients [10, 11].

The relationship between hypertension and the body mass index (BMI) is well established in immunocompetent subjects with a tendency towards a higher prevalence of hypertension with increasing BMI [12, 13]. The metabolic and immunologic changes associated with the chronic-disease state in HIV-infected patients, not on treatment, predispose them to having suboptimal BMIs. However, there is a significant increase in BMI following initiation of treatment [14–16]. This implies that the association between the CD4 cell count and hypertension could be different across the various BMI categories. This creates an imperative for further exploration of this relationship as it may represent an avenue for intervention in HIV/AIDS patients to reduce adverse outcomes associated with noncommunicable diseases and also to improve the quality of life of these patients.

The aim of this study was therefore to assess if there is an independent relationship between CD4 cell count and hypertension in HIV/AIDS patients and if this association is modified or confounded by the BMI. Specifically we had as objectives to determine if there is a linear association between blood pressure (BP) values and CD4 cell count and to determine if there is an association between hypertension and CD4 cell count categories after controlling for BMI and other important confounders.

2. Methods

2.1. Study Design and Participants Selection. This was a secondary analysis of data from a cross-sectional study conducted at the Limbe Regional Hospital in Cameroon involving HIV-infected patients receiving care at the HIV treatment center of this health facility [17]. The selection of study participants, study procedures, data sources, and measurements are described in detail in a previous report [17].

2.2. Participants and Sampling. Patients coming for regular care and follow-up at this HIV treatment center were recruited randomly (HAART-naïve group) and by consecutive convenient sampling (HAART group matched by age and sex to the HAART-naïve group) to take part in the study. Patients were selected if they were aged 21 and above, had been on HAART for at least 12 months (HAART group), and are with no known previous history of hypertension, diabetes, or renal disease (based on patients' self-reports and medical records). Patients with nonadherence to HAART for more than 6 months and those on medications known to affect blood pressure, corticosteroids, and oral contraceptives were excluded.

2.3. Study Procedures and Variables. A face-to-face interview and a physical examination were done for all participants who consented to take part in the study. A structured questionnaire was used for data collection on participants' sociodemographic and clinical characteristics. Data on HIV infection status and duration, previous and most recent CD4 counts less than 3 months old, and lifestyle habits such as smoking, alcohol consumption, and physical activity were collected from the patients and complemented by recorded parameters from their medical records. The physical exam consisted of measuring patient blood pressures, body mass indices, and waist and hip circumferences.

2.4. Data Sources and Measurements. Blood pressure was measured on the right arm for all participants while seated using an electronic automated BP monitor (Omron M2, HEM-7121-E) of an appropriate cuff size (22–34 cm). Two measurements were taken at an average interval of 5 minutes and a mean blood pressure was calculated from the two readings. Hypertension was diagnosed according to the World Health Organization (WHO) criteria as systolic BP $\geq$ 140 mmHg and/or diastolic BP $\geq$ 90 mmHg [18]. A CD4 cell count below 350 was considered as low based on the WHO recommended threshold for initiation of HAART at the time. CD4 cell count as a continuous variable was thus transformed into a binary variable with categories < 350 cells/μL and $\geq$ 350 cells/μL. Weight was measured with a scale (BRN 9311) to the nearest half kilogram and patients were allowed to wear just light clothing unlikely to considerably affect the overall weight read. Height was measured with a stadiometer to the nearest half centimeter. Body mass index, calculated as weight (kg)/[height (m) $\times$ height (m)], was reported to 2 decimal places in Kg/m^2. Conventional cut-offs were used to define the various BMI categories as follows: below 18.5 as underweight, 18.5 to 24.9 as normal, 25 to 29.9 as overweight, and above 30 as obesity. Waist and hip circumferences were measured midway between the iliac crest and the lower rib margin and at the intertrochanteric level, respectively. Waist-to-hip ratio, calculated as waist (cm)/hip (cm) circumferences, was reported to the 2 decimal places. Conventional ranges were used to define abdominal obesity derived from the WHR as a WHR > 0.9 in men and WHR > 0.85 in women. Intake of more than three (two for women) standard glasses of wine per day or more than ten (five for women) local beers (1 local beer contains 28 g of alcohol) per week was considered as excessive alcohol consumption. At least 30 minutes of intense physical activity once a week or more was considered as regular physical activity.

2.5. Data Management and Data Analysis. STATA version 14.1 statistical software was used to perform the analysis. For objective 1, the CD4 cell count value was log transformed due to its skewed distribution, and a linear regression model was built to assess the association between blood pressure (systolic and diastolic) and log CD4 cell count, both as continuous variables. Linear regression analyses were also done in subgroups of the Log CD4 cell count to identify possible group-specific trends. For objective 2, the Wilcoxon rank sum (Mann–Whitney) test was used to compare the median CD4 cell count in patients with and without hypertension. Also, the Chi-square test was used to assess for any association between hypertension and CD4 cell count as a binary variable across each BMI category, except in situations where Fisher's exact test was most appropriate. For objective 3, a logistic regression model was built to assess the association between hypertension and CD4 cell count while adjusting for BMI, and other confounders. Low p values were suggestive of strong evidence of an association between variables, with statistical significance set at a value of $p < 0.05$.

Table 1: Sociodemographic and clinical characteristics of the participants.

Characteristic	Participants (n = 200)
Age in years (mean ± SD)	39.1 ± 9.4
Females, n (%)	140 (70%)
Married, n (%)	89 (44.5%)
Unskilled occupation, n (%)	26 (13%)
Northwest region, n (%)	88 (44%)
BMI in Kg/m^2 (mean ± SD)	24.1 ± 2.9
BMI-defined overweight and obesity (prevalence, %)	40.5%
BMI categories	
Underweight	2 (1.0%)
Normal	117 (58.5%)
Overweight	81 (40.5%)
WHR (mean ± SD)	0.86 ± 0.06
WHR-defined abdominal obesity (prevalence, %)	44.5%
Hypertension in mmHg (prevalence, % (95%CI))	28.5% (22.4–35.3)
Systolic blood pressure (mean ± SD)	128 ± 20
Diastolic blood pressure (mean ± SD)	79 ± 13
Duration of HIV infection in months, median (IQR)	22 (1–68)
CD4 cell count in cells/μL, median (IQR)	271 (130–408)
WHO clinical stage, n (%)	
Stage I	23 (11.5%)
Stage II	62 (31.0%)
Stage III	98 (49.0%)
Stage IV	17 (8.5%)

2.6. Ethical Considerations. Ethical approval for the primary study was obtained from the Institutional Review Board of the Faculty of Health Sciences of the University of Buea (approval number: 2013/0083/UB/FHS/IRB) and in accordance with the Helsinki Declaration on ethical principles. No ethical clearance was required for the secondary data analysis. All participants found to have elevated blood pressure values were referred to the medical team of the same hospital for further investigation on the possibility of hypertension and management as appropriate. The "Strengthening the Reporting of Observational Studies in Epidemiology" (STROBE) guidelines were used for reporting this study.

3. Results

3.1. Sociodemographic and Clinical Characteristics of the Study Population. Two hundred eligible participants who consented to participate were recruited. The participants had a mean age of 39.1 ± 9.4 years and 70% were female. The sociodemographic characteristics of the participants are summarized on Table 1. The mean BMI of the participants was 24.1 ± 2.9 Kg/m^2 with a prevalence of BMI-defined overweight and obesity of 40.5%. The mean WHR was 0.86 ± 0.06 and the median duration of HIV infection in months was 22 months (IQR: 1–68). Fifty percent of the participants had been on first-line antiretroviral therapy for a median duration of 58.6 ± 28.5 months. Fifty-seven participants (28.5%) had hypertension and the median CD4 cell count of this study population was 271 cells/μL (IQR: 130–408). The clinical characteristics of the participants are presented on Table 1.

There was a statistically significant association between BMI as a categorical variable and both hypertension (Fisher's exact, p = 0.010) and CD4 cell count (Fisher's exact, p = 0.012). The observed trend was an increasing prevalence of hypertension across increasing BMI and a higher BMI with higher CD4 cell count. Factors found to have an association with hypertension were age above 40, male gender, BMI-defined overweight/obesity, HAART use, and HIV infection duration above 30 months (Table 2).

3.2. Association between Blood Pressure and CD4 Cell Count. Scatter plots for systolic and diastolic blood pressure values against the log CD4 cell count were produced (Figures 1 and 2). From the built linear regression model, there was no linear relationship between the systolic blood pressure (p = 0.200, correlation coefficient = 0.12) or the diastolic blood pressure (p = 0.123, correlation coefficient = 0.14) and the log CD4 cell count. No significant linear associations were identified between these variables in the subgroups of the log CD4 cell count (Table 3).

3.3. Association between Hypertension and CD4 Cell Count across BMI Categories. There was no significant difference in the median CD4 cell count in those with (356 cells/μL (IQR: 182–505)) and those without hypertension (242 cells/μL (IQR: 111–377)), p = 0.069. Participants with CD4 cell counts ≥ 350 cells/μL were three times more likely to have

TABLE 2: Factors associated with hypertension in the study population.

Factor	Participants ($n = 200$)	Participants with HTN ($n = 57$)	p value
Age (in years)			
>40	78	35 (44.9%)	**<0.001**
≤40	122	22 (18.0%)	
Gender			
Male	60	26 (44.3%)	**0.002**
Female	140	31 (22.1%)	
Family history of HTN			
Yes	11	1 (9.1%)	0.142
No	189	56 (29.6%)	
Smoking			
Yes	11	6 (54.6%)	**0.049**
No	189	51 (27.0%)	
Alcohol consumption			
Yes	52	14 (26.9%)	0.767
No	148	43 (29.1%)	
Physical exercise			
Yes	42	12 (28.6%)	0.990
No	158	45 (28.5%)	
BMI-defined overweight/obesity			
Yes	81	32 (39.5%)	**0.004**
No	119	25 (21.0%)	
WHR-defined overweight/obesity			
Yes	89	24 (27.0%)	0.667
No	111	33 (29.7%)	
HAART use			
Yes	100	38 (38.0%)	**0.003**
No	100	19 (19.0%)	
Duration of HIV infection (months)			
>30	92	35 (38.0%)	**0.006**
≤30	108	22 (20.4%)	

BMI: body mass Index, HTN: hypertension, and WHR: waist-to-hip ratio.

TABLE 3: Linear regression model for systolic and diastolic blood pressures and log CD4 cell count.

Parameter	Regression coefficient	Intercept	p value	R-square	Correlation coefficient
Overall ($n = 123$)					
Systolic BP	2.55	115.17	0.200	0.0136	0.1165
Diastolic BP	2.01	63.30	0.123	0.0196	0.1398
Log CD4: >3-4 ($n = 16$)					
Systolic BP	−28.70	225.84	0.121	0.1632	−0.4039
Diastolic BP	−0.24	78.20	0.981	0.0	−0.0066
Log CD4: >4-5 ($n = 19$)					
Systolic BP	−11.73	180.13	0.466	0.0317	−0.1779
Diastolic BP	−4.62	97.64	0.664	0.0114	−0.1067
Log CD4: >5-6 ($n = 56$)					
Systolic BP	4.23	106.57	0.682	0.0031	0.0559
Diastolic BP	5.47	48.10	0.400	0.0132	0.1147
Log CD4: >6-7 ($n = 32$)					
Systolic BP	8.47	76.62	0.504	0.0150	0.1227
Diastolic BP	5.75	45.51	0.555	0.0117	0.1084

TABLE 4: Association between CD4 and hypertension across BMI categories, $n = 123$.

BMI groups and CD4 categories	Hypertension	Odds ratios (95% CI)	p value*
All participants			
<350	15/78 (19%)	1	**0.006**
≥350	19/45 (42%)	3.07 (1.32–7.16)**	
Normal BMI			
<350	8/55 (15%)	1	0.066
≥350	7/21 (33%)	2.94 (0.87–9.87)	
Overweight			
<350	7/22 (32%)	1	0.211
≥350	12/24 (50%)	2.14 (0.62–7.38)	
MH controlled for BMI	-	2.50 (1.05–5.93)***	0.032

*Chi-square test. **Crude odds ratio. ***Mantel Haenszel pooled odds ratios, the test of homogeneity of odds ratios, and $p = 0.721$.

TABLE 5: Association between CD4 cell count and hypertension after controlling for confounders.

Factor and categories	Adjusted odds ratio*	95% confidence interval	p value**
CD4 cell count (≥350/<350)	1.66	0.48–5.71	0.419
Age (>40/≤40 years)	1.76	0.70–4.39	0.229
Gender (Male/Female)	2.77	1.09–7.03	**0.032**
Family History of HTN (Yes/No)	0.34	0.03–3.69	0.373
BMI-defined obesity (Yes/No)	2.75	1.09–6.91	**0.031**
HAART (Yes/No)	1.32	0.21–8.29	0.765
HIV duration (>30/≤30)	1.30	0.21–7.96	0.773

*Odds ratio adjusting for all variables on the table; **p values for the Wald test statistic. BMI: body mass index, HAART: highly active antiretroviral therapy, and HTN: hypertension.

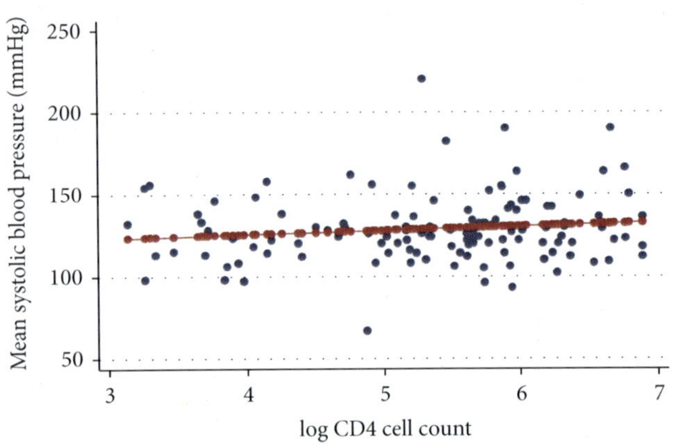

FIGURE 1: Scatter plot for mean systolic blood pressure and log CD4 cell count. *The red line represents the prediction line of the regression model.*

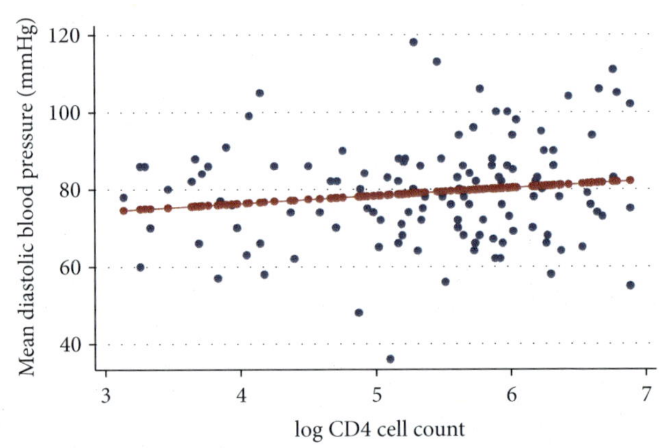

FIGURE 2: Scatter plot for mean diastolic blood pressure and log CD4 cell count. *The red line represents the prediction line of the regression model.*

hypertension than those with CD4 cell counts < 350 cells/μL (OR: 3.07; 95% CI: 1.32–7.16; $p = 0.006$). There was a reduction in the strength of association between CD4 cell count and hypertension after adjusting for BMI, suggestive of a positive confounding effect by BMI (Mantel Haenszel pooled odds ratio: 2.50) (95% CI: 1.05–5.93, $p = 0.032$) (Table 4). There was no effect modification of this association by BMI (test of homogeneity $p = 0.721$).

On logistic regression adjusted for age, sex, family history of hypertension, BMI-defined overweight, HAART use, and duration of HIV infection, we found no significant association between CD4 cell count and hypertension (AOR: 1.66; 95% CI: 0.48–5.71; $p = 0.419$) (Table 5).

4. Discussion

In this study, we aimed to determine if there is an association between blood pressure, hypertension, and CD4 cell count and investigate if this association could vary with changes in BMI. We found no linear association between the log CD4 cell count and blood pressure. A CD4 cell count ≥ 350 cells/μL was associated with higher odds of hypertension, and the strength of this association decreased after adjusting for BMI. This association was completely lost when several other risk factors of hypertension were adjusted for.

There was no linear association between the CD4 cell count and both the systolic and diastolic blood pressure values. Also, there was no statistically significant difference between the median CD4 cell count among participants with and without hypertension. Likewise, the subgroup analysis within intervals of the log CD4 cell count did not identify any linear relationship between these variables. It is worth noting, however, that the nonexistence of an association between the CD4 cell count and blood pressure values from the linear regression model simply means that a change in the CD4 cell count is not associated with a proportional change in the blood pressure, but this does not exclude the possibility of other nonlinear associations between them. This is confirmed by the fact that we later on found an association between the CD4 cell count as a binary variable and hypertension, with CD4 cell counts of 350 cells/μL and above found to be associated with hypertension. The observed association of a higher prevalence of hypertension among patients with high CD4 cell counts is contrary to the findings of the studies by De Socio et al. [3] and Manner et al. [4] in which an independent and significant association was observed between hypertension and nadir CD4 cell count. Nevertheless, the majority of participant in both studies were of a different ethnicity from that of our participants. Even though the prevalence of hypertension in our study was similar to that reported by De Socio et al., half of those hypertension patients in their study were on antihypertensive medications with a third of them being well controlled, and a just small proportion of their participants were on HAART [3]. All these factors could potentially account for the differences in mean blood pressure values and underlying associations between blood pressure and CD4 cell count in these studies and ours.

HIV infection results in a chronic inflammatory, endothelial dysfunction and subsequent impaired elasticity of arteries [19, 20]. HIV infection with and without HAART has been directly associated with aortic stiffness as well [21, 22]. Furthermore, Kaplan et al. reported that a low CD4 cell count is a strong risk factor for carotid atherosclerosis through its association with subclinical carotid artery lesions, even after adjusting for antiretroviral therapy which could be a major confounder of this association [23]. These are all in favor of an association between nadir CD4 cell count and hypertension. Nevertheless, we do note that the possibility of participants in our study having developed hypertension when their CD4 cell counts were low does exist but cannot be ascertained given the study design. On the other hand, Bloomfield et al. [24] in a large retrospective study reported findings similar to ours, as they observed a higher prevalence of hypertension with higher CD4 cell counts among participants aged 35 and below.

Raised BMI, which is associated with hypertension, was found to also have an association with higher CD4 cell counts, making it a potential confounder of the association between hypertension and CD4 cell count. Adjusting for BMI reduced the strength of the association between hypertension and CD4 cell count, indicating a positive confounding effect from BMI. This is understandable given the fact that the risk of having hypertension increases as the BMI increases. A close analysis of the stratum specific odd ratios of the association between hypertension and CD4 cell count across the BMI categories reveals a stronger association among patients with normal BMI compared to overweight patients (Table 4). This finding is, however, as a result of chance given the nonsignificant test of homogeneity of the compared odds ratios.

These observed discrepancies in the study findings suggest hypertension results from a more complex interplay of several environmental and genetic predisposing factors. In this study, older age, male gender, BMI overweight, HAART, and prolonged HIV infection were all found to significantly contribute to having hypertension. As such, any attempt to fully elucidate the direct link between hypertension and CD4 cell count should therefore take into consideration the effect of all these important factors associated with hypertension.

The logistic regression model revealed no association between hypertension and CD4 cell count after adjusting for age, sex, family history of hypertension, BMI-defined obesity, antiretroviral therapy, and duration of HIV infection. This means that the association between hypertension and CD4 cell could exist due to some important confounding.

The interpretation of our results should, however, take into considerations some important limitations of the study. As with all cross-sectional studies, causality cannot be ascertained since, inasmuch as a given CD4 threshold could predispose to hypertension, the presence of hypertension as a comorbidity in HIV-infected patients could predispose them to poor or delayed immune recovery and consequently lower than expected CD4 cell count levels. However, we aimed to study if there existed an association irrespective of its being causal. Nevertheless, prospective cohorts will be better designs to study this association between CD4 cell count and hypertension as serial blood pressure and CD4 cell count measurements over time will enable us to determine at what CD4 cell count values hypertension is most likely to set in. Also the generalizability of these results to settings demographically different from the settings of this study may not be entirely possible. Despite these limitations, this study reiterates the importance of factors associated with hypertension while investigating the effect of HIV infection and CD4 cell count on hypertension.

5. Conclusion

This study found no linear association between CD4 cell count and blood pressure. There is no independent relationship between CD4 cell count and hypertension after adjusting for important confounders such as BMI, age, sex, HAART use, and duration of HIV infection. Large prospective studies are therefore recommended to explore this relationship.

Authors' Contributions

Christian Akem Dimala designed the study, conducted the data analysis, and produced the manuscript. Benjamin Momo Kadia, Ben-Lawrence Kemah, Maxime Tindong, and Simeon-Pierre Choukem edited and reviewed the manuscript for technical and scientific coherence.

Acknowledgments

The authors thank all the participants of this study.

References

[1] World Health organization, Joint United Nations Programme on HIV/AIDS. FAst facts about HIV treatment. Geneva; 2009.

[2] J. F. Palella, K. M. Delaney, A. C. Moorman et al., "Declining morbidity and mortality among patients with advanced human immunodeficiency virus infection," *The New England Journal of Medicine*, vol. 338, no. 13, pp. 853–860, 1998.

[3] G. V. De Socio, E. Ricci, P. Maggi et al., "Prevalence, awareness, treatment, and control rate of hypertension in HIV-infected patients: The HIV-HY study," *American Journal of Hypertension*, vol. 27, no. 2, pp. 222–228, 2014.

[4] I. W. Manner, M. Trøseid, O. Oektedalen, M. Baekken, and I. Os, "Low nadir CD4 cell count predicts sustained hypertension in HIV-infected individuals," *The Journal of Clinical Hypertension*, vol. 15, no. 2, pp. 101–106, 2013.

[5] W. Ngatchou, D. Lemogoum, P. Ndobo et al., "Increased burden and severity of metabolic syndrome and arterial stiffness in treatment-naive HIV+ patients from Cameroon," *Vascular Health and Risk Management*, vol. 9, no. 1, pp. 509–516, 2013.

[6] J. E. Ho and P. Y. Hsue, "Cardiovascular manifestations of HIV infection," *Heart*, vol. 95, no. 14, pp. 1193–1202, 2009.

[7] I. W. Manner, M. Baekken, D. Kvale et al., "Markers of microbial translocation predict hypertension in HIV-infected individuals," *HIV Medicine*, vol. 14, no. 6, pp. 354–361, 2013.

[8] F. F. Rönsholt, H. Ullum, T. L. Katzenstein, J. Gerstoft, and S. R. Ostrowski, "Persistent inflammation and endothelial activation in HIV-1 infected patients after 12 years of antiretroviral therapy," *PLoS ONE*, vol. 8, no. 6, Article ID e65182, 2013.

[9] J. H. Stein and P. Y. Hsue, "Inflammation, immune activation, and CVD risk in individuals with HIV infection," *Journal of the American Medical Association*, vol. 308, no. 4, pp. 405-406, 2012.

[10] A. Carr, K. Samaras, A. Thorisdottir, G. R. Kaufmann, D. J. Chisholm, and D. A. Cooper, "Diagnosis, prediction, and natural course of HIV-1 protease-inhibitor-associated lipodystrophy, hyperlipidaemia, and diabetes mellitus: a cohort study," *The Lancet*, vol. 353, no. 9170, pp. 2093–2099, 1999.

[11] A. M. Cattelan, M. Trevenzoli, L. Sasset, L. Rinaldi, V. Balasso, and P. Cadrobbi, "Indinavir and systemic hypertension," *AIDS*, vol. 15, no. 6, pp. 805–807, 2001.

[12] R. Roka, A. Michimi, and G. Macy, "Associations between hypertension and body mass index and waist circumference in U.S. adults: a comparative analysis by gender," *High Blood Pressure & Cardiovascular Prevention*, vol. 22, no. 3, pp. 265–273, 2015.

[13] S. Dua, M. Bhuker, P. Sharma, M. Dhall, and S. Kapoor, "Body mass index relates to blood pressure among adults," *North American Journal of Medical Sciences*, vol. 6, no. 2, pp. 89–95, 2014.

[14] T. Tate, A. L. Willig, J. H. Willig et al., "HIV infection and obesity: where did all the wasting go?" *Antiviral Therapy*, vol. 17, no. 7, pp. 1281–1289, 2012.

[15] A. Sharma, S. A. Bynum, M. F. Schneider et al., "Changes in body mass index following haart initiation among HIV-infected women in the women's interagency HIV study," *Journal of AIDS & Clinical Research*, vol. 5, no. 7, pp. 2–8, 2014.

[16] O. J. Ogunmola, O. Y. Oladosu, and A. M. Olamoyegun, "Association of hypertension and obesity with HIV and antiretroviral therapy in a rural tertiary health center in Nigeria: a cross-sectional cohort study," *Vascular Health and Risk Management*, vol. 10, pp. 129–137, 2014.

[17] C. A. Dimala, J. Atashili, J. C. Mbuagbaw, A. Wilfred, and G. L. Monekosso, "Prevalence of hypertension in HIV/AIDS patients on highly active antiretroviral therapy (HAART) compared with HAART-naïve patients at the limbe regional hospital, Cameroon," *PLoS ONE*, vol. 11, no. 2, Article ID e0148100, 2016.

[18] O. Khatib and M. El-Guindy, "Clinical guidelines for the management of hypertension," Tech. Rep., World Health Organisation, Cairo, 2005.

[19] J. V. Baker, D. Duprez, J. Rapkin et al., "Untreated HIV infection and large and small artery elasticity," *Journal of Acquired Immune Deficiency Syndromes*, vol. 52, no. 1, pp. 25–31, 2009.

[20] P. Y. Hsue, P. W. Hunt, A. Schnell et al., "Role of viral replication, antiretroviral therapy, and immunodeficiency in HIV-associated atherosclerosis," *AIDS*, vol. 23, no. 9, pp. 1059–1067, 2009.

[21] G. Schillaci, G. V. L. De Socio, G. Pucci et al., "Aortic stiffness in untreated adult patients with human immunodeficiency virus infection," *Hypertension*, vol. 52, no. 2, pp. 308–313, 2008.

[22] G. Schillaci, G. V. L. De Socio, M. Pirro et al., "Impact of treatment with protease inhibitors on aortic stiffness in adult patients with human immunodeficiency virus infection," *Arteriosclerosis, Thrombosis, and Vascular Biology*, vol. 25, no. 11, pp. 2381–2385, 2005.

[23] R. C. Kaplan, L. A. Kingsley, S. J. Gange et al., "Low CD4+ T cell count as a major atherosclerosis risk factor in HIV-infected women and men," *AIDS*, vol. 22, no. 13, pp. 1615–1624, 2008.

[24] G. S. Bloomfield, J. W. Hogan, A. Keter et al., "Hypertension and obesity as cardiovascular risk factors among HIV seropositive patients in Western Kenya," *PLoS ONE*, vol. 6, no. 7, Article ID e22288, 2011.

6

Preeclampsia Is Associated with Increased Central Aortic Pressure, Elastic Arteries Stiffness and Wave Reflections, and Resting and Recruitable Endothelial Dysfunction

Juan Torrado,[1] Ignacio Farro,[1] Yanina Zócalo,[1] Federico Farro,[1] Claudio Sosa,[2] Santiago Scasso,[2] Justo Alonso,[2] and Daniel Bia[1]

[1]*Centro Universitario de Investigación, Innovación y Diagnóstico Arterial (CUiiDARTE), Physiology Department, Faculty of Medicine, Republic University, 2125 General Flores, 11800 Montevideo, Uruguay*
[2]*Department of Obstetrics and Gynecology "C", Pereira Rossell Hospital, Faculty of Medicine, Republic University, 1550 Bulevar Artigas, 11600 Montevideo, Uruguay*

Correspondence should be addressed to Daniel Bia; dbia@fmed.edu.uy

Academic Editor: Francesco Cappuccio

Introduction. An altered endothelial function (EF) could be associated with preeclampsia (PE). However, more specific and complementary analyses are required to confirm this topic. Flow-mediated dilation (FMD), low-flow-mediated constriction (L-FMC), and hyperemic-related changes in carotid-radial pulse wave velocity (PWVcr) offer complementary information about "recruitability" of EF. *Objectives.* To evaluate, in healthy and hypertensive pregnant women (with and without PE), central arterial parameters in conjunction with "basal and recruitable" EF. *Methods.* Nonhypertensive (HP) and hypertensive pregnant women (gestational hypertension, GH; preeclampsia, PE) were included. Aortic blood pressure (BP), wave reflection parameters (AIx@75), aortic pulse wave velocity (PWVcf) and PWVcr, and brachial and common carotid stiffness and intima-media thickness were measured. Brachial FMD and L-FMC and hyperemic-related change in PWVcr were measured. *Results.* Aortic BP and AIx@75 were elevated in PE. PE showed stiffer elastic but not muscular arteries. After cuff deflation, PWVcr decreased in HP, while GH showed a blunted PWVcr response and PE showed a tendency to increase. Maximal FMD and L-FMC were observed in HP followed by GH; PE did not reach significant arterial constriction. *Conclusion.* Aortic BP and wave reflections as well as elastic arteries stiffness are increased in PE. PE showed both "resting and recruitable" endothelial dysfunctions.

1. Introduction

Preeclampsia/eclampsia (PE) syndrome, defined as new onset and persistent hypertension after 20 weeks of gestation in association with significant proteinuria [1], is a major cause of maternal-fetal morbidity and mortality worldwide. The pathophysiology of PE remains incompletely understood, and anticipation and appropriate management of this disorder are frequently insufficient [2]. The prevalent pathogenic theory of PE includes the manifestation of two characteristic and sequential processes considered to be of paramount importance. The first corresponds to an insufficient placentation, which drives an increase in the resistance of the uteroplacental circulation, and the second involves the maternal reaction through the activation of an inappropriate inflammatory response with a (proposed) globally impaired endothelial function (EF) [3]. Structural and functional alterations in large arteries have also been reported accompanying PE syndrome [4, 5].

Impaired EF and arterial damage could occur for a certain time before significant proteinuria and clinical manifestations of PE become apparent [3, 6]. Thus, the possibility of identifying early subclinical endothelial dysfunction, as well as structural and/or functional arterial alterations during pregnancy, could be of value in recognizing and classifying the different hypertensive disorders of pregnancy. Hopefully, this will have a positive impact on the understanding of this syndrome, as well as on the appropriate and early management of these patients.

Celermajer et al.'s technique, commonly known as *flow-mediated dilation* (FMD), utilizes the vascular (or vaso-) reactivity test (VRT) and has become the most popular method to assess EF [7]. The VRT consists of positioning a pneumatic cuff around the upper arm and provoking an arterial occlusion for five minutes (transient ischemia, TI). This maneuver elicits an increase in blood flow in the brachial artery once the cuff is deflated (i.e., reactive hyperemia, RH), which subsequently stimulates endothelium to release nitric oxide (NO). Finally, locally produced NO results in a dilation of the brachial artery (assessed by B-Mode ultrasound) [7] and a reduction of arterial stiffness (changes in pulse wave velocity (PWV) assessed by mechanotransducers [8]). The magnitude of the arterial dilation is used as an indicator of EF, and healthy pregnant women show an enhanced vascular response evaluated by this method compared with healthy nonpregnant women [9, 10]. Whereas FMD provides information about the "recruitability" of EF (i.e., its responsiveness to a specific stimulus), it does not provide information concerning basal/tonic EF (i.e., release of endothelial autacoids before FMD measures are initiated) [11]. In this context, Gori et al. described a novel index for assessing the response of the artery to low flow, which utilizes data obtained from the cuff occlusion period of an FMD test [12]. Synonymous to FMD, the vasoconstriction observed under conditions of reduced flow has been named low-flow-mediated vasoconstriction (L-FMC) [12]. Inclusion of L-FMC data to traditional measurement of FMD could provide additional and/or complementary information, which, they propose, may improve the detection of patients with cardiovascular disease and profile the vascular response to exercise among healthy volunteers [13]. Whether the integration of L-FMC into traditional FMD studies will provide additional/complementary information among patients with hypertensive disorders in pregnancy is unknown.

In addition, changes in arterial stiffness assessed by means of carotid-to-radial pulse wave velocity (PWVcr) due to the same test (VRT) have been proposed as an alternative tool for the evaluation of EF [8, 14]. PWV, in particular carotid-to-femoral PWV, is recognized as the "gold standard" parameter for the evaluation of regional aortic stiffness having a wide biomedical application [15]. A reduction in PWVcr values (i.e., upper limb region) in response to VRT has been evidenced in healthy young adults, whereas a blunted reduction has been reported in pathophysiological circumstances such as hypertension [16] and congestive heart failure [14]. However, the impaired EF (which could follow hypertensive disorders of pregnancy) can be assessed by using PWVcr changes and if it provides additional or complementary information to those of brachial diameter assessment has not been studied yet.

In this context, the aims of this work were as follows: firstly, to determine noninvasive central and peripheral arterial parameters in a group of healthy and hypertensive pregnant women, through the use of validated techniques and parameters; secondly, to determine and analyze "basal and recruitable" EF through the measurement of FMD, L-FMC, and PWVcr changes.

2. Methods

2.1. Subjects. This was a cross-sectional study involving 26 pregnant women. The normotensive subjects (healthy pregnant women, HP; $n = 10$) were recruited from the routine antenatal clinic. They were all healthy and without family history of premature heart disease. All women had uncomplicated pregnancies before and during the study. Women with preeclampsia (PE; $n = 8$) and with gestational hypertension (GH; $n = 8$) were recruited from the antenatal hospital ward, where they were admitted due to mild hypertension (140/90 to 149/109 mmHg).

The definitions used followed the classification of the gestational hypertensive disorders, as recommended by the report of the National Collaborating Centre for Women's and Children's Health, hypertension in pregnancy, of the National Institute for Health and Clinical Excellence [1]. Under this classification, PE was defined as BP greater than 140/90 mmHg on two consecutive occasions more than 4 h apart, in combination with significant proteinuria (>300 mg total protein in a 24 h urine collection) developing after 20 weeks of gestation in previously normotensive women. The same hemodynamic conditions without significant proteinuria defined gestational hypertension.

All PE included in the study were *mild* in terms of the severity of the syndrome. None of them received any vasoactive drugs. Participants were asked to abstain from physical activity and vitamin supplementation for at least 4 hours prior to the examination. Baseline demographic data were obtained by an obstetrician during a clinical interview and laboratory samples were extracted prior to the examination. The study protocol was approved by the Ethics Research Committee of the School of Medicine (Republic University, Uruguay) and all participants gave written informed consent.

2.2. Baseline Noninvasive Arterial Evaluation. After recompilation of clinical and laboratory data, subjects were instructed to lie in a left lateral position (to avoid vena cava compression by the uterus) in a temperature-controlled (21°–23°C) room, for at least 15 minutes, in order to establish stable hemodynamic conditions. Heart rate (HR) and right brachial (peripheral) systolic and diastolic blood pressure (pSBP and pDBP, resp.) were measured using an oscillometric device (Omron HEM-433INT Oscillometric System; Omron Healthcare Inc., Illinois, USA) at 2-minute intervals during the whole procedure. Mean blood pressure (MBP) was derived from the standard equation usually employed at the peripheral level: MBP = pDBP + 1/3(pSBP − pDBP).

2.2.1. Carotid-to-Femoral Pulse Wave Velocity and Pulse Wave Analysis. The carotid-to-femoral pulse wave velocity (PWVcf) was measured to analyze aortic regional stiffness. To this end, carotid and femoral artery waveforms were consecutively obtained with a high-fidelity applanation tonometer from the carotid and femoral regions simultaneously with continuous ECG monitoring (SphygmoCor 7.01, AtCor Medical, Sydney, Australia) (Figure 1) [15]. Then, carotid-femoral propagation time (Δt_3) was determined by subtracting the time delay between the peak of R wave of the ECG recording

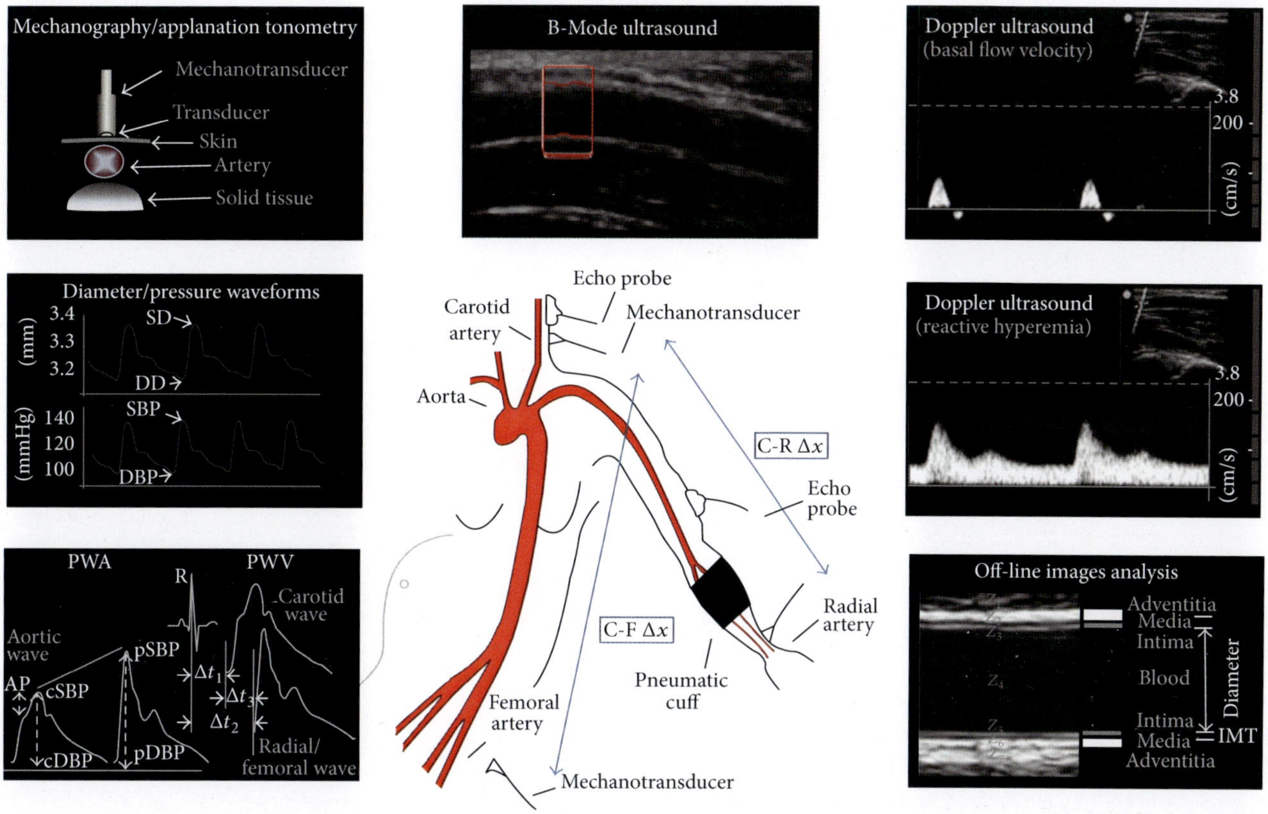

Figure 1: Schema of the instrumental approach employed to assess noninvasive arterial structure and function in basal and post-VRT conditions. Employed techniques are as follows: carotid-to-femoral and carotid-to-radial PWV (applanation tonometry and mechanography), PWA (applanation tonometry), arterial diameters and CIMT (B-Mode ultrasound), and blood flow velocities (Doppler ultrasound). PWA: pulse wave analysis; PWV: pulse wave velocity; AP: augmentation pressure; Δt_1, Δt_2: time delay between R wave from ECG and carotid foot wave and femoral/radial foot wave, respectively; Δt_3: time delay between carotid foot wave and femoral/radial foot wave; cSBP/pSBP: central/peripheral systolic blood pressure; cDBP/pDBP: central/peripheral diastolic blood pressure; DD: diastolic diameter; SD: systolic diameter; CIMT: carotid intima-media thickness; Z: acoustic impedance; C-F and C-R Δx: carotid-to-femoral and carotid-to-radial distance, respectively.

to femoral foot of the pressure waveform (Δt_2) of the corresponding cardiac cycle and the time delay between the peaks of R wave to carotid foot of the pressure waveform (Δt_1) [15]. The algorithm utilized to detect the so-called "foot of the wave" was the *intersecting tangents*. Straight distance between the recording sites (carotid-to-femoral distance (C-F Δx)) was then carefully measured using tape on the body surface to reduce the influence of altered body contour in pregnancy. Finally, PWVcf was automatically calculated as the quotient between C-F Δx and Δt_3 (Figure 1) [15]. The reported value of PWVcf for a subject was always the average of at least eight consecutive beats.

Pulse wave analysis (PWA) was used to assess central hemodynamics as well as systemic arterial stiffness and wave reflections [15]. For this purpose, mean radial artery waveform was obtained (through the acquisition of many cycles) with the applanation tonometer from the wrist, and a corresponding mean ascending aortic pressure waveform was generated with a validated generalized transfer function using the same mentioned customized software (SphygmoCor 7.01, AtCor Medical, Sydney, Australia). The radial pulse waveform was then calibrated using the diastolic and mean arterial pressure obtained at the brachial artery [15]. Central systolic, diastolic, and pulse blood pressure (cSBP, cDBP, and cPP, resp.), heart rate (HR) corrected central augmentation index (AP/cPP × 100[%] heart rate adjusted to a HR of 75 bpm; AIx@75), and amplification ratio (pPP/cPP) were determined with the integrated software.

2.2.2. Carotid Artery Studies. Ultrasound assessment of carotid arteries was based on the techniques and recommendations described in international consensus [17]. High-resolution B-Mode ultrasound images of both (right and left) common carotid arteries (CCAs) were obtained using a 10 MHz linear-array transducer connected to a portable ultrasound system (SonoSite, MicroMaxx, SonoSite Inc., 21919 30th Drive SE, Bothell, WA 98021, USA). Measurements (still images and video clips/cine loops) were digitally stored for off-line analysis (Figure 1). Near and far walls were analyzed and images were obtained from anterior, lateral, and posterior angles. At first, a carotid plaque screening was performed, for which the definition used was a focal structure that encroaches into the arterial lumen of at least 0.5 mm or 50% of the surrounding intima-media thickness or demonstrated a thickness of greater than or equal to 1.5 mm [17]. Then, longitudinal views of the CCAs were acquired and a video (cine-loop) of at least 10 seconds was recorded and stored. The CIMT and beat-to-beat diameter waveforms were obtained and analyzed off-line using a step-by-step border detection algorithm (based on changes in acoustic impedance (Z)), applied to each digitized image (Hemodyn-4M software, Buenos Aires, Argentina). A region of 1.0 cm proximal to the carotid bulb was identified, and the far wall CIMT was determined as the distance between the lumen-intima and the media-adventitia interfaces (Figure 1). The software performs multiple automated or semiautomated measurements along the centimeter and averages them, increasing the accuracy of the measures.

The instantaneous diameter (from the leading edge of the near wall intima-media interface to the intima-media interface of the far wall) waveform was obtained during pulsation in order to obtain diastolic and systolic arterial diameter. Then, complementary biomechanical parameters such as Peterson's elastic modulus (E_P) and beta stiffness-index (β) were calculated relating these measures with central blood pressure as follows:

$$E_P = \frac{(\text{cSBP} - \text{cDBP})}{(\text{SD} - \text{DD})/\text{DD}},$$
$$\beta = \frac{\text{Ln}(\text{cSBP}/\text{cDBP})}{(\text{SD} - \text{DD})/\text{DD}}, \quad (1)$$

where cSBP, cDBP, SD, and DD are central systolic and diastolic blood pressure and carotid systolic and diastolic diameter, respectively (Figure 1). E_P measures the ability of the arteries to change their dimensions in response to the pulse pressure caused by cardiac pulsatile ejection (pressure change required for (theoretic) 100% increase in diameter), whereas β is considered to be relatively independent of blood pressure levels [15].

2.3. Vascular Reactivity and Endothelial Function. Once baseline noninvasive arterial evaluation was carried out, we utilized the theoretical basis, general protocol, and methodological aspects of the VRT recommended by the guidelines for the ultrasound assessment of endothelial-dependent flow-mediated vasodilation of the brachial artery [7, 18]. For this purpose, participants were submitted to five minutes of ischemia by occluding left radial and cubital arteries using a pneumatic cuff placed around the left forearm (just below the elbow to at least 50 mmHg above pSBP) and several parameters of vascular reactivity were measured before, during, and after ischemia (Figure 1). The parameters used for the evaluation of EF are listed below.

2.3.1. FMD, L-FMC, Brachial Biomechanics, and Shear Rate. Taking into account "gold standard" accepted methodology for the evaluation of EF ("recruitability") and simultaneously for PWVcr measurement (see later), left brachial artery was visualized longitudinally above the antecubital crease using same high-resolution B-Mode ultrasound device mentioned earlier (Sonosite; MicroMaxx; USA) (Figure 1). Similarly, video sequences were recorded at rest, during forearm occlusion and after cuff deflation. Subsequently and similarly to the processing of carotid images, recordings were analyzed off-line using same automated step-by-step algorithm applied to each digitalized image that allows the brachial diameter waveform obtainment and FMD and L-FMC calculation [19]. Brachial local stiffness (E_P and β) was also determined by relating brachial arterial pressure and brachial diameters, as was explained earlier for carotid measurements.

FMD was quantified as the percentage of change in brachial DD, considering the basal levels and those measured one minute after cuff deflation:

$$\text{FMD\%} = \frac{\text{DD}_{\text{after cuff deflation}} - \text{DD}_{\text{baseline}}}{\text{DD}_{\text{baseline}}} \times 100. \quad (2)$$

In addition, Doppler signals were performed to acquire blood flow velocity in baseline conditions and at specific moments during the reactive hyperemia period. Doppler signals were used to obtain the brachial *shear rate* (and its percentage of change), relating mean blood flow velocity (Vm (cm/s)) to brachial mean diameter (Dm) according to the following equations:

$$\text{SR} = \frac{\text{Vm}}{\text{Dm}},$$
$$\text{SR\%} = \frac{\text{SR}_{\text{after cuff deflation}} - \text{SR}_{\text{baseline}}}{\text{SR}_{\text{baseline}}} \times 100. \quad (3)$$

SR is an estimate of *shear stress* without accounting for blood viscosity [20] and was obtained for the characterization of the endothelial stimulus. The study protocol is represented in Figure 2.

2.3.2. Carotid-to-Radial Pulse Wave Velocity. Noninvasive, carotid, and radial pressure waveforms were simultaneously obtained using strain gauge mechanotransducers (Motorola MPX 2050, Motorola Inc., Corporate 1303 E. Algonquin Road, Schaumburg, Illinois 60196, USA) by placing them on the skin over the carotid and radial sites (left hemibody). PWVcr was determined taking into account the given distance between these arterial sites (C-R Δx) and the time delay (Δt) between the carotid and radial waveforms onset (Figure 1). The algorithm used for the detection of the foot waves was described and explained in previous work [8]. Although a four-minute recording after cuff release was obtained, one minute after ischemia was the specific moment where the analysis was especially taken, according to previous reports [8, 16] (Figure 2). The PWVcr accepted variation coefficient was less than 7%.

PWVcr levels corresponding to baseline and to postischemia period were determined by averaging eight consecutive beats. After that, percent of change of PWVcr (with respect to basal levels) was quantified as follows:

$$\Delta\text{PWVcr\%} = \frac{\text{PWVcr}_{\text{after cuff deflation}} - \text{PWVcr}_{\text{baseline}}}{\text{PWVcr}_{\text{baseline}}} \times 100. \quad (4)$$

All structural and function arterial evaluations were done by the same trained operator.

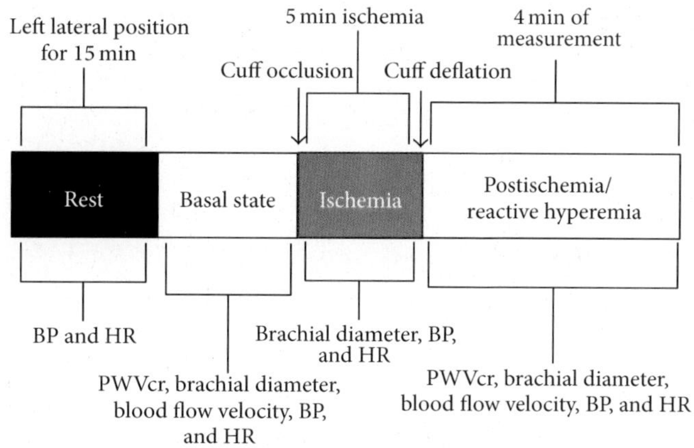

FIGURE 2: Representative diagram of the study protocol applied to evaluate changes in arterial parameters. PWVcr: carotid-to-radial pulse wave velocity; BP: blood pressure; HR: heart rate.

2.4. Statistics. The statistical analyses were performed using the Statistical Package for Social Sciences (version 22.0). Normality of the distribution of the data was examined using the Shapiro-Wilk test and Q-Q plot. All studied variables followed a normal distribution. All data are presented as mean value (MV) ± standard deviation (SD). Two-way analysis of variance (ANOVA) was employed for the evaluation of differences in variables within and between hypertensive and control pregnant women. Post hoc comparisons were done with the Bonferroni test. Differences in percentage of change of variables determined before and after the VRT (arterial diameter, PWV, and shear rate) were evaluated using two-tailed paired Student's t-test. Linear regression analyses were used to assess relationship between variables. $P < 0.05$ indicates significant statistical differences.

3. Results

Recordings were successfully obtained from all women and all studies were included in the analysis. The mean duration of the studies was 1 hour approximately and they were all well tolerated (without symptoms and/or complications).

The mean gestational age at examination of all the pregnant women was 35 ± 3 weeks. Demographic and anthropometric features and laboratory samples are shown in Table 1. Significant proteinuria in the daily urine collection could divide the group of hypertensive pregnant women in those with preeclampsia (with significant proteinuria >300 mg/24 hours, PE) and those with gestational hypertension (without or with only traces of proteinuria, GH). No significant proteinuria was found in HP. Maternal age, gestational age, and number of previous gestations were similar between study groups. Body weight and body mass index (BMI) were significantly higher in PE compared with HP and GH ($P < 0.05$). Uric acid levels were within normal values in HP and GH, while in PE they were abnormally increased [21].

Baseline cardiovascular characteristics are given and compared in Table 2. Baseline peripheral SBP, DBP, and MAP levels were significantly higher in PE and GH in comparison with HP ($P < 0.001$). No peripheral BP differences were found among groups with hypertension (GH versus PE). However, differences were found in these groups when central hemodynamics is analyzed. For example, cPP was different between study groups. In addition, PE showed higher values of cSBP compared with GH ($P = 0.004$), without differences in cPP and cDBP. When compared with HP women, levels of cSBP and cDBP in women with PE and GH were higher.

AIx@75 and the amplification ratio, two composite measures of systemic arterial stiffness and wave reflection amplitude, were analyzed and are presented in Table 2. AIx@75 was significantly higher in PE with respect to GH and HP (24.3 ± 5.7% versus 11.8 ± 7.6 and 12.2 ± 12.4%, resp.; $P = 0.05$). No significant differences were found in this parameter between GH and HP. On the other hand, amplification ratio (cPP/pPP) was only statistically different between PE and GH, with PE having the lowest values.

When analyzing muscular peripheral arteries (i.e., brachial artery) by local (E_P and β) and regional arterial stiffness parameters (PWVcr), no differences were found among groups. However, CCA and aorta (i.e., elastic arteries) showed meaningful differences in stiffness. In general, PE showed stiffer elastic arteries with respect to other groups. For example, right CCA E_P was significantly increased (duplicating approximately its values) in PE with respect to HP and GH ($P < 0.001$ and $P = 0.004$, resp.). Similar tendencies were noticed in β from the right CCA but not reaching statistical differences, indicating that changes in carotid artery stiffness in PE and GH are pressure-dependent. On the left side, differences were observed in E_P comparing PE and HP, and similar tendencies were maintained for β.

Finally, hypertensive pregnant women showed higher values of PWVcf (regional aortic stiffness) compared with HP women. However, no differences were found between the groups with hypertension, although women with PE had a tendency to show higher values ($P = 0.14$).

None of the groups (HP, GH, or PE) presented atherosclerotic plaques. However, structural differences were noticed on the right common carotid artery. Right, but not left, CIMT

Table 1: Demographic and laboratory samples characteristics of the study populations according to pregnancy status.

	Healthy pregnant (HP) MV ± SD	Gestational hypertension (GH) MV ± SD	Preeclampsia (PE) MV ± SD	P value*
n	10	8	8	
Age (years)	29.4 ± 6.2	30.9 ± 6.7	33.6 ± 5.9	0.373
Gestational age (weeks)	34.6 ± 3.7	34.9 ± 2.9	36.3 ± 2.2	0.502
Number of gestations (n)	1.8 ± 2.1	4.5 ± 3.8	3.5 ± 4.5	0.286
Weight (kg)	67.1 ± 7.3	76.5 ± 10.9	97.0 ± 12.6^{a,b}	<0.001
Height (cm)	157.6 ± 6.8	159.6 ± 5.3	160.3 ± 8.6	0.703
BMI (kg/m^2)	27.1 ± 3.6	30.2 ± 5.4	38.1 ± 6.6^{a,b}	0.001
Creatinine (mg/dL)	0.7 ± 0.1	0.6 ± 0.1	0.6 ± 0.1	0.664
Uric acid (mg/dL)	3.2 ± 1.1	4.1 ± 1.4	6.7 ± 2.5^{a,b}	0.001
24-hour proteinuria (g)	0.0 ± 0.1	0.2 ± 0.1^{a}	0.5 ± 0.1^{a,b}	<0.001
SGOT (UI/L)	12.2 ± 3.2	15.7 ± 5.9	14.5 ± 2.5	0.722
SGPT (UI/L)	11.5 ± 5.2	13.7 ± 6.0	11.8 ± 4.1	0.587
LDH (UI/L)	320.5 ± 59.7	347.8 ± 49.8	386.9 ± 93.3	0.846
Hematocrit (%)	31.7 ± 3.7	34.2 ± 2.9	33.7 ± 2.0	0.681
Platelets (μL^{-1})	213.0 ± 78.0	195.4 ± 60.0	202.6 ± 45.6	0.862

Values are expressed as mean value (MV) ± standard deviation (SD). Post hoc test with multiple comparisons: a and b indicate $P < 0.05$ with respect to HP and GH, respectively. All comparisons were determined using ANOVA + Bonferroni test. HP: healthy pregnancies; GH: gestational hypertension; PE: preeclamptic pregnancies; BMI: body mass index; SGOT: serum glutamic-oxaloacetic transaminase; SGPT: serum glutamic-pyruvic transaminase; LDH: lactate dehydrogenase. *Between groups.

was significantly elevated in PE with respect to HP women ($P = 0.010$).

Taking into account the VRT (vascular reactivity test), all groups evoked endothelial stimulus (reactive hyperemia) evaluated by changes in shear rate before and after cuff deflation ($P < 0.001$). In addition, peak SR and ΔSR% were the same among groups ($P = 0.86$ and $P = 0.39$, resp.) (Table 3). No significant changes were found in heart rate or blood pressure intra- and intergroup before and after cuff deflation, ensuring stable hemodynamic conditions during the maneuver (data not shown).

Regarding the FMD, all of them showed a dilatation of the brachial artery with respect to the basal state but without statistical significance in women with PE. As was expected, HP women showed quantitatively the highest FMD response (9.4 ± 3.0%; $P < 0.001$), while women with GH and PE reached the lowest values (3.6 ± 3.3%; $P = 0.021$; 2.2 ± 2.9%; $P = 0.081$, resp.). FMD mean values of GH and PE compared to HP were significantly different ($P < 0.001$). As was mentioned above, baseline PWVcr were similar among groups. One minute after the cuff deflation, PWVcr decreased only in HP (7.0 ± 1.6 to 5.9 ± 0.8 m/s, $P < 0.01$). However, GH showed a blunted hyperemic PWVcr response (7.1 ± 0.9 to 7.0 ± 0.8 m/s; $P = 0.627$), while PE showed a tendency to increase arterial stiffness (6.0 ± 1.1 to 6.4 ± 1.3 m/s; $P = 0.06$). PWVcr percentage changes [ΔPWVcr (%)] differed comparing HP women with women with GH (−13.9% versus −0.9%; $P < 0.01$) and with PE (−13.9% versus +7.0%; $P < 0.01$). No differences were found between GH and PE ($P = 0.221$).

L-FMC of the brachial artery was different according to the pregnancy status ($P < 0.001$). Maximal vasoconstriction (negative values) was observed in HP women (−7.8 ± 3.7%, $P < 0.001$) followed by women with GH (−4.5 ± 2.1%, $P < 0.001$), while women with PE did not reach significant arterial constriction during the cuff inflation (−0.7 ± 3.5; $P = 0.576$) (Table 3). There were no differences in L-FMC between PE and GH.

Demographic, anthropometric, and laboratory variables shown in Table 1 did not significantly correlate with any of the arterial parameters. In addition, there was no significant correlation between parameters of EF (i.e., FMD, L-FMC, and ΔPWVcr%) and AIx@75 or amplification ratio (data not shown). However, a low but statistically significant correlation was found between baseline PWVcf and L-FMC ($r = 0.45$, $P = 0.04$), without reaching statistical significance with other EF parameters. A significant correlation between FMD, L-FMC, and ΔPWVcr% was seen among these parameters in the whole study population (Figure 3).

4. Discussion

The present study is, to our knowledge, the first one to determine and assess simultaneously, in a group of healthy and hypertensive pregnant women, the vascular reactivity or EF by using three different but complementary methods in conjunction with the determination of central and peripheral arterial structural and functional parameters.

The main results of this work were as follows: (1) central aortic blood pressure and wave reflections as well as elastic (aortic and carotid) arteries stiffness are increased in PE, with respect to peripheral blood pressure-matched GH and HP, and (2) PE showed both resting (L-FMC) and recruitable (FMD and ΔPWVcr%) endothelial dysfunction.

Among the methods that allow measurement of vascular reactivity or EF in the clinical setting, FMD has rapidly

TABLE 2: Baseline cardiovascular characteristics of the study populations according to pregnancy status.

	Healthy pregnant (HP) MV ± SD	Gestational hypertension (GH) MV ± SD	Preeclampsia (PE) MV ± SD	P value*
Heart rate (bpm)	81.8 ± 15.9	84.8 ± 9.7	85.3 ± 14.0	0.844
Peripheral SBP (mmHg)	111.8 ± 8.2	139.4 ± 6.0[a]	145.5 ± 7.5[a]	<0.001
Peripheral DBP (mmHg)	63.5 ± 9.5	78.9 ± 11.9[a]	84.6 ± 8.8[a]	<0.001
MBP (mmHg)	79.6 ± 5.8	99.0 ± 6.3[a]	105.9 ± 7.3[a]	<0.001
Peripheral PP (mmHg)	50.7 ± 18.6	58.6 ± 11.4	58.0 ± 12.7	0.571
Central SBP (mmHg)	96.7 ± 6.7	118.9 ± 3.9[a]	130.3 ± 5.8[a,b]	<0.001
Central DBP (mmHg)	63.5 ± 9.5	80.4 ± 11.2[a]	85.6 ± 10.0[a]	<0.001
Central PP (mmHg)	33.2 ± 11.4	35.5 ± 7.1	42.8 ± 10.8	0.041
Amplification ratio	1.5 ± 0.2	1.7 ± 0.2	1.4 ± 0.2[b]	<0.001
AIx@75 (%)	12.2 ± 12.4	11.8 ± 7.6	24.3 ± 5.7[a,b]	0.018
Carotid-to-femoral PWV (m/s)	5.6 ± 0.8	7.1 ± 0.8[a]	8.2 ± 1.2[a]	<0.001
Carotid-to-radial PWV (m/s)	7.0 ± 1.6	7.1 ± 0.9	6.0 ± 1.1	0.159
Brachial SR (s^{-1})	117.9 ± 43.1	102.8 ± 26.7	93.4 ± 43.5	0.417
Brachial SD (mm)	3.8 ± 0.3	3.9 ± 0.4	4.3 ± 0.5	0.149
Brachial DD (mm)	3.7 ± 0.3	3.7 ± 0.4	4.1 ± 0.4	0.210
Brachial E_P (mmHg)	1010 ± 464	1188 ± 832	1183 ± 350	0.754
Brachial β	11.4 ± 5.0	11.1 ± 8.3	11.3 ± 3.4	0.953
Right CCA SD (mm)	7.1 ± 0.6	7.1 ± 0.6	7.1 ± 0.5	0.988
Right CCA DD (mm)	6.5 ± 0.6	6.5 ± 0.6	6.7 ± 0.5	0.749
Right E_P (mmHg)	355 ± 102	434 ± 161	709 ± 185[a,b]	<0.001
Right CCA β	4.56 ± 1.47	5.24 ± 3.07	6.95 ± 1.58	0.073
Right CIMT (mm)	0.47 ± 0.10	0.55 ± 0.08	0.66 ± 0.21[a]	0.036
Left CCA SD (mm)	7.1 ± 0.4	7.2 ± 0.3	7.1 ± 0.7	0.932
Left CCA DD (mm)	6.5 ± 0.4	6.6 ± 0.2	6.7 ± 0.6	0.637
Left CCA E_P (mmHg)	376 ± 153	471 ± 182	714 ± 256[a]	0.005
Left CCA β	4.8 ± 2.0	5.6 ± 3.1	7.0 ± 2.4	0.205
Left CIMT (mm)	0.51 ± 0.09	0.55 ± 0.08	0.59 ± 0.10	0.162

Values are expressed as mean value (MV) ± standard deviation (SD). Post hoc test with multiple comparisons: a and b indicate $P < 0.05$ with respect to HP and GH, respectively. All comparisons were determined using ANOVA + Bonferroni test. HP: healthy pregnancies; GH: gestational hypertension; PE: preeclamptic pregnancies; SBP: systolic blood pressure; DBP: diastolic blood pressure; MBP: mean blood pressure; PP: pulse pressure; AIx@75: augmentation index adjusted to a heart rate of 75 bpm; PWV: pulse wave velocity; SR: shear rate; SD and DD: systolic and diastolic diameter, respectively; E_P: Peterson's elastic modulus; β: stiffness index; CCA: common carotid artery; CIMT: carotid intima-media thickness. *Between groups.

TABLE 3: VRT-related changes in vascular parameters of the study groups according to pregnancy status.

	Healthy pregnant (HP) MV ± SD	Gestational hypertension (GH) MV ± SD	Preeclampsia (PE) MV ± SD	P value*
FMD (%)	9.4 ± 3.0	3.6 ± 3.3[a]	2.2 ± 2.9[a]	<0.001
L-FMC (%)	−7.8 ± 3.7	−4.5 ± 2.1	−0.7 ± 3.5[a]	<0.001
ΔPWVcr (%)	−13.9 ± 9.4	−0.9 ± 6.9[a]	7.0 ± 8.5[a]	<0.001
Peak shear rate (s^{-1})	231.7 ± 72.6	237.6 ± 67.5	219.5 ± 59.5	0.86
ΔShear rate (%)	113.8 ± 87.4	131.2 ± 53.7	168.6 ± 97.1	0.39

Values are expressed as mean value (MV) ± standard deviation (SD). Post hoc test with multiple comparisons: a indicate $P < 0.05$ with respect to HP and GH, respectively. All comparisons were determined using ANOVA + Bonferroni test. HP: healthy pregnancies; GH: gestational hypertension; PE: preeclamptic pregnancies; FMD: flow-mediated dilation; L-FMC: low-flow-mediated constriction; PWVcr: carotid-to-radial pulse wave velocity. *Between groups.

gained popularity because of its simplicity, reproducibility, and noninvasiveness [7, 18]. However, as was mentioned earlier, one important limitation of FMD is that it only provides information about the "recruitability" of EF (i.e., its responsiveness to a specific stimulus) and not about concerning "resting" EF (i.e., release of endothelial autacoids before FMD measures are initiated) [11]. We here analyze in hypertensive pregnant women both types of functional aspects of EF: "endothelial recruitability" through FMD and PWVcr changes and "resting endothelial tone" through L-FMC. The magnitude of FMD observed in HP in response to VRT was similar to that described in previous reports

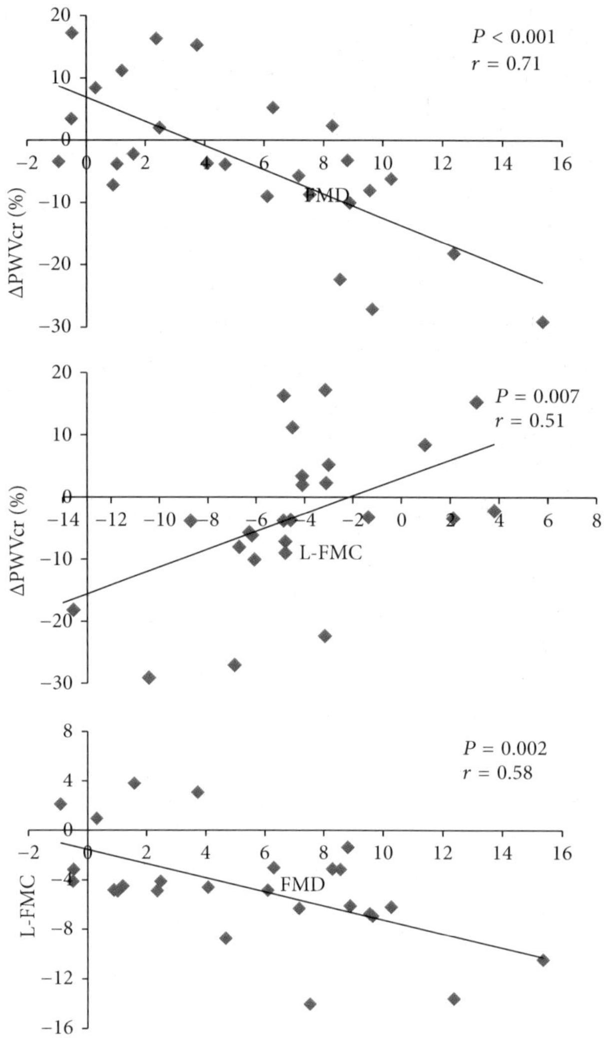

FIGURE 3: Correlation analysis between EF parameters. FMD: flow-mediated dilation; L-FMC: low-flow-mediated constriction; ΔPWVcr%: percentage of change in carotid-to-radial pulse wave velocity.

[9, 10]. As it was expected, hypertensive pregnant women showed a reduction in FMD with respect to HP, in coherence with greater degrees of endothelial dysfunction [22, 23]. It is noteworthy that only PE did not reach statistical significance in the dilation of the brachial artery, obtaining a more complete blunted response. Although the FMD of PE was numerically lower than those from GH, this difference did not reach statistical significance. This could be attributed or not attributed to the magnitude of the standards deviation of the mean due to the low sample size. Nevertheless, approximately 25% of women initially diagnosed with GH will develop PE [24]. Therefore, the vascular profile from pregnant women with GH who might develop PE could be quite similar to those women with PE. However, there is a lack of information that compares FMD between groups with PE and GH and only few studies directly analyze this issue. According to Quinton et al., the FMD at one minute of the cuff deflation was not different between the GH and PE in women who were not receiving any medication, while there were statistical differences between these groups when women were receiving medical treatment [25]. Nevertheless, in a prospective study conducted by Filho et al., they did not find differences in FMD of the brachial artery in patients with two different forms of hypertensive disorders of pregnancy [26].

When analyzing changes in arterial stiffness due to VRT, HP showed the major reduction in PWVcr values. On the other hand, women with hypertension showed not only a blunted response in PWVcr changes but also, in PE, a tendency to increase arterial stiffness one minute after the cuff deflation was evidenced. Indeed, by means of this method, changes of PWVcr in PE tended to be higher in comparison to GH, indicating probably greater degree of impairment of EF. It is noteworthy that all participants showed the same increase in blood flow velocity with respect to basal conditions after cuff deflation ("endothelial stimulus"), and variables such as baseline levels of PWVcr, basal brachial diameter, blood pressure, and gestational age were similar among the groups.

Taking into account "resting" endothelial tone, our results show that, during cuff inflation, brachial artery responses varied between the studied groups. L-FMC of the brachial artery was significant only in HP and GH, without any constriction in PE, suggesting that PE develop also basal endothelial dysfunction. Although L-FMC was firstly described and assessed at the radial artery, Spiro et al. evidenced later that this phenomenon also occurs in healthy subjects at the brachial artery and it can be measured reliably [27]. Studies agree that radial artery vasoconstriction occurs during cuff inflation in nonpregnant women [12, 28, 29], whereas recent studies examining the brachial diameter during occlusion demonstrate conflicting results [27, 28, 30–32]. Weissgerber et al. did not evidence L-FMC in the brachial artery in pregnant women [29]. Differences in cardiovascular profile, methodological issues, and interobserver variability could explain the widely variable results. For example, we here measure L-FMC of the brachial artery in a regimen of low but not zero blood flow (as it occurs in the radial artery) in a level that is upstream of the occlusion site. Therefore, the magnitude of reduced blood flow in the brachial artery and its relationship with the basal levels (endothelial "negative" stimulus for vasoconstriction) should surely yield different brachial responses.

As it was previously reported, we found that women with PE showed marked structural and functional alterations in peripheral and central hemodynamics [4, 33–35]. PE had a strong tendency to present higher values in practically all studied parameters related to central hemodynamics. For instance, central SBP, AIx@75, CCA E_P, and PWVcf were significantly higher in PE with respect to HP. We also found differences in central hemodynamics between women with hypertension, but this was not the rule as it was for PE versus HP. Only cSBP, AIx@75, and right CCA E_P were markedly augmented in comparison to GH. These findings were not due to differences in peripheral blood pressure, which was elevated to a similar degree in both types of hypertensive states. These pieces of information analyzed together indicate that women with hypertensive disorders in pregnancy (mainly PE) have increased central BP overload, central arterial stiffness, and amount of wave reflections, probably related to a vasoconstriction state due to endothelial dysfunction [35]. Altered central hemodynamics in PE may signify an inadequately increased left ventricle afterload and myocardial oxygen demand in the mother circulation, as well as hemodynamic disturbances transmitted to the fetal circulation [36].

Blunted FMD, L-FMC, and PWVcr changes evidenced in PE are in consonance with the plasma uric acid levels that were found elevated only in this group. In previous reports, hyperuricemia was associated with an increase of plasma xanthine oxidase activity and/or a reduction in antioxidant systems [37] related to increased formation of reactive oxygen species and endothelial dysfunction [38]. Differences in BMI were found among the groups. Increased BMI in PE could reflect an associated overweight/obesity state, differences in Na^+ and body fluid retention by the hemodynamic overload due to the hypertensive condition, or a combination of both.

We found a significant correlation between the EF parameters. Our results indicate that brachial artery responses to inflation and deflation of the cuff related to endothelial dynamics could share some vascular mechanism. However, there are confusing results around the FMD and L-FMC correlation, with variable results depending on the analyzed artery (brachial versus radial) and type of physiological or pathophysiological circumstance [11–13, 27]. This emphasizes again the complexity of the study of "endothelial functions." Although both L-FMC and FMD are an expression of the vascular reactivity in response to changes in blood flow, their relationship is neither conceptually simple nor mathematically linear [13]. On the other hand, when analyzing the relationship between FMD and PWVcr the analysis can also be a little more complex. According to Moens and Korteweg equation, PWV is determined by arterial diameter and also by the elastic modulus [5]. If post-VRT changes in PWVcr in PE and GH would have followed only the changes in brachial diameter (FMD), the obtained changes in PWVcr would have shown an equal behavior to the geometrical change (change in diameter) [39]. However, in accordance with the obtained values in the groups with hypertension, a dissociation among these variables was evidenced, with an increase of arterial diameter (which would reduce the levels of PWVcr) without significant changes in PWVcr levels (or even a trend to increase in PE) after the cuff deflation period. This discordance between parameters behavior in response to the VRT indicates an increase in the elastic modulus in parallel with changes in the arterial diameter. Thus, at least in PE, we evidenced a reciprocal and simultaneous change in the vascular wall intrinsic properties and the brachial diameter.

An impaired response to changes in blood flow in a concrete vascular ledge (e.g., brachial artery), without simultaneous adequate change both in brachial diameter and in arterial stiffness, could have important hemodynamic consequences. At first, a reduction in the vasodilator reserve related to endothelial dysfunction as it was seen in other pathophysiological circumstances [40] could implicate an incapacity of the arterial system to determine an appropriate vascular adjustment against hemodynamic changes in the long (fetal growth) and even in the short term (exercise, change of position, etc.). Second, an impaired capability of response to hemodynamic changes due to endothelial dysfunction could yield other functional cardiovascular alterations that was seen in PE, like increased left ventricle afterload and diastolic dysfunction [41]. This point is in consonance with altered values of central parameters found in PE mentioned above. The important additional information brought by introduction changes in PWVcr and L-FMC, together with the information of central and peripheral hemodynamics, is that these variables provide information concerning a different aspect of vascular reactivity and EF, therefore complementing (and not overlapping with) the information provided by FMD. This vascular approach may provide a more comprehensive assessment of vascular state and endothelial function in hypertensive disease of pregnancy.

The sample size of our study was relatively small. However, our findings were statistically significant and, by definition, this indicates that the study was adequately statistically powered. Our technical approaches including the use of both multiple automated and semiautomated edge-detection/point software in ultrasound image and pressure wave assessment are largely operator-independent and also empower our findings [28]. Given the means of the different variables and SDs observed in previous works and in the present sample, twenty-five subjects ($n = 25$) of the total sample size (the sum of the sizes of comparison groups) would be required to detect a statistically significant effect of the pregnancy status with at least 80% of power [42].

The detection of pregnant women who finally will develop PE remains a clinical challenge. There is no isolated technique which satisfies completely this purpose with enough accuracy. At the present time, different combinations of clinical risk factors, biochemical markers, and Doppler ultrasound of the uterine arteries are recommended [43]. The detection rate of PE using only one clinical model of screening that includes risk factors (e.g., nulliparity, maternal age, family history of PE, etc.) is 45.3%, while only with Doppler ultrasound of uterine arteries at the second trimester it is 63.1% and with a combined approach it reaches 67.5%, with a 25% of false positive rate [5]. The clinical importance of improving detection of PE can also be stressed when confidential enquiries are analyzed, showing that in a substantial proportion of cases of fetal death due to preeclampsia a different management might have altered the outcome [44]. Moreover, the evidence demonstrates that administration of antiplatelet agents (primarily low dose of aspirin in different trials) to well-selected women leads to a significant reduction in the risk of developing preeclampsia and its serious consequences [45]. For these reasons, an accurate prediction of preeclampsia or early diagnosis may, therefore, allow more efficient allocation of resources for monitoring and improving maternal and perinatal outcomes [1, 2]. On the other hand, the extensive and growing information that links endothelial dysfunction/arterial damage with pathophysiology of PE motivates researchers and clinicians to evaluate arterial parameters (including endothelial function) in this clinical setting. Additionally, there is a need to count with a more comprehensive assessing EF in a patient in concrete. In that sense, the inclusion of validated arterial parameters and a more complete EF evaluation in the contemporary assessment of preeclampsia into multiparametric models could improve prediction of PE [43]. In this small study, which addresses the feasibility of measuring these parameters simultaneously, simply, and noninvasively, we found encouraging results that we believe warrant further investigation in order to contribute to the early recognition of preeclampsia.

5. Conclusion

This is the first study that measures and analyzes, in the same pregnant women, central and peripheral hemodynamics and EF by using different parameters that offer additional and complementary information. "Resting and recruitable" EF from pregnant women can be assessed by using PWVcr changes and L-FMC, respectively. Impaired EF which follows hypertensive disorder of pregnancy, mainly PE, showed both "resting and recruitable" endothelial dysfunctions.

Central aortic pressure and wave reflections as well as stiffness of elastic arteries are improperly increased in PE. Future studies will have to determine if incorporation of these pieces of information together, assessing basal state and functional reserve or capability of response of the vascular system into multiparametric models that include clinical, obstetric, and laboratory variables and Doppler ultrasound of uterine arteries, will be able to improve contemporary prediction of preeclampsia (from healthy pregnancy and from gestational hypertension). Hopefully, this could change the clinical management and prognosis of the pregnant women with PE. The clinical impact of these results remains uncertain but merits further investigation.

Acknowledgments

The authors wish to acknowledge Elbio Agote and Manuela Pereira for their technical assistance.

References

[1] National Collaborating Centre for Women's and Children's Health, "Hypertension in pregnancy. The management of hypertensive disorders during pregnancy," Clinical Guideline 107, National Institute for Health and Clinical Excellence (NICE), London, UK, 2010.

[2] E. Scazzocchio and F. Figueras, "Contemporary prediction of preeclampsia," *Current Opinion in Obstetrics & Gynecology*, vol. 23, no. 2, pp. 65–71, 2011.

[3] J. M. Roberts and C. A. Hubel, "The two stage model of preeclampsia: variations on the theme," *Placenta*, vol. 30, supplement A, pp. 532–537, 2009.

[4] C. Kaihura, M. D. Savvidou, J. M. Anderson, C. M. McEniery, and K. H. Nicolaides, "Maternal arterial stiffness in pregnancies affected by preeclampsia," *The American Journal of Physiology—Heart and Circulatory Physiology*, vol. 297, no. 2, pp. H759–H764, 2009.

[5] A. T. Papageorghiou, C. K. H. Yu, I. E. Erasmus, H. S. Cuckle, and K. H. Nicolaides, "Assessment of risk for the development of pre-eclampsia by maternal characteristics and uterine artery Doppler," *BJOG: An International Journal of Obstetrics & Gynaecology*, vol. 112, no. 6, pp. 703–709, 2005.

[6] F. Khan, J. J. F. Belch, M. MacLeod, and G. Mires, "Changes in endothelial function precede the clinical disease in women in whom preeclampsia develops," *Hypertension*, vol. 46, no. 5, pp. 1123–1128, 2005.

[7] M. C. Corretti, T. J. Anderson, E. J. Benjamin et al., "Guidelines for the ultrasound assessment of endothelial-dependent flow-mediated vasodilation of the brachial artery: a report of the international brachial artery reactivity task force," *Journal of the American College of Cardiology*, vol. 39, no. 2, pp. 257–265, 2002.

[8] J. Torrado, D. Bia, Y. Zócalo, I. Farro, F. Farro, and R. L. Armentano, "Hyperemia-related changes in arterial stiffness:

comparison between pulse wave velocity and stiffness index in the vascular reactivity assessment," *International Journal of Vascular Medicine*, vol. 2012, Article ID 490742, 7 pages, 2012.

[9] I. Dørup, K. Skajaa, and K. E. Sørensen, "Normal pregnancy is associated with enhanced endothelium-dependent flow-mediated vasodilation," *The American Journal of Physiology—Heart and Circulatory Physiology*, vol. 276, no. 3, pp. H821–H825, 1999.

[10] M. D. Savvidou, N. A. Kametas, A. E. Donald, and K. H. Nicolaides, "Non-invasive assessment of endothelial function in normal pregnancy," *Ultrasound in Obstetrics and Gynecology*, vol. 15, no. 6, pp. 502–507, 2000.

[11] T. Gori, J. D. Parker, and T. Mnzel, "Flow-mediated constriction: further insight into a new measure of vascular function," *European Heart Journal*, vol. 32, no. 7, pp. 784–787, 2011.

[12] T. Gori, S. Dragoni, M. Lisi et al., "Conduit artery constriction mediated by low flow : a novel noninvasive method for the assessment of vascular function," *Journal of the American College of Cardiology*, vol. 51, no. 20, pp. 1953–1958, 2008.

[13] T. Gori, S. Grotti, S. Dragoni et al., "Assessment of vascular function: flow-mediated constriction complements the information of flow-mediated dilatation," *Heart*, vol. 96, no. 2, pp. 141–147, 2010.

[14] K. K. Naka, A. C. Tweddel, S. N. Doshi, J. Goodfellow, and A. H. Henderson, "Flow-mediated changes in pulse wave velocity: a new clinical measure of endothelial function," *European Heart Journal*, vol. 27, no. 3, pp. 302–309, 2006.

[15] S. Laurent, J. Cockcroft, L. Van Bortel et al., "Expert consensus document on arterial stiffness: methodological issues and clinical applications," *European Heart Journal*, vol. 27, no. 21, pp. 2588–2605, 2006.

[16] H. Kamran, L. Salciccioli, G. Qureshi, H. Kazmi, J. Kassotis, and J. Lazar, "Effect of reactive hyperemia on carotid-radial pulse wave velocity in hypertensive participants and direct comparison with flow-mediated dilation: a pilot study," *Angiology*, vol. 61, no. 1, pp. 100–106, 2010.

[17] J. H. Stein, C. E. Korcarz, R. T. Hurst et al., "Use of carotid ultrasound to identify subclinical vascular disease and evaluate cardiovascular disease risk: a consensus statement from the American Society of Echocardiography Carotid Intima-Media Thickness Task Force. Endorsed by the Society for Vascular Medicine," *Journal of the American Society of Echocardiography*, vol. 21, no. 2, pp. 93–111, 2008.

[18] D. H. J. Thijssen, M. A. Black, K. E. Pyke et al., "Assessment of flow-mediated dilation in humans: a methodological and physiological guideline," *American Journal of Physiology—Heart and Circulatory Physiology*, vol. 300, no. 1, pp. H2–H12, 2011.

[19] D. Craiem, G. Chironi, A. Simon, and J. Levenson, "New assessment of endothelium-dependent flow-mediated vasodilation to characterize endothelium dysfunction," *American Journal of Therapeutics*, vol. 15, no. 4, pp. 340–344, 2008.

[20] K. E. Pyke, E. M. Dwyer, and M. E. Tschakovsky, "Impact of controlling shear rate on flow-mediated dilation responses in the brachial artery of humans," *Journal of Applied Physiology*, vol. 97, no. 2, pp. 499–508, 2004.

[21] M. Abbassi-Ghanavati, L. G. Greer, and F. G. Cunningham, "Pregnancy and laboratory studies: a reference table for clinicians," *Obstetrics and Gynecology*, vol. 114, no. 6, pp. 1326–1331, 2009.

[22] A. P. Cockell and L. Poston, "Flow-mediated vasodilatation is enhanced in normal pregnancy but reduced in preeclampsia," *Hypertension*, vol. 30, no. 2, pp. 247–251, 1997.

[23] B. Takase, T. Goto, A. Hamabe et al., "Flow-mediated dilation in brachial artery in the second half of pregnancy and prediction of pre-eclampsia," *Journal of Human Hypertension*, vol. 17, no. 10, pp. 697–704, 2003.

[24] P. Saudan, M. A. Brown, M. L. Buddle, and M. Jones, "Does gestational hypertension become pre-eclampsia?" *British Journal of Obstetrics and Gynaecology*, vol. 105, no. 11, pp. 1177–1184, 1998.

[25] A. E. Quinton, M. J. Peek, C.-M. Cook, and A. Kirby, "Flow-mediated dilatation assessment in women with preeclampsia compared to women with gestational hypertension," *Hypertension in Pregnancy*, vol. 31, no. 4, pp. 377–386, 2012.

[26] E. V. D. C. Filho, C. Mohr, B. J. A. Filho et al., "Flow-mediated dilatation in the differential diagnosis of preeclampsia syndrome," *Arquivos Brasileiros de Cardiologia*, vol. 94, no. 2, pp. 182–186, 2010.

[27] J. R. Spiro, J. E. Digby, G. Ghimire et al., "Brachial artery low-flow-mediated constriction is increased early after coronary intervention and reduces during recovery after acute coronary syndrome: characterization of a recently described index of vascular function," *European Heart Journal*, vol. 32, no. 7, pp. 856–866, 2011.

[28] E. A. Dawson, A. Alkarmi, D. H. J. Thijssen et al., "Low-flow mediated constriction is endothelium-dependent: effects of exercise training after radial artery catheterization," *Circulation: Cardiovascular Interventions*, vol. 5, no. 5, pp. 713–719, 2012.

[29] T. L. Weissgerber, G. A. L. Davies, and M. E. Tschakovsky, "Low flow-mediated constriction occurs in the radial but not the brachial artery in healthy pregnant and nonpregnant women," *Journal of Applied Physiology*, vol. 108, no. 5, pp. 1097–1105, 2010.

[30] K. E. Pyke and M. E. Tschakovsky, "Peak vs. total reactive hyperemia: which determines the magnitude of flow-mediated dilation?" *Journal of Applied Physiology*, vol. 102, no. 4, pp. 1510–1519, 2007.

[31] B. A. Parker, S. J. Ridout, and D. N. Proctor, "Age and flow-mediated dilation: a comparison of dilatory responsiveness in the brachial and popliteal arteries," *The American Journal of Physiology—Heart and Circulatory Physiology*, vol. 291, no. 6, pp. H3043–H3049, 2006.

[32] D. H. J. Thijssen, M. M. Van Bemmel, L. M. Bullens et al., "The impact of baseline diameter on flow-mediated dilation differs in young and older humans," *The American Journal of Physiology—Heart and Circulatory Physiology*, vol. 295, no. 4, pp. H1594–H1598, 2008.

[33] A. Elvan-Taşpinar, A. Franx, M. L. Bots, H. W. Bruinse, and H. A. Koomans, "Central hemodynamics of hypertensive disorders in pregnancy," *American Journal of Hypertension*, vol. 17, no. 10, pp. 941–946, 2004.

[34] A. Hausvater, T. Giannone, Y.-H. G. Sandoval et al., "The association between preeclampsia and arterial stiffness," *Journal of Hypertension*, vol. 30, no. 1, pp. 17–33, 2012.

[35] M. Spasojevic, S. A. Smith, J. M. Morris, and E. D. M. Gallery, "Peripheral arterial pulse wave analysis in women with pre-eclampsia and gestational hypertension," *BJOG: An International Journal of Obstetrics & Gynaecology*, vol. 112, no. 11, pp. 1475–1478, 2005.

[36] J. P. van den Wijngaard, B. E. Westerhof, D. J. Faber, M. M. Ramsay, N. Westerhof, and M. J. van Gemert, "Abnormal arterial flows by a distributed model of the fetal circulation," *American Journal of Physiology—Regulatory, Integrative and Comparative Physiology*, vol. 291, no. 5, pp. R1222–R1233, 2006, Erratum in: *American Journal of Physiology—Regulatory, Integrative and Comparative Physiology*, vol. 292, no. 1, p. R663, 2007.

[37] A. Yildirim, K. Altinkaynak, H. Aksoy, Y. N. Sahin, and F. Akcay, "Plasma xanthine oxidase, superoxide dismutase and glutathione peroxidase activities and uric acid levels in severe and mild pre-eclampsia," *Cell Biochemistry and Function*, vol. 22, no. 4, pp. 213–217, 2004.

[38] U. M. Khosla, S. Zharikov, J. L. Finch et al., "Hyperuricemia induces endothelial dysfunction," *Kidney International*, vol. 67, no. 5, pp. 1739–1742, 2005.

[39] J. Torrado, D. Bia, Y. Zocalo et al., "Reactive hyperemia-related changes in carotid-radial pulse wave velocity as a potential tool to characterize the endothelial dynamics," in *Proceedings of the Annual International Conference of the IEEE Engineering in Medicine and Biology Society*, pp. 1800–1803, Minneapolis, Minn, USA, 2009.

[40] S. H. Kubo, T. S. Rector, A. J. Bank, R. E. Williams, and S. M. Heifetz, "Endothelium-dependent vasodilation is attenuated in patients with heart failure," *Circulation*, vol. 84, no. 4, pp. 1589–1596, 1991.

[41] E. V. Tyldum, B. Backe, A. Støylen, and S. A. Slørdahl, "Maternal left ventricular and endothelial functions in preeclampsia," *Acta Obstetricia et Gynecologica Scandinavica*, vol. 91, no. 5, pp. 566–573, 2012.

[42] J. Eng, "Sample size estimation: how many individuals should be studied?" *Radiology*, vol. 227, no. 2, pp. 309–313, 2003.

[43] K. H. Nicolaides, R. Bindra, O. M. Turan et al., "A novel approach to first-trimester screening for early pre-eclampsia combining serum PP-13 and Doppler ultrasound," *Ultrasound in Obstetrics and Gynecology*, vol. 27, no. 1, pp. 13–17, 2006.

[44] Maternal and Child Health Research Consortium, *Confidential Enquiry into Stillbirths and Deaths in Infancy: 8th Annual Report, 1 January–31 December 1999*, Maternal and Child Health Research Consortium, London, UK, 2001.

[45] L. Duley, D. J. Henderson-Smart, S. Meher, and J. F. King, "Antiplatelet agents for preventing pre-eclampsia and its complications," *Cochrane Database of Systematic Reviews*, no. 2, Article ID CD004659, 2007.

7

Target Organ Damage and the Long Term Effect of Nonadherence to Clinical Practice Guidelines in Patients with Hypertension: A Retrospective Cohort Study

Tadesse Melaku Abegaz, Yonas Getaye Tefera, and Tamrat Befekadu Abebe

College of Medicine and Health Sciences, School of Pharmacy, Department of Clinical Pharmacy, University of Gondar, Gondar, Ethiopia

Correspondence should be addressed to Tadesse Melaku Abegaz; abegaztadesse981@gmail.com

Academic Editor: Tomohiro Katsuya

Background. There was limited published data on target organ damage (TOD) and the effect of nonadherence to practice guidelines in Ethiopia. This study determined TOD and the long term effect of nonadherence to clinical guidelines on hypertensive patients. *Methods.* An open level retrospective cohort study has been employed at cardiac clinic of Gondar university hospital for a mean follow-up period of 78 months. Multivariate Cox regression was conducted to test associating factors of TOD. *Results.* Of the total number of 612 patients examined, the overall prevalence of hypertensive TOD was 40.3%. The presence of comorbidities, COR = 1.073 [1.01–1.437], AOR = 1.196 [1.174–1.637], and nonadherence to clinical practice guidelines, COR = 1.537 [1.167–2.024], AOR = 1.636 [1.189–2.251], were found to be predicting factors for TOD. According to Kaplan-Meier analysis patients who were initiated on appropriate medication tended to develop TOD very late: Log Rank [11.975 ($p = 0.01$)]. *Conclusion.* More than forty percent of patients acquired TOD which is more significant. Presence of comorbidities and nonadherence to practice guidelines were correlated with the incidence of TOD. Appropriate management of hypertension and modification of triggering factors are essential to prevent complications.

1. Background

Hypertension (HTN) is deemed the major cause of morbidity and mortality worldwide. It affects approximately 1 billion individuals globally [1]. HTN ranked as the leading single factor for Global Burden of Diseases, most notably in Sub-Saharan Africa and South Asia regions where a substantial proportion of the world's population resides. In Sub-Saharan Africa, prevalence of raised blood pressure was around 30% [2]. A recent systematic review showed that the prevalence of hypertension among Ethiopian population was estimated to be 19.6%. Its burden is supposed to be increasing due to the growth and aging of the population around the world [3, 4]. Death from hypertension arises from target organ damage (TOD) such as cardiovascular, cerebrovascular, and renovascular accidents. TOD is the structural and functional impairment of major body organs due to elevated blood pressure (BP). These vital organ impairments including left ventricular hypertrophy (LVH), proteinuria, retinopathy, and vascular dementia are collectively referred as target organ damage [5]. The heart, brain, and kidney are the main target of elevated blood pressure because these organs take the large share of the blood circulating in the vasculature [6]. The cardiovascular complications include left ventricular hypertrophy (LVH), heart failure (HF), ischemic heart disease (IHD), and cardiac arrhythmias. Cerebrovascular injury resulted in the form of ischemic and hemorrhagic stroke events, whereas the renal effect ranges from asymptomatic structural damage to end stage renal disease with massive protein urea. Hypertensive patient also occasionally presented with retinopathy, peripheral vascular disease, and sexual dysfunction [7].

Globally, about 62% of cerebrovascular diseases and 49% of ischemic heart disease are attributable to elevated blood pressure (BP) [8]. In developing countries, its morbidity and mortality are increasing due to a change in life style.

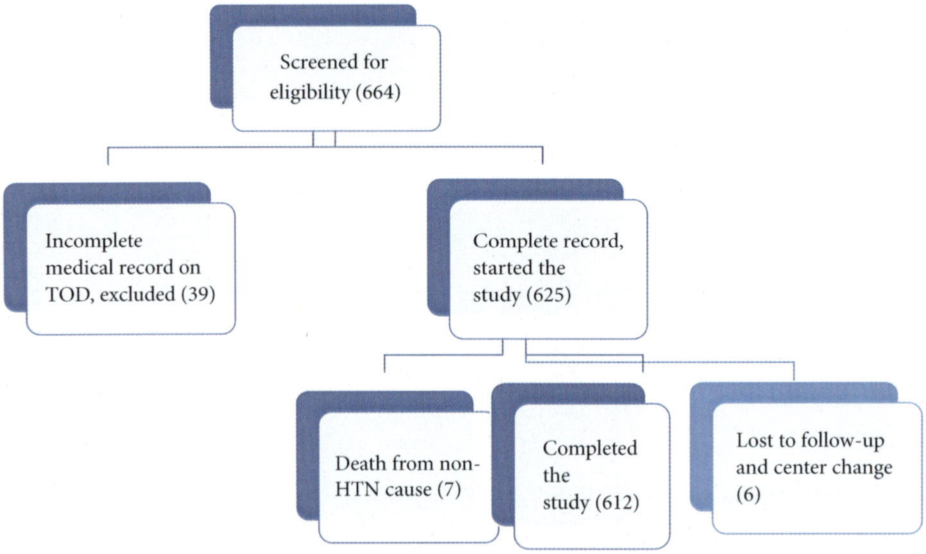

FIGURE 1: The inclusion of subjects in the cohort study.

Patients with uncontrolled blood pressure (UBP) are the most at risk for TOD. A cohort study has reported that poorly controlled hypertension is independently associated with mortality, cardiovascular risk, and disease progression [9]. Some other factors such as advanced age (longevity), overweight, and obesity were also found to be related to the incidence of cardiovascular complications in hypertensive patients [10].

The burden of TOD could be modified by early diagnosis, treatment, and close follow-up of HTN. Periodic review of treatment modalities has been tried globally so as to bring the best treatment approach [11]. New diagnostic maneuvers and treatments are being introduced every year to get blood pressure lower. Other interventions like combination therapy are frequently practiced to achieve optimal control of BP [12]. These measures achieve effective reduction of TOD through blood pressure (BP) control [13]. Despite these efforts, the incidence TOD is dramatically increasing worldwide due, partially, to the lack of implementation of clinical practice guidelines (CPGs). Estimation of the magnitude of TOD among HTN patients and investigation of potential risk factors for TOD will enable us to reduce or modify the burden of TOD [14]. The current study has been expected to address epidemiologic nihilism of TOD. To the researchers' knowledge, there was limited published data on the determinants of TOD in developing countries including Ethiopia. This study focused on the prevalence and predicting factors of TOD on hypertensive patients attending tertiary care hospital, north Ethiopia, during the year 2015-2016.

2. Methodology

2.1. Study Area and Study Population. Gondar university hospital (GUH) is a teaching referral hospital that serves 5 million people in northwest Ethiopia. It has both in-patient and outpatient departments (OPDs). The medical OPD comprised the newly established 1000-bed medical ward including chronic diseases. Chronic disease follow-up is given at this hospital for hypertensive, diabetic, asthmatic, and heart failure patients from the area. The follow-up period is arranged between weeks and months based on the choice of the patient and appointment for further investigations by senior physicians. All hypertensive patients that do have follow-up at GUH were our source population. Patients who had complete documentation were included under the study population. All age groups were considered for the study.

2.2. Study Design and Study Period. An open level retrospective cohort study has been applied by which all eligible patients are enrolled in the study as soon as they are registered to cardiac clinic till the completion of the study. Patients were retrospectively followed for a mean period of 78 months. During this time patients might develop TOD, be lost to follow-up, or remain without complications. TOD at the time of presentation was also included. Patients on treatment were particularly evaluated for appropriateness of their therapy versus the incidence of TOD.

2.3. Sample Size Determination and Sampling Technique. About 664 hypertensive patients that return to clinic at their appointment dates were evaluated for eligibility. Figure 1 illustrated the stepwise enrollment of study subjects.

2.4. Inclusion and Exclusion Criteria. Patients who have had a complete medical record and who have a routine and regular follow-up were included in our study. Patients who were lost to follow-up and death from nonhypertension cause were excluded.

2.5. Variables. The types of complications were our dependent variables while date of appointment, BP level, concordance with the national treatment guidelines and the eighth joint national conference (JNC-8), regimen change, age, sex, and type of therapy were the independent variables.

2.6. Data Entry and Analysis. Data was entered to and analyzed by SPSS software for windows version 21. A person-time method was taken to calculate the incidence rate of TOD. Cox regression was conducted to test associating factors of target organ damage. Kaplan analysis was done to evaluate the effect of inappropriate drug selections on TOD. p value was set at 0.05 with 95% confidence interval. Incidence rate (IR) of each TOD was determined by taking into account the actual observation time of each subject during the study period. It was calculated based on the following formula:

$$\text{IR} = \frac{\text{number of new cases addedd each year}}{\text{total person} - \text{time of observtion in poplaton at risk}},$$

$$\text{IR} = \frac{\text{number of new hypertensive cases addedd each year}}{\text{total person} - \text{time of observation in hypertensive patients}}. \quad (1)$$

2.7. Data Collection Procedure. Data was collected by trained data collectors who have been working at University of Gondar, School of Pharmacy. A structured questionnaire containing sociodemographic data, type of complication, year of complication, and follow-up period was designed by the investigators. Data collectors directly fill the questionnaire by searching the relevant information available on patients' medical card. Echocardiography and electrocardiography results were referred during our data collection. Blood pressure measurement took place during the last follow-up. Each subject underwent further physical examination to determine clinical features of LVH, HF, stroke, renal failure, and fundoscopy for hypertensive retinopathy. Hypertensive cardiac damage was defined by the presence of electrocardiographic LVH based on the voltage criteria [15]. Abnormal heart rhythms, wall motions, and tension were taken from echocardiographic results using M-mode and two-dimensional (2D) echocardiography. Renal damage was confirmed based on the presence of microalbuminuria as determined by spot urine albumin-to creatinine ratio. CT scan results were investigated to distinguish stroke events [13]. Erectile dysfunction was evaluated with the International Index for Erectile Function questionnaire.

Ethical Considerations. Permission from School of Pharmacy was obtained in the form of written consent. Ethical clearance was requested and obtained from clinical director of University of Gondar hospital.

3. Results

3.1. Sociodemographic and Clinical Characteristics of Respondents. Of the total 664 patients, 612 who fulfilled the inclusion criteria were enrolled for the study which gives a response rate of 92.2%. The mean age of the participants was 52.43 ± 13.2. The mean follow-up period was 78 months. About 341 (55.72%) study subjects were females. Majority of the participants were having both systolic and diastolic hypertension (70.7%). Nearly forty-five percent (44.94%) of the respondents were appointed to rerun to clinic for the next visit every two months. About forty percent of the study participants encountered TOD (40.35) Table 1.

TABLE 1: The sociodemographic and clinical characteristics of participants ($N = 612$).

Clinical characteristics	N (%)
Age (mean ± SD)	52.43 ± 13.2
Sex	
Females	341 (55.72)
Males	271 (44.28)
Residence	
Urban	459 (75)
Rural	153 (25)
Type of hypertension	
Systolic	160 (26.14)
Diastolic	50 (8.17)
Both	402 (65.69)
Duration of appointment	
One month	236 (38.56)
Two months	264 (43.14)
≥three months	112 (18.30)
Comorbidities	
Yes	222 (36.27)
No	390 (63.73)
Target organ damage (TOD)	
Yes	247 (40.36)
No	365 (59.64)

Most of the complications found to be appeared at the time of presentation (22.8%). Complications declined 1 to 3 years after diagnosis (11.9%). But, after five years of diagnosis the complication became more common again (18.7%) (Figure 2).

3.2. Incidence Rate of Hypertensive TOD. The incidence rate of HF was around 30.8 cases/1000/person per year (PY). The second most common TOD is IHD (22 cases/1000/PY). Significant number of patients also experienced hypertensive urgencies (17.55/1000/PY). Sexual dysfunction is the least reported organ damage (0.49/1000/PY) each year (Table 2).

The most prevalent TOD was HF (11.6) followed by ischemic heart disease (8.3). The least common TOD was sexual dysfunction (0.67), retinopathy (0.9), and AF (0.9) (Table 3).

A Cox regression result indicated that several factors were associated with the occurrence of TOD in hypertensive patients. Physicians nonadherence to clinical practice guidelines (CPGs) was associated with the occurrence of TOD, COR = 1.537 [1.167–2.024], AOR = 1.636 [1.189–2.251]. Absence of regimen change, COR = 1.702 [1.240–2.336], AOR = 1.857 [1.325–2.602], and the presence of comorbidities, COR = 1.073 [1.01–1.437], AOR = 1.196 [1.174–1.637], increased the risk of TOD. In addition, patients with seven-year duration of hypertension were nearly three times more likely to

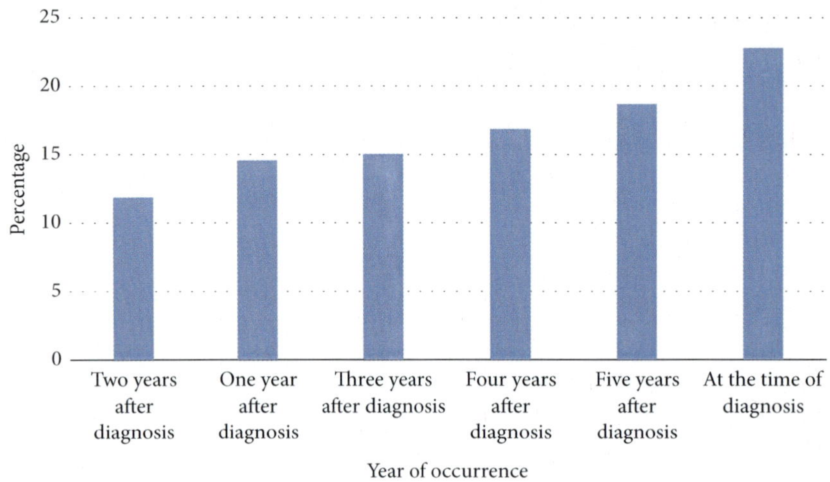

FIGURE 2: The occurrence of hypertensive complications each year.

TABLE 2: The incidence rate of TOD in hypertensive patients' 1000/person/year. A person-time analysis.

Complication	Incidence/1000 person/year
CKD	9
Retinopathy	2.44
LVH	5.4
IHD	22
HF	30.8
Valvular heart disease	1.46
Stroke	14.65
Atrial fibrillation	2.44
Hypertensive urgencies	17.55
Sexual dysfunction	0.49

TABLE 3: The overall prevalence of TOD in hypertensive patients.

Type of complication	Prevalence N (%)
Retinopathy	6 (0.9)
LVH	12 (2)
IHD	51 (8.3)
HF	75 (12.2)
CKD	20 (3.3)
Hypertensive urgency	39 (6.4)
Sexual dysfunction	4 (0.67)
Stroke	34 (5.5)
AF	6 (0.9)
Total TOD	247 (100.0)

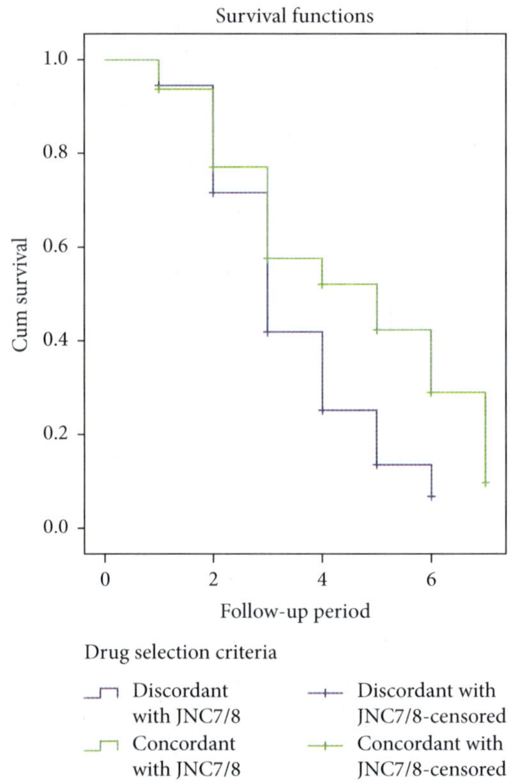

FIGURE 3: Kaplan Meier analysis curve of TOD based on the concordance of prescribed medications: a 78-month follow-up.

develop complications, COR: 2.951 [2.651–5.535], AOR: 2.974 [2.631–7.072]. Moreover, monotherapy with beta-blockers was found to increase the incidence of TOD COR: 2.951 [2.651–5.535] and AOR: 2.974 [2.631–7.072]. However, sex, age, type of therapy, and residence were not significantly associated with the rate of TOD (Table 4).

When patients were followed for a period of 78 months in terms of treatment concordant with guidelines, there was significant difference in the rate of TOD among patients: Log Rank 11.975 ($p = 0.01$). Concordant patients develop TOD very late as compared to those who receive medication without the standard treatment guideline. The mean progression free period for discordant patients was shorter than concordant patients (Figure 3).

4. Discussion

Hypertensive complications manifested as end organ damage are the major indicator of advanced disease. The timing of

TABLE 4: Predictors of the target organ damage due to hypertension: multivariate cox regression.

Variables	Complication (yes)	Complication (no)	CHR (95%)	AHR (95% CI)
Sex (Male)	126 (20.59)	145 (23.69)	0.902 (0.693–1.174)	0.768 (0.563–1.145)
Residence (rural)	78 (12.75)	75 (12.25)	1.245 (0.923–1.679)	1.261 (0.824–1.759)
Presence of comorbidities	118 (19.3)	104 (16.99)	1.073 (1.01–1.437)	1.596 (1.174–1.637)*
HTN (diastolic)	21 (3.43)	29 (4.74)	0.782 (0.57–1.087)	0.635 (0.448–1.536)
Both	179 (29.25)	223 (36.44)	0.713 (0.387–1.831)	0.526 (0.327–1.725)
Duration of appointment				
Two months	118 (19.28)	146 (23.6)	2.167 (0.295–5.19)	4.548 (0.591–6.423)
≥Three months	35 (5.72)	77 (12.58)	1.176 (0.776–1.781)	1.094 (0.709–1.689)
Controlled BP	199 (32.52)	282 (46.10)	0.605 (0.411–0.839)	0.771 (0.507–0.974)*
Discordant with JNC	176 (28.76)	279 (45.59)	1.537 (1.167–2.024)*	1.636 (1.189–2.251)*
Absence of regimen change	191 (31.21)	312 (50.98)	1.702 (1.240–2.336)**	1.857 (1.325–2.602)**
Therapy				
Dual therapy	138 (22.55)	153 (25.0)	0.832 (0.642–1.080)	0.79 (0.473–1.786)
Triple therapy	56 (9.15)	53 (8.66)	0.715 (0.511–1.001)	1.317 (0.629–1.852)
Age				
31–40	32 (5.23)	41 (6.70)	0.75 (0.349–1.612)	0.732 (0.332–1.617)
41–50	44 (7.19)	53 (8.66)	0.995 (0.621–1.594)	0.975 (0.599–1.587)
51–60	60 (9.80)	98 (16.01)	0.89 (0.573–1.382)	0.745 (0.587–1.536)
61–70	64 (10.46)	82 (13.40)	0.797 (0.534–1.190)	0.862 (0.512–1.163)
≥70	47 (7.68)	53 (8.66)	0.904 (0.607–1.347)	0.836 (0.477–1.421)
Duration of hypertension				
Three years and below	19 (3.10)	41 (6.70)	1	1
Four years	14 (2.29)	25 (4.10)	1.216 [0.823–2.572]	1.211 [0.584–2.635]
Five years	70 (11.44)	108 (17.65)	1.276 [0.815–3.265]	1.355 [0.674–3.481]
Six years	105 (17.16)	136 (22.22)	1.241 [0.736–2.341]	1.316 [0.622–2.415]
Seven years	39 (6.37)	55 (8.99)	2.592 [2.35–6.332]	2.716 [1.632–7.082]*
Class of hypertensive medications				
ACIES	15 (2.45)	27 (4.41)	1	1
BBCs	20 (3.27)	24 (3.92)	2.951 [2.651–5.535]	2.974 [2.631–7.072]*
CCBs	17 (2.78)	21 (3.43)	0.614 [0.143–2.639]	0.517 [0.137–2.174]
Diuretics	14 (2.29)	25 (4.08)	1.654 [0.727–3.974]	1.521 [0.689–3.454]
Diuretics + ACEIs	70 (11.44)	80 (13.07)	1.375 [0.146–3.369]	1.528 [0.636–3.158]
Diuretics + β-blocker	68 (11.11)	73 (11.93)	1.146 [0.765–2.321]	1.256 [0.674–2.117]
B-blockers + ACEIs + diuretics	56 (9.15)	53 (8.66)	1.248 [0.436–2.773]	1.210 [0.481–2.576]
Other combinations	21 (3.43)	28 (4.57)	1.431 [0.726–2.372]	1.431 [0.783–2.541]

ACEIS: angiotensin convertase inhibitors, CCBs: calcium channel blockers, BBCs: beta-blockers, CHR: crude hazard ratio, and AHR: adjusted hazard ratio, *significant at 0.05 level. Female, urban residence, absence of comorbidity, systolic hypertension, one-month duration of appointment, uncontrolled BP, concordance with guidelines, presence of regimen change, monotherapy, and age between 21 and 30 were our reference variables. ** indicates significance at 0.01 level.

appearance of organ damage was dependent on the presence of triggering factors. This study aimed to evaluate the burden and determinants of TOD in hypertensive patients attending GUH. It was found that the overall cases of TOD were 40.3%. Comparative result (43.1%) was reported in Nigerian hypertensive patients [7]. Another study revealed 44.5% TOD in hypertension patients attending primary care [16]. In the present study most of the complications were found to appear at the time of presentation (22.8%). This might be due to the late presentation of patients and underdiagnosis of cases [17–19]. Complications declined 1 to 3 years after diagnosis due to the initiation of therapy and life style modifications [20]. But after five years the complication became common again; this might be due to the fact that the therapy is overcome due to the progression of the disease in resistance to HTN and aging of the patients [21, 22].

The cumulative incidence of HF was 30.8% which was relatively higher rate as compared to a finding reported by Sahle et al. 6.26/1000/year [23]. The high incidence of HF in our study might be due to the lack of adherence to CPGs in order to prescribe medications with compelling indication which could have reduced the progression of structural heart disease into overt HF [24]. Moreover the regression of LVH might be delayed if appropriate medicine is not initiated because antihypertensive drugs have different effect on ventricular regression [25]. In addition the high rate of IHD could contribute to the presence of HF as IHD might gradually progress to HF [26]. The prevalence of LVH was 2.2% in the present study. High magnitude of LVH was reported in Spain (22.9%), Nigeria (27.9%), and Greece (33%) [7, 16, 27]. The lower finding of LVH in our study could be attributed to the rapid progression of LVH into HF which diminishes the number of LVH cases [28]. The rate of hypertensive retinopathy was below one percent in the present study and it was nearly 2% in Nigerian patients [6]. On the contrary, it was significantly higher (39.9%) in Iranian hypertensive patients (HPs); this might be due to the high level of sever BP pressure, in Iranian population which might directly impose with the occurrence of complications. Moreover, there was a significant difference in the study design and period between the two studies [29].

In this study, nearly 5.5% of hypertensive patients encountered stroke events. Almost similar result (6.3%) was observed in multicenter study from Greece [16]. Choi and Park reported a relatively higher rate of stroke in Korean HPs. This might be due to the longer follow-up period and nearly one-half of the respondents were having AF which is the major risk factor for stroke in Korean HPs [30]. Our studies revealed nearly one percent prevalence of AF. A nationwide study from Thailand stated that prevalence of AF in hypertensive individuals was found to be (3.46%) [31]. The prevalence of atrial fibrillation was 16.4% in Nigerian population. This disparity could be attributed to low rate of BP control and comorbid peripheral vascular disease in Nigerian HPs [7].

It was found that multiple factors were found to be implicated with the incidence of TOD to long standing hypertensive patients. The frequency of regimen changes independently affects the occurrence of TOD. Periodic regimen changes were associated with low incidence of TOD. This might be due to the initiation of a single therapeutic agent at subtherapeutic dose [11]. Hence, the regimen change might allow new and appropriate therapeutic options including combination therapies [32]. Sex was not correlated with higher incidence of TOD. However, Papazafiropoulou et al. has reported that TOD was more prevalent in males than in females [16]. Other studies identified that male gender was associated with the incidence of stroke [33] and AF [20]. A large survey from Chinese HTN population has discovered that older age, male gender, and SBP were independently associated with cardiovascular, coronary, and renal complications [34]. However, in this study any age group and type of HTN was not related with cardiovascular or cerebrovascular damage.

The present study has also found that the coincidence of comorbidities increased the risk of TOD nearly 1.5 times. This is due to the fact that these special populations predisposed for other noncommunicable disease states which might independently cause TOD [35]. Moreover, when patients acquire more than one disease state at the same time, they are forced to take multiple medications which is commonly referred polypharmacy. The effect of polypharmacy is escaping of one or more doses of a certain drug due to pill burden and suffering from side effects which leads to uncontrolled HTN. Previous studies indicated that polypharmacy was independently correlated with uncontrolled HTN which in turn determines the incidence of TOD [35–37]. Medication recommendations to the national standards guidelines were found to substantially reduce the number of TOD. It is true that the provision of medications as per national standard treatment guidelines enables adequate control of blood pressure and regression of TOD through the administration of the right therapeutic agent for the right patient [38]. This 78-month follow-up of subjects indicated that patients that took appropriate medications develop TOD very late as compared to those who receive medication without the standard treatment guideline. The mean progression free period for discordant patients was shorter than concordant patients. A study compared treatment guidelines and BP control also stated that patients who were prescribed an antihypertensive regimen that is JNC concordant were having optimal control of BP [39]. The basic aim of adherence to standard treatment guidelines in the treatment of hypertension is to achieve adequate disease control, since controlled hypertension results delayed complications and progression of target organ damage.

Overall, this study has provided a baseline evidence on the burden and determinants of TOD in Ethiopia. However, it did not investigate the impact of obesity, metabolic syndrome, and social habits such as smoking history on TOD. It is also carried out in a single center with limited number of patients. Hence, a thorough investigation of these factors is warranted nationwide.

5. Conclusion

More than forty percent of patients acquired target organ damage which is more significant. Heart failure is the most common form TOD in hypertensive patients. Factors such as presence of comorbidities, nonadherence to practice guidelines, and failing to change regimen were correlated with the incidence of target organ damage. Patient who receive medications according to standard treatment develop TOD very late as compared to those who took medication without the standard treatment guideline. Early diagnosis and management of hypertension and modification of triggering factors are essential to prevent complications. Moreover, drug prescription should be based on the standard treatment guidelines.

Abbreviations

AOR: Adjusted odds ratio
BP: Blood pressure
COR: Crude odds ratio
GUH: Gondar university hospital
HF: Heart failure
HPs: Hypertensive patients
HTN: Hypertension
IHD: Ischemic heart disease
IR: Incident rate
JNC: Joint national committee

LVH: Left ventricular hypertrophy
SPSS: Statistical package for social sciences
TOD: Target organ damage
UBP: Uncontrolled blood pressure.

Data Access

The datasets used during the current study are available from the corresponding author on reasonable request.

Ethical Approval

Permission was obtained from School of Pharmacy, College of Medicine and Health Sciences, University of Gondar. Ethical approval was given from the clinical director of Gondar university hospital.

Authors' Contributions

Tadesse Melaku Abegaz conceived the study, prepared the manuscript, and supervised the study and Tamrat Befekadu Abebe and Yonas Getaye Tefera collected the necessary data, analyzed the raw data, and proofread the manuscript. All authors read and approved the final manuscript.

Acknowledgments

The researchers would like to thank University of Gondar, College of Medicine and Health Sciences for facilitating and allowing conducting of the study. The authors' gratitude also goes to all physicians and nurses who work at chronic clinic of University of Gondar referral hospital.

References

[1] H. G. Pacheco, N. M. Victorino, J. P. N. Urquiza et al., "Patients with hypertensive crises who are admitted to a coronary care unit: clinical characteristics and outcomes," *Journal of Clinical Hypertension*, vol. 15, no. 3, pp. 210–214, 2013.

[2] F. Ataklte, S. Erqou, S. Kaptoge, B. Taye, J. B. Echouffo-Tcheugui, and A. P. Kengne, "Burden of undiagnosed hypertension in sub-saharan africa: a systematic review and meta-analysis," *Hypertension*, vol. 65, no. 2, pp. 291–298, 2015.

[3] K. T. Kibret and Y. M. Mesfin, "Prevalence of hypertension in Ethiopia: a systematic meta-analysis," *Public Health Reviews*, vol. 36, no. 1, article 14, 2015.

[4] S. Bromfield and P. Muntner, "High blood pressure: the leading global burden of disease risk factor and the need for worldwide prevention programs," *Current Hypertension Reports*, vol. 15, no. 3, pp. 134–136, 2013.

[5] S. K. Nadar, M. H. Tayebjee, F. Messerli, and G. Y. H. Lip, "Target organ damage in hypertension: pathophysiology and implications for drug therapy," *Current Pharmaceutical Design*, vol. 12, no. 13, pp. 1581–1592, 2006.

[6] A. Ramli, N. S. Ahmad, and T. Paraidathathu, "Medication adherence among hypertensive patients of primary health clinics in Malaysia," *Patient Preference and Adherence*, vol. 6, pp. 613–622, 2012.

[7] O. O. Oladapo, L. Salako, L. Sadiq, K. Shoyinka, K. Adedapo, and A. O. Falase, "Target-organ damage and cardiovascular complications in hypertensive Nigerian Yoruba adults: a cross-sectional study," *Cardiovascular Journal of Africa*, vol. 23, no. 7, pp. 379–384, 2012.

[8] F. Bonsa, E. K. Gudina, and K. W. Hajito, "Prevalence of hypertension and associated factors in Bedele Town, Southwest Ethiopia," *Ethiopian Journal of Health Sciences*, vol. 24, no. 1, pp. 21–26, 2014.

[9] S. D. S. Fraser, P. J. Roderick, N. J. McIntyre et al., "Suboptimal blood pressure control in chronic kidney disease stage 3: baseline data from a cohort study in primary care," *BMC Family Practice*, vol. 14, article 88, 2013.

[10] B. Moges, B. Amare, B. Fantahun, and A. Kassu, "High prevalence of overweight, obesity, and hypertension with increased risk to cardiovascular disorders among adults in northwest Ethiopia: a cross sectional study," *BMC Cardiovascular Disorders*, vol. 14, article 155, 2014.

[11] P. A. James, S. Oparil, B. L. Carter et al., "2014 evidence-based guideline for the management of high blood pressure in adults: report from the panel members appointed to the Eighth Joint National Committee (JNC 8)," *Journal of the American Medical Association*, vol. 311, no. 5, pp. 507–520, 2014.

[12] M. Zhang, Y. Meng, Y. Yang et al., "Major inducing factors of hypertensive complications and the interventions required to reduce their prevalence: an epidemiological study of hypertension in a rural population in China," *BMC Public Health*, vol. 11, article 301, 2011.

[13] G. Shlomai, G. Grassi, E. Grossman, and G. Mancia, "Assessment of target organ damage in the evaluation and follow-up of hypertensive patients: where do we stand?" *Journal of Clinical Hypertension*, vol. 15, no. 10, pp. 742–747, 2013.

[14] T. Almgren, B. Persson, L. Wilhelmsen, A. Rosengren, and O. K. Andersson, "Stroke and coronary heart disease in treated hypertension—a prospective cohort study over three decades," *Journal of Internal Medicine*, vol. 257, no. 6, pp. 496–502, 2005.

[15] R. L. Antikainen, T. Grodzicki, A. J. Palmer, D. G. Beevers, J. Webster, and C. J. Bulpitt, "Left ventricular hypertrophy determined by Sokolow-Lyon criteria: a different predictor in women than in men?" *Journal of Human Hypertension*, vol. 20, no. 6, pp. 451–459, 2006.

[16] A. Papazafiropoulou, E. Skliros, A. Sotiropoulos et al., "Prevalence of target organ damage in hypertensive subjects attending primary care: C.V.P.C. study (epidemiological cardio-vascular study in primary care)," *BMC Family Practice*, vol. 12, article 75, 2011.

[17] O. E. Ayodele, C. O. Alebiosu, P. O. Akinwusi, A. Akinsola, and A. Mejiuni, "Target organ damage and associated clinical conditions in newly diagnosed hypertensives attending a tertiary health facility.," *Nigerian Journal of Clinical Practice*, vol. 10, no. 4, pp. 319–325, 2007.

[18] B. Waebera, A. De La Sierra, and L. M. Ruilope, "Target organ damage: how to detect it and how to treat it?" *Journal of Hypertension*, vol. 27, no. 3, pp. S13–S18, 2009.

[19] C. Sierra and A. de la Sierra, "Early detection and management of the high-risk patient with elevated blood pressure," *Vascular Health and Risk Management*, vol. 4, no. 2, pp. 289–296, 2008.

[20] R. A. Dickey and J. J. Janick, "Lifestyle modifications in the prevention and treatment of hypertension," *Endocrine Practice*, vol. 7, no. 5, pp. 392–399, 2001.

[21] E. S. Muxfeldt, F. de Souza, V. S. Margallo, and G. F. Salles, "Cardiovascular and renal complications in patients with resistant hypertension," *Current Hypertension Reports*, vol. 16, article 471, 2014.

[22] M. Allen, K. Kelly, and I. Fleming, "Hypertension in elderly patients: recommended systolic targets are not evidence based," *Canadian Family Physician*, vol. 59, no. 1, pp. 19–24, 2013.

[23] B. W. Sahle, A. J. Owen, H. Krum, and C. M. Reid, "Incidence of heart failure in 6083 elderly hypertensive patients: the Second Australian National Blood Pressure Study (ANBP2)," *European Journal of Heart Failure*, vol. 18, no. 1, pp. 38–45, 2016.

[24] H. Getachew, A. S. Bhagavathula, T. B. Abebe, and S. A. Belachew, "Inappropriate prescribing of antithrombotic therapy in ethiopian elderly population using updated 2015 STOPP/START criteria: a cross-sectional study," *Clinical Interventions in Aging*, vol. 11, pp. 819–827, 2016.

[25] C. F. Filho, L. C. de Abreu, V. E. Valenti et al., "Anti-hypertensive drugs have different effects on ventricular hypertrophy regression," *Clinics*, vol. 65, no. 7, pp. 723–728, 2010.

[26] A. L. Bui, T. B. Horwich, and G. C. Fonarow, "Epidemiology and risk profile of heart failure," *Nature Reviews Cardiology*, vol. 8, no. 1, pp. 30–41, 2011.

[27] L. Cea-Calvo, P. Conthe, P. Gómez-Fernández et al., "Target organ damage and cardiovascular complications in patients with hypertension and type 2 diabetes in Spain: a cross-sectional study," *Cardiovascular Diabetology*, vol. 5, article 23, 2006.

[28] A. H. Gradman and F. Alfayoumi, "From left ventricular hypertrophy to congestive heart failure: management of hypertensive heart disease," *Progress in Cardiovascular Diseases*, vol. 48, no. 5, pp. 326–341, 2006.

[29] M. R. Besharati, A. Rastegar, M. R. Shoja, and M. E. Maybodi, "Prevalence of retinopathy in hypertensive patients," *Saudi Medical Journal*, vol. 27, no. 11, pp. 1725–1728, 2006.

[30] C. U. Choi and C. G. Park, "Estimating the probability of stroke in Korean hypertensive patients visiting tertiary hospitals using a risk profile from the framingham study," *BMC Neurology*, vol. 9, article 16, 2009.

[31] R. Krittayaphong, R. Rangsin, B. Thinkhamrop et al., "Prevalence and associating factors of atrial fibrillation in patients with hypertension: a nation-wide study," *BMC Cardiovascular Disorders*, vol. 16, article 57, 2016.

[32] J. Frank, "Managing hypertension using combination therapy," *American Family Physician*, vol. 77, no. 9, pp. 1279–1289, 2008.

[33] A. C. Beisl Noblat, M. Barreto Lopes, G. Barreto Lopes, and A. A. Lopes, "Complications of hypertension in men and women seen in a referral outpatient care unit," *Arquivos Brasileiros de Cardiologia*, vol. 83, no. 4, pp. 308–319, 2004.

[34] F. Wang, H. Cui, L. Fan, Y. Hu, G. Hu, and L. Liu, "Association factors of target organ damage: analysis of 17682 older hypertensive patients in China," *Heart*, vol. 97, no. 3, pp. A95–A95, 2011.

[35] R. Izzo, G. De Simone, V. Trimarco et al., "Hypertensive target organ damage predicts incident diabetes mellitus," *European Heart Journal*, vol. 34, no. 44, pp. 3419–3426, 2013.

[36] M. Brunström and B. Carlberg, "Effect of antihypertensive treatment at different blood pressure levels in patients with diabetes mellitus: systematic review and meta-analyses," *BMJ*, vol. 352, article i717, 2016.

[37] B. N. Mukete and K. C. Ferdinand, "Polypharmacy in older adults with hypertension: a comprehensive review," *Journal of Clinical Hypertension*, vol. 18, no. 1, pp. 10–18, 2016.

[38] M. Litwin, A. Niemirska, J. Śladowska-Kozlowska et al., "Regression of target organ damage in children and adolescents with primary hypertension," *Pediatric Nephrology*, vol. 25, no. 12, pp. 2489–2499, 2010.

[39] C. G. Rowan, J. R. Turner, A. Shah, and J. A. Spaeder, "Antihypertensive treatment and blood pressure control relative to hypertension treatment guidelines," *Pharmacoepidemiology and Drug Safety*, vol. 23, no. 12, pp. 1294–1302, 2014.

8

The Association between Intradialytic Hypertension and Metabolic Disorders in End Stage Renal Disease

Vaia D. Raikou[1] **and Despina Kyriaki**[2]

[1]*Department of Nephrology, Doctors' Hospital, Athens, Greece*
[2]*Department of Nuclear Medicine, General Hospital "Laïko", Athens, Greece*

Correspondence should be addressed to Vaia D. Raikou; vraikou@med.uoa.gr

Academic Editor: Tomohiro Katsuya

Background. Intradialytic hypertension was associated with a high mortality risk. We examined the relationship between intradialytic hypertension and metabolic disorders in hemodialysis treatment patients. *Methods.* We studied 76 patients in online hemodiafiltration. Dialysis adequacy was defined by Kt/V for urea. Normalized protein catabolic rate (nPCR), as a marker of protein intake, was calculated. Sodium removal was determined as percent sodium removal. Metabolic acidosis was determined by serum bicarbonate less than 22 mmol/L. Interdialytic urine volume more than 100 ml was recorded. Intradialytic hypertension was defined by an increase in systolic blood pressure equal to 10 mmHg from pre- to posthemodialysis. Arterial stiffness was assessed as carotid-femoral pulse wave velocity (c-fPWV) and carotid augmentation index (AIx). Chi-square tests and logistic regression analysis were applied for intradialytic hypertension prediction. *Results.* Patients with intradialytic hypertension were older and had significantly lower hemoglobin, nPCR, urine output, and serum bicarbonate and significantly higher c-fPWV, though similar Kt/V for urea, than patients without intradialytic hypertension. They also had increased sodium removal and pulse pressure related to less urine output. Serum bicarbonate was inversely associated with c-fPWV ($r = -0.377$, $p = 0.001$). Chi-square test showed significant association between intradialytic hypertension and serum bicarbonate < 22 mmol/L ($x^2 = 5.6$, $p = 0.01$), which was supported by an adjusted model. *Conclusion.* The intradialytic hypertension was significantly associated with metabolic disorders including malnutrition/inflammation and uncontrolled metabolic acidosis in hemodialysis treatment patients. Severe metabolic acidosis may reflect sodium imbalance and hemodynamic instability of these patients resulting in volume overload and increased vascular resistance.

1. Introduction

In chronic kidney disease, hypertension is influenced by both blood pressure (BP) and the progression of renal disease. In end stage renal disease (ESRD) on maintenance hemodialysis, hypertension is a main feature and more than 85% of new patients with ESRD present with hypertension [1].

Hypertension in these patients is multifactorial. Significant implicating factors include persistent hypervolemia and elevated peripheral vascular resistance. In patients with 3 hemodialysis sessions per week, blood pressure increases during the interdialytic interval according to weight gain, particularly in older patients and those with higher dry weight. The main goal of hemodialysis treatment is the control of extracellular volume (ECV), because inadequate sodium and fluid removal results in fluid overload, increased BP, and increased mortality [2]. Elevated peripheral resistance can be attributable to inappropriate activation of the sympathetic nervous system due to higher plasma angiotensin II and norepinephrine concentrations [1, 3].

The association of hypertension with adverse outcomes has been demonstrated, due mainly to its relationship with abnormalities in cardiac structure and cardiac function including left ventricular hypertrophy, diastolic dysfunction, and arterial stiffness [4–6].

However, BP shows a dynamic nature during dialysis procedures, including modest decreases, a common phenomenon, and intradialytic hypotension and hypertension, which are two special situations significantly related to an increased risk of mortality in these patients [7, 8]. It has been shown that intradialytic hypertension, which is a phenomenon where the blood pressure increases during and immediately after hemodialysis, was associated with a higher mortality risk than the most often intradialytic hypotension [9, 10].

In this study, we examined the relationship between intradialytic hypertension and metabolic disorders in permanent hemodialysis treatment patients.

2. Materials and Methods

2.1. Subjects. This is a dual-center observational cross-sectional study, which was reviewed and approved by the "Laïko, University General Hospital of Athens" and the Renal Unit of "Diagnostic and Therapeutic Center of Athens Hygeia SA" Institutional Review Board. 76 patients (47 men and 29 women, mean age: 62,2 ± 15 years) were included in the study, and they or their legal guardian provided informed oral consent prior to study enrolment.

The applied hemodialysis modality was online-predilution hemodiafiltration (onl-HDF) in all subjects. The median time in hemodiafiltration therapy was 5 years ± interquartile range 3–10.

The hemodiafiltration treatment was performed 3 times weekly with a dialysis time of 4 h per session. We used a filter of 1.5–2 m^2 surface area by high-flux synthetic membrane, defined by an ultrafiltration coefficient > 20 ml/h [11] in all participants. We also used the same volume of replacement liquid equal to 20 liters, a blood flow of 350–400 ml/min, and a dialysate flow rate of 500–600 ml/min. A bicarbonate-based ultrapure buffer dialysis solution was used and the final concentration of bicarbonate in the dialysate was 32 mmol/L. A dialysate calcium concentration of 1.50–1.75 mmol/L and a sodium concentration of 138–145 mmol/L were applied. Dialysis dose was defined by spKt/V/session (single pool, K: dialyzer clearance; t: time; V: urea distribution volume) [12]. We excluded from the study subjects whose calculated spKt/V/session was less than 1.2.

We also excluded patients <18 years of age at initiation of dialysis treatment and patients with less than 6 months of follow-up or those without regular vascular hemodialysis access. Subjects with autoimmune diseases, infections, and atrial fibrillation malignancy and those with interdialytic weight gain of more than 5% of total body weight were not included in the study. Interdialytic weight gain was calculated as the mean value over the exposure period of one treatment month.

The enrolled patients were on a free regular diet and they did not apparently have interdialytic peripheral edema or extradialytic orthostatic hypotension. Nineteen of the participants were current smokers (a ratio of 25%). Twenty of the enrolled patients disposed residual renal function defined by an interdialytic urine volume of more than 100 ml (a ratio of 26.3%).

Only calcium-free phosphate binders including sevelamer carbonate, lanthanum, and/or aluminium hydroxide were prescribed in combination with vitamin D derivatives for the regulation of bone disease (a ratio of 44.7%). None of our participants was receiving $NaHCO_3$ per os or warfarin therapy. All the included patients were treated by erythropoietin α or β agents.

In our data, the cause of renal failure included hypertensive nephrosclerosis at a ratio of 32.9%, chronic glomerulonephritis at a ratio of 28.9%, polycystic disease at a ratio of 11.8%, diabetic nephropathy at a ratio equal to 9.2%, and other causes at a ratio of 17.1%.

2.2. Blood Pressure Measurements: Definitions. Blood pressure data were considered over a treatment month, as the exposure period, which typically included 12 dialysis sessions per patient. Systolic blood pressure (SBP) was measured with the patient in the seated position using automated oscillometric devices immediately before, after, and during (at 30-minute intervals) all treatment sessions. We excluded treatments in which SBP was measured <3 times.

We defined intradialytic hypertension as an increase in SBP equal to 10 mmHg from pre- to posthemodialysis according to previous reports [7]. Participants who had an average change in SBP from pre- to immediately posthemodialysis equal to or more than 10 mmHg throughout the study period were considered to have intradialytic hypertension (n = 15, a ratio 19.7%).

On the other hand, the measurement of blood pressure at home was requested using an automatic sphygmomanometer Omron M4-I (Omron Co. Ltd., Kyoto, Japan). The blood pressure was doubly measured two times per day, in the morning after rising and in the evening in a fasting, calming, and resting state, and two means were recorded per day. Their average was used for statistical analysis. Mean peripheral blood pressure (MBP) was calculated as MBP = DBP + 1/3 (SBP − DBP).

We also used a 24-hour ambulatory blood pressure monitor with the Mobil-O-Graph device for verification of measurements and whether the mean blood pressure values significantly differed from home recorded values; the means of 24-hour monitoring were used for statistical analysis rather than the means by home measurements.

In accordance with the KDOQI hypertension threshold [13], the participants with mean blood pressure > 130/80 mmHg (n = 29, a prevalence of 38.2%) assessed by 24-hour monitoring and/or home measured according to recommended standard protocol or subjects with an individual hypertension history were considered hypertensive and every one of them was regularly receiving antihypertensive therapy including calcium channel blockers, beta-blockers, or inhibitors of angiotensin II AT1 receptors.

2.3. Hemodynamic Measurements. Before the midweek dialysis session, the participants rested for at least 10 minutes and hemodynamic measurements were performed. Arterial stiffness was measured as carotid-femoral pulse wave velocity (c-fPWV) and carotid augmentation index (AIx) using the SphygmoCor System® (AtCor Medical Pty. Ltd., Sydney, Australia) according to the manufacturer's specifications [14]. In each subject, two sequences of measurements were performed, and their mean was used for statistical analysis. Pulse pressure (PP) was derived.

2.4. Blood Collection. Blood samples were obtained just before the start of the mean weekly dialysis session in a twelve-hour fasting state from the vascular access of enrolled subjects and serum was separated and processed for various assays. At the end of the session, blood samples was drawn at 2 min after dialysis from the arterial dialysis tubing after the reduction of blood pump speed to less than 80 ml/min in order for the dose of dialysis session to be calculated using sp Kt/V for urea [14]. The mean of 12 calculations for sp Kt/V for urea per dialysis session during a treatment month was used for statistical analysis.

In each subject, four sequences of samples (every week within the exposure period) were obtained for the serum bicarbonate measurements, and their average was used for statistical analysis. We paid attention thus to the low serum bicarbonate level to be combined with low arterial pH (acidemia) and decreased PCO_2, which determines the metabolic acidosis presence, rather than respiratory alkalosis, which is another clinical condition that causes decreased bicarbonate level, but without acidemia [15].

2.5. Laboratory Measurements. Albumin, calcium (Ca) corrected for the albumin levels, phosphate (P), high-density lipoproteins (HDL), and low-density lipoproteins (LDL) were measured by photometric biochemical analysis (MINDRAY BS-200, Diamond Diagnostics, USA). The ratios of LDL/HDL and Ca × P products were calculated. Sodium (Na^+) levels both at the start and at the end of the treatment session were also measured by biochemical analysis. Sodium removal was determined as percent sodium removal (PSR) using the following formula: (Na^+ pre – Na^+ post/Na^+ pre) × 100.

The evaluation of sodium removal was used for the estimation of extracellular volume (ECV) assuming that the change in body weight during a dialysis session represents the change in extracellular volume due to ultrafiltration, in combination with clinical characteristics related to an incorrect dry body weight including the presence of interdialytic peripheral edema, interdialytic orthostatic hypotension, or extradialytic uncontrolled blood pressure.

Hematological analyzer (Sysmex, xt-4000i, Roche, Germany) was used for hemoglobin (Hb).

The concentration of intact parathormone (i-PTH) was measured by radioimmunoassay (CIS Bio International, France).

High sensitivity C-reactive protein (hsCRP) serum concentrations were measured using enzyme-linked immunosorbent assay (ELISA, Immundiagnostik AG, Germany) according to the manufacturer's specifications.

Metabolic acidosis was defined by serum bicarbonate concentrations less than 22.0 mmol/L, which were measured in gas machine (Roche, cobas b 121) by an electrode-based method taking care of the blood specimens [16].

Normalized protein catabolic rate for dry body mass (nPCR) was calculated from the urea generation rate [17]. Body mass index (BMI) was obtained from height and postdialysis body weight.

3. Data Analysis

Data were analyzed using SPSS 15.0 statistical package for Windows (SPSS Inc., Chicago, Illinois) and expressed as mean ± standard deviation or as median value (interquartile range) for data that showed skewed distribution. Differences between mean values were assessed using unpaired t-test for two groups and data that showed skewed distributions were compared with Mann–Whitney U test.

Correlations between variables were defined by Spearman's coefficient and the relationships between categorical variables were defined by chi-square tests. p values less than 0.05 were considered significant. We built a model using logistic regression analysis by enter method in order to define the risk factors which could impact the installation of intradialytic hypertension in our data using traditional and specific variables for these patients.

4. Results

In Table 1, the differences between the groups of patients with ($n = 15$) and without ($n = 61$) intradialytic hypertension are shown.

We observed that the patients with intradialytic hypertension were older and had significantly lower Hb, nPCR, urine output, and bicarbonate serum concentrations than patients without intradialytic hypertension. However, they had significantly higher c-fPWV and AIx in comparison with patients without intradialytic hypertension. They also had higher sodium removal, Ca × P products, PP, dialysis vintage, and hsCRP, but lower i-PTH than patients without intradialytic hypertension. Both groups of patients had similar BMI, albumin, dialysis sufficiency, and interdialytic weight gain.

Chi-square tests showed significant association between the prevalence of intradialytic hypertension and both serum bicarbonate concentrations < 22 mmol/L and extradialytic hypertension ($x^2 = 5.6$, $p = 0.01$ and $x^2 = 4.2$, $p = 0.04$, resp.) (Figures 1 and 2). The association between intradialytic hypertension and preservation or not of residual renal function defined by urine output was found to be nonsignificant.

In the built adjusted model for the factors which could impact the manifestation of intradialytic hypertension, we found the old age, the bigger dialysis vintage, the elevated sodium removal, and the lower serum bicarbonate to be significant risk factors adjusting to diabetes mellitus, extradialytic hypertension, Hb, nPCR, hsCRP, and dialysis sufficiency defined by spKt/V for urea (Table 2).

Bivariate correlations showed significant association between c-fPWV and hsCRP, i-PTH, and serum bicarbonate ($r = 0.399$, $p = 0.001$; $r = 0.361$, $p = 0.02$; and $r = -0.377$, $p = 0.001$, Figure 3, resp.). We also did note significantly inverse association between urine output and pulse pressure ($r = -0.481$, $p = 0.03$, Figure 4).

5. Discussion

The variability of BP during hemodialysis treatment, which is defined by either intradialytic hypotension or intradialytic

TABLE 1: Differences between groups of patients according to the manifestation of intradialytic hypertension in a total of 76 subjects in hemodiafiltration ($^*p \leq 0.05$).

Characteristic	Patients with intradialytic hypertension ($n = 15$) *Mean ± SD/mean rank*	Patients without intradialytic hypertension ($n = 61$) *Mean ± SD/mean rank*	*p value*
Age (years)	70.2 ± 14.3*	60.3 ± 14.6	*0.02*
Dialysis vintage (years)	/45.2	/36.9	0.2
Kt/V for urea	/40.9	/37.9	0.6
nPCR (g/Kg/day)	2.1 ± 0.6*	2.4 ± 0.5	*0.03*
Urine volume (ml/day)	100.5 ± 0*	238.7 ± 147.7	*0.002*
BMI (Kg/m^2)	23.9 ± 3.7	24.6 ± 2.8	0.4
Serum bicarbonate (mmol/L)	/24.03*	/42.06	*0.005*
i-PTH (pg/ml)	/35.7	/39.2	0.6
Calcium corrected to albumin (mg/dl)	9.7 ± 0.7	9.4 ± 0.6	0.2
P (mg/dl)	5.5 ± 1.8	5.4 ± 1.9	0.8
Ca × P products	53.7 ± 17.1	50.9 ± 18.1	0.6
Interdialytic weight gain (liters)	2.05 ± 0.9	2.2 ± 0.9	0.5
Hb (gr/dl)	11.3 ± 1.6*	12.5 ± 1.2	*0.05*
Albumin (gr/dl)	/35.6	/39.2	0.5
LDL/HDL	2.06 ± 0.8	2.4 ± 0.9	0.1
c-fPWV (m/s)	12.3 ± 2.03*	11.08 ± 1.7	*0.02*
Augmentation index (AIx, %)	26 ± 2.2*	23.7 ± 1.9	*0.001*
Pulse pressure (PP, mmHg)	65.2 ± 23.8	56.5 ± 17.8	0.1
Percent sodium removal (PSR, %)	/46.8	/36.5	0.08
hsCRP (mg/L)	8.3 ± 5.6	7.9 ± 5.9	0.8

TABLE 2: Logistic regression model by enter method showing risk factors for demonstration of intradialytic hypertension in our data.

Characteristic	*p* value	Odds ratio	Confidence interval
Age	**0.007**	**1.2**	**1.04–1.3**
Diabetes mellitus	0.9	1.06	0.006–183.8
Extradialytic hypertension	0.7	1.4	0.2–10.1
Dialysis vintage	**0.02**	**1.3**	**1.03–1.6**
Hemoglobin	0.6	0.8	0.3–2.0
nPCR	0.1	0.2	0.02–1.5
hsCRP	0.1	0.9	0.7–1.04
Kt/V for urea	0.2	0.02	0.0–13.5
Percent sodium removal	**0.02**	**1.9**	**1.09–3.2**
Serum bicarbonate	**0.006**	**0.5**	**0.3–0.8**

hypertension, may be attributed in hemodynamic abnormalities or/and in a paradoxical response to the dialysis procedure in a subset of hemodialysis patients [8]. Although intradialytic hypotension occurs more often compared to intradialytic hypertension, it has been reported that intradialytic hypertension confers a higher mortality risk than hypotension [9]. Recently, it has been shown that frequent intradialytic hypertension was associated with increased 30-day morbidity and mortality considering the intradialytic hypertension as a short-term risk marker additionally to long-term mortality [18].

The prevalence of intradialytic hypertension has been described in 5–20% of hemodialysis treatments [9, 18]. In our data, the prevalence of this phenomenon reached 19.7%.

The history of hypertension is the cause for the phenomenon of intradialytic hypertension in a number of dialysis patients [19, 20]. Indeed, in this study, we noted a significant unadjusted association between intradialytic BP rise and extradialytic hypertension. The removal of antihypertensive medications during hemodialysis treatment may be also a contributor to intradialytic BP rise. However, a previous study demonstrated that the antihypertensive number, class,

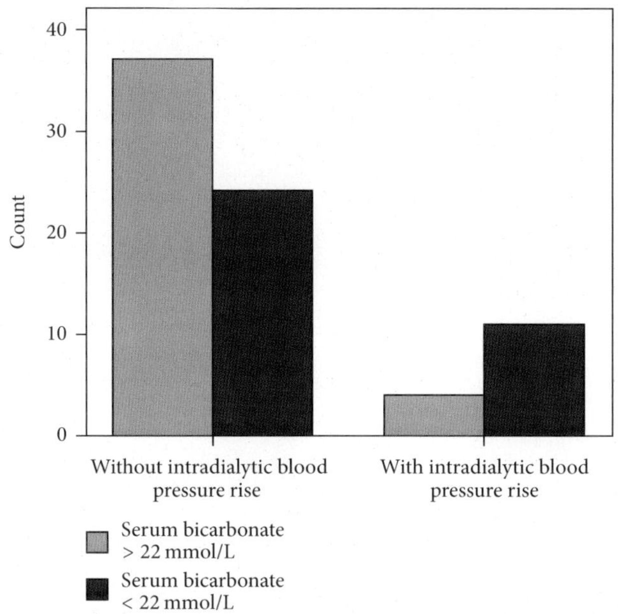

Figure 1: Bar chart for the association between intradialytic hypertension and metabolic acidosis state defined by serum bicarbonate less than 22 mmol/L ($x^2 = 5.6$, $p = 0.01$).

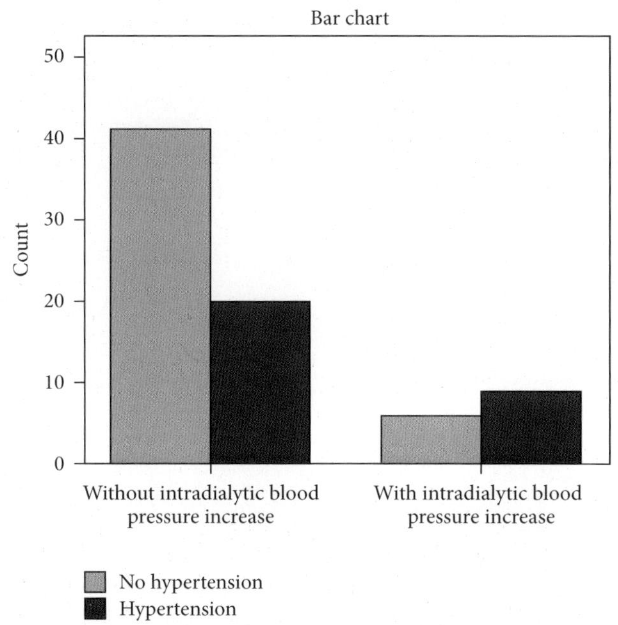

Figure 2: The prevalence of intradialytic hypertension in participants with extradialytic hypertension ($x^2 = 4.2$, $p = 0.04$).

and dialyzability status were not significantly associated with intradialytic BP variability [21].

The pathophysiology of intradialytic hypertension is poorly explained, even though the mechanisms and management of this phenomenon have been investigated in numerous studies over the past few years. A conjunction among positive sodium balance, volume overload, activation of the renin-angiotensin aldosterone (RAAS) and sympathetic nervous system, endothelial cell dysfunction, erythropoiesis-stimulating agents, and bone mineral disease abnormalities has been suggested.

Hypervolemia is a well-recognized risk factor for hypertension among dialysis patients. Patients with intradialytic hypertension have been found to be more chronically volume-overloaded than other hemodialysis patients, although they typically may have small interdialytic weight gain and clinically do not appear to be volume-overloaded [9, 22]. Indeed, in this study, patients with intradialytic hypertension had no apparent peripheral edema or uncontrolled extradialytic hypertension and they had similar interdialytic weight gain to those without intradialytic hypertension. However, they had significantly lower urine output in conjunction with higher sodium removal, higher PP, and increased arterial stiffness markers including c-fPWV and AIx in comparison to the patients without intradialytic hypertension. We also did note significantly inverse association between urine volume and PP.

To obtain a good BP control in dialysis patients, we must define the correct dry weight and individualize the adequate sodium concentration in dialysate, thus to achieve a zero intradialytic sodium balance [23]. Elevated sodium removal may be due to our trying to reach a dry weight lower than the correct one, which may have, as a consequence, intradialytic hypotensive episodes and muscle cramps, which can lead to the need for an increase in dialysate sodium concentration, thirst, and eventually greater interdialytic weight gain causing as a final result an ECV increase and hypertension [24]. Such a phenomenon is particularly exciting when a lower urine volume is combined, such as in our subjects with intradialytic hypertension. Moreover, in our previous study, PP was found to be influenced by volume overload rather than by arterial stiffness [25] and this finding may be confirmed by the found significantly inverse association between urine output and PP in present study. In the meantime, it has been already reported that fluid overload plays an important role in the development of arterial stiffness in dialysis patients and PWV varies during dialysis due to alterations in hydration status [26, 27]. All the above could suggest that our participants with intradialytic hypertension were fluid-overloaded even though they apparently were not.

On the other hand, although a causal role of volume overload has not been established, factors beyond volume overload are important mediators of intradialytic hypertension in many patients [22]. A link between volume overload and endothelial dysfunction markers has been suggested, which may be also stimulated by a greater sodium concentration in dialysate [28]. Recent investigations have established endothelial cell dysfunction as a key mediator in intradialytic hypertension and elevated vascular resistance, which remains the main driving force for BP increases [7, 9, 10]. Endothelial cells contribute to BP homeostasis by producing and releasing factors such as nitric oxide, a smooth muscle vasodilator, and endothelin-1, a vasoconstrictor. Among patients with intradialytic hypertension, studies have demonstrated that endothelin-1 levels rise during dialysis while systemic nitric oxide levels remain inappropriately low [29, 30]. Erythropoietin stimulating agents may contribute to intradialytic

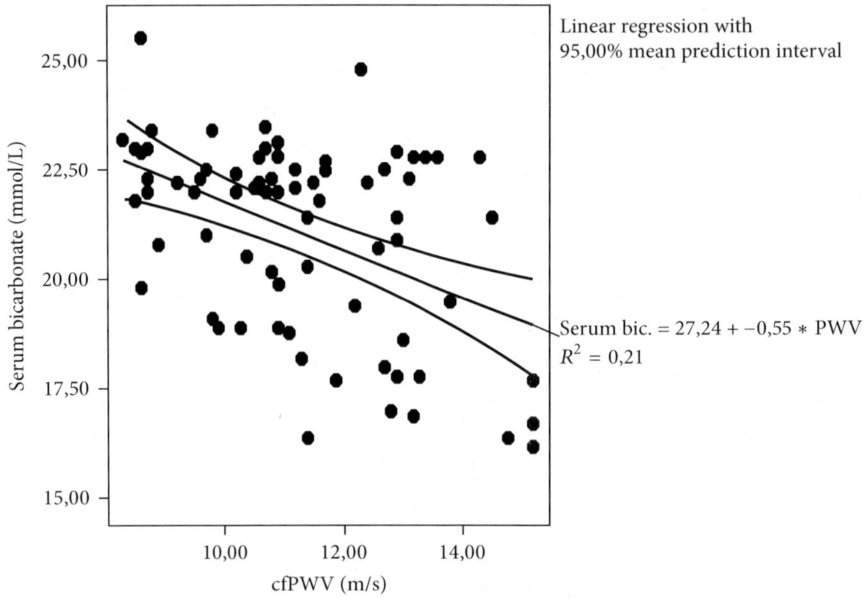

Figure 3: The correlation between carotid-femoral pulse wave velocity (c-fPWV) and serum bicarbonate concentrations ($r = -0.377$, $p = 0.001$).

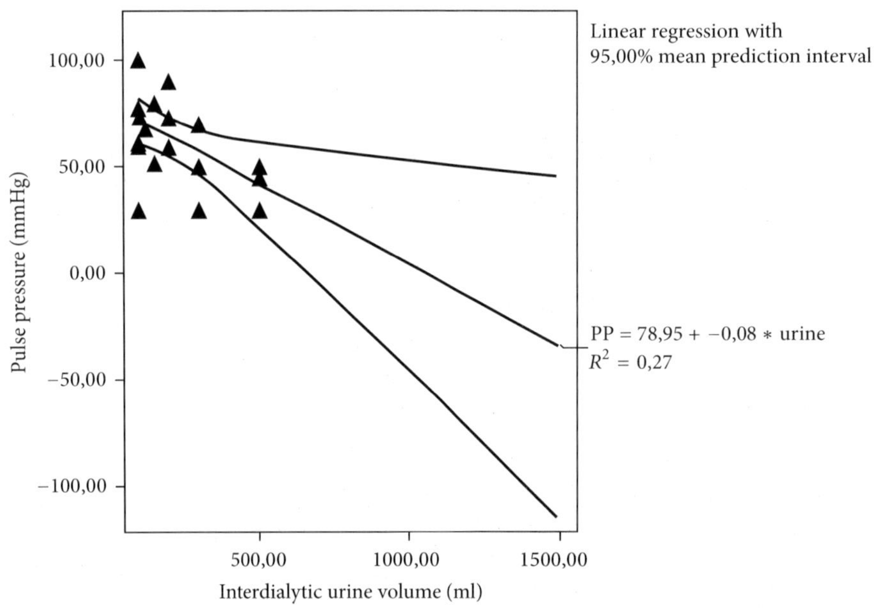

Figure 4: The correlation between pulse pressure and interdialytic urine volume ($r = -0.481$, $p = 0.03$).

hypertension via this mechanism [31]. However, it has been suggested that mediators other than endothelin-1 may be responsible for increased intradialytic vascular resistance [9]. Our recent previous study showed that the loss of residual renal function related to fluid overload was associated with cardiovascular outcomes in dialysis patients, due additionally to the coexistence of increased levels of monocyte chemoattractant protein-1 (MCP-1), a chemokine, which may reflect a progressive inflammation/oxidative stress condition [14].

Clinical characteristics associated with intradialytic BP rise include older age, lower body weight, lower serum creatinine and albumin, and utilization of more antihypertensive medications [32, 33]. Lower albumin and predialysis urea nitrogen levels may contribute to small reductions in osmolarity during dialysis and this prevents the blood pressure from falling. In this study, subjects with intradialytic hypertension were older and had significantly lower hemoglobin, lower nPCR as a marker of protein intake and malnutrition, and lower i-PTH, although they had higher hsCRP resulting in the cooccurrence of malnutrition, inflammation, and atherosclerosis (MIA syndrome), in comparison to the patients without intradialytic hypertension. In agreement, previously, it has been reported that low, rather than high, i-PTH was associated with inflammation and oxidative stress, as a result of MIA syndrome [34].

Malnutrition and anemia have already been reported as specific cardiovascular risk factors for dialysis patients and each of the MIA syndrome components worsens the survival of these patients [35, 36]. Malnutrition may be related to metabolic acidosis due to increased protein catabolism, decreased protein synthesis, endocrine abnormalities, and inflammation among dialysis patients [37]. Metabolic acidosis defined by low serum bicarbonate (<22 mmol/L) is a common condition in end stage renal disease patients resulting in inflammatory stimulation, lipids oxidation, and oxidative stress [38, 39]. Maintenance dialysis therapies are often unable to completely correct the base deficit. Previously, the association of uremic acidosis with arterial pressure has been reported in hypertensive patients [40].

In this study, we observed that our subjects with intradialytic BP rise had significantly lower serum bicarbonate levels than the other patients. This finding cannot be attributed to reduced dialysis treatment adequacy or other treatment related conditions, because both groups of patients had obtained a similar spKt/V for urea and they followed the same therapy rules. However, the older age, the cooccurrence of malnutrition/inflammation, the bigger dialysis vintage, and the lower urine output may contribute to a higher metabolic acidosis state in intradialytic hypertension patients. The unadjusted association between uncorrected metabolic acidosis and intradialytic hypertension was found to be significant in our data, as a confirming finding.

Interestingly, our subjects with intradialytic hypertension and higher metabolic acidosis state had simultaneously less urine output and increased arterial stiffness markers, which also reflect fluid overload apart from vascular injury, as it was explained above. Moreover, we did note significantly inverse association between c-fPWV and serum bicarbonate concentrations. In support, our adjusted model discovered that the low serum bicarbonate in conjunction with high sodium removal, older age, and a long dialysis time were important risk factors for manifested intradialytic hypertension adjusting for diabetes mellitus, dialysis adequacy, extradialytic hypertension, and MIA syndrome components. Particularly, the high sodium removal increased the risk for intradialytic BP rise to 1.9-fold (1.09–3.2) in our data.

These findings could suggest that uncorrected metabolic acidosis results in intradialytic BP rise in hemodialysis patients, due to its relationship with sodium imbalance and volume overload in these patients, even if clinically nonapparent, apart from its role in the increased ionized plasma calcium, which is already associated with hypertension [41]. Previously, we and others showed that patients with severe acidosis had less diuresis and they presented with important fluid overload and cardiovascular morbidity, in agreement with the findings of the present study [15, 42]. Furthermore, we could support that multiple products, other than endothelin-1, derived by severe acidosis, possibly contribute to endothelial dysfunction, resulting in elevated vascular resistance and intradialytic hypertension.

6. Conclusion

The manifestation of intradialytic hypertension was significantly associated with metabolic disorders including malnutrition/inflammation and uncontrolled metabolic acidosis in permanent hemodialysis treatment patients. Severe metabolic acidosis may reflect sodium imbalance and hemodynamic instability of these patients resulting in volume overload, despite being clinically nonapparent and despite the increased vascular resistance.

Additional Points

Limitations. The main limitation of this study is the small number of included patients in combination with its cross-sectional nature. The measurement of the total serum anions for actual metabolic acidosis calculation was also unavailable in this study.

Ethical Approval

This study was approved by the ethics committee of the hospitals "Laïko, University General Hospital of Athens" and the Renal Unit of "Diagnostic and Therapeutic Center of Athens Hygeia SA." All procedures performed in studies involving human participants were in accordance with the ethical standards of the institutional and/or national research committee and with the 1964 Helsinki Declaration and its later amendments or comparable ethical standards.

Authors' Contributions

Vaia D. Raikou was responsible for the research plan, statistics, data collection, and manuscript writing and Despina Kyriaki was responsible for biochemical analyses and radioimmunoassays.

References

[1] G. L. Bakris, J. M. Burkart, E. D. Weinhandl, P. A. McCullough, and M. A. Kraus, "Intensive hemodialysis, blood pressure, and antihypertensive medication use," *American Journal of Kidney Diseases*, vol. 68, no. 5, pp. S15–S23, 2016.

[2] B. Charra and C. Chazot, "Volume control, blood pressure and cardiovascular function: lessons from hemodialysis treatment," *Nephron*, vol. 93, no. 4, pp. p94–p101, 2003.

[3] D. Harrison, "Inflammation, immunity and hypertension," in *Journal of Hypertension*, vol. 34, supplement 1, 2016, ISH 2016 Abstract Book:e535.

[4] P. A. McCullough, C. T. Chan, E. D. Weinhandl, J. M. Burkart, and G. L. Bakris, "Intensive hemodialysis, left ventricular hypertrophy, and cardiovascular disease," *American Journal of Kidney Diseases*, vol. 68, no. 5, pp. S5–S14, 2016.

[5] T. Ogawa, M. Koeda, and K. Nitta, "Left ventricular diastolic dysfunction in end-stage kidney disease: pathogenesis, diagnosis, and treatment," *Therapeutic Apheresis and Dialysis*, vol. 19, no. 5, pp. 427–435, 2015.

[6] R. Kheder-Elfekih, A. Yannoutsos, J. Blacher, G. M. London, and M. E. Safar, "Hypertension and chronic kidney disease: respective contribution of mean and pulse pressure and arterial stiffness," *Journal of Hypertension*, vol. 33, no. 10, pp. 2010–2015, 2015.

[7] P. N. Van Buren, C. Kim, R. D. Toto, and J. K. Inrig, "The prevalence of persistent intradialytic hypertension in a hemodialysis population with extended follow-up," *The International Journal of Artificial Organs*, vol. 35, no. 12, pp. 1031–1038, 2012.

[8] P. N. Van Buren and J. K. Inrig, "Special situations: intradialytic hypertension/chronic hypertension and intradialytic hypotension," *Seminars in Dialysis*, 30, Jun 2017.

[9] P. N. Van Buren, "Pathophysiology and implications of intradialytic hypertension," *Current Opinion in Nephrology and Hypertension*, vol. 26, no. 4, pp. 303–310, 2017.

[10] M. M. Assimon and J. E. Flythe, "Intradialytic blood pressure abnormalities: the highs, the lows and all that lies between," *American Journal of Nephrology*, vol. 42, no. 5, pp. 337–350, 2015.

[11] P. Chauveau, H. Nguyen, C. Combe et al., "Dialyzer membrane permeability and survival in hemodialysis patients," *American Journal of Kidney Diseases*, vol. 45, no. 3, pp. 565–571, 2005.

[12] J. T. Daugirdas, "Second generation logarithmic estimates of single-pool variable volume Kt/V: an analysis of error," *Journal of the American Society of Nephrology*, vol. 4, no. 5, pp. 1205–1213, 1993.

[13] J. K. Inrig, "Intradialytic hypertension: a less-recognized cardiovascular complication of hemodialysis," *American Journal of Kidney Diseases*, vol. 55, no. 3, pp. 580–589, 2010.

[14] V. D. Raikou, V. Kardalinos, and D. Kyriaki, "The relationship of residual renal function with cardiovascular morbidity in hemodialysis patients and the potential role of monocyte chemoattractant protein-1," *Kidney Diseases*, vol. 4, no. 1, pp. 20–28, 2018.

[15] V. Raikou and D. Kyriaki, "Association between low serum bicarbonate concentrations and cardiovascular disease in patients in the end-stage of renal disease," *Diseases*, vol. 4, no. 4, p. 36, 2016.

[16] B. Kirschbaum, "Spurious metabolic acidosis in hemodialysis patients," *American Journal of Kidney Diseases*, vol. 35, no. 6, pp. 1068–1071, 2000.

[17] J. T. Daugirdas, "Simplified equations for monitoring Kt/V, PCRn, eKt/V, and ePCRn," *Advances in Chronic Kidney Disease*, vol. 2, no. 4, pp. 295–304, 1995.

[18] M. M. Assimon, L. Wang, and J. E. Flythe, "Intradialytic hypertension frequency and short-term clinical outcomes among individuals receiving maintenance hemodialysis," *American Journal of Hypertension*, vol. 31, no. 3, pp. 329–339, 2018.

[19] M. Cirit, F. Akçiçek, E. Terzioğlu et al., ""Paradoxical" rise in blood pressure during ultrafiltration in dialysis patients," *Nephrology Dialysis Transplantation*, vol. 10, pp. 1417–1420, 1995.

[20] R. Agarwal and R. P. Light, "Intradialytic hypertension is a marker of volume excess," *Nephrology Dialysis Transplantation*, vol. 25, no. 10, pp. 3355–3361, 2010.

[21] J. E. Flythe, S. Kunaparaju, K. Dinesh, K. Cape, H. I. Feldman, and S. M. Brunelli, "Factors associated with intradialytic systolic blood pressure variability," *American Journal of Kidney Diseases*, vol. 59, no. 3, pp. 409–418, 2012.

[22] P. N. Van Buren and J. K. Inrig, "Mechanisms and treatment of intradialytic hypertension," *Blood Purification*, vol. 41, no. 1-3, pp. 188–193, 2016.

[23] F. Locatelli, S. Colzani, M. D'Amico, C. Manzoni, and S. Di Filippo, "Dry weight and sodium balance," *Seminars in Nephrology*, vol. 21, no. 3, pp. 291–297, 2001.

[24] S. Di Filippo, C. Manzoni, S. Andrulli, F. Tentori, and F. Locatelli, "Sodium removal during pre-dilution haemofiltration," *Nephrology Dialysis Transplantation*, vol. 18, pp. vii31–vii36, 2003.

[25] V. D. Raikou, N. Tentolouris, D. Kyriaki, A. Evaggelatou, and H. Tzanatou, "β 2-microglobulin, pulse pressure and metabolic alterations in hemodialysis patients," *Nephron Clinical Practice*, vol. 117, no. 3, pp. c237–c245, 2011.

[26] D. Zheng, L.-T. Cheng, Z. Zhuang, Y. Gu, L.-J. Tang, and T. Wang, "Correlation between pulse wave velocity and fluid distribution in hemodialysis patients," *Blood Purification*, vol. 27, no. 3, pp. 248–252, 2009.

[27] B. Di Iorio, P. Nazzaro, E. Cucciniello, and V. Bellizzi, "Influence of haemodialysis on variability of pulse wave velocity in chronic haemodialysis patients," *Nephrology Dialysis Transplantation*, vol. 25, no. 5, pp. 1579–1583, 2010.

[28] N. Mitsides, T. Cornelis, N. J. H. Broers et al., "Extracellular overhydration linked with endothelial dysfunction in the context of inflammation in haemodialysis dependent chronic kidney disease," *PLoS ONE*, vol. 12, no. 8, Article ID e0183281, 2017.

[29] K.-J. Chou, P.-T. Lee, C.-L. Chen et al., "Physiological changes during hemodialysis in patients with intradialysis hypertension," *Kidney International*, vol. 69, no. 10, pp. 1833–1838, 2006.

[30] E. M. El-Shafey, G. F. El-Nagar, M. F. Selim, H. A. El-Sorogy, and A. A. Sabry, "Is there a role for endothelin-1 in the hemodynamic changes during hemodialysis?" *Clinical and Experimental Nephrology*, vol. 12, no. 5, pp. 370–375, 2008.

[31] P. A. Abraham and M. G. Macres, "Blood pressure in hemodialysis patients during amelioration of anemia with erythropoietin," *Journal of the American Society of Nephrology*, vol. 2, pp. 927–936, 1991.

[32] J. K. Inrig, E. Z. Oddone, V. Hasselblad et al., "Association of intradialytic blood pressure changes with hospitalization and mortality rates in prevalent ESRD patients," *Kidney International*, vol. 71, no. 5, pp. 454–461, 2007.

[33] J. K. Inrig, U. D. Patel, R. D. Toto, and L. A. Szczech, "Association of blood pressure increases during hemodialysis with 2-year mortality in incident hemodialysis patients: a secondary analysis of the dialysis morbidity and mortality wave 2 study," *American Journal of Kidney Diseases*, vol. 54, no. 5, pp. 881–890, 2009.

[34] R. Pecoits-Filho, B. Lindholm, and P. Stenvinkel, "The malnutrition, inflammation, and atherosclerosis (MIA) syndrome—the heart of the matter," *Nephrology Dialysis Transplantation*, vol. 17, supplement 11, pp. 28–31, 2002.

[35] S. R. Jahromi, S. Hosseini, E. Razeghi, A. P. Meysamie, and H. Sadrzadeh, "Malnutrition predicting factors in hemodialysis patients.," *Saudi journal of kidney diseases and transplantation : an official publication of the Saudi Center for Organ Transplantation, Saudi Arabia*, vol. 21, no. 5, pp. 846–851, 2010.

[36] P. Stenvinkel, "Inflammatory and atherosclerotic interactions in the depleted uremic patient," *Blood Purification*, vol. 19, no. 1, pp. 53–61, 2001.

[37] C. M. C. de Oliveira, C. L. D. C. Vidal, E. F. Cristino, F. M. L. Pinheiro, and M. Kubrusly, "Metabolic acidosis and its association with nutritional status in hemodialysis," *Jornal brasileiro de nefrologia : ̓orgao oficial de Sociedades Brasileira e Latino-Americana de Nefrologia*, vol. 37, no. 4, pp. 458–466, 2015.

[38] K. Kalantar-Zadeh, R. Mehrotra, D. Fouque, and J. D. Kopple, "Metabolic acidosis and malnutrition-inflammation complex syndrome in chronic renal failure," *Seminars in Dialysis*, vol. 17, no. 6, pp. 455–465, 2004.

[39] N. D. Vaziri, "Dyslipidemia of chronic renal failure: the nature, mechanisms, and potential consequences," *American Journal of Physiology-Renal Physiology*, vol. 290, no. 2, pp. F262–F272, 2006.

[40] V. Kovacic, L. Roguljic, and V. Kovacic, "Metabolic acidosis of chronically hemodialyzed patients," *American Journal of Nephrology*, vol. 23, no. 3, pp. 158–164, 2003.

[41] K. M. L. Leunissen, B. W. Van den Berg, and J. P. Van Hooff, "Ionized calcium plays a pivotal role in controlling blood pressure during haemodialysis," *Blood Purification*, vol. 7, no. 5, pp. 233–239, 1989.

[42] I. A. Checherita, C. David, A. Ciocalteu, I. Lascar, and L. Budala, "Oral treatment of metabolic acidosis in hemodialyzed patients and the implications on the hemodynamic status," *Romanian Journal of Morphology and Embryology*, vol. 54, pp. 539–543, 2013.

9

Prevalence and Sociodemographic Determinants of Hypertension History among Women in Reproductive Age in Ghana

Samuel H. Nyarko

Department of Population and Behavioural Sciences, School of Public Health, University of Health and Allied Sciences, Hohoe, Ghana

Correspondence should be addressed to Samuel H. Nyarko; samharrenson@gmail.com

Academic Editor: Franco Veglio

Background. Hypertension is a global health problem. Yet, studies on hypertension rarely focus on women in Ghana. The purpose of this study is to ascertain the prevalence and sociodemographic determinants of hypertension history among Ghanaian women in reproductive age. *Methods.* This study used data from the 2014 Ghana Demographic and Health Survey. Bivariate and logistic regression analyses were carried out to ascertain the prevalence and determinants of hypertension history among the respondents. *Results.* The study found that the overall prevalence of hypertension history among the respondents was 7.5%; however, there were vast variations within most of the sociodemographic categories. Age, level of education, marital status, work status, and wealth status had a significant relationship with hypertension history among the respondents. Women in advanced age groups, highly educated, married, and widowed/divorced/separated, nonworking women, and women from wealthy households were at higher risk of having hypertension history. *Conclusion.* Myriads of sociodemographic factors determine the hypertension history of women in Ghana. It is therefore essential to target medical and psychosocial hypertension interventions at Ghanaian women in the higher risk groups.

1. Background

Hypertension is the constant pumping of blood through blood vessels with excessive force [1]. It is a major public health problem that is associated with relatively low levels of awareness, drug treatment, and blood pressure control [2, 3]. It is a "silent killer" because it often has no warning signs or symptoms, and many people do not realize they have it [1]. It can cause serious damage to health by hardening the arteries, decreasing the flow of blood and oxygen to the heart which in turn can cause chest pain, heart failure, heart attack, and stroke [1].

Worldwide, the overall prevalence of hypertension in adults aged 25 and above in 2008 was around 40 percent. Even though the proportion of the world's population with hypertension decreased slightly between 1980 and 2008, because of population growth and ageing, the number of people with uncontrolled hypertension rose from 600 million to nearly 1 billion between 1980 and 2008 [4]. Hypertension is estimated to cause 7.5 million deaths, about 12.8 percent of the total of all global deaths, accounting for 57 million disability adjusted life years (DALYS) [4]. Across the World Health Organisation regions, the prevalence of hypertension was highest in Africa, where it was 46 percent for both sexes. The lowest prevalence was in the Americas at 35 percent for both sexes [4].

In Ghana, the prevalence of adult hypertension has been found to be consistently high in both urban and rural areas ranging from 19 to 48 percent [5]. The awareness, treatment experience, and effective control of hypertension were also found to be low [3, 5], with treatment levels ranging from 6.9 to 52.5 percent while control levels range from 1.7 to 12.7 percent [5]. Hypertension has been found to be a significant cause of renal and heart failure in Ghana [6, 7] and has been one of the root causes of higher levels of cardiovascular diseases in Africa [8]. It is quite obvious that inadequate population-based studies on hypertension have been conducted in Ghana, with virtually all of them focused on subpopulations. It has also been observed that albeit population-based prevention strategies including reduction in salt intake and integration of hypertension care into primary care may prove beneficial, the determinants of hypertension remain to be ascertained [2]. This paper therefore sought to ascertain the prevalence and sociodemographic determinants of hypertension history among women in reproductive age (15–49) in Ghana.

2. Materials and Methods

Data for this study were obtained from the 2014 Ghana Demographic and Health Survey (2014 GDHS), implemented by the Ghana Statistical Service (GSS), the Ghana Health Service (GHS), and the National Public Health Reference Laboratory (NPHRL) of the GHS. It is the sixth and latest in a series of population and health surveys conducted in Ghana as part of the global Demographic and Health Surveys (DHS) Program. A nationally representative survey of 9,396 women aged 15–49 from 11,835 households was conducted [9]. Ethical approval for the survey was catered for by the Ghana Health Service Ethical Review Committee; therefore, further ethical approval is not applicable in this case.

The outcome variable of the study is history of hypertension among women. In determining this, respondents were asked about their hypertension history, as to whether they had ever been told by a doctor or any health personnel that they had high blood pressure. This generated a binary response from the respondents in terms of yes or no. The independent variables therefore were a number of sociodemographic factors that may have the potential to influence hypertension history of respondents. These comprised age, education level, religious affiliation, ethnicity, wealth, marital and work status, and type and region of residence.

The data were extracted and processed using Stata version 13. Some variables were therefore recoded to suit the purpose of the study. To adjust for clustering during sampling and for that reason ensure national representation of the findings, all results were weighted using the generated sample weight for the dataset. In this sense, prevalence of hypertension history was computed and presented in the form of proportions by selected sociodemographic characteristics of respondents. In order to ascertain the sociodemographic factors that determined hypertension history among the respondents, logistic regression analysis was applied. Consequently, odds ratios, P values, and confidence intervals were computed and presented in Tables 1 and 2 for analysis and discussion.

3. Results

3.1. Sociodemographic Characteristics of Respondents. Table 1 presents a summary of the sociodemographic characteristics of respondents and prevalence of hypertension history. As indicated in the table, more than one-third (34.2%) of the respondents who participated in the study were from 20 to 29 years while about one-fifth (20.1%) were from 40 to 49 years and 17.3 percent were from 15 to 19 years. About 63 percent had secondary education or higher while 17.8 percent had primary education.

With regard to religious affiliation, about 80 percent were Christians and 15.2 percent were Muslims while only 2 percent were traditionalists. More than half (52.4%) were Akans while 14.8 percent were Mole-Dagbanis and less than one-tenth (7.7%) were Ga-Dangmes. In terms of household wealth, about 46 percent were from rich households while about one-third (33.5%) were from poor households. Also, about 57 percent were married or living together while 33 percent were never married or living together. The majority (73.4%) were working while 26.6 percent were not working. For type of residence, more than half (53.7%) were from the urban settings while 46.3 were from rural settings. In relation to region of residence, about one-fifth (20.2%) and close to one-fifth (19.1%) were from the Greater Accra and Ashanti Regions, respectively, while only 3.8 and 2.3 percent were from the Upper East and West regions, respectively.

3.2. Prevalence of Hypertension History among Women in Reproductive Age. During the survey, respondents were asked whether they had been told by a doctor or any health professional that they had high blood pressure. A summary of this has been presented by the sociodemographic characteristics of respondents (Table 1). Overall, 7.5 percent of the respondents reported ever being told by a health professional that they had hypertension. The highest percentage of hypertension history was reported among women aged 40–49 (18.4%) while the lowest percentage was reported among women aged 15–19.

Women who had primary school education reported higher percentage (7.8%) of hypertension history than their counterparts who had secondary school education or higher (7.7%) and no formal education (6.6%). The prevalence of hypertension history was also highest among Christian women (7.6%) but lowest among traditional women (5.4%). With regard to ethnicity, the highest percentages were reported among Ga-Dangme (12.6%) and Ewe women (10.6%) while the lowest were reported among Mole-Dagbani (6.2%) and other groups of women (4.3%). Further, the percentage of hypertension history was highest among women from rich households but lowest among their counterparts from poor households. Apparently, the prevalence of hypertension increased greatly with wealth status of the respondents. Working women at the time of the survey also reported higher percentage (8.5%) of hypertension history than their counterparts who were not working (4.7%). There were also some spatial variations in hypertension history among the respondents. For instance, women from urban settings reported higher percentage (9.7%) of hypertension history than those from rural settings (5.0%). Also, women from the Greater Accra Region (13.1%) reported the highest prevalence of hypertension history, followed by women from the Volta Region (9.3%) and Eastern Region (8.3%). However, the lowest prevalence was reported among women from the Upper West Region (3.2%).

3.3. Determinants of Hypertension History among Women in Reproductive Age. In order to ascertain the potential determinants of hypertension history among the respondents, a logistic regression analysis including odds ratios was applied (Table 2). A cursory look at the table shows that age of woman, level of education, and marital, work, and wealth status

TABLE 1: Prevalence of hypertension history by sociodemographic characteristics.

Sociodemographic characteristics	Percentage with hypertension history	Number and percent of women
Age		
15–19	0.4	1,625 (17.3)
20–29	3.2	3,217 (34.2)
30–39	9.2	2,667 (28.4)
40–49	18.4	1,887 (20.1)
Education level		
No formal education	6.6	1,792 (19.1)
Primary education	7.8	1,672 (17.8)
Secondary/higher education	7.7	5,932 (63.1)
Religious affiliation		
Christian	7.6	7,529 (80.1)
Muslim	7.3	1,424 (15.2)
Traditionalist	5.4	189 (2.0)
No religion	5.7	254 (2.7)
Ethnicity		
Akan	7.0	4,920 (54.4)
Ga-Dangme	12.6	727 (7.7)
Ewe	10.6	1,267 (13.5)
Mole-Dagbani	6.2	1,389 (14.8)
Others	4.3	1,093 (11.6)
Wealth status		
Poor	4.1	3,147 (33.5)
Middle	7.0	1,938 (20.6)
Rich	10.3	4,311 (45.9)
Marital status		
Never married	1.7	3,094 (33.0)
Married/living together	9.7	5,321 (56.6)
Widowed/divorced/separated	13.5	981 (10.4)
Work status		
Not working	4.7	2,495 (73.4)
Working	8.5	6,901 (26.6)
Type of residence		
Urban	9.7	5,051 (53.7)
Rural	5.0	4,345 (46.3)
Region		
Western	5.6	1,038 (11.0)
Central	3.3	937 (10.0)
Greater Accra	13.1	1,898 (20.2)
Volta	9.3	720 (7.7)
Eastern	8.3	877 (9.3)
Ashanti	6.6	1,798 (19.1)
Brong Ahafo	5.5	769 (8.2)
Northern	5.6	786 (8.4)
Upper East	4.1	358 (3.8)
Upper West	3.2	215 (2.3)
Total 15–49	7.5	9,396

TABLE 2: Logistic regression of hypertension history among women aged 15–49.

Variables	Odds ratio (OR)	*P* value	95% conf. interval
Age of woman			
15–19 (Ref.)	1		
20–29	5.14	0.000***	2.19–2.75
30–39	13.11	0.000***	1.42–1.71
40–49	34.41	0.000***	1.14–3.71
Level of education			
No formal education (Ref.)	1		
Primary	1.45	0.023*	1.05–2.09
Secondary/higher	1.48	0.026*	1.04–2.02
Religious affiliation			
Christian (Ref.)	1		
Muslim	1.31	0.105	0.94–1.84
Traditional/spiritualist	0.83	0.676	0.35–1.95
No religion	0.76	0.390	0.41–1.40
Ethnicity			
Akan (Ref.)	1		
Ga/Dangme	1.16	0.427	0.79–1.69
Ewe	1.32	0.119	0.92–1.88
Mole-Dagbani	0.13	0.596	0.70–1.82
Other	0.77	0.250	0.50–1.19
Marital status			
Never married (Ref.)	1		
Married/living together	2.08	0.001***	1.36–3.18
Widowed/divorced/separated	2.21	0.001***	1.35–3.58
Work status			
Not working (Ref.)	1		
Working	0.77	0.050*	0.58–1.02
Wealth status			
Poor	1		
Average	1.69	0.001***	1.22–2.33
Rich	2.41	0.000***	1.66–3.51
Place of residence			
Urban (Ref.)	1		
Rural	0.90	0.481	0.69–1.19
Region of residence			
Western	1		
Central	0.54	0.010**	0.34–0.86
Greater Accra	1.73	0.007**	1.16–2.60
Volta	1.65	0.043*	1.01–2.68
Eastern	1.40	0.101	0.93–2.09
Ashanti	0.94	0.781	0.63–1.41
Brong Ahafo	1.16	0.499	0.74–1.83
Northern	1.68	0.052	0.99–2.84
Upper East	1.18	0.556	0.67–2.09
Upper West	0.82	0.538	0.44–1.51

Ref. = reference category.
*$P \leq 0.05$; **$P \leq 0.01$; and ***$P \leq 0.001$.

had a significant relationship with hypertension history, unlike religious affiliation, ethnicity, and place and region of residence. With regard to risk of hypertension history, it was found that the odds were higher among women aged 40–49 (OR = 34.41), 30–39 (OR = 13.11), and 20–29 (OR = 5.14) compared to women aged 15–19. The odds were also higher among women who had primary school education (OR = 1.45) and secondary school or higher education (OR = 1.48) compared to women who had no formal education.

Women who were married or living together (OR = 2.08) and women who were widowed, divorced, or separated (OR = 2.21) also had higher odds of hypertension history compared to their counterparts who were never married or living together. The odds were however lower among working women (OR = 0.77) compared to nonworking women. Concerning wealth status, women from rich (OR = 2.41) and average (OR = 1.69) households had higher odds of hypertension history compared to their counterparts from poor households. Even though region of residence, on the whole, had no significant relationship with hypertension history, the Central (P = 0.010), Greater Accra (P = 0.007), and Volta (P = 0.043) Regions had significant influence on the regional variations among the respondents.

4. Discussion

In this study, about 8 percent of women in reproductive age in Ghana were found to have hypertension history. Age, education, and marital, work, and wealth status were found to be associated with hypertension history among the respondents. In view of this, the risk of hypertension history had increased considerably with increasing age among respondents. A number of studies across the globe have also found that increasing age is a determining factor of hypertension status among respondents [5, 10–14]. The reason for the high risk of hypertension among women in advanced age may be subject to a number of interpretations. For instance, unlike younger women, women in advanced age groups may not have the physical energy, the cardiovascular resistance, or the zeal needed to perform regular aerobic exercises which may help maintain optimum blood pressure level. Besides, some women in advanced age groups may prefer sedentary lifestyles or jobs which in itself may be a risk factor for hypertension [13], while some may even be prone to thinking too much about "trivial circumstances" in their lives. These among others may likely render women in advanced age groups more susceptible to high blood pressure or hypertension.

Level of education was also found to have a significant influence on hypertension history among the respondents. Thus, the risk of hypertension history increased marginally with increasing level of education among the respondents. It has also been reported by a number of studies that educational level or literacy is significantly associated with hypertension [13–16]. Like this study, some of these studies have found higher risk of hypertension among the highly educated compared to the uneducated while others have also reported the reverse. However, none of them has been able to provide possible reasons for their findings. This may be as a result of the fact that the factors that made highly educated women more susceptible to hypertension may be unclear and for that matter difficult to assert.

The study further found that married or cohabiting women and widows, divorcees, or separated women were more likely to have hypertension history than women who were never married. It was observed that existing studies that examined determinants of hypertension among a number of different populations hardly considered marital status of respondents. Even though it is quite unclear why married and widowed, divorced, or separated women were more susceptible to hypertension history, it is possible that this may be due to the inevitable "vicissitudes of marriage."

Additionally, working women were found to be less likely to have hypertension history compared to their counterparts who were not working. Even though the prevalence of hypertension history was higher among working women, the risk of hypertension history was higher among nonworking women. The influence of working status on the hypertension history of respondents has been scarcely investigated by studies. Nevertheless, it may be fair to presume that higher risk of hypertension history among nonworking women may be due to "inactivity" or "sedentary life" [13, 16, 17] and its concomitant social and economic pressures.

The effect of household wealth status on hypertension history has also been established in this study. The risk of hypertension history was therefore found to increase appreciably with increasing household wealth status of respondents. A number of reports have indicated that household wealth index or socioeconomic status has a significant relationship with hypertension history among people [12, 13, 18]. Like this study, some reports have indicated a positive relationship between wealth index and hypertension whereas others have found a negative relationship between the two. However, it is not clear which factors might have subjected women from rich households to higher risk of hypertension history in this study. Perhaps, one of the reasons may be that women from households with higher wealth index in Ghana may mostly be using vehicles or gadgets for their daily duties instead of performing physical activities such as regular walking and manual work which may be a protective factor against hypertension. This may render women from rich households vulnerable to hypertension compared to their poor counterparts.

5. Conclusion

Hypertension history, even though not quite high on the whole, is still a health problem among women in reproductive age in Ghana, following the vast variations found within the subcategories of the sociodemographic characteristics of respondents. Age of respondent, level of education, marital status, work status, and household wealth status were therefore the sociodemographic factors that determined hypertension history among women in reproductive age group in Ghana for the study period. Consequently, it becomes necessary to target medical and psychosocial hypertension interventions towards Ghanaian women who are in advanced age groups, highly educated, married, widowed/divorced/separated, and not working as well as women from wealthy households.

Disclosure

Data for this study were obtained from the DHS Program.

Competing Interests

The author declares that there are no competing interests.

References

[1] World Health Organization, *Hypertension*, World Health Organization, Geneva, Switzerland, 2011, http://www.searo.who.int/entity/noncommunicable_diseases/media/non_communicable_diseases_hypertension_fs.pdf.

[2] A. G. B. Amoah, "Hypertension in Ghana: a cross-sectional community prevalence study in Greater Accra," *Ethnicity & Disease*, vol. 13, no. 3, pp. 310–315, 2003.

[3] J. Addo, C. Agyemang, L. A. Smeeth, A. de-Graft Aikins, A. K. Edusei, and O. Ogedegbe, "A review of population-based studies on hypertension in Ghana," *Ghana Medical Journal*, vol. 46, no. 2, pp. 4–11, 2012.

[4] World Health Organization, *Raised Blood Pressure: Situation and Trends*, World Health Organization, Geneva, Switzerland, 2016, http://www.who.int/gho/ncd/risk_factors/blood_pressure_prevalence_text/en/.

[5] W. K. Bosu, "Epidemic of hypertension in Ghana: a systematic review," *BMC Public Health*, vol. 10, article 418, 2010.

[6] J. Plange-Rhule, R. Phillips, J. W. Acheampong, A. K. Saggar-Malik, F. P. Cappuccio, and J. B. Eastwood, "Hypertension and renal failure in Kumasi, Ghana," *Journal of Human Hypertension*, vol. 13, no. 1, pp. 37–40, 1999.

[7] I. Owusu, "Causes of heart failure as seen in Kumasi, Ghana," *The Internet Journal of Third World Medicine*, vol. 5, no. 1, 2006.

[8] R. S. Cooper, A. G. B. Amoah, and G. A. Mensah, "High blood pressure: the foundation for epidemic cardiovascular disease in African populations," *Ethnicity and Disease*, vol. 13, supplement 2, pp. S48–S52, 2003.

[9] Ghana Statistical Service (GSS), Ghana Health Service (GHS), and ICF International, *Ghana Demographic and Health Survey 2014*, GSS, GHS, and ICF International, Rockville, Md, USA, 2015.

[10] N. van den Berg, C. Meinke-Franze, T. Fiss, S. E. Baumeister, and W. Hoffmann, "Prevalence and determinants of controlled hypertension in a German population cohort," *BMC Public Health*, vol. 13, article 594, 2013.

[11] E. I. Ugwuja, U. S. Ezenkwa, A. N. Nwibo, M. Ogbanshi, O. Idoko, and R. Nnabu, "Prevalence and determinants of hypertension in an agrarian rural community in Southeast Nigeria," *Annals of Medical and Health Sciences Research*, vol. 5, no. 1, pp. 45–49, 2015.

[12] M. Alam, G. P. Soni, K. K. Jain, S. Verma, and P. Panda, "Prevalence and determinants of hypertension in elderly population of Raipur city, Chhattisgarh," *International Journal of Research in Medical Sciences*, vol. 3, no. 3, pp. 568–573, 2015.

[13] A. Laxmaiah, I. I. Meshram, N. Arlappa et al., "Socio-economic & demographic determinants of hypertension & knowledge, practices & risk behaviour of tribals in India," *Indian Journal of Medical Research*, vol. 141, pp. 697–708, 2015.

[14] E. A. Williams, K. E. Keenan, D. Ansong et al., "The burden and correlates of hypertension in rural Ghana: a cross-sectional study," *Diabetes & Metabolic Syndrome: Clinical Research & Reviews*, vol. 7, no. 3, pp. 123–128, 2013.

[15] M. Temmar, C. Labat, S. Benkhedda et al., "Prevalence and determinants of hypertension in the Algerian Sahara," *Journal of Hypertension*, vol. 25, no. 11, pp. 2218–2226, 2007.

[16] J. Addo, A. G. B. Amoah, and K. A. Kwadwo, "The changing patterns of hypertension in Ghana: a study of four rural communities in the Ga district," *Ethnicity & Disease*, vol. 16, no. 4, pp. 894–899, 2006.

[17] M. R. Maracy, A. Feizi, and M. Bagherynejad, "The prevalence and correlated determinants of hypertension and type 2 diabetes: a large community-based study in Isfahan, Iran," *Pakistan Journal of Medical Sciences*, vol. 28, no. 2, pp. 247–252, 2012.

[18] P. Lloyd-Sherlock, J. Beard, N. Minicuci, S. Ebrahim, and S. Chatterji, "Hypertension among older adults in low and middle-income countries: prevalence, awareness and control," *International Journal of Epidemiology*, vol. 43, no. 1, pp. 116–128, 2014.

10

Impact of Resistance Exercise under Hypoxia on Postexercise Hemodynamics in Healthy Young Males

Masahiro Horiuchi, [1] **Arisa Ni-i-nou,** [2] **Mitsuhiro Miyazaki,** [2] **Daisuke Ando,** [3] **and Katsuhiro Koyama** [3]

[1] *Division of Human Environmental Science, Mt. Fuji Research Institute, Japan*
[2] *Faculty of Education and Human Sciences, University of Yamanashi, Japan*
[3] *Graduate School Department of Interdisciplinary Research, University of Yamanashi, Japan*

Correspondence should be addressed to Masahiro Horiuchi; mhoriuchi@mfri.pref.yamanashi.jp

Academic Editor: Omotayo O. Erejuwa

We investigated the effects of resistance exercise under hypoxia on postexercise hemodynamics in eight healthy young males. The subjects belonged to a track & field club (sprinters, hurdlers, and long jumpers) and engage in regular physical training (1-2 h per day, 3-5 days per week). Each participant performed eight sets of bilateral leg squats with a one-minute interval under normoxia (room air) and hypoxia (13 % FiO_2). During a 60-minute recovery, we set normoxic condition either after normoxic or hypoxic exercise. These two experimental protocols (normoxia and hypoxia) were performed in a random order with a one-week washout period. The leg squat exercise consists of 50 % 1-RM (14 repetitions) × 5 sets and 50% 1-RM (repetitions max; 7 repetitions) × 3 sets. The resting period between each set was 1 min, and a total of 91 repetitions were performed. Blood pressure, heart rate (HR), and several biomarkers were measured pre- and postexercise. The mean arterial pressure (MAP) significantly decreased after exercise compared to the pre-exercise values under both conditions ($P < 0.05$). The MAP at 20 and 30 min of recovery in hypoxia was significantly lower than in normoxia ($P < 0.05$, respectively). The antidiuretic hormone significantly increased after 60 min of recovery in both conditions; moreover, the values in hypoxia were significantly higher than those in normoxia ($P < 0.05$). The delta changes in MAP from baseline (pre-exercise) were significantly related to changes in HR from baseline in normoxia ($r = 0.560$, $P < 0.001$) but not in hypoxia. These results suggest that the hypoxic condition elicits greater hypotension after resistance exercise in comparison to normoxia. Moreover, the underlying mechanisms for the attenuation of hypotension after resistance exercise may differ between normoxia and hypoxia.

1. Introduction

In healthy individuals, an acute single bout of physical exercise elicits reductions in arterial blood pressure for approximately 2 h when compared to the baseline (pre-exercise) levels; this phenomenon is so-called postexercise hypotension (PEH) [1–3]. In addition, recent findings suggest that the magnitude of reductions in blood pressure (BP) with acute exercise may be associated with chronic reductions in the resting BP caused by exercise training [4, 5]. These results suggest that PEH with acute exercise may be relevant for predicting the long-term effects of BP changes.

Although these studies were conducted with aerobic exercise [4, 5], several studies have observed the occurrence of PEH after acute resistance exercise [6–10]. Moreover, a recent meta-analysis revealed that a single bout of resistance exercise can lower the BP in normotensive and hypertensive populations and the use of larger muscle groups resulted in greater BP reductions after resistance exercise [11]. Resistance exercise may exert some additional advantages; for example, resistance exercise is recommended for prevention of sarcopenia, wherein age-induced muscular degeneration often leads to compromised performance in activities of daily living [12]. Moreover, it has been suggested that resistance exercise in hypoxia reportedly has beneficial effects in terms of increased muscle strength and size [13, 14]. However, it should be noted that greater PEH may frequently cause syncope after exercise [15] and higher intensity exercise induces a postexercise syncope compared to lower intensity exercise [16]. These results suggest that negative effects of PEH should also be considered, in particular, higher exercise intensity (e.g., high intensity aerobic or resistance exercise). Indeed, it was reported that the arterial blood pressure reached 320/250 mmHg during the maximal bilateral leg press [17] but the pressure subsequently fell rapidly after lifting [18]. As a result, the cerebral perfusion pressure falls below the pre-exercise levels, leading to an increased risk of syncope [18, 19]. Indeed, we reported that, after prolonged leg cycling, there was a greater reduction in the mean arterial blood pressure (MAP), and the decrease in MAP was positively related to decreases in cerebral oxygenation only in hypoxia [20]. These results suggest that resistance exercise in hypoxia may involve an increased risk of syncope even for healthy individuals, indicating that clarification of the mechanisms of PEH after resistance exercise in hypoxia is important. However, little is known about how resistance exercise in hypoxia may affect postexercise hemodynamics.

The aim of this study, therefore, was to investigate the influence of resistance exercise in hypoxia on postexercise hemodynamics in healthy young males. We hypothesized that resistance exercise in hypoxia elicits greater reductions in arterial blood pressure than in normoxia. To test this hypothesis, we used bilateral leg squats at 50% 1-RM (repetition max) with the inspiration of oxygen (FiO_2) at ~13% based on a previous study [21]. In addition, we measured several potent vasoconstrictors (antidiuretic hormone and aldosterone) and vasodilators (human atrial natriuretic peptide and adenosine) that may influence BP regulation.

2. Methods

2.1. Participants. This study was approved by the Ethical Committee of the University of Yamanashi in Japan and was performed in accordance with the guidelines of the Declaration of Helsinki (No: 201606). Eight healthy male subjects with a mean age of 19.9 ± 0.8 years, a height of 170.0 ± 3.1 cm, and a body mass of 65.1 ± 11.3 kg (mean ± standard deviation [SD]) participated in this study. The subjects belonged to the track & field club at the University of Yamanashi (sprinters, hurdlers, and long jumpers) and engage in regular physical activity (1-2 h per day, 3-5 days per week). None of the subjects had been exposed to an altitude higher than 1500 m within the six months prior to the study. All subjects were nonsmokers and had no prior history of cardiovascular disease (i.e., hypertension, diabetes, or hyperlipidemia) or orthopedic disease. After receiving a detailed explanation of the study, including the procedures, possible risks, and benefits of participation, each subject signed an informed consent form.

2.2. Control of Diet and Physical Activity. Throughout the study, including the washout period (*please refer to the experimental procedures*), the subjects were asked to avoid alcohol consumption and were only allowed to drink water. The diets consumed by the subjects on the night before the day of the study and the breakfast on the day of the study (when resistance exercise was performed in normoxia or hypoxia) were controlled. Briefly, the same dinner (containing: energy 967 kcal, protein 27 g, fat 30.5 g, carbohydrate 146 g, and sodium 1457 mg) and breakfast (energy 320 kcal, protein 3 g, fat 0 g, carbohydrate 80 g, and sodium 112 mg) were prepared for all the subjects. Strenuous exercise was prohibited 48 h before each main study session.

2.3. Experimental Procedures. The subjects were requested to abstain from caffeinated beverages for 12 h before each session and from strenuous exercise and alcohol for 24 h before each session. Throughout all the study sessions, we carefully controlled the room temperature at 20 ± 1°C to prevent the effects of change in BP, and external stimuli were minimized. All subjects performed two trials: (a) normobaric normoxic exercise (room air; equivalent altitude to 400 m) and (b) normobaric hypoxic exercise (fraction of inspired oxygen: $FiO_2 = 0.13$). These two trials were performed in a random order and at the same time (8:30 -11:30) of the day to avoid the effect of the circadian rhythm, with at least a 1-week washout period. During this washout period, the subjects were asked to maintain their usual life and to avoid strenuous exercise. In the hypoxic trial, a 5-minute normoxic sitting rest condition was set while breathing room air. After this period, a 10-minute sitting and a 5-minute standing rest, followed by the bilateral leg squat exercise, was set while breathing hypoxic gas ($FiO_2 = 0.13$). Thereafter, a 60-minute sitting recovery was set while breathing room air (Figure 1). Hypoxic gas was supplied via a 200 liter Douglas bag reservoir through a two-way, nonrebreathing valve and face mask using a hypoxic generator system (Hypoxico Everest Summit II: Will Co., Ltd., Tokyo, Japan), as previously reported in our recent study [22]. The inspired oxygen concentration was verified before and after each experiment (AE-310; Minato Medical Science, Osaka, Japan). In the normoxic trial, the same protocol as the hypoxic trial was adopted, but the subjects breathed room air throughout the study. The resistance exercise consisted of bilateral leg squats (1 repetition/2 sec) at 50% of 1-RM for eight sets with 1-minute intervals based on a previous study [21] and preliminary test in our laboratory. During the first five sets, they performed 14 reps, while during the last three sets, they performed seven reps. Thus, there was a total of 91 reps for the leg squats (14 reps × 5 sets plus 7 reps × 3 sets). The 1-RM trials were designed using increments of 10 kg until 60–80% of the perceived maximum was reached. The load was then gradually increased by small weights (2.5–5 kg) until lift fail, which was defined as the participant's failure to maintain proper form or to completely lift the weight. Proper technique and a complete range of motion were required for each successful 1-RM trial [23]. For further confirmation, each subject repeated the 1-RM trails, and we confirmed the same 1-RM for all the subjects. No injuries were observed during the 1-RM testing. This test was performed 1 week before the main study. The last acceptable lift with the highest possible load was determined as 1-RM.

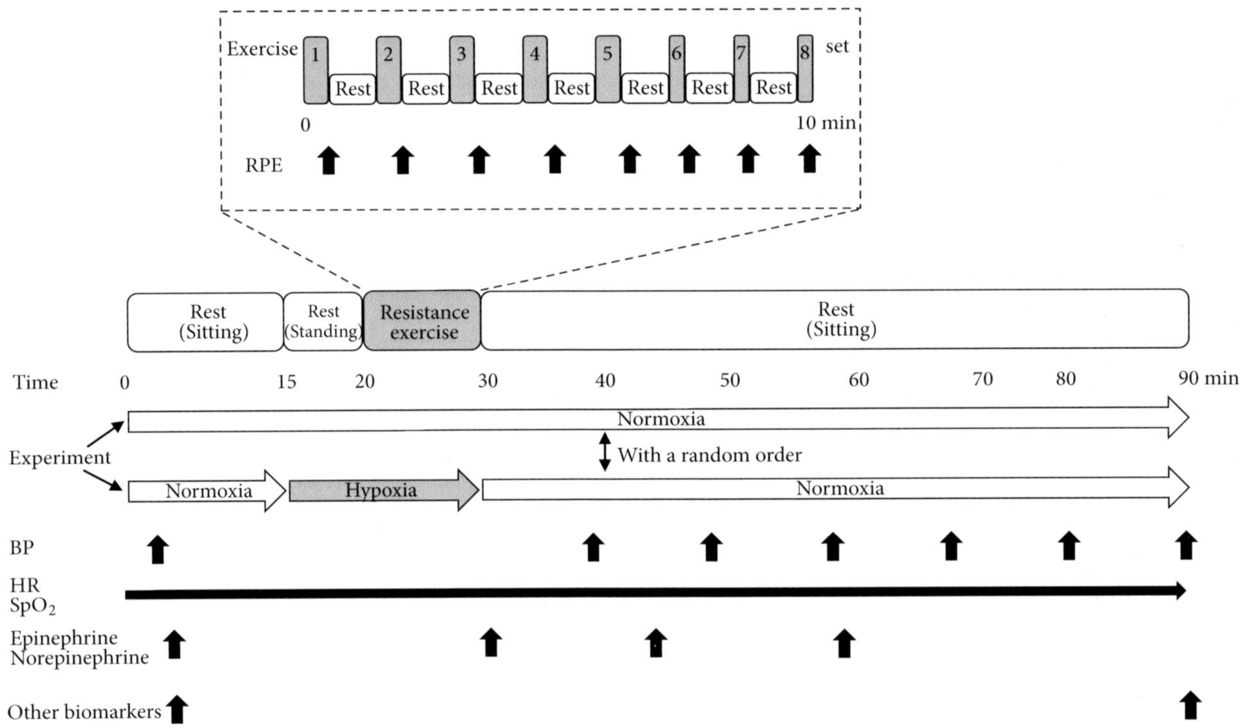

FIGURE 1: Experimental protocol of the present study. BP: blood pressure, HR: heart rate, and SpO_2: arterial oxygen saturation. RPE: rate of perceived exertion. Black arrows indicate measuring points and periods.

2.4. Measurements. BP was measured by the oscillometric method (HEM-907, OMRON, Tokyo, Japan) at baseline (pre-exercise) and at 10, 20, 30, 40, 50, and 60 min after exercise. At rest, BP was measured twice, and the average BP of the two measurements was considered as the subject's BP value. We also confirmed that the difference in the SBP or DBP was < 5mmHg compared to the values of one before measurement at rest [24]. According to the technical details provided by the manufacture (Omron, Co., Ltd., Tokyo, Japan), this device can adjust for different arm circumference (e.g., using different width of cuffs). Indeed, the validity of this device (e.g., the values of repeated measurements were different by < 5 mmHg) has been confirmed in previous studies [25–27]. During 60 min recovery period, BP was measured once to minimize the time course effect. Heart rate (HR) and arterial oxygen saturation (SpO_2) were continuously monitored using a wireless HR monitor (RS 800CX, Polar Electro, Japan) and automatic vital sensor (TM-256, A&D, Tokyo, Japan), respectively, throughout the experiment.

2.5. Blood Sampling and Analysis. Venous blood samples (20 ml) were taken from the antecubital vein at baseline and after 60 min of recovery. Samples were immediately centrifuged at 3000 rpm for 15 min at 4°C (MX-300 Tomy Seiko Co, Ltd., Tokyo, Japan) to separate the plasma and serum and were then frozen at -80°C for further analysis of the antidiuretic hormone (ADH), aldosterone, human atrial natriuretic peptide (hANP), adenosine, osmotic pressure (OSM), and free fatty acid (FFA) by SRL Co. Ltd. (Tokyo, Japan).

2.6. Data Analysis. The mean arterial pressure (MAP) was calculated using the following:

$$\text{MAP} = \frac{[\text{systolic BP (SBP)} - \text{diastolic BP (DBP)}]}{3} + \text{DBP} \quad (1)$$

The values of HR and SpO_2 were adopted at baseline, immediately after each set of leg squats and after 1, 2, 5, 10, 20, 30, 40, 50, and 60 min of recovery for further analysis. These values were averaged during the last 1 min at sitting baseline and during the 10 s immediately after each exercise and each recovery period.

2.7. Statistics. The values are expressed as the mean ± SD. Two-way repeated-measures with pairwise (Dunnet) post hoc tests were used to evaluate the changes in all physiological variables across different oxygen levels. First, as these variables were continuous variables, we analyzed them as parametric dataset. However, the sample size was small; therefore, equal variance failed in the variables, and Friedman nonparametric and pairwise (Scheffe) post hoc tests were used. The Spearman correlation coefficient was used for the relationship between changes in the MAP and HR from baseline to the values during recovery periods. A P value of less than 0.05 was considered statistically significant. Statistical analyses were performed using commercial software packages (Sigma Stat 3.5; Hulinks, Chicago, IL, USA).

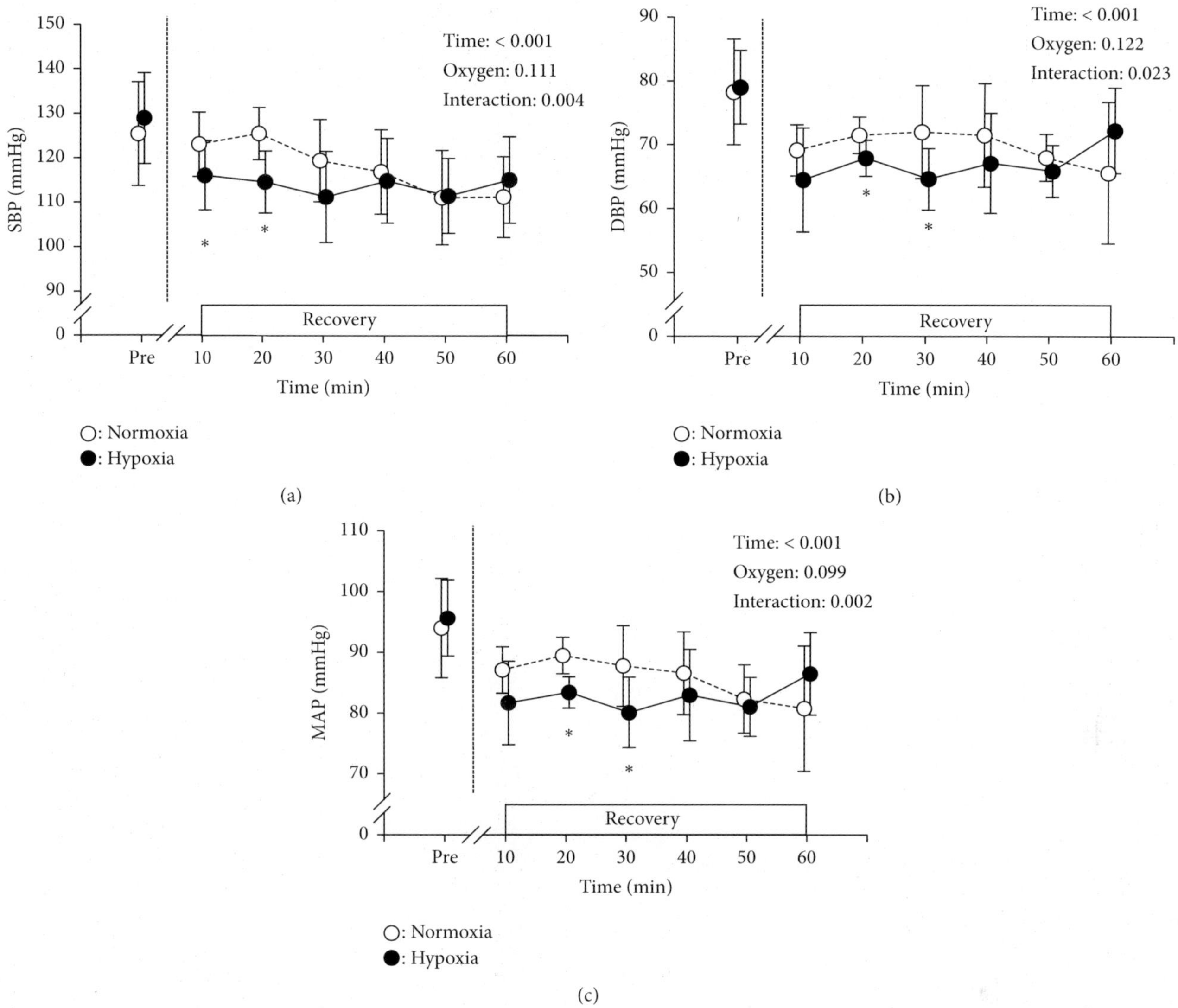

FIGURE 2: Changes in systolic blood pressure (SBP: panel (a)), diastolic blood pressure (DBP: panel (b)), and mean arterial blood pressure (MAP: panel (c)) at baseline (pre) and during 60 min recovery under normoxia (open circles) and hypoxia (closed circles). * indicates a significant difference between normoxia and hypoxia within the same time period.

3. Results

The changes in BP variables are shown in Figure 2. There were no significant differences in the pre-exercise values of SBP, DBP, and MAP between normoxia and hypoxia. Significant main effect for time and interaction (time × oxygen) was observed for all BP variables. The SBP after 10 and 20 min of recovery in hypoxia was significantly lower than in normoxia ($P < 0.05$). Similarly, the DBP and MAP after 20 and 30 min of recovery in hypoxia were also lower than in normoxia ($P < 0.05$). Moreover, the SBP after 30 min and the MAP after 10 min of recovery in hypoxia showed lower values than in normoxia ($P < 0.1$).

The HR during the first five sets of exercise increased from about 150 bpm to 175 bpm, while they decreased slightly during the last three sets to ~160 bpm. After eight sets of exercise, the HR decreased acutely within the first 2 min and then decreased gradually until 60 min after exercise. There were no significant differences in HR at any of the time points between normoxia and hypoxia (Figure 3(a)). SpO_2 decreased ~10% during exercise in the normoxic trial and ~20% in the hypoxic trial. During recovery, the SpO_2 in both trials recovered to baseline values within 1 min. There were significant differences in SpO_2 between trials for each exercise set, but no differences were observed at baseline or during recovery (Figure 3(b)).

Table 1 shows the biomarker changes between normoxia and hypoxia. A significant main effect for time (pre vs. post) was observed in ADH, aldosterone, hANP, and OSM ($P < 0.05$). Additionally, a significant main effect for the condition (normoxia vs. hypoxia) was observed in ADH, resulting in the values for ADH after exercise in hypoxia being significantly higher than in normoxia.

The baseline values (pre-exercise) for both epinephrine and norepinephrine showed similar values between conditions. Immediately after exercise, both values remarkably

Table 1: Blood biomarkers between pre- and poststudy in two different oxygen conditions.

		Normoxia	Hypoxia	Time	Oxygen	Interaction
ADH, pg ml^{-1}	Pre	1.48 ± 1.56	1.59 ± 1.16	0.015	0.023	0.220
	Post	2.35 ± 1.39†	3.44 ± 2.27*†			
Aldosterone, pg ml^{-1}	Pre	153 ± 38	161 ± 26	<0.001	0.401	0.336
	Post	267 ± 83†	313 ± 87†			
hANP, pg ml^{-1}	Pre	16.5 ± 7.6	16.1 ± 7.4	0.024	0.966	0.456
	Post	11.8 ± 3.1†	12.5 ± 4.6†			
Adenosine, u l^{-1}	Pre	20.6 ± 8.7	19.3 ± 7.0	0.844	0.350	0.429
	Post	20.9 ± 8.2	19.2 ± 6.1			
OSM, mOsm kgH20^{-1}	Pre	283 ± 1	285 ± 2	0.007	0.361	0.402
	Post	280 ± 2†	280 ± 4†			
Free fatty acid, μEq L^{-1}	Pre	100.4 ± 52.8	94.8 ± 74.0	0.104	0.071	0.204
	Post	207.4 ± 151.5	126.1 ± 61.9			

Values are mean ± standard deviation. ADH: antidiuretic hormone (vasopressin); hANP: human atrial natriuretic peptide. OSM: osmotic pressure. $^{*}P < 0.05$ between normoxia and hypoxia within the post.
$^{\dagger}P < 0.05$ between pre and post within the same condition.

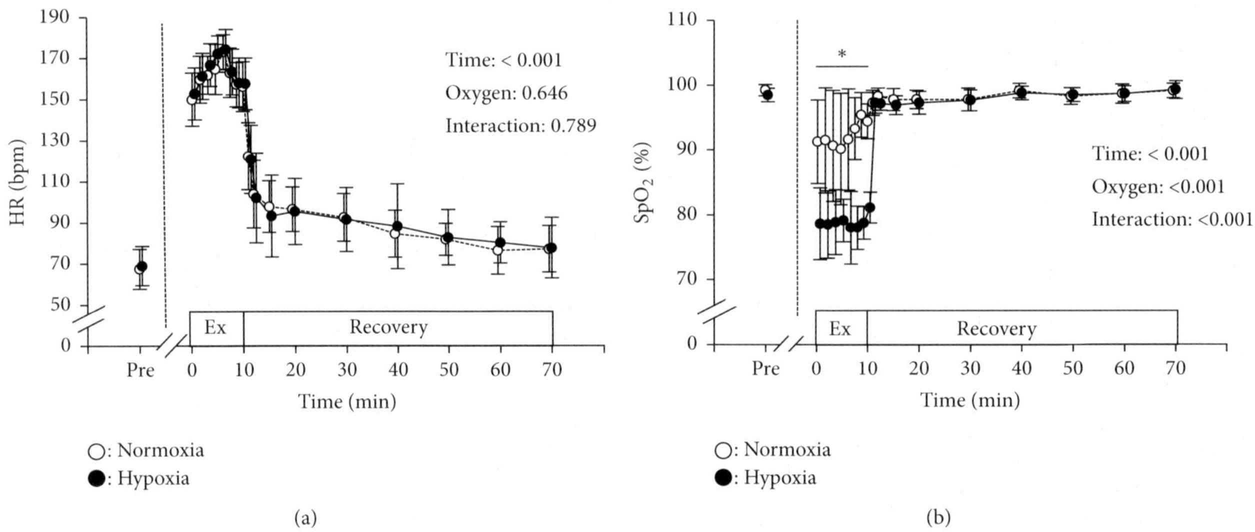

Figure 3: Changes in HR (panel (a)) and SpO_2 (panel (b)) at baseline (pre) and during exercise and recovery. Circles indicate the same as in Figure 2. * indicates a significant difference between normoxia and hypoxia within the same time period.

increased fourfold over the pre-exercise values; thereafter, both parameters decreased in accordance with time changes. No significant differences were observed between trials at any point (Figure 4). Summarized results of the statistical analysis [i.e., F values, effect size (partial η^2) and statistical power (1-β)] of the biomarkers and BP variables are shown in Table 2.

Changes in the MAP from the baseline values during recovery were related to the changes in HR from the baseline values during recovery in normoxia when all data were included (6 points during recovery × 8 participants = 48 plots, Figure 5(a)); however, this correlation was not statistically significant in hypoxia (Figure 5(b)).

4. Discussion

To the best of our knowledge, this is the first study to investigate the influence of resistance exercise under hypoxia on postexercise hemodynamics. The major findings of the present study were threefold: (1) the reductions in BP and the increases in ADH responses during recovery after resistance exercise were greater in hypoxia than in normoxia, (2) the HR responses throughout the study were similar between normoxia and hypoxia, and (3) the changes in HR from the baseline values during the recovery period were associated with the MAP changes in normoxia, but this relationship was not observed in hypoxia. Collectively, these results suggest

TABLE 2: Summarized results of statistical analysis in the subset of outcomes.

		F value			Effect size (partial η^2)			Power (1-β)		
	df	Time	Oxygen	Interaction	Time	Oxygen	Interaction	Time	Oxygen	Interaction
ADH	(1, 7)	8.408	10.365	1.815	0.546	0.597	0.206	0.702	0.788	0.215
Aldosterone	(1, 7)	44.125	0.800	1.066	0.863	0.103	0.132	0.999	0.122	0.146
hANP	(1, 7)	8.262	0.002	0.622	0.541	0.000	0.082	0.695	0.050	0.105
Adenosine	(1, 7)	0.042	1.001	0.704	0.006	0.125	0.091	0.054	0.140	0.113
OSM	(1, 7)	14.044	0.955	0.798	0.667	0.120	0.102	0.893	0.136	0.121
Free fatty acid	(1, 7)	3.495	4.542	1.966	0.333	0.394	0.219	0.366	0.452	0.229
Epinephrine	(3, 21)	18.527	1.327	1.045	0.726	0.159	0.130	1.000	0.170	0.243
Norepinephrine	(3, 21)	92.469	0.035	0.078	0.930	0.005	0.011	1.000	0.053	0.062
SBP	(6, 42)	9.464	3.316	3.761	0.575	0.321	0.350	1.000	0.350	0.933
DBP	(6, 42)	6.451	3.088	2.768	0.480	0.306	0.283	0.997	0.330	0.824
MAP	(6, 42)	8.661	3.629	4.370	0.553	0.341	0.384	1.000	0.377	0.966

df: degree of freedom.

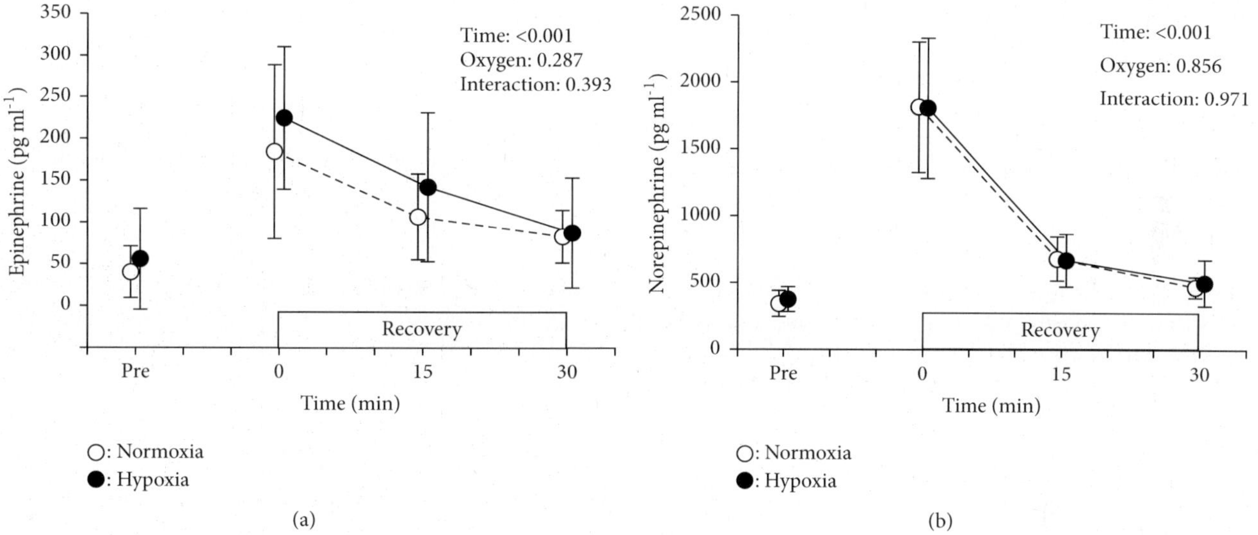

FIGURE 4: Changes in plasma epinephrine (panel (a)) and norepinephrine (panel (b)) at baseline (pre), immediately after resistance exercise (time = 0) and during the first 30 min of recovery. Circles indicate the same as in Figure 2.

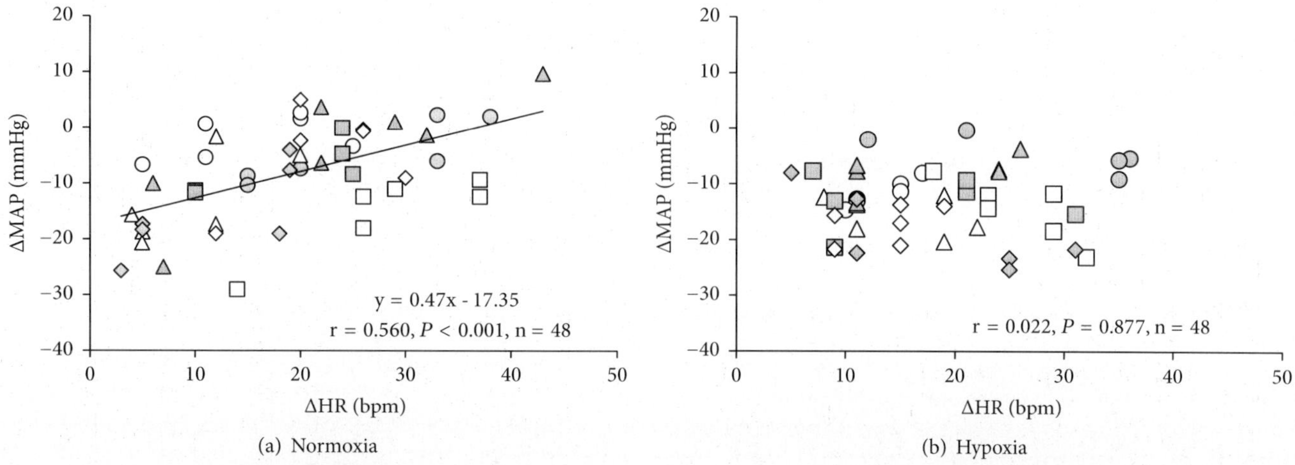

FIGURE 5: Relationship between changes in MAP and HR under normoxia (panel (a)) and hypoxia (panel (b)) when all data points during the recovery period are pooled. The changes in MAP and HR were calculated between the baseline values and each recovery period (10, 20, 30, 40, 50, and 60 min). Different symbols indicate each subject.

that hypoxic resistance exercise caused greater hypotension after exercise and increased in ADH responses. From observing the results of the relation between HR and MAP during recovery periods, the underlying mechanisms of PEH after resistance exercise may be different between normoxia and hypoxia.

Since MAP is a functional product of cardiac output (HR × stroke volume [SV]) and systemic vascular resistance (SVR), it may at first be reasonable to focus on these two basic components (three parameters). Previous studies have demonstrated controversial findings regarding how these parameters (i.e., cardiac output [CO], SV, and SVR) change after resistance exercise. Some studies found that CO decreased [6, 7, 9, 10], probably due to reductions in SV [7, 9, 10], while one study showed unchanged CO [8]. On the other hand, it was reported that SVR increased [6], remained unchanged [8, 10], or decreased [7] after resistance exercise. Unfortunately, these previous studies were conducted in normoxia and not hypoxia [6–10]; in the present study, we assessed only HR and did not find any differences between trials. Therefore, it is uncertain whether reductions in CO (including SV) and/or SVR caused greater hypotension in hypoxia. However, a previous study reported that there were no differences in HR, SV, and CO between normoxia and hypoxia after exercise [28]. Additionally, it has been reported that endothelial mediated vasodilation was greater in hypoxia than in normoxia after exercise [29]. Although we did not measure blood flow, meaning without parameters of SVR (i.e., MAP/blood flow), there may be a possibility that the greater postexercise hypotension in hypoxia in the present study might be induced by reductions in SVR. It may be worth mentioning that the relationship between the changes in MAP and HR differed between trials despite similar HR responses *per se* in both trials. All the previously mentioned studies above found increases in HR during recovery after resistance exercise, which suggests that this increased HR during the hypotensive period may play an important role in maintaining BP, namely, the prevention of syncope after exercise. A positive relation between these parameters, which was observed in the normoxia trial, may indicate that reductions in MAP are compensated for by a higher HR, while other mechanisms should be considered in the hypoxia trial. Our analysis included all data (i.e., all the subjects and time points); however, interindividual and intraindividual variations should be considered in future studies.

The hypoxia trial led to greater ADH secretion than the normoxia trial. A classic hemodynamics study reported that ADH increased to about two times the pre-exercise level after treadmill walking [30]. Furthermore, it has been reported that acute hypoxic exposure may produce significant hypotension with consequent increased plasma arginine vasopressin (i.e., increased ADH) [31]. Therefore, our results may be partly supported by these studies. In contrast, a subsequent study reported that release of arginine vasopressin was unaffected by hypoxia *per se* (i.e., at resting condition); moreover, arginine vasopressin increased during exercise, and its release was primarily stimulated by increased OSM [32]. Although the study settings of previous studies and the present study were completely different, the results of OSM in the preset study that showed significant decreases from the prevalues in both normoxia and hypoxia seemed inconsistent. We must acknowledge that measured points were only before exercise and 60 min after exercise and, therefore, further explanation about the relationship among changes in MAP, ADH, and OSM during this longer period (more than 60 min) cannot be obtained at this stage. Another concern is the longer exposure in hypoxia. In the present study, the subjects were exposed to hypoxia for ~ 90 min (13% FiO_2). Similar long exposure to hypoxia ~60 min (10.5% FiO_2) was present in a previous study [31], while a relatively shorter period of exposure to hypoxia with exercise ~20 min (13% FiO_2) was reported in another study [32]. Therefore, our results indicated that longer exposure to hypoxia could be a secondary effect of hypoxia, including greater release of ADH and greater reductions in BP after resistance exercise that was in the previous study [31]. Nonetheless, we did not find any significant association or causal relationship between changes in the BP and ADH; therefore, future studies that explore this subject are warranted.

With regard to other biomarkers, we obtained confusing findings. Previous hemodynamic studies highlighted the potential role of exaggerated circulating epinephrine levels in syncope under hypoxia [33, 34]. Indeed, fourfold higher epinephrine levels were found at the onset of hypotension in hypoxia [35]. Moreover, exaggerated circulating epinephrine levels may have been linked with skeletal muscle vasodilation and/or vasodilation or splanchnic circulation [36, 37]. In the present study, the epinephrine and norepinephrine levels immediately after exercise were fourfold higher than the baseline values, but there were no statistical differences between normoxia and hypoxia.

One difficulty in interpreting our results against the previous studies is that we did not assess orthostatic tolerance and no subjects claimed (pre) syncope symptoms throughout the study. By contrast, hANP and adenosine, which are potent vasodilators, decreased or remained unchanged and there were no differences between the trials. These may also be difficulties in interpreting the BP responses during recovery in the present study. However, as the circulating half-life of ANP is only 2-3 min, it is questionable whether hANP release may relate to BP responses [38]. In addition, a previous study reported that decreased BP after exercise was not directly related to the release of ANP [39]. It was also reported that adenosine is responsible for vasodilation during the initial phase after ischemic exercise in dogs, but the re-uptake of adenosine is very rapid following exercise [40]. It is well known that the renin–angiotensin–aldosterone system is a hormone system that regulates BP and fluid balance. Briefly, renin is released from the kidneys during low perfusion pressure; thereafter, it converts angiotensin to angiotensin I, followed by angiotensin II, which is a powerful vasoconstrictor. Angiotensin II also stimulates the secretion of the hormone aldosterone [41]. We found significant increases in aldosterone after 60 min of recovery, but there were no differences in the aldosterone levels between the trials. A classic hemodynamic study found that aldosterone levels increased ~twofold at 15 min after exercise [30]. Therefore, although this is highly speculative with regard to the hypotension period, decreased hANP and increased aldosterone levels may prevent further reductions in BP (i.e., the prevention of syncope).

However, these biomarker results (i.e., epinephrine, norepinephrine, hANP, adenosine, and aldosterone responses) may not account for the different BP regulation between normoxia and hypoxia; therefore, further results are required. Since higher levels of FFA in rats, following acute infusion into the portal vein, mediate the pressor response [42], there may be a possibility that the FFA levels affected the BP response during recovery in the present study. Indeed, a previous study demonstrated that both the FFA and the BP variables increased in parallel after a heparin infusion activated lipoprotein lipase activity and facilitated the turnover of triglycerides to FFAs [43]. In the present study, we found that oxygen, time, and, interaction had no significant effect on the FFA levels; however, the FFA in both trials increased slightly and showed a lower trend in hypoxia 60 min post-recovery. Therefore, our results for BP can be partly explained by previous studies. We must acknowledge that this is also speculative, and we should assesse glucose and lipid metabolism directly in future studies.

4.1. Methodological Considerations. There are several limitations in interpreting the results of the present study. First, the relatively small sample size should be considered. Thus, based on our previous study [24], we also conducted post hoc power analysis for pairwise comparisons that were observed with significant differences in variables (i.e., SBP, DBP, MAP, and ADH) as the standard of 80% power with a two-sided significance level of 0.05 (G Power 3.1). We estimated that a sample size of eight would have been necessary to achieve the appropriate statistical power for BP comparisons (SBP at 10 min and 20 min and DBP and MAP at 20 min and 30 min), while 13 subjects would have been required for ADH values postexercise. However, 7 of the 8 subjects showed higher ADH values in hypoxia than in normoxia, and the statistical power was high enough for the BP variables. Although future studies are required, it is unlikely that additional data will strongly affect our conclusions. Second, we recruited only young males in this study. It is therefore uncertain whether our results can be generalized to other populations, such as females and aged people. Similarly, the lack of differences in the physical fitness level of the study subjects should be considered to account for individual differences in future studies. Finally, the precise mechanisms causing greater hypotension after hypoxic resistance exercise than after normoxic resistance exercise are still unclear. We cannot account for this, and therefore the assessment of other potential candidates for influencing BP regulation (e.g., cardiac output, vascular resistance, baroreflex sensitivity, and various vasodilator substances [e.g., nitric oxide, prostaglandins, ATP, and histamine]), alterations in muscle metabolism, and the promotion of angiogenesis may be required in future studies [2, 44].

5. Conclusion

Our results demonstrate that bilateral leg squats in hypoxia elicit greater hypotension during recovery than in normoxia. Moreover, ADH release was greater during the recovery period in hypoxia than in normoxia. Changes in HR from baseline during recovery from baseline were related to changes in MAP only in normoxia. These results suggest that the higher HR values during recovery may compensate for hypotension only in normoxia; thus, the underlying mechanisms for the attenuation of hypotension after resistance exercise may differ between normoxia and hypoxia. These findings could help explain the increased risk of syncope after resistance exercise at high-altitudes.

Acknowledgments

The authors thank all participants for their time and effort. They also offer thanks to Miss Yumi Asakawa and Mr. Masataka Kiuchi for their technical assistance. This study was financially supported in part by Japan Society for the Promotion of Science (26440268JP to Masahiro Horiuchi, 17K01757 to Katsuhiro Koyama).

References

[1] J. R. MacDonald, "Potential causes, mechanisms, and implications of post exercise hypotension," *Journal of Human Hypertension*, vol. 16, no. 4, pp. 225–236, 2002.

[2] J. R. Halliwill, "Mechanisms and Clinical Implications of Post-exercise Hypotension in Humans," *Exercise and Sport Sciences Reviews*, vol. 29, no. 2, pp. 65–70, 2001.

[3] M. J. Kenney and D. R. Scals, "Postexercise hypotension: Key features, mechanisms, and clinical significance," *Hypertension*, vol. 22, no. 5, pp. 653–664, 1993.

[4] A. Hecksteden, T. Grütters, and T. Meyer, "Association between postexercise hypotension and long-term training-induced blood pressure reduction: A pilot study," *Clinical Journal of Sport Medicine: Official Journal of the Canadian Academy of Sport Medicine*, vol. 23, no. 1, pp. 58–63, 2013.

[5] S. A. M. Liu, J. Goodman, R. Nolan, S. Lacombe, and S. G. Thomas, "Blood pressure responses to acute and chronic exercise are related in prehypertension," *Medicine & Science in Sports & Exercise*, vol. 44, no. 9, pp. 1644–1652, 2012.

[6] L. Teixeira, R. M. Ritti-Dias, T. Tinucci, D. Mion Jr., and C. L. De Moraes Forjaz, "Post-concurrent exercise hemodynamics and cardiac autonomic modulation," *European Journal of Applied Physiology*, vol. 111, no. 9, pp. 2069–2078, 2011.

[7] A. C. C. Queiroz, J. C. S. Sousa, N. D. Silva et al., "Captopril does not Potentiate Post-Exercise Hypotension: A Randomized Crossover Study," *International Journal of Sports Medicine*, vol. 38, no. 4, pp. 270–277, 2017.

[8] A. C. Queiroz, J. C. Sousa, A. A. Cavalli et al., "Post-resistance exercise hemodynamic and autonomic responses: Comparison between normotensive and hypertensive men," *Scandinavian Journal of Medicine & Science in Sports*, vol. 25, pp. 486–494, 2015.

[9] A. C. C. Queiroz, C. C. Rezk, L. Teixeira, T. Tinucci, D. Mion, and C. L. M. Forjaz, "Gender influence on post-resistance exercise hypotension and hemodynamics," *International Journal of Sports Medicine*, vol. 34, no. 11, pp. 939–944, 2013.

[10] C. C. Rezk, R. C. B. Marrache, T. Tinucci, D. Mion Jr., and C. L. M. Forjaz, "Post-resistance exercise hypotension, hemodynamics, and heart rate variability: Influence of exercise intensity," *European Journal of Applied Physiology*, vol. 98, no. 1, pp. 105–112, 2006.

[11] J. Casonatto, K. F. Goessler, V. A. Cornelissen, J. R. Cardoso, and M. D. Polito, "The blood pressure-lowering effect of a single bout of resistance exercise: A systematic review and meta-analysis of randomised controlled trials," *European Journal of Preventive Cardiology*, vol. 23, no. 16, pp. 1700–1714, 2016.

[12] American College of Sports M, "American College of Sports Medicine position stand. Progression models in resistance training for healthy adults," *Medicine and Science in Sports and Exercise*, vol. 41, pp. 687–708, 2009.

[13] B. Yan, X. Lai, L. Yi, Y. Wang, and Y. Hu, "Effects of Five-Week Resistance Training in Hypoxia on Hormones and Muscle Strength," *The Journal of Strength and Conditioning Research*, vol. 30, no. 1, pp. 184–193, 2016.

[14] M. Kon, N. Ohiwa, A. Honda et al., "Effects of systemic hypoxia on human muscular adaptations to resistance exercise training," *Physiological Reports*, vol. 2, article e12033, 2014.

[15] J. R. Halliwill, D. C. Sieck, S. A. Romero, T. M. Buck, and M. R. Ely, "Blood pressure regulation X: What happens when the muscle pump is lost? Post-exercise hypotension and syncope," *European Journal of Applied Physiology*, vol. 114, no. 3, pp. 561–578, 2014.

[16] T. Mündel, B. G. Perry, P. N. Ainslie et al., "Postexercise orthostatic intolerance: Influence of exercise intensity," *Experimental Physiology*, vol. 100, no. 8, pp. 915–925, 2015.

[17] J. D. MacDougall, D. Tuxen, D. G. Sale, J. R. Moroz, and J. R. Sutton, "Arterial blood pressure response to heavy resistance exercise," *Journal of Applied Physiology*, vol. 58, no. 3, pp. 785–790, 1985.

[18] M. R. Edwards, D. H. Martin, and R. L. Hughson, "Cerebral hemodynamics and resistance exercise," *Medicine & Science in Sports & Exercise*, vol. 34, no. 7, pp. 1207–1211, 2002.

[19] S. A. Romero and W. H. Cooke, "Hyperventilation before resistance exercise: Cerebral hemodynamics and orthostasis," *Medicine & Science in Sports & Exercise*, vol. 39, no. 8, pp. 1302–1307, 2007.

[20] M. Horiuchi, S. Dobash, M. Kiuchi, J. Endo, K. Koyama, and A. W. Subudhi, "Reduction in cerebral oxygenation after prolonged exercise in hypoxia is related to changes in blood pressure," *Advances in Experimental Medicine and Biology*, vol. 876, pp. 95–100, 2016.

[21] M. Kon, T. Ikeda, T. Homma, and Y. Suzuki, "Effects of low-intensity resistance exercise under acute systemic hypoxia on hormonal responses," *The Journal of Strength and Conditioning Research*, vol. 26, no. 3, pp. 611–617, 2012.

[22] M. Horiuchi, Y. Fukuoka, Y. Handa, D. Abe, and H. Pontzer, "Measuring the Energy of Ventilation and Circulation during Human Walking using Induced Hypoxia," *Scientific Reports*, vol. 7, article e4938, 2017.

[23] T. Suga, K. Okita, N. Morita et al., "Intramuscular metabolism during low-intensity resistance exercise with blood flow restriction," *Journal of Applied Physiology*, vol. 106, no. 4, pp. 1119–1124, 2009.

[24] M. Horiuchi, S. Oda, T. Uno, J. Endo, Y. Handa, and Y. Fukuoka, "Effects of short-term acclimatization at the summit of Mt. Fuji (3776 m) on sleep efficacy, cardiovascular responses, and ventilatory responses," *High Altitude Medicine & Biology*, vol. 18, no. 2, pp. 171–178, 2017.

[25] K. Gurpreet, G. H. Tee, and C. Karuthan, "Evaluation of the accuracy of the Omron Hem - 907 blood pressure device," *Medical Journal of Malaysia*, vol. 63, no. 3, pp. 239–243, 2008.

[26] S. Omboni, I. Riva, A. Giglio, G. Caldara, A. Groppelli, and G. Parati, "Validation of the Omron M5-I, R5-I and HEM-907 automated blood pressure monitors in elderly individuals according to the international protocol of the European society of hypertension," *Blood Pressure Monitoring*, vol. 12, no. 4, pp. 233–242, 2007.

[27] W. B. White and Y. A. Anwar, "Evaluation of the overall efficacy of the Omron office digital blood pressure HEM-907 monitor in adults," *Blood Pressure Monitoring*, vol. 6, no. 2, pp. 107–110, 2001.

[28] E. M. Snyder, T. P. Olson, B. D. Johnson, and R. P. Frantz, "Influence of sildenafil on lung diffusion during exposure to acute hypoxia at rest and during exercise in healthy humans," *European Journal of Applied Physiology*, vol. 103, no. 4, pp. 421–430, 2008.

[29] K. Katayama, O. Fujita, M. Iemitsu et al., "The effect of acute exercise in hypoxia on flow-mediated vasodilation," *European Journal of Applied Physiology*, vol. 113, no. 2, pp. 349–357, 2013.

[30] R. Wilcox, T. Bennett, I. Macdonald, B. F. Pipkin, and P. Baylis, "Post-exercise hypotension: the effects of epanolol or atenolol on some hormonal and cardiovascular variables in hypertensive men," *British Journal of Clinical Pharmacology*, vol. 24, no. 2, pp. 151–162, 1987.

[31] M. P. Heyes, M. O. Farber, F. Manfredi et al., "Acute effects of hypoxia on renal and endocrine function in normal humans," *The American Journal of Physiology*, vol. 243, no. 3, pp. R265–R270, 1982.

[32] A. Takamata, H. Nose, T. Kinoshita, M. Hirose, T. Itoh, and T. Morimoto, "Effect of acute hypoxia on vasopressin release and intravascular fluid during dynamic exercise in humans," *American Journal of Physiology-Regulatory, Integrative and Comparative Physiology*, vol. 279, no. 1, pp. R161–R168, 2000.

[33] J. R. Halliwill, "Hypoxic regulation of blood flow in humans: Skeletal muscle circulation and the role of epinephrine," *Advances in Experimental Medicine and Biology*, vol. 543, pp. 223–236, 2003.

[34] J. R. Halliwill and C. T. Minson, "Cardiovagal regulation during combined hypoxic and orthostatic stress: Fainters vs. nonfainters," *Journal of Applied Physiology*, vol. 98, no. 3, pp. 1050–1056, 2005.

[35] F. A. Dinenno, M. J. Joyner, and J. R. Halliwill, "Failure of systemic hypoxia to blunt α-adrenergic vasoconstriction in the human forearm," *The Journal of Physiology*, vol. 549, no. 3, pp. 985–994, 2003.

[36] L. B. Rowell and J. R. Blackmon, "Hypotension induced by central hypovolaemia and hypoxaemia," *Clinical Physiology*, vol. 9, no. 3, pp. 269–277, 1989.

[37] R. G. J. Westendorp, G. J. Blauw, M. Frölich, and R. Simons, "Hypoxic syncope," *Aviation, Space, and Environmental Medicine*, vol. 68, no. 5, pp. 410–414, 1997.

[38] A. L. Davis, "Atrial natriuretic factor.," *Advances in Pediatrics*, vol. 36, pp. 137–150, 1989.

[39] J. R. MacDonald, J. D. MacDougall, S. A. Interisano et al., "Hypotension following mild bouts of resistance exercise and submaximal dynamic exercise," *European Journal of Applied Physiology and Occupational Physiology*, vol. 79, no. 2, pp. 148–154, 1999.

[40] H. V. Sparks, "Mechanism of vasodilation during and after ischemic exercise," *Federation Proceedings*, vol. 39, no. 5, pp. 1487–1490, 1980.

[41] M. Paul, A. P. Mehr, and R. Kreutz, "Physiology of local renin-angiotensin systems," *Physiological Reviews*, vol. 86, no. 3, pp. 747–803, 2006.

[42] R. J. Grekin, A. P. Vollmer, and R. S. Sider, "Pressor effects of portal venous oleate infusion: a proposed mechanism for obesity hypertension," *Hypertension*, vol. 26, no. 1, pp. 193–198, 1995.

[43] K. D. Monahan, D. J. Dyckman, and C. A. Ray, "Effect of acute hyperlipidemia on autonomic and cardiovascular control in humans," *Journal of Applied Physiology*, vol. 103, no. 1, pp. 162–169, 2007.

[44] J. R. Halliwill, T. M. Buck, A. N. Lacewell, and S. A. Romero, "Postexercise hypotension and sustained postexercise vasodilatation: What happens after we exercise?" *Experimental Physiology*, vol. 98, no. 1, pp. 7–18, 2013.

11

A Concept Mapping Study of Physicians' Perceptions of Factors Influencing Management and Control of Hypertension in Sub-Saharan Africa

Juliet Iwelunmor,[1] Sarah Blackstone,[1] Joyce Gyamfi,[2] Collins Airhihenbuwa,[3] Jacob Plange-Rhule,[4] Bamidele Tayo,[5] Richard Adanu,[4] and Gbenga Ogedegbe[2]

[1] *University of Illinois, Urbana-Champaign, Champaign, IL 61872, USA*
[2] *New York University, New York, NY 10016, USA*
[3] *Pennsylvania State University, State College, PA 16802, USA*
[4] *University of Ghana, Legon, Accra, Ghana*
[5] *Loyola University Chicago, Chicago, IL 60660, USA*

Correspondence should be addressed to Juliet Iwelunmor; jiwez@illinois.edu and Sarah Blackstone; blackst1@illinois.edu

Academic Editor: Roberto Pontremoli

Hypertension, once a rare problem in Sub-Saharan Africa (SSA), is predicted to be a major cause of death by 2020 with mortality rates as high as 75%. However, comprehensive knowledge of provider-level factors that influence optimal management is limited. The objective of the current study was to discover physicians' perceptions of factors influencing optimal management and control of hypertension in SSA. Twelve physicians attending the Cardiovascular Research Training (CaRT) Institute at the University of Ghana, College of Health Sciences, were invited to complete a concept mapping process that included brainstorming the factors influencing optimal management and control of hypertension in patients, sorting and organizing the factors into similar domains, and rating the importance and feasibility of efforts to address these factors. The highest ranked important and feasible factors include helping patients accept their condition and availability of adequate equipment to enable the provision of needed care. The findings suggest that patient self-efficacy and support, physician-related factors, policy factors, and economic factors are important aspects that must be addressed to achieve optimal hypertension management. Given the work demands identified by physicians, future research should investigate cost-effective strategies of shifting physician responsibilities to well-trained no-physician clinicians in order to improve hypertension management.

1. Introduction

Shortages in the health care workforce in Sub-Saharan Africa (SSA) have reached a crisis point [1–3], limiting effective reduction of hypertension related morbidity and mortality rates in patients [4]. In SSA, there are 2.4 million doctors and nurses, which translates to 2 doctors and 11 nursing/midwifery personnel per 10,000 people, compared to 19 doctors and 49 nursing/midwifery personnel per 10,000 in North America [5]. The shortage of health workers is partly due to brain drain or the movement of health personnel in search of a better standard of living, higher salaries, professional advancement opportunities, ready access to advanced technology, and more stable political conditions [2]. These shortages are a multifaceted problem, and improvements are needed if reduction in hypertension related morbidity in SSA is to be achieved.

By the year 2020, available evidence estimates that 75% of all deaths in SSA will be attributable to hypertension [6]. This startling statistic raises important questions about how to best mitigate barriers to optimal hypertension control in the region [7–11]. In SSA countries like Ghana, hypertension is now a major public health concern and the second leading cause of outpatient morbidity in adults aged 45 and above [7, 12–14]. The magnitude of the hypertension problem, including in-depth knowledge of underlying risk factors, remains incompletely understood [4]. Moreover, hypertension is increasing at alarming rates for reasons including urbanization, rapid migration from rural to urban areas, changes in dietary habits, aging of population, and social stress [9, 12, 15, 16]. Poorly managed hypertension also exacerbates the burden of chronic diseases such as stroke, end-stage renal disease, and heart failure, leading to increased morbidity and mortality rates in Africa [17, 18]. Also, knowledge and awareness of hypertension in SSA are alarmingly low, with only 6%–34% of hypertensive adults showing awareness of their status [12, 19, 20]. Although rates of hypertension treatment range from 28% in Ghana [12, 19] to roughly 80% in Nigeria [21, 22], actual rates of patients with maintained blood pressure control are as low as 2% [20].

Most of the existing literature to date in SSA related to hypertension management focuses exclusively on patients [23–25] and sheds little light on physicians' factors or attitudes likely to influence poor patient outcomes. Yet published literature conducted elsewhere suggests that physicians and patients differ substantially in their perceptions, knowledge, and/or attitudes which may lead to conflict or poor patient outcomes [26]. As a result, a better understanding of physicians' perceptions is needed to improve hypertension management in the region and improve quality of care. The purpose of the current study was to determine perceived physician-related barriers and/or facilitators to optimal management and control of hypertension in the region.

2. Methods

2.1. Participants. A group of physicians attending the Cardiovascular Research Training (CaRT) Institute at the University of Ghana, College of Health Sciences, was invited to participate in this study. The mission of CaRT is to train the next generation of researchers with expertise in cardiovascular epidemiology in SSA, social determinants of cardiovascular disease (CVD), comparative effectiveness research, community-based participatory research, and dissemination and implementation of community- and practice-based interventions targeted at cardiovascular risk reduction. The investigators met with physicians attending CaRT and explained that the goal of the project was to identify factors that influence optimal hypertension control in patients in Sub-Saharan Africa. Following consent, the investigative team asked participants to complete the concept mapping steps below using the Concept Systems Global Max software (Concept Systems, Inc., Ithaca, NY). Inclusion criteria for the study were participants being at least 18 years of age and participating in the CaRT training program. Twelve physicians participated in this study (nine from Nigeria and three from Ghana). Of these, ten were males and two were females. Number of years in practice ranged from six years to sixteen years. Smaller groups are more conducive to concept mapping methods, detailed below, which is the rationale for the small sample size [27].

2.2. Concept Mapping Methods. Concept mapping, a structured, participatory mixed-methods approach to data collection, was used to gather and interpret the ideas generated from physicians in the region. The main steps of concept mapping have been described extensively in the literature [27, 28]. It is a six-step process that integrates group process activities on a topic of interest with several multivariate quantitative analytical tools (multidimensional scaling and hierarchical cluster analysis) to yield both statistical and graphical representation of a conceptual domain [28]. Concept mapping procedures consist of five steps and then utilization of results as follows. (1) Preparation: the researchers outline the research goals and describe that the primary focus is participants' perceptions of factors influencing blood pressure management and control. (2) Generation: the researchers present participants with a focus prompt (e.g., a specific factor that influences blood pressure control is...). Participants generate several items that they believe are relevant to the focus prompt. The investigative team reviews the list to remove duplicates to create a final list of generated ideas. (3) Structuring: participants engage in sorting sessions, in which statements are grouped based on similarities into clusters identified and created by the participants. The sorting provides the data needed to generate clusters of factors that influence hypertension management. (4) Representation: computerized analyses are run and the data are summarized into concept maps. The results of the analysis are shared with participants to be examined and discussed. (5) Interpretation: participants are invited back to interpret the final cluster maps. These interpretation group discussions are designed to address the research goal of exploring factors that influence optimal management of blood pressure control in West Africa. See Figure 1 for an outlined process of concept mapping. Concept mapping is a unique approach that promotes "trustworthiness" in the analysis of qualitative data as it includes participants in all aspects of the research process [28, 29]. Also, the application of the quantitative tools provides structure and reliability to data generated through qualitative techniques [27, 29].

2.2.1. Brainstorming. The following prompt was used to elicit ideas from physicians: "*As a health care provider, a specific factor that affects your ability to control high blood pressure is...*"; brainstorming sessions were conducted online in order to promote candid responses and reduce potential desirability effects. In response to the focus statement, participants were asked to provide concise statements that described factors related to optimal hypertension management and control in patients. A total of 81 statements were generated by participants. The investigative team then distilled these into 54 distinct statements by eliminating duplicate statements, editing statements for clarity, or combining similar statements that reflected physicians' perceptions of factors influencing optimal management of hypertension.

2.2.2. Sorting and Rating. The statements from the brainstorming session were then randomly reordered for concept mapping sorting and rating steps. Physicians worked on

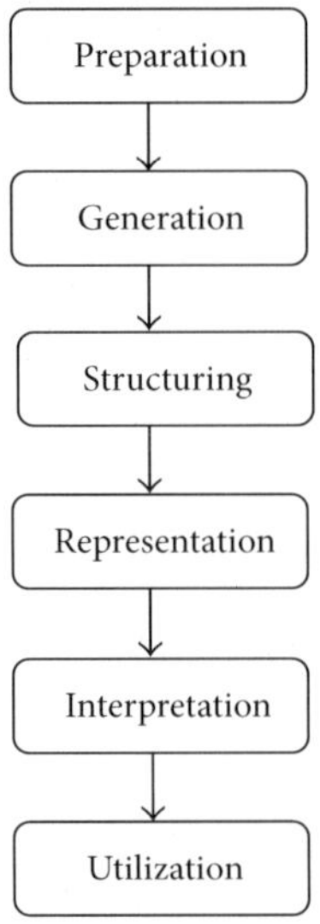

Figure 1: Steps involved in concept mapping procedures.

an individual basis to sort the statements into conceptually similar groups and were asked to rate the importance and feasibility of statements separately on a 5-point scale. Importance and feasibility were rated on a 5-point scale that ranged from, for importance, 1: relatively unimportant, to 5: extremely important, and, for feasibility, 1: not at all feasible, to 5: extremely feasible, compared to all other statements. For instance, for each statement physicians were asked, "how important is this to hypertension management" and "how feasible is this to address?" See Figure 2 for sample sorting.

2.3. Analysis. Concept Systems software was also used for analyzing data generated from the sorting and rating exercise. The software used multidimensional scaling (MDS) to create a two-dimensional "point map" that illustrates the distances between the statements generated for each set of sort data [27]. Aside from being used to structure the sort data, MDS does not independently influence the interpretation of results [29]. The MDS analysis is based on the measurement model that assumes that the relative similarity of objects can be represented in terms of the relative distance between pairs of points [30]. The two-dimensional "point map" is chosen for its ease and interpretability [31]. On the point map, items that are more similar based on participant appear closer together. We also calculated the "stress value" of the point map, which is a measure of how well the MDS solution maps the original data. A lower stress value indicates a better fit of the MDS point map to the original data [29]. Subsequently, we conducted hierarchical cluster analysis of the MDS coordinates and computed average rates of each statement and cluster of statements. This created a cluster map that partitions the statements on the point map into conceptual domains [27]. The maps that result show the individual statements in two-dimensional (x, y) space with more similar statements located nearer to each other and also show how the clusters partition the space on the map [28, 29]. Since there are no criteria by which a final number of clusters can be selected [29], investigators independently evaluated potential solutions (i.e., 6 clusters and 9 clusters) and agreed on the final model.

2.4. Interpretation. In the interpretation phase of concept mapping, we asked physicians to examine different cluster solutions to determine the best number of clusters and grouping of the statements. Clusters were created by participant feedback, based on the distance between items. Items that are closer together illustrate greater degrees of similarity and were sorted together by more people. Each cluster's content was examined for each cluster and discussed amongst participants. The process of determining final clusters was based on participants' subjective preferences. A seven-cluster solution was initially presented to the physicians because the statements within the clusters were conceptually similar to each other. Following further discussion, a four-cluster solution was considered to be visually superior in summarizing the results of the concept mapping. Finally, Go Zone matrices were created based on the final cluster map [27]. Go Zone matrices assign x- and y-axes to sets of data rated by the physicians where each statement is assigned coordinates based on its respective mean rating. Lines in the Go Zone matrix, which correspond to the mean rating for each axis, divide the graph into four quadrants (low/low, low/high, high/low, and high/high). For instance, items in the top right quadrant are those that were rated as highly important to hypertension management and feasible to address. Following the assumption that high ratings are ideal, the high/high quadrant is considered the Go Zone as it contains those ideas rated most highly on both criteria [32] (i.e., importance and feasibility for addressing patients' blood pressure).

3. Results

3.1. Cluster Map Solution and Interpretation. The four-cluster concept map generated is presented in Figure 1. Clusters include patient self-efficacy and support factors (20 statements), physician-related factors (14 statements), policy level factors (15 statements), and economic factors (5 statements). See Figure 3. The statements in the clusters are denoted by numbers in the figure and they correspond to the item numbers in Table 1.

Salient statements from the patient self-efficacy clusters included "*lack of patient compliance to therapies: diet, medication, physical activity, and stress management (workplace, home, etc.)*" (item number 3) and "*patients think hypertension is curable after some time on medication*" (item number 43). These statements also reflect physicians' doubt of patients' treatment efficacy. The cluster of physician-related factors reflects barriers and facilitators that physicians themselves may face with helping patients manage and control their hypertension. Two salient statements in the cluster: "*we do not adequately counsel our patients on ways to control their blood pressure*" (item number 9) and "*the failure of physicians to adopt a patient centered model in educating*

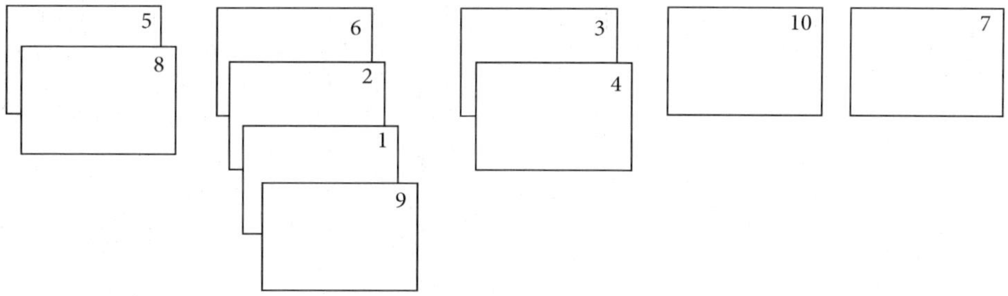

FIGURE 2: Hypothetical sorting exercise. Participants group statements into different piles based on similarities.

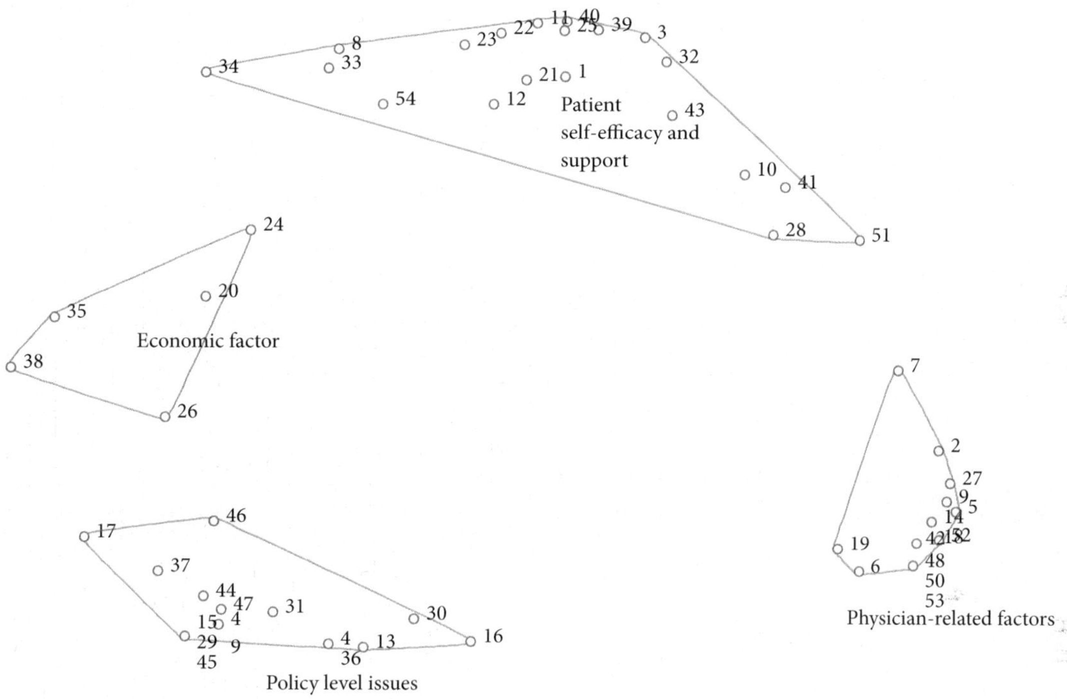

FIGURE 3: Final cluster map based on participant sorting. Each of the four clusters identified by physicians is represented. Numbers correspond to statements that were sorted into each category. Items that are closer together indicate higher degrees of similarity based on sorting.

patients about their conditions" (item number 14), highlight that physicians' attitudes towards hypertension management may be more important than their actual knowledge of the disease. Furthermore, statements in relation to workload (item number 46 "*high patient burden at hypertension clinics*") may also make it difficult to have good doctor-patient communication or engage in strategies such as patient counseling which would contribute to reduction in high blood pressure rates.

Policy level factors and economic factors reflect physician perceptions of barriers to hypertension management and control operating at the systems level which patients may have little or no control over [33]. For example, statements, such as "*primary healthcare systems are nonfunctional*" (item number 31) and "*the cost and availability of blood pressure drugs*" (item number 38), may affect the hypertension care outcome in patients or contribute to physician inertia that may have anticipated or unanticipated effects with hypertension awareness, treatment, control, and medication adherence in the region [33].

3.2. Go Zones. Figure 4 provides the Go Zones matrices for each of the four clusters. These statements were rated either above or below the mean for both importance and feasibility by the physicians. Of all the statements, the one rated highest for importance was item number 1: "*our patients are in denial and they fail to accept their condition,*" and the highest for feasibility is item number 13: "*we do not have the required equipment to provide the needed care for the management of high blood pressure.*" The statement that was ranked among the lowest for importance is item number 7: "*the age of the patient influences physicians ability to discuss blood pressure management.*" Two items were ranked as not feasible; both were patient related issues and they include item number 22: "*patients experience stress of modern day life,*" and item number 24: "*patients lack resources for follow-up care.*"

TABLE 1: Brainstorming statements sorted into their final clusters.

Cluster	Number	Statement (number corresponds to item number on cluster map)
(1) Patient self-efficacy and support	1	Our patients are in denial and they fail to accept their condition
	3	Lack of patient compliance to therapies: diet, medication, physical activity, and stress management (workplace, home, etc.)
	8	The influence of peers or other patients with hypertension
	10	Patients take multiple drugs
	11	Our patients are not conscious of the amount of salt in their diet
	12	The low educational level of our patients
	21	Patients use alternative medication such as herbal, traditional, and spiritual interventions for blood pressure
	22	Poor diet by patients
	23	Patients experience stress of modern day life
	25	Patient adoption of sedentary lifestyle
	28	Our patients do not understand the severity of the disease
	32	Patient nonadherence to medication
	33	Cultural and religious barriers to medication use
	34	Patients lack of family support with hypertension management
	39	The health behaviors of the patients themselves
	40	Patients increasingly patronize fast food
	41	Patients experience side effects of high blood pressure medications
	43	Patients think hypertension is curable after some time on medication
	51	Patients are unable to take the different types of medication given because they are many
	54	The preference for alternative medicines whose providers promise a cure rather than the control and lifetime management offered by physicians
(2) Physician-related issues	2	We do not address medication adherence with our patients
	5	We do not discuss lifestyle activities like physical activity with our patients for blood pressure control
	6	The inability of the physician to empathize and relate to/with his/her clients/patients
	7	The age of the patient influences physicians ability to discuss blood pressure management
	9	We do not adequately counsel our patients on ways to control their blood pressure
	14	The failure of physicians to adopt a patient centered model in educating patients about their conditions
	18	Our communication skills with our patients are poor which makes it difficult for them to comply with our instructions on blood pressure control
	19	Not involving patients in decisions on modalities of treatments
	27	We do not educate patients on the complications of hypertension
	42	Health workers knowledge of blood pressure control is limited
	48	The inability of physicians to identify comorbidities
	50	Physicians lack knowledge and skills which probably will result in lack of confidence to treat these conditions in patients
	52	Not taking into account patients opinion with regard to options for managing their blood pressure
	53	Inertia on the part of clinicians to alter medications to achieve blood pressure control targets
(3) Policy level issues	4	Lack of comprehensive treatment protocols in most centers
	13	We do not have the required equipment to provide the needed care for the management of high blood pressure
	15	The healthcare institutions do not have adequate facilities to provide proper blood pressure services
	16	Lack of adequate hospital follow-up
	17	The long distance between the patient's home and the hospital makes it difficult for follow-up

TABLE 1: Continued.

Cluster	Number	Statement (number corresponds to item number on cluster map)
	29	The use of inaccurate BP monitoring machine
	30	Lack of curricula as the ones available are largely based on infectious disease and little on conditions like hypertension
	31	Primary healthcare systems are nonfunctional
	36	The lack of standard protocol on blood pressure management in our primary health care systems
	37	The availability of the right medication
	44	The nonenforcement of standards of blood pressure treatment
	45	Sometimes, equipment required to measure the blood pressure is either not available or not functional
	46	High patient burden at hypertension clinics
	47	Lack of policy or protocol by the Nigerian health sector on blood pressure control
	49	Lack of standardization of blood pressure measurement in health care settings
	20	Patients paying out of pocket
	24	Patients lack resources for follow-up care
(4) Economic factors	26	Patients use fake drugs
	35	Patients cannot afford the required medication
	38	The cost and availability of blood pressure drugs

Statement numbers correspond to numbered items on cluster map.

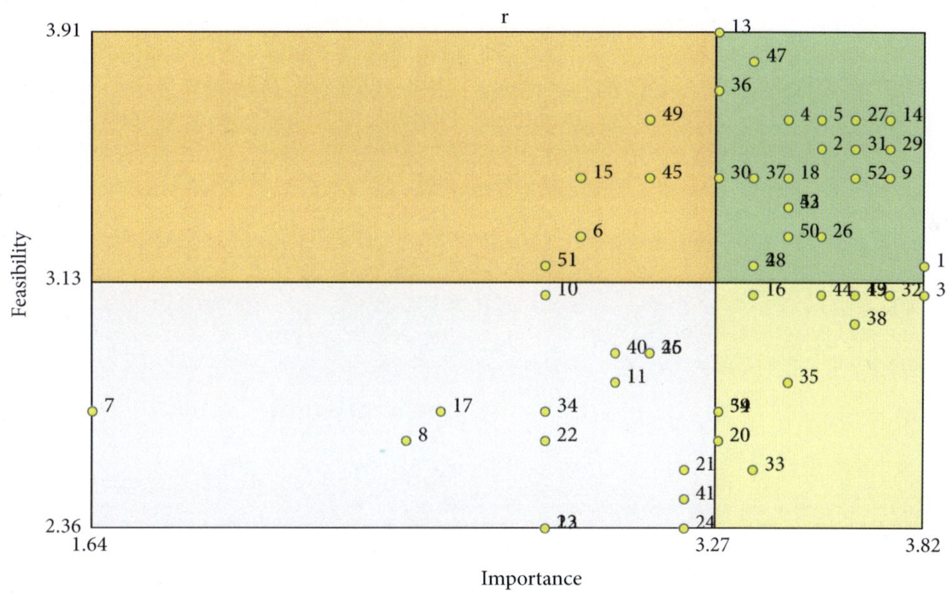

FIGURE 4: Go Zone analysis on importance and feasibility ratings by physicians. Items in the upper right quadrant represent those ranked highly in terms of importance and feasibility. Items in the lower right quadrant were ranked highly important, but not feasible. Each item number corresponds to the statement number in Table 1.

4. Discussion

Using concept mapping, this study examined physicians' perceptions of factors influencing hypertension management and control in patients in Sub-Saharan Africa. Unlike other methods of qualitative inquiry such as focus groups, concept mapping allows for a shared understanding of factors influencing optimal management and control of hypertension in patients through a wide range of physician generated statements and ideas. In total, 54 statements were generated and grouped into four clusters that reflect patient self-efficacy and support factors, physician-related factors, policy level factors, and economic factors.

Although physicians generally agreed on the importance and feasibility of these statements, it can be surmised from their ratings that two specific factors, namely, patient-related factors (i.e., the patient's ability to come to terms with their diagnosis of hypertension) and economic factors (access to medical resources/equipment for the management of hypertension), were regarded as the most important hurdles that are not too difficult or too costly to surmount. Particularly with regard to patients, failure to accept their condition and denial of hypertension were noted as the most important factor influencing patient adherence to medication and behavioral changes. This may be in part due to the lack of adequate patient counseling on blood pressure management as well as the failure to adopt a patient centered model, which were both noted as barriers to optimal blood pressure management in this study. It might also be inferred that high workload may preclude their engagement of ineffective hypertension management strategies. Indeed, this result complements those of other studies examining chronic disease in Sub-Saharan Africa. Murphy and colleagues [34] found that negative provider interactions affected patients' ability to accept their condition as well as their motivation to engage with providers about behavioral and lifestyle changes needed to manage diabetes. Patients also noted the lack of sufficient counselling and discussed that they wanted providers to spend more time educating them on the disease and management, as they felt ill-equipped to handle it themselves. Additionally, our study found that lack of a functional primary health care mechanism and patients' lack of resources for follow-up care, including regular access to medication, greatly hamper efforts to control blood pressure. This complements the work of Goudge et al. [35], in South Africa, in which the authors found that over half of the households surveyed could not afford regular follow-up care; in some cases families had no income and depended on gifts from friends and other family members to afford health care. Majority of these cases received intermittent treatment at best. Even among households with the means to seek care, only half of the participants were treated regularly for a chronic condition. Weaknesses at the health systems level including poor referral systems, interrupted medication supply, and poor provider-patient interactions were primary barriers to consistent treatment. Interventions addressing these barriers at the provider and health systems level are needed to facilitate optimal maintenance and treatment of hypertension.

Though there is ample evidence that hypertension is an increasing problem in SSA, there is a lack of evidence regarding health care workers' perceptions of factors that influence optimal disease management. Our results complement the few studies that have investigated this topic and are similar to those reported in a recent review of systems level factors influencing hypertension control in SSA [3]. In many parts of SSA, workforce shortage has reached a crisis point and severely limits the ability of physicians to effectively reduce hypertension related morbidity and mortality rates. Workforce shortage and overworked physicians were also noted as barriers in this study. In Parker et al. [32], a survey of 16 health practitioners also identified medical staff shortage as a challenge to the effective management of hypertension at primary care facilities in South Africa. Similarly, an analysis of interviews conducted among patients from 18 community health centers in Cape Town suggested that "*doctors and nurses were working under increasingly difficult circumstances and staff shortages are the main barriers to effectively managing patients with chronic conditions such as hypertension*" 37 g [36]. Similarly, a nurse-led protocol for the management of hypertension in 454 patients over a 26-month period led to a drop of systolic pressure (11.7 mmHg) and diastolic pressure in patients (7.8 mmHg) between baseline and final visits [37]. Task-shifting is one possible solution to the noted barriers by physicians in this study as it would (1) reduce the workload for currently practicing physicians and (2) allow patients to receive more time with health care providers discussing how to properly manage hypertension through appropriate lifestyle changes [38]. As providers in this study noted that patient self-efficacy factors related to acceptance and management of their condition were among the several barriers to optimal hypertension control, more in-depth and longer sessions with health care providers could help patients improve self-efficacy and address concerns related to disease management.

Despite the implications for policy and practice, there are limitations to the current study. The relatively low sample size makes it difficult to generalize findings to other physicians in the region. Furthermore, the concept mapping process itself was very intensive, requiring several hours of participation for brainstorming, sorting of statements, and rating of those statements. The use of the Cardiovascular Research Training Program (CaRT) was extremely helpful as coordinators allocated time during the training which enabled physicians to finish the various concept mapping steps on time. However, the time demand of concept mapping may have prohibited more physicians from participating due to their high workload.

5. Conclusion

The findings of our study suggest that hypertension management and control as reflected in the perceptions of physicians is a multifaceted problem. Patient self-efficacy and support, physician-related factors, policy factors, and economic factors are important aspects that must be addressed if reduction in hypertension related morbidity and mortality rate in Sub-Saharan Africa is to be achieved. The strength of this study is the focus on key stakeholders (i.e., physicians) in Sub-Saharan Africa who are often left out of discussions of ways to mitigate the worldwide rising problem of hypertension. Their practical experience allows them insight into a wide range of factors that may impede efforts to reduce hypertension related morbidity and mortality not only at a local but also on a regional and global level. Given the work demands for physicians, future research should explore viable and cost-effective strategies such as task-shifting or the rational distribution of tasks among health care workforce teams in Sub-Saharan Africa.

Acknowledgments

The investigators would like to acknowledge the physicians attending the Cardiovascular Research Training (CaRT) Institute at the University of Ghana, College of Health Sciences, for their support for this project and participation in the concept mapping process. This project is supported by a research initiation grant from the UIUC Research Board and by NIH/FIC 5D43TW009140-04 (PI Ogedegbe) and R03TW010081 (PI Iwelunmor).

References

[1] M. Chopra, J. E. Lawn, D. Sanders et al., "Achieving the health Millennium Development Goals for South Africa: challenges and priorities," *The Lancet*, vol. 374, no. 9694, pp. 1023–1031, 2009.

[2] E. Kalipeni, L. L. Semu, and M. A. Mbilizi, "The brain drain of health care professionals from sub-Saharan Africa: a geographic perspective," *Progress in Development Studies*, vol. 12, no. 2-3, pp. 153–171, 2012.

[3] S. Naicker, J. Plange-Rhule, R. C. Tutt, and J. B. Eastwood, "Shortage of healthcare workers in developing countries—Africa," *Ethnicity & Disease*, vol. 19, no. 1, supplement 1, p. S1-60-4, 2009.

[4] G. Ogedegbe, J. Gyamfi, J. Plange-Rhule et al., "Task shifting interventions for cardiovascular risk reduction in low-income and middle-income countries: a systematic review of randomised controlled trials," *BMJ Open*, vol. 4, no. 10, Article ID e005983, 2014.

[5] B. M. Mayosi, "The 10 'Best Buys' to combat heart disease, diabetes and stroke in Africa," *Heart*, vol. 99, no. 14, pp. 973–974, 2013.

[6] P. M. Kearney, M. Whelton, K. Reynolds, P. Muntner, P. K. Whelton, and J. He, "Global burden of hypertension: analysis of worldwide data," *The Lancet*, vol. 365, no. 9455, pp. 217–223, 2005.

[7] J. Addo, C. Agyemang, L. Smeeth, A. de-Graft Aikins, A. K. Edusei, and O. Ogedegbe, "A review of population-based studies on hypertension in Ghana," *Ghana Medical Journal*, vol. 46, supplement, no. 2, pp. 4–11, 2012.

[8] R. S. Cooper, C. N. Rotimi, J. S. Kauftnan, W. F. T. Muna, and G. A. Mensah, "Hypertension treatment and control in sub-Saharan Africa: the epidemiological basis for policy," *British Medical Journal*, vol. 316, no. 7131, pp. 614–617, 1998.

[9] M. M. Ibrahim and A. Damasceno, "Hypertension in developing countries," *The Lancet*, vol. 380, no. 9841, pp. 611–619, 2012.

[10] J. Iwelunmor, C. O. Airhihenbuwa, R. Cooper et al., "Prevalence, determinants and systems-thinking approaches to optimal hypertension control in West Africa," *Globalization and Health*, vol. 10, no. 1, article 42, 2014.

[11] N. Unwin, P. Setel, S. Rashid et al., "Noncommunicable diseases in sub-Saharan Africa: where do they feature in the health research agenda?" *Bulletin of the World Health Organization*, vol. 79, no. 10, pp. 947–953, 2001.

[12] W. K. Bosu, "Epidemic of hypertension in Ghana: a systematic review," *BMC Public Health*, vol. 10, article 418, 2010.

[13] M. Cook-Huynh, D. Ansong, R. C. Steckelberg et al., "Prevalence of hypertension and diabetes mellitus in adults from a rural community in Ghana," *Ethnicity and Disease*, vol. 22, no. 3, pp. 347–352, 2012.

[14] J. Plange-Rhule, R. Phillips, J. W. Acheampong, A. K. Saggar-Malik, F. P. Cappuccio, and J. B. Eastwood, "Hypertension and renal failure in Kumasi, Ghana," *Journal of Human Hypertension*, vol. 13, no. 1, pp. 37–40, 1999.

[15] P. Duboz, E. Macla, N. Chapuis-Lucciani, G. Boëtsch, and L. Gueye, "Migration and hypertension in Dakar, Senegal," *American Journal of Physical Anthropology*, vol. 149, no. 2, pp. 250–258, 2012.

[16] M. E. Hendriks, F. W. N. M. Wit, M. T. L. Roos et al., "Hypertension in Sub-Saharan Africa: cross-sectional surveys in four rural and urban communities," *PLoS ONE*, vol. 7, no. 3, Article ID e32638, 2012.

[17] E. S. le Blanc, E. O'Connor, E. P. Whitlock, C. D. Patnode, and T. Kapka, "Effectiveness of primary care-relevant treatments for obesity in adults: a systematic evidence review for the U.S. Preventive services task force," *Annals of Internal Medicine*, vol. 155, no. 7, pp. 434–447, 2011.

[18] D. Lemogoum, J.-P. Degaute, and P. Bovet, "Stroke prevention, treatment, and rehabilitation in Sub-Saharan Africa," *American Journal of Preventive Medicine*, vol. 29, no. 5, supplement 1, pp. 95–101, 2005.

[19] C. Agyemang, M. A. Bruijnzeels, and E. Owusu-Dabo, "Factors associated with hypertension awareness, treatment, and control in Ghana, West Africa," *Journal of Human Hypertension*, vol. 20, no. 1, pp. 67–71, 2006.

[20] D. S. Houinato, A. R. Gbary, Y. C. Houehanou et al., "Prevalence of hypertension and associated risk factors in Benin," *Revue d'Epidemiologie et de Sante Publique*, vol. 60, no. 2, pp. 95–102, 2012.

[21] S. A. Isezuo, A. A. Sabir, A. E. Ohwovorilole, and O. A. Fasanmade, "Prevalence, associated factors and relationship between prehypertension and hypertension: a study of two ethnic African populations in Northern Nigeria," *Journal of Human Hypertension*, vol. 25, no. 4, pp. 224–230, 2011.

[22] V. O. Omuemu, O. H. Okojie, and C. E. Omuemu, "Awareness of high blood pressure status, treatment and control in a rural community in Edo State," *Nigerian Journal of Clinical Practice*, vol. 10, no. 3, pp. 208–212, 2007.

[23] O. J. Daniel, O. A. Adejumo, E. N. Adejumo, R. S. Owolabi, and R. W. Braimoh, "Prevalence of hypertension among urban slum dwellers in Lagos, Nigeria," *Journal of Urban Health*, vol. 90, no. 6, pp. 1016–1025, 2013.

[24] T. H. Harries, V. Twumasi-Abosi, J. Plange-Rhule, and F. P. Cappuccio, "Hypertension management in Kumasi: barriers and prejudice?" *Journal of Human Hypertension*, vol. 19, no. 12, pp. 975–977, 2005.

[25] E. Macia, P. Duboz, and L. Gueye, "Prevalence, awareness, treatment and control of hypertension among adults 50 years and older in Dakar, Senegal," *Cardiovascular Journal of Africa*, vol. 23, no. 5, pp. 265–269, 2012.

[26] S. Nam, C. Chesla, N. A. Stotts, L. Kroon, and S. L. Janson, "Barriers to diabetes management: patient and provider factors," *Diabetes Research and Clinical Practice*, vol. 93, no. 1, pp. 1–9, 2011.

[27] M. K. Trochim, *Concept Mapping for Planning and Evaluation*, SAGE Publications, Thousand Oaks, Calif, USA, 2007.

[28] S. M. Burke, A. V. Carron, and M. A. Eys, "Physical activity context: preferences of university students," *Psychology of Sport and Exercise*, vol. 7, no. 1, pp. 1–13, 2006.

[29] S. R. Rosas and M. Kane, "Quality and rigor of the concept mapping methodology: a pooled study analysis," *Evaluation and Program Planning*, vol. 35, no. 2, pp. 236–245, 2012.

[30] J. B. Kruskal, "Multidimensional scaling by optimizing goodness of fit to a nonmetric hypothesis," *Psychometrika*, vol. 29, no. 1, pp. 1–27, 1964.

[31] J. B. Kruskal and M. Wish, *Multidimensional Scaling*, SAGE Publications, Newbury Park, Calif, USA, 2009.

[32] A. Parker, B. Nagar, G. Thomas, M. Badri, and N. B. A. Ntusi, "Health practitioners' state of knowledge and challenges to effective management of hypertension at primary level," *Cardiovascular Journal of Africa*, vol. 22, no. 4, pp. 186–190, 2011.

[33] J. Iwelunmor, J. Plange-Rhule, C. O. Airhihenbuwa, C. Ezepue, and O. Ogedegbe, "A narrative synthesis of the health systems factors influencing optimal hypertension control in Sub-Saharan Africa," *PLoS ONE*, vol. 10, no. 7, Article ID e0130193, 2015.

[34] K. Murphy, T. Chuma, C. Mathews, K. Steyn, and N. Levitt, "A qualitative study of the experiences of care and motivation for effective self-management among diabetic and hypertensive patients attending public sector primary health care services in South Africa," *BMC Health Services Research*, vol. 15, article 303, 2015.

[35] J. Goudge, L. Gilson, S. Russell, T. Gumede, and A. Mills, "Affordability, availability and acceptability barriers to health care for the chronically ill: longitudinal case studies from South Africa," *BMC Health Services Research*, vol. 9, article 75, 2009.

[36] N. D. Labhardt, J.-R. Balo, M. Ndam, J.-J. Grimm, and E. Manga, "Task shifting to non-physician clinicians for integrated management of hypertension and diabetes in rural Cameroon: a programme assessment at two years," *BMC Health Services Research*, vol. 10, no. 1, article 339, 2010.

[37] A. P. Kengne, P. K. Awah, L. L. Fezeu, E. Sobngwi, and J.-C. Mbanya, "Primary health care for hypertension by nurses in rural and urban sub-Saharan Africa," *Journal of Clinical Hypertension*, vol. 11, no. 10, pp. 564–572, 2009.

[38] A. Lekoubou, P. Awah, L. Fezeu, E. Sobngwi, and A. P. Kengne, "Hypertension, diabetes mellitus and task shifting in their management in sub-Saharan Africa," *International Journal of Environmental Research and Public Health*, vol. 7, no. 2, pp. 353–363, 2010.

12

Socioeconomic Status and Hypertension among Teachers and Bankers in Addis Ababa, Ethiopia

Girma Fikadu and Seblewengel Lemma

Addis Continental Institute of Public Health, P.O. Box 26751/1000, Addis Ababa, Ethiopia

Correspondence should be addressed to Girma Fikadu; girmafikadu23@yahoo.com

Academic Editor: John M. Flack

Background. The social and economic changes taking place in developing countries are influencing the pace at which hypertension and its risk factors are expanding. As opposed to the already established inverse association in developed nations, the association between socioeconomic status and hypertension in developing countries is poor and inconsistent. This study aims to determine the association between socioeconomic status and hypertension among teachers and bankers in Addis Ababa, Ethiopia. *Methods.* This study is based on a cross-sectional study conducted to assess the prevalence of NCDs in Addis Ababa, Ethiopia. The study was undertaken among workers of the Commercial Bank of Ethiopia and teachers of public schools in 2010. *Results.* Majority of participants were teachers (70.3%). Most of the respondents (54.1%) earn an annual income between 15,000 ETB and 48,000 ETB, and 51.9% of them have educational status of first degree and above. Among the socioeconomic factors income was strongly associated with the odds of having hypertension (AOR: 2.17 with 95% CI: 1.58–2.98). *Conclusions.* Higher burden of hypertension is observed among teachers and bankers in Addis Ababa, Ethiopia. Promotion of healthy behaviors and interventions that target higher income groups needs to be put in place.

1. Introduction

Recently, in addition to the high prevalence of infectious diseases, the incidence of noncommunicable disease is alarmingly increasing in the developing countries [1]. Although there are some more recent studies indicating the decline of CVD in Africa, NCDs are generally showing rapid rise in these countries [2]. One of the explanations for the increase is the economic and social transformation taking place in these countries, and the lifestyle changes resulted from such transformation [3].

Hypertension is one of the noncommunicable diseases that is advancing at fast pace in African countries [4]. The trend is unexpected given the socioeconomic status of people in these countries, as the disease is believed to be disease of the rich and developed nations [5].

Besides being a major cause of death, hypertension is a major risk factor for many chronic diseases like coronary heart disease, stroke, heart failure, kidney disease, and others [6]. It is responsible for about 6% (9 million) of deaths worldwide and affects about one billion people globally [5]. Hypertension is enormously affecting the working groups. Its global prevalence among older adults aged 25 and over is around 40% in 2008 [6]. The highest of this effect falls on the people in middle and low income countries [6]. Low income countries like Sub-Saharan Africa are experiencing unexpected rise in the incidence of hypertension [1]. The few studies conducted in Ethiopia are also showing high prevalence of the disease in the country. According to one study, 10.5% of the Ethiopian population has been estimated to have hypertension [7]. Another more recent study conducted in the capital shows that approximately 30% of adults in Addis Ababa have hypertension [8]. Added to the silent nature of the disease and the poor health seeking behavior of the people, as the country is going through a rapid economic development, and social and behavioral change, the figure is estimated to be higher.

Income, education, and occupation are the most commonly used indicators or measures of the socioeconomic status of an individual. Although its measurement is difficult in the developing countries, household income has shown consistent association to the general measures of health [9]. Educational status is also widely used as a measure of socioeconomic status and is related to many health outcomes [10]. Educational attainment reflects a household's ability to avoid risky behaviors and practice good health. Occupation is another common measure of socioeconomic status linking economic factors to health outcomes. It reflects health risks and protection factors related to the occupation and provision of source of income to practice good health behavior [11].

There are significant evidences indicating an inverse association between socioeconomic status and hypertension in the developed countries [12–14]. This is because in the developed countries individuals with high socioeconomic status may be the early adopters of healthy lifestyles that help to lower the risk of hypertension. But, in the developing countries, these groups are early adopters of harmful lifestyles characterized by smoking, diets with high energy and fats, and sedentary lifestyles [15]. The inverse association of socioeconomic status with hypertension is not evident in the developing countries.

The results from the few studies conducted in the developing countries have shown inconsistent results. For instance a study from Nigeria among adults aged 30–60 years found an inverse association between socioeconomic status and hypertension [16]. In contrary to this finding, a study on civil servants in the same nation found that those at higher occupational levels had higher hypertension when compared with those at lower occupational levels [15]. Another cross sectional home to home study conducted in urban population in Dar es Salaam, Tanzania, aged 25 to 64 came up with a result similar to that of the developed countries [17]. However, the use of different measurement of socioeconomic status and the stages of their economic development in these countries have made comparisons across other literatures difficult.

The results from many middle income countries are also showing positive association between socioeconomic status and hypertension. A study in rural Indian adults shows the highest socioeconomic group had almost double the prevalence of hypertension as those from the lowest socioeconomic group [18]. Another study within the same country has also showed a significantly positive relationship between socioeconomic status and hypertension [19]. In study undertaken among Jamaican women, the prevalence of hypertension is highest among the wealthiest women compared with the poorest [14].

There are significant study results indicating the high prevalence of hypertension among the bank workers [19, 20]. In contrast some studies undertaken in Africa are showing the prevalence of hypertension being higher among teachers compared to the bankers. In Ethiopia little is known about how socioeconomic factors may influence the distribution of hypertension. Therefore the current study aims to examine the association between socioeconomic status and hypertension among the bankers and teachers in the capital, Addis Ababa.

2. Materials and Methods

2.1. Study Design and Population. This study is based on a cross sectional study conducted for the purpose of assessing the prevalence of noncommunicable diseases among working adults in Addis Ababa, Ethiopia. The study was conducted by Addis Continental Institute of Public Health in collaboration with University of Washington Multidisciplinary International Research Training Program. Study populations are permanent employees of the Commercial Bank of Ethiopia and teachers in government schools in Addis Ababa.

A multistage probabilistic sampling strategy was used to identify and recruit participants [21]. First two study sites, the commercial bank of Ethiopia and public schools, were purposefully selected based on their work force stability. Then probability proportional to size sampling procedures was used to select both Commercial Bank of Ethiopia branch offices and government schools. From each of the selected locations, all employees were invited to participate. More details of the methodology are described elsewhere [21, 22].

2.2. Data Collection and Measurements. The study was conducted in accordance with the WHO's STEP wise approach for noncommunicable disease surveillance in the developing countries [21, 23]. Additional questions were also added to reflect better the context of Ethiopia [21].

2.3. Socioeconomic Status. Socioeconomic status is commonly conceptualized as the social class of an individual or group. It is often measured as a combination of education, income, and occupation [10, 12].

Education. Questions on completed education levels or grades were asked. The responses were grouped into two wider categories: diploma and below and degree and above.

Occupation. It refers to the institutions in which the study populations are employed.

Income. Three income categories are identified based on the 50% median income classification and used for analysis [24, 25].

Blood Pressure. It was measured using a digital measuring device (Microlife BP A50, Microlife AG, Switzerland) with the participant sitting after resting for at least 5 minutes. Blood pressure was measured 3 times, with at least 3 minutes between consecutive measurements. In accordance with the WHO recommendation the mean systolic and diastolic blood pressure from the second and third measurements were considered for analysis [26]. For the purpose of this study people with systolic blood pressure greater than or equal to 140 mmHg, or diastolic pressure greater than or equal to 90 mmHg, or people with normal blood pressure who are taking antihypertensive drug therapy were classified as hypertensive. Classification of hypertension was determined according to Joint National Committee on Prevention, Detection, Evaluation and Treatment of High Blood Pressure [27] (see Table 1).

Table 1

High blood pressure (HBP)	Systolic blood pressure (mmHg)	Diastolic blood pressure (mmHg)
Normal	<120	<80
Prehypertension	120–139	or 80–89
Stage 1 hypertension	140–159	or 90–99
Stage 2 hypertension	≥160	or ≥100

Weight and Height. Participants were weighed using a solar-powered scale with an accuracy of ±100 grams. Their height was measured using an adjustable wooden measuring board, specifically designed to provide accurate measurements [22, 23].

Body Mass Index. Body mass index (BMI) was calculated as weight in kilograms divided by the square of height in meters. Classifications of BMI groups were done based on WHO recommendation. BMI < 18.5 represents underweight, 18.5 to <25 stands for normal weight, ≥25 to <30 refers to overweight, and obesity is decided when BMI ≥ 30 [28].

2.4. Statistical Analysis. SPSS (version 20.0) was used for statistical analysis. Data completeness and consistency were checked by running frequency on each variable. After excluding participants with missing BP measurement data and pregnant women ($n = 339$) from the original study sample, a total of 1866 study subjects were considered for the analysis. Frequencies and percentages were used for descriptive statistics to see the distribution of the different variables. Bivariate and multivariate logistic regressions were conducted to see the association between the measures of socioeconomic status and hypertension. Adjusted odds ratios (AOR) with 95% confidence interval were reported.

Table 2: Distribution of socioeconomic and demographic characteristics among teachers and bankers in Addis Ababa, Ethiopia.

Characteristics	Frequency	Percent
Sex		
Male	1,124	60.2
Female	742	39.8
Mean age, years (±SD)	36.03 (11.91)	
Age (years)		
≤24	358	19.2
25–34	660	35.4
35–44	311	16.7
45–54	367	19.7
≥55	170	9.1
Religion		
Orthodox	1,455	78
Muslim	74	4
Protestant	284	15.2
Catholic	16	0.9
Others	37	2
Marital status		
Single	933	50
Married	813	43.6
Other	120	6.4
Occupation		
Bankers	554	29.7
Teachers	1,312	70.3
Educational status		
Diploma and below	897	48.1
Degree and above	969	51.9
Income		
Low (≤15000)	460	24.7
Medium (15001–48000)	1010	54.1
High (>48000)	396	21.2

3. Results

3.1. Characteristics of the Study Population. A total of 51 schools and CBE's branch offices participated in the study. As the study has collected data on all the variables related to NCDs, for this study participants with no BP measurement data ($n = 318$) and pregnant women ($n = 21$) were excluded from the original study sample. Accordingly a total of 1866 study subjects (1124 men and 742 women) with complete data on all the variables were included in the study.

As Table 2 indicates, the majority, 1,124 (60.2%), of the participants were male and 742 (39.8%) were female with the male to female sex ratio of 1.5 : 1. The mean age of the participants was 36.03 with a standard deviation of 11.91 years. Table 2 shows the socioeconomic and demographic characteristics of the study population.

3.2. Socioeconomic Status. More than seventy percent of the participants were teachers by occupation. Majority of the respondents (54.1%) were in the middle income category earning between 15,000 and 48,000 Ethiopian birr per year. Slightly more than half (51.9%) of the participants had first degree and above and the other half (48.1%) are diploma and below, making educational status normally distributed (Table 3).

3.3. Lifestyle and Behavioral Risk Factors. As Table 3 indicates, the majority (55.3%) of the participants had a normal BMI, while 26.3% were overweight. The prevalence of obesity was 5.8% and underweight was 12.6%. 83 (4.4) of the participants are current smokers and 9.1% were previous smokers. 14.4% and 2.5% of the study participants are moderate and heavy drinkers, respectively. About 61% of the participants are not physically active. 4.8% of participants were diabetic and 13.9% of them have mental distress. Thirty percent of the participants have family history of hypertension.

The prevalence of hypertension in the study is 21% (95% CI = 19.15, 22.85). 127 (6.8%) of the hypertensive participants are currently receiving BP treatment. Only 278 (14.9%) of the participants are aware of their hypertension status before the interview.

TABLE 3: Distribution of behavioral risk factors among teachers and bankers in Addis Ababa, Ethiopia.

Characteristics	Frequency	Percent
BMI		
Underweight	235	12.6
Normal	1032	55.3
Overweight	490	26.3
Obese	109	5.8
Smoking status		
Nonsmoker	1614	86.5
Pervious smoker	169	9.1
Current smoker	83	4.4
Alcohol consumption		
Nondrinker	582	31.2
Low drinker	969	51.9
Moderate drinker	269	14.4
Heavy drinker	46	2.5
Physical exercise		
Yes	728	39
No	1138	61
Diabetes status		
Yes	90	4.8
No	1776	95.2
Mental distress status		
Yes	259	13.9
No	1607	86.1
Family history of hypertension		
Yes	563	30.2
No	1138	61
Not known	165	8.8

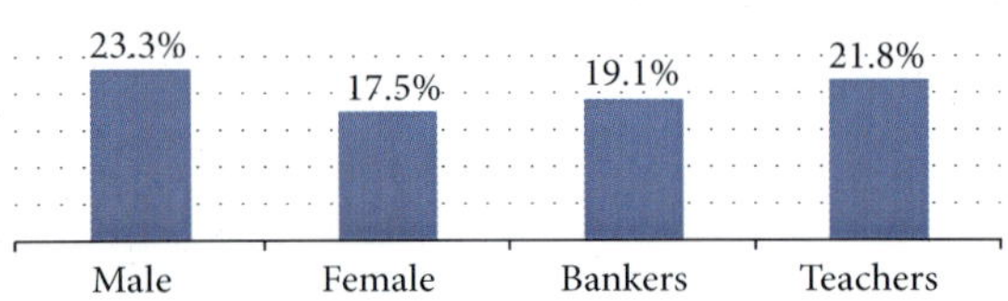

FIGURE 1: Prevalence of hypertension by sex and occupation among study participants in Addis Ababa, Ethiopia.

The results from the bivariate logistic regression indicate that males tend to be more hypertensive than females (OR: 1.43, 95% CI: 1.13–1.81) (Figure 1). The odds of hypertension increases with increase in age: 35–44 (OR: 3.11, 95% CI: 1.94–4.99), 44–55 (OR: 7.786, 95% CI: 5.021–12.075), and above 50 (OR: 14.23, 95% CI: 8.72–23.23).

A higher prevalence of hypertension was observed among middle income groups (OR: 2.26, 95% CI: 1.66–3.07); a statistically significant prevalence is also observed among the higher income groups (OR: 1.75, 95% CI: 1.21–2.52). However, as Table 4 shows, there was no statically significant difference in prevalence of hypertension among the educational categories (P value = 0.536) and occupation of the participants (P value = 0.197).

4. Discussion

This study identified hypertension as a significant health problem among bankers and teachers in Addis Ababa. 21% of the participants are found to be hypertensive. The study populations have showed a high prevalence of hypertension. The prevalence is 19.13% and 21.8% for bankers and teachers, respectively. These figures are higher compared with the 10.5% prevalence among the general population of Ethiopia [7] and lower than the 30% prevalence among adults in Addis Ababa in previous studies [8]. The prevalence of hypertension in this study is consistent with 19.3% reported in Nigeria [29] and 21.8% for Uganda [30].

All the significant factors which have proven to be related with the incidence of hypertension were entered into the multivariate regression model. In addition checks were conducted and no multicollinearity was found among the variables used for measuring socioeconomic status.

From the socioeconomic status measures used, only income has shown strong positive association with hypertension. Even after adjustment is made educational status and occupation have shown no significant association with the prevalence of hypertension.

The association of income with hypertension in this study is consistent with the findings from many low and middle income countries [1, 12, 31]. The middle and high income groups have shown higher odds of having hypertension. This finding indicates that in the context of the developing country having a higher income is not necessarily protective of health as it is in the developed world. This is probably due to the lifestyle of this group of people in these countries. These groups may use this income to provide more resources that may be used mostly for purchasing calorie-dense foods and excessive drinking, and in some instances it is a cause of sedentary lifestyles which are the underlying risk factors of hypertension.

Among this study population no significant association between education and hypertension was found. The absence of the association in this study may be due to the nature of the study population. In this study there is little variation in terms of educational status of the participants. However, studies done in the developing countries like Tanzania, Nigeria, and Ghana found out that education is inversely associated with the odds of developing hypertension [16, 31]. Similar findings were also documented in China [32], Iran [33], and Jamaica [14].

Occupation also has shown no statistically significant association with hypertension. Although there is a lack of studies that compared the two population groups, in studies conducted independently, the odds of developing hypertension is higher among the bank workers [19, 20]. In those studies it is explained that bankers' job is more stressful and sedentary (Table 5).

4.1. Additional Points. To the best of our knowledge this is the first study that assessed the association between socioeconomic status and hypertension in Ethiopia. The study adds

TABLE 4: Bivariate analysis for the association between socioeconomic status and hypertension among teachers and bankers in Addis Ababa, Ethiopia.

Variables	Hypertension		OR (95% CI)	*P* value
	Yes	No		
Sex				
Male	262	862	1.431 (1.132–1.809)	0.003
Female	130	612	1	
Age				
≤24	28	330	1	
25–34	60	600	1.179 (0.738–1.882)	0.492
35–44	65	246	3.114 (1.941–4.997)	<0.001
45–54	146	221	7.786 (5.021–12.075)	<0.001
≥55	93	77	14.235 (8.721–23.234)	<0.001
Income				
Low (≤15000)	59	401	1	
Medium (15001–48000)	252	758	2.260 (1.660–3.075)	<0.001
High (>48000)	81	315	1.748 (1.211–2.521)	0.003
Education				
Diploma and below	183	714	0.932 (0.746–1.165)	0.536
Degree and above	209	760	1	
Occupation				
Bank workers	106	448	1.178 (0.918–1.511)	0.197
Teachers	286	1026	1	

TABLE 5: Multivariate logistic regression analysis: association between socioeconomic status and hypertension among teachers and bankers in Addis Ababa, Ethiopia.

Variables	Adjusted OR	95% CI for AOR	*P* value
Income			
Low (≤15000)	1		
Medium (15001–48000)	2.168	1.579–2.978	<0.001
High (>48000)	1.955	1.312–2.913	0.001
Education			
Diploma and below	1.042	0.825–1.317	0.728
Degree and above	1		
Occupation			
Bank workers	0.750	0.569–0.989	0.042
Teachers	1		

to the scarce study results in this aspect. Even though the study has come up with important findings, there are certain limitations worth mentioning here. First of all, the fact that our study participants are all working professionals who are urban residents and fairly well educated makes the generalizing of the result to the larger population difficult.

Secondly as the study is based on secondary data the problem of social desirability bias is mentioned in the original study. Participants may withhold information regarding their life-style habits that may not be generally acceptable for working adults (smoking, drinking, etc.) which may result in an underestimation of these behaviors [34].

5. Conclusions

This study highlights the high prevalence of hypertension in the study population. As in many other developing countries hypertension is becoming a serious public health concern among working adults like teachers and bankers in Ethiopia. Like many developing and middle income countries, in this study better income is positively associated with higher odds of having hypertension. However, no association between hypertension and measures of socioeconomic status like education and occupation was found in this study.

6. Recommendation

As hypertension is becoming a serious public health concern in Ethiopia, it has to be given due concern in the health agenda of the country as one of top priority. Income does not play a direct role in increasing the odds of hypertension. It rather influences the practice of risky behavioral factors that are responsible for hypertension. Therefore promoting healthy lifestyles and interventions in lifestyle modifications related to the behavioral risk factors is recommended in reducing and controlling the prevalence of hypertension [27].

Awareness creation and promotion of healthy behaviors have to be widely conducted, especially in the better income groups so that they will make rational decision in choosing their behaviors. Particularly, the long term consequences that arise from these lifestyles have to be stressed to the society in general and these groups in particular.

Future studies are also highly recommended to confirm these findings in general population with varying measures of socioeconomic status.

Ethical Approval

All study participants provided informed consent. The participants were told about their right to withdraw from the study period at any time. Additionally, the Commercial Bank of Ethiopia and Addis Ababa Education Bureau were requested officially to give permission to conduct the study. Ethical clearance was obtained from Institutional Review Boards of Addis Continental Institute of Public Health, Addis Ababa, Ethiopia. The permission to use the data set was also obtained from Addis Continental Institute of Public Health.

Competing Interests

The authors declared that they have no competing interests.

Authors' Contributions

Girma Fikadu initiated the research, wrote the research proposal, conducted the research, did data analysis, and wrote the paper. Seblewengel Lemma was involved in reviewing the proposal, guiding the analysis, and directing the write-up of the paper and advised the study from the inception to the end. Both authors read and approved the final paper.

Acknowledgments

This research was completed while Girma Fikadu was postgraduate student at Addis Continental Institute of Public Health. The authors thank Addis Continental Institute of Public Health for providing permission to work on the data. The authors also thank the Commercial Bank of Ethiopia and Addis Ababa Education Office for granting access to conduct the study and Internal Clinical Laboratories for completing all laboratory analyses.

References

[1] O. S. Ogah and B. L. Rayner, "Recent advances in hypertension in sub-Saharan Africa," *Heart*, vol. 99, no. 19, pp. 1390–1397, 2013.

[2] R. S. Cooper and P. Bovet, "Measures of health and disease in Africa: are current methods giving us useful information about trends in cardiovascular diseases?" *Progress in Cardiovascular Diseases*, vol. 56, no. 3, pp. 270–277, 2013.

[3] M. E. Hendriks, F. W. N. M. Wit, M. T. L. Roos et al., "Hypertension in Sub-Saharan Africa: cross-sectional surveys in four rural and urban communities," *PLoS ONE*, vol. 7, no. 3, Article ID e32638, 2012.

[4] K. S. Reddy and S. Yusuf, "Emerging epidemic of cardiovascular disease in developing countries," *Circulation*, vol. 97, no. 6, pp. 596–601, 1998.

[5] World Health Organiation, *Global Brief on Hypertension: Silent Killer, Global Public Health Crisis*, World Health Organiation, Genève, Switzerland, 2013.

[6] WHO, "Global status report on noncommunicable diseases 2014," 2014, http://www.who.int/nmh/publications/ncd-status-report-2014/en/.

[7] F. Tesfaye, N. G. Nawi, H. Van Minh et al., "Association between body mass index and blood pressure across three populations in Africa and Asia," *Journal of Human Hypertension*, vol. 21, no. 1, pp. 28–37, 2007.

[8] M. Molla, "Systematic reviews of prevalence and associated factors of hypertension in Ethiopia: finding the evidence," *Science Journal of Public Health*, vol. 3, no. 4, pp. 514–519, 2015.

[9] S. Macintyre, L. McKay, G. Der, and R. Hiscock, "Socio-economic position and health: what you observe depends on how you measure it," *Journal of Public Health Medicine*, vol. 25, no. 4, pp. 288–294, 2003.

[10] J.-C. Fotso and B. Kuate-Defo, "Measuring socioeconomic status in health research in developing countries: should we be focusing on households, communities or both?" *Social Indicators Research*, vol. 72, no. 2, pp. 189–237, 2005.

[11] M. A. Winkleby, D. E. Jatulis, E. Frank, and S. P. Fortmann, "Socioeconomic status and health: how education, income, and occupation contribute to risk factors for cardiovascular disease," *American Journal of Public Health*, vol. 82, no. 6, pp. 816–820, 1992.

[12] Z. Yu, A. Nissinen, E. Vartiainen et al., "Associations between socioeconomic status and cardiovascular risk factors in an urban population in China," *Bulletin of the World Health Organization*, vol. 78, no. 11, pp. 1296–1305, 2000.

[13] G. A. Kaplan and J. E. Keil, "Socioeconomic factors and cardiovascular disease: a review of the literature," *Circulation*, vol. 88, no. 4, part 1, pp. 1973–1998, 1993.

[14] M. A. Mendez, R. Cooper, R. Wilks, A. Luke, and T. Forrester, "Income, education, and blood pressure in adults in Jamaica, a middle-income developing country," *International Journal of Epidemiology*, vol. 32, no. 3, pp. 400–408, 2003.

[15] C. H. Bunker, F. I. Okoro, N. Markovic et al., "Relationship of hypertension to socioeconomic status in a west African population," *Ethnicity & Health*, vol. 1, no. 1, pp. 33–45, 1996.

[16] R. A. Adedoyin, C. E. Mbada, O. O. Awofolu, and O. M. Oyebami, "The influence of socio-economic status on casual blood pressures of the adult Nigerians," *European Journal of Cardiovascular Prevention and Rehabilitation: Official Journal of the European Society of Cardiology, Working Groups on Epidemiology & Prevention and Cardiac Rehabilitation and Exercise Physiology*, vol. 12, no. 3, pp. 71–83, 2005.

[17] P. Bovet, A. G. Ross, J.-P. Gervasoni et al., "Distribution of blood pressure, body mass index and smoking habits in the urban population of Dar es Salaam, Tanzania, and associations with socioeconomic status," *International Journal of Epidemiology*, vol. 31, no. 1, pp. 240–247, 2002.

[18] E. C. A. M. Gilberts, M. J. C. W. J. Arnold, and D. E. Grobbee, "Hypertension and determinants of blood pressure with special reference to socioeconomic status in a rural south Indian community," *Journal of Epidemiology and Community Health*, vol. 48, no. 3, pp. 258–261, 1994.

[19] M. B. Soudarssanane, M. Karthigeyan, and S. Stephen, "Key predictors of high blood pressure and hypertension among adolescents: a simple prescription for prevention," *Indian Journal of Community Medicine*, vol. 31, no. 3, p. 164, 2006.

[20] A. Undhad, P. J. Bharodiya, and R. P. Sonani, "Correlates of hypertension among the bank employees of Surat city of Gujarat," *National Journal of Community Medicine*, vol. 2, no. 1, pp. 123–125, 2011.

[21] *Preliminary Results Survey of Non Communicable Diseases among Bank Employees and Teachers in Addis Ababa, Ethiopia*, 2010, http://www.addiscontinental.edu.et/files/aciph_communicable_disease.pdf.

[22] K. S. Ganesh and S. N. Deivanai, "Prevalence and risk factors of hypertension among bank employees in urban Puducherry, India," *International Journal of Occupational and Environmental Medicine*, vol. 5, no. 2, pp. 94–100, 2014.

[23] W. S. Wai, R. S. Dhami, B. Gelaye et al., "Comparison of measures of adiposity in identifying cardiovascular disease risk among Ethiopian adults," *Obesity*, vol. 20, no. 9, pp. 1887–1895, 2012.

[24] WHO, *WHO STEPwise Approach to Chronic Disease Risk Factor Surveillance (STEPS)*, World Health Organ, 2008.

[25] S. Danziger, *Understanding Poverty*, Harvard University Press, Cambridge, Mass, USA, 2009.

[26] African Development Bank, *The Middle of the Pyramid: Dynamics of Middle Class in Africa*, AfDB, 2011.

[27] National High Blood Pressure Education Program, *The Seventh Report of the Joint National Committee on Prevention, Detection, Evaluation, and Treatment of High Blood Pressure*, National Heart, Lung, and Blood Institute, Bethesda, Md, USA, 2004, http://www.ncbi.nlm.nih.gov/books/NBK9630/.

[28] WHO, *Physical Status: The Use and Interpretation of Anthropometry*, World Health Organisation, Geneva, Switzerland, 1995.

[29] S. Isezuo, A. Sabir, A. Ohwovorilole, and O. Fasanmade, "Prevalence, associated factors and relationship between prehypertension and hypertension: a study of two ethnic African populations in Northern Nigeria," *Journal of Human Hypertension*, vol. 25, pp. 224–230, 2011.

[30] G. Musinguzi and F. Nuwaha, "Prevalence, awareness and control of hypertension in Uganda," *PLoS ONE*, vol. 8, no. 4, Article ID e62236, 2013.

[31] A. Cois and R. Ehrlich, "Analysing the socioeconomic determinants of hypertension in South Africa: a structural equation modelling approach," *BMC Public Health*, vol. 14, article 414, 2014.

[32] A. Jenson, A. L. Omar, M. A. Omar, A. S. Rishad, and K. Khoshnood, "Assessment of hypertension control in a district of Mombasa, Kenya," *Global Public Health*, vol. 6, no. 3, pp. 293–306, 2011.

[33] H. R. Anbarlo and S. A. Irvanlo, "Correlation between education and effect on increase knowledge high blood pressure patients referral to hospital," *International Journal of Current Research and Academic Review*, vol. 3, no. 1, pp. 60–64, 2015.

[34] A. Tran, B. Gelaye, B. Girma et al., "Prevalence of metabolic syndrome among working adults in Ethiopia," *International Journal of Hypertension*, vol. 2011, Article ID 193719, 8 pages, 2011.

13

Reference Intervals of Central Aortic Blood Pressure and Augmentation Index Assessed with an Oscillometric Device in Healthy Children, Adolescents, and Young Adults from Argentina

Alejandro Diaz,[1] **Yanina Zócalo**,[2] **Daniel Bia**,[2] **and Edmundo Cabrera Fischer**[3]

[1]*Instituto de Investigación en Ciencias de la Salud, UNICEN, CONICET, Tandil, Argentina*
[2]*Physiology Department, School of Medicine, Centro Universitario de Investigación, Innovación y Diagnóstico Arterial (CUiiDARTE), Republic University, General Flores 2125, 11800 Montevideo, Uruguay*
[3]*Instituto de Medicina Traslacional, Trasplante y Bioingeniería (IMTTyB), Universidad Favaloro, CONICET, Buenos Aires, Argentina*

Correspondence should be addressed to Alejandro Diaz; alejandrounicen@gmail.com

Academic Editor: Claudio Borghi

Age-related reference intervals (RIs) of central (aortic) systolic blood pressure (cSBP) and augmentation index (cAIx) obtained from large healthy population are lacking in Argentina (South America). *Aims.* To analyze the existence of associations among cSBP and cAIx with demographic, anthropometric, and hemodynamic parameters and to generate percentile curves and RIs adjusted to each level of age and gender and/or body height. cSBP and cAIx were measured in 1038 healthy children, adolescents, and young adults. First, we evaluated if RIs for males and females were necessary using correlation and covariate analysis. Second, mean (M) and standard deviation (SD) age-related equations were obtained for cSBP and cAIx, using parametric regression methods based on fractional polynomials. Third, age specific percentiles curves were generated. Fourth, body height specific percentiles curves were generated using a similar procedure. The obtained equations (considering age as independent variable) for all subjects ($cSBP^{0.26}$ and $(cAIx + 12.001)^{0.5}$) were as follows: cSBP Mean = 3.0581 + 0.2189 log(Age) − 0.001044Age; cSBP SD = −0.03919 + 0.1535 log(Age) − 0.004564Age; cAIx mean = 9.5226 − 6.1599 log(Age) + 0.1450Age; cAIx SD = 1.3880 − 0.8468 log(Age) + 0.03212Age. This study, performed in Argentinean healthy children, adolescents, and young adults with ages of 5 to 22 years, provides the first RIs and percentile curves of cSBP and cAIx. Additionally, specific body height-related cAIx percentiles are reported for the analyzed population. The RIs and percentiles contribute to the knowledge of arterial dynamic evolution along the normal aging process and the interpretation of data obtained in clinical research and daily clinical practice.

1. Introduction

The analysis and monitoring of vessels morphology and function in young people have become of major interest for both pediatricians and adult specialists in order to preserve and optimize cardiovascular health from childhood to adulthood [1]. The noninvasive assessment of arterial stiffness (AS) provides valuable information of structural and functional state of the vascular system, beyond that of the conventional blood pressure (BP) measurements [2]. For instance, increases in AS in adolescents and young adults are associated with left ventricular mass index, independently of traditional cardiovascular risk factors (CRFs) [3]. Screening for AS may be useful to identify subjects with cardiovascular risk in children, adolescents, and young adults' populations [3].

There are several parameters to assess AS being frequently used the aortic pulse wave velocity (PWV) and augmentation index (AIx) of the aorta and the brachial artery. PWV and AIx increase with the arterial aging process [4–6]. Is important to take into account the fact that PWV is widely considered a direct marker of AS [7], while the AIx is a well-known modality to express arterial wave reflections, often considered as a surrogate index of AS [6–8].

Linked to AIx assessment, central (aortic) systolic blood pressure (cSBP) is a parameter that strongly reflects vascular changes of central elastic arteries compared to peripheral (brachial) BP, both in adults and children and adolescents [9, 10]. Moreover, changes in cSBP levels affect the heart, brain, and kidneys which are directly exposed to them [11].

Central arterial and haemodynamic parameters (cAIx and cSBP) can be estimated noninvasively using a good number of techniques. They include Doppler ultrasound, applanation tonometry, oscillometry, and magnetic resonance imaging; all of them are associated with its own strengths and weaknesses [2, 12]. Oscillometric devices have been suggested to be especially adequate in children and adolescents, since the methodology includes the use of a simple pressure cuff and have the advantages of being relatively fast, operator independent and require minimal cooperation of the patient [13, 14].

Independently of the technique or device used to assess the arterial properties, there are several gaps in the approach of cSBP and cAIx measurements [1], performed in pediatric clinical practice such as (a) what are the interval references (RIs) of cSBP and cAIx values for each measurement? And (b) do they differ by gender and/or body height?

The 2016 European Society of Hypertension guidelines for the management of high BP in children and adolescents do not recommend the routine assessment of arterial parameters and cSBP, however, highlights the need to increase knowledge in the field of arterial parameters as markers of function of the vascular system [15]. Furthermore, the 2013 ESH/ESC guidelines for the management of arterial hypertension considered that cSBP can provide useful information in young patients with isolated systolic hypertension [16]. Moreover, cSBP may be especially relevant in asymptomatic children and adolescents incidentally found to have isolated systolic hypertension without target organ damage [15].

Unfortunately, at present few epidemiological studies in healthy pediatric populations are available, in which RIs of cSBP and cAIx were obtained using brachial oscillometric cuff method [17, 18]. To the best of our knowledge, the largest databases of RIs of cSBP and cAIx in pediatrics come from Hungary [17] and Germany, in which the Arteriograph and Mobil-O-Graph System were respectively used [18].

Considering the lack of knowledge in terms of cSBP and cAIx reference values for children, adolescents, and young adults from Argentina, our research purposes were as follows:

(1) to analyze the existence of associations among cSBP and cAIx with demographic, anthropometric, and hemodynamic parameters,

(2) to generate percentile curves and RIs adjusted to each level of age and (if required) gender and/or body height.

2. Materials and Methods

This study is part of a project started in 2014 in Tandil city (Buenos Aires Province), Argentina, aimed at investigating the prevalence of CRFs. Preliminary data obtained in this location have been previously reported [19–21]. Tandil is located 360 Km south of Buenos Aires City (37°19′08″S-9°08′05″W).

The study protocol was approved by the Institutional Ethics Committee and was carried on in agreement with the Declaration of Helsinki and the Good Clinical Practice Guidelines. Written informed consent was obtained from the participants or authorized person.

Asymptomatic children, adolescents, and young adults (5–22 years old) from the Tandil community were considered for enrolment in this study. Subjects were submitted to clinical interview, blood sampling evaluation, and anthropometric assessment, carried out in all cases by the same group of physicians. Blood samples were obtained after 9–12 hours of fasting. Glycaemia, lipid profile, and kidney functional parameters were determined. Anthropometric evaluation and a brief clinical interview allowed assessing CRFs exposure. Asymptomatic subjects included in the study met the following criteria: (1) none had history of cardiovascular, pulmonary, or renal disease; (2) normal peripheral BP at the time of examination (BP $\leq$ 140/90 mmHg in adults and BP $<$ 90th percentile in subjects $<$ 16 years old) [15]; (3) none were taking medications (antihypertensive, antihyperlipidemic, or antidiabetic drugs); (4) all included subjects had glycaemia $<$ 6.11 mmol/L ($<$110 mg/dl), total blood cholesterol levels $<$ 5.17 mmol/L ($<$200 mg/dl) [16], and normal serum triglycerides levels $<$ 1.69 mmol/L ($<$150 mg/dl), $\leq$1.5 mmol/L ($<$130 mg/dl), and $\leq$1.13 mmol/L ($<$100 mg/dl) for subjects older than 18 years, subjects between 10 to 17 years, and children under 10 years, respectively [15, 22].

Current and past smokers, diabetic, obese subjects (body mass index [BMI] $\geq$ 30 kg/m^2 for adults or BMI $\geq$ 97th percentile for subjects under 18 years old), hypertensive subjects, or subjects with averaged high brachial BP levels at the time of the study were excluded. To this end, peripheral (brachial) BP measurements were obtained using fully automatic sphygmomanometers, operating on oscillometric principle (705IT, Omron Healthcare Inc., USA). Adults' BP levels were classified following guidelines for the management of arterial hypertension [16]. Thus, hypertension was defined as peripheral systolic BP (pSBP) $\geq$ 140 mmHg and/or peripheral diastolic BP (pDBP) $\geq$ 90 mmHg. In turn, brachial BP levels in children and adolescents were categorized, taking into account sex, age, and body height, according to criteria of the American Pediatrics Association and the European Society of Hypertension report [15].

2.1. Augmentation Index and Blood Pressure Measurements. All measurements were performed using the Arteriogrph system (Arteriograph; TensioMed Ltd, Budapest, Hungary) after 10 minutes of rest in a quiet room with stable temperature (22 ± 1°C). The Arteriograph system is an operator-independent noninvasive device that applies an oscillometric, occlusive technique by use of an upper-arm cuff to register brachial pressure waves.

The mentioned device was used to assess simultaneously central (aortic) systolic and pulse pressure (cSBP, cPP) and peripheral (brachial) systolic, diastolic, pulse, and mean BP levels (pSBP, pDBP, pPP and MAP, resp.). The measurement procedure takes approximately 3 minutes and is operatively comparable to an automatic digital BP oscillometric measurement. In this study, the same device was used for all measurements. The working principle and the invasive validations of this method have been detailed previously [6, 23]. The method is based on the physiological fact that the early ($P1$) systolic pulse pressure wave of the aorta, generated by the left ventricle ejection, travels along the aorta and is reflected ($P2$) from the area of the aortic bifurcation. Occluding the brachial artery by pressurizing the cuff 35–40 mmHg above the actual SBP creates easily distinguished, pronounced pressure peaks in the cuff. Separated in this way, early and late systolic waves can be recorded. The time lapses between the peaks of $P1$ and $P2$ are equal to the travel time of the aortic pressure wave from the aortic root to the bifurcation and back. By halving this time and measuring the sternal notch, pubic bone distance (which is rather close to the true aortic length [24], the Ao-PWV can be calculated (Ao-PWV = jugulum-symphysis distance/transit time). Additionally, the Arteriography system calculates the brachial augmentation index (bAIx) using the formula: bAIx (%) = ($P2$ − $P1$/PP) × 100. The cAIx was calculated based on invasive measurements previously reported [23], which showed a very strong linear correlation between bAIx and cAIx ($R = 0.94$, $p < 0.001$). These studies showed a strong and significant correlation between the invasively obtained values and oscillometrically measured cAIx, cSBP, and aortic PWV. Taking into account the influence of heart rate on cAIx [25], in each subject the mentioned index was calculated corresponding to 75 beats by minute (cAIx-HR75).

2.2. Data Analysis. In this research, a step-wise data analysis was done as is described in the following.

First, aiming at determining whether RIs analysis for cAIx and cAIx-HR75 was necessaries, we separately assessed the degree of association (correlation) and equivalence (agreement) between cAIx and cAIx-HR75 levels, by studying potential mean and/or proportional differences (errors) between measurements and constructing limits of agreement (correlation and Bland-Altman analysis). As a first result, specific RIs for cAIx and cAIx-HR75 were defined as not necessaries. About this, both variables showed a great association (cAIx = −0.2753 + 0.9957 · cAIx-HR75; $R^2 = 0.9953$). However, despite a statistically significant difference between both variables (mean error = −0.3167%, $p < 0.0001$; mean error 95% confidence interval = −0.3522% to −0.2811%; mean error standard deviation (SD) = 0.5836%, 95% confidence interval = −1.4605% to 0.8272%), the difference was not considered clinically significant, as to force the generation of RIs separately (for cAIx and cAIx-HR75).

Second, we evaluated if RIs for males and females were necessary. To this end, bivariate and point-biserial correlations were done (Table 2), and after that gender influence was examined before and after adjustment for cofactors (i.e., age, BP) applying covariance analysis (ANCOVA) (Table 3). ANCOVA allows comparing one variable (i.e., cSBP or cAIx) in two or more groups (i.e., males versus females) taking into account (or to correct for) variability of other variables, called covariates or cofactors. With this purpose, correlations were done to identify demographic, anthropometric (i.e., body height, body weight) and/or hemodynamic (i.e., heart rate, pSBP, and pDBP) variables that in theory could be considered as cofactors in covariate analysis. Once the variables significantly associated with cSBP and cAIx were identified, ANCOVA analysis was done adjusting for them (Table 3). With this purpose, several models (cofactors combinations) were analyzed. Always, prior to the ANCOVA test, Levene's test for equality of variances and homogeneity of regression slopes test were performed. If Levene's test is positive ($p < 0.05$) then the variances in the groups are different (the groups are not homogeneous), and therefore the assumptions for ANCOVA are not met. Additionally, the interpretation of ANCOVA and the associated adjusted (or marginal) means relies on the assumption of homogeneous regression slopes for the compared groups (i.e., males and females); if this assumption is not met ($p < 0.05$) the ANCOVA results are unreliable. After statistical analysis, as a result, generation of specific cSBP and cAIx RIs for males and females was considered as necessaries.

Third, the mean value and SD age-related equations (for males and females) were obtained for cSBP and cAIx. With this purpose, parametric regression methods based on fractional polynomials (FPs), as described by Royston and Wright [26] and previously used to generate RIs for arterial parameters in the European Arterial Stiffness Collaboration Group methodological strategy [27, 28], were implemented using MedCalc Software (MedCalc, Ostend, Belgium). Briefly, fitting FPs for age specific cSBP and cAIx mean value and SD regression curves were defined using iterative procedure (generalized least squares, GLS). The obtained results enabled estimating age specific mean and SD for both parameters (cSBP and cAIx). For instance, cAIx mean equation could be cAIx = $a + b * \text{age}^p + c * \text{age}^q + \cdots$, where $a, b, c, \ldots$ are the coefficients, and $p, q, \ldots$ are the powers, with numbers selected from the set [−2, −1, −0.5, 0, 0.5, 1, 2, 3] estimated from the regression for the mean cAIx curve and likewise from the regression for the SD curve. Continuing the example, FPs with powers [1, 2], that is, with $p = 1$ and $q = 2$, illustrate an equation with the form $a + b*\ \text{age} + c * \text{age}^2$ [26]. The residuals were used to assess the model fit, which was deemed appropriate if the scores were normally distributed, with a mean of 0 and a SD of 1, randomly scattered above and below 0 when plotted against age. The best fitted curves, considering visual and mathematical criteria (Kurtosis and Skewness coefficients), were selected. Then, using the equations obtained for mean and SD, age specific percentiles were defined using the standard normal distribution (Z) (Tables 4, 5, and 6 for cSBP and Tables 7, 8, and 9 for cAIx). Age specific 1th, 2.5th, 5th, 10th, 25th, 50th, 75th, 90th, 95th, 97.5th, and 99th percentile curves were calculated as mean cAIx + Zp ∗ SD, where Zp assumed the values of −2.3263, −1.9599, −1.6448, −1.2815, −0.6755, 0, 0.6755, 1.2815, 1.6448, 1.9599, and 2.3263, respectively. The obtained equations were as follows:

(i) For all subjects ($cSBP^{0.26}$ and $(cAIx + 12.001)^{0.5}$),

$$\begin{aligned} \text{cSBP Mean} &= 3.0581 + 0.2189 \log(\text{Age}) \\ &\quad - 0.001044\text{Age} \\ \text{cSBP SD} &= -0.03919 + 0.1535 \log(\text{Age}) \\ &\quad - 0.004564\text{Age} \\ \text{cAIx Mean} &= 9.5226 - 6.1599 \log(\text{Age}) + 0.1450\text{Age} \\ \text{cAIx SD} &= 1.3880 - 0.8468 \log(\text{Age}) \\ &\quad + 0.03212\text{Age}. \end{aligned} \tag{1}$$

(ii) For males ($cSBP^{1.13}$ and $(cAIx + 7.001)^{0.53}$),

$$\begin{aligned} \text{cSBP Mean} &= 146.7373 + 5.4105 \log(\text{Age}) \\ &\quad + 1.7801\text{Age} \\ \text{cSBP SD} &= -10.3739 + 39.2556 \log(\text{Age}) \\ &\quad - 1.2532\text{Age} \\ \text{cAIx Mean} &= 7.4365 - 3.7152 \log(\text{Age}) \\ &\quad + 0.05135\text{Age} \\ \text{cAIx SD} &= -1.2276 + 3.4356 \log(\text{Age}) \\ &\quad - 0.1113\text{Age}. \end{aligned} \tag{2}$$

(iii) For females ($cSBP^{0.26}$ and $(cAIx + 12.001)^{0.66}$),

$$\begin{aligned} \text{cSBP Mean} &= 2.9920 + 0.3501 \log(\text{Age}) \\ &\quad - 0.007039\text{Age} \\ \text{cSBP SD} &= -0.07844 + 0.2039 \log(\text{Age}) \\ &\quad - 0.005824\text{Age} \\ \text{cAIx Mean} &= 21.8535 - 18.4253 \log(\text{Age}) \\ &\quad + 0.5115\text{Age} \\ \text{cAIx SD} &= 3.2466 - 1.6274 \log(\text{Age}) \\ &\quad + 0.03122\text{Age}. \end{aligned} \tag{3}$$

Finally, a similar procedure was performed to obtain cAIx RIs considering the body height (BH) [17]. The obtained equations were as follows:

For males $(cAIx + 7.001)^{0.53}$,

$$\begin{aligned} \text{cAIx Mean} &= -16.3756 + 13.9683 \log(\text{BH}) \\ &\quad - 0.06468\text{BH} \\ \text{cAIx SD} &= -14.8123 + 8.6667 \log(\text{BH}) \\ &\quad - 0.02016\text{BH}. \end{aligned} \tag{4}$$

For females $(cAIx + 12.001)^{0.66}$,

$$\begin{aligned} \text{cAIx Mean} &= -46.6729 + 35.8589 \log(\text{BH}) \\ &\quad - 0.1523\text{BH} \\ \text{cAIx SD} &= 38.0202 - 21.0915 \log(\text{BH}) \\ &\quad + 0.06424\text{BH}. \end{aligned} \tag{5}$$

In the equations detailed above, always cSBP, cAIx, Age, and BH were expressed in mmHg, %, years, and centimeters, respectively.

Limit of statistical signification was considered when a p value < 0.05 was found. Calculus of the minimum sample size required was calculated taken into account a normal distribution of the covariate (age) in the sample (in a conservative way) and a 95% and 90% limit of reference and confidence interval (two sided), respectively, with a 95% and 10% reference range and relative margin of error, respectively. In this research, the minimum required sample size for RIs construction (i.e., for males or females) was 377 subjects [29].

3. Results

3.1. General Characteristics of the Analyzed Population. In this research 1038 healthy subjects (576 males and 462 females) were included. In Table 1 the characteristics of all children, adolescents, and young adults are summarized, discriminating values obtained for males and females. Mean age for the whole population was 15.35 ± 3.15 years (range 5.00–21.92 y.o.) and no significant age differences were found (Table 1). In this cohort, males showed the highest body weight, body height, and BMI values ($p < 0.001$). Also, males exhibit significant higher jugulum-symphysis distance than females ($p < 0.001$). Mean values of pSBP and pPP obtained in males were significantly higher than those obtained in females ($p < 0.001$); on the contrary pDBP and HR were significantly lower in males compared with females. No significant differences related to gender in terms of pMAP values were observed. Moreover, males have higher mean values of cSBP and cPP than females ($p < 0.05$ and $p < 0.001$, resp.). See Table 1.

No significant gender differences in peripheral AIx, ejection duration, and Ao-PWV mean values were observed in the analyzed population. Obtained mean values of cAIx and cAIx-HR75 were always higher in females than in males ($p < 0.001$). See Table 1.

3.2. Analysis of cSBP and cAIx Associations. As was mentioned significant differences between cAIx and cAIx-HR75 were found; however absolutely values of these differences were really minimal (mean error = −0.3167, $p < 0.0001$; mean error 95% confidence interval = −0.3522 to −0.2811; mean error SD = 0.5836, 95% confidence interval = −1.4605 to 0.8272). Consequently, taking into account the RIs generated in terms of cAIx, it was evidenced that it was not necessary to generate RIs using cAIx-HR75 obtained values. That is to say, percentiles generated using cAIx or cAIx-HR75

Table 1: Children and adolescents characteristics.

	All (1038)				Male (n = 576)				Female (n = 462)				p value (male versus female)
	MV	SD	Min	Max	MV	SD	Min	Max	MV	SD	Min	Max	
Age (years)	15.35	3.15	5.00	21.92	15.51	2.84	5.00	21.75	15.15	3.49	5.17	21.92	0.068
Body height (cm)	162.67	13.98	102.00	191.00	167.15	13.72	104.00	191.00	157.09	12.20	102.00	178.00	<0.001
Body weight (Kg)	57.00	14.14	15.00	96.00	61.39	14.70	15.00	96.00	51.51	11.22	18.00	75.00	<0.001
BMI (Kg./m^2)	21.17	3.11	7.90	29.40	21.60	3.14	13.60	29.40	20.64	2.98	7.90	27.82	<0.001
Jugulo -symphysis distance (cm)	47.48	4.96	28.00	74.00	49.13	4.87	28.00	74.00	45.44	4.27	28.00	56.00	<0.001
Heart rate (b.p.m.)	68.43	12.17	44.00	113.00	65.49	11.83	44.00	104.00	72.09	11.60	44.00	113.00	<0.001
Peripheral SBP (mmHg)	111.81	9.58	81.00	135.00	114.01	9.64	89.00	135.00	109.06	8.78	81.00	134.00	<0.001
Peripheral MBP (mmHg)	79.07	7.49	8.00	102.00	79.24	7.68	8.00	98.00	78.86	7.25	61.00	102.00	0.412
Peripheral DBP (mmHg)	62.71	7.51	3.00	89.00	61.97	7.17	36.00	82.00	63.63	7.84	3.00	89.00	<0.001
Peripheral PP (mmHg)	48.96	8.29	.49	86.00	51.99	8.12	31.00	86.00	45.17	6.81	.49	70.00	<0.001
Central (aortic) SBP (mmHg)	98.86	8.39	75.20	124.90	99.35	8.40	78.00	124.90	98.24	8.36	75.20	121.00	0.035
Central (aortic) PP (mmHg)	36.26	5.88	21.80	62.90	37.43	5.72	21.80	62.90	34.78	5.75	23.20	58.60	<0.001
Peripheral (brachial) AIx (%)	−1.34	7.01	−85.00	.60	−1.64	8.12	−85.00	.29	−.96	5.31	−84.00	.60	0.122
cAIx (%)	9.20	8.46	−12.00	45.90	6.67	7.40	−7.00	36.00	12.35	8.64	−12.00	45.90	<0.001
cAIx HR75 (%)	9.51	8.49	−12.34	45.61	7.12	7.45	−7.82	36.53	12.49	8.76	−12.34	45.61	<0.001
Return time (ms)	173.47	21.17	14.00	310.00	178.91	19.43	85.00	230.00	166.68	21.32	14.00	310.00	<0.001
Ejection duration (ms)	299.06	22.73	185.00	385.00	297.90	21.09	185.00	360.00	300.49	24.59	190.00	385.00	0.068
Ao-PWV (m/s)	5.50	.63	3.40	7.70	5.51	.64	3.40	7.70	5.48	.62	3.90	7.70	0.607

BMI: body mass index. SBP, MBP, DBP, and PP: systolic, mean, diastolic, and pulse blood pressure, respectively. AIx: augmentation index. cAIx and cAIx HR75: central (aortic) augmentation index net value and normalized for heart rate equal 75 beats/minute, respectively. Ao-PWV: Aortic pulse wave velocity. Min and Max: minimal and maximal value, respectively. A $p < 0.05$ was considered statistically significant.

were very similar and observed differences were lack of clinical relevance. In other words, the difference was not considered clinically significant, as to force the generation of RIs separately (for cAIx and cAIx-HR75).

Table 2 show the bivariate and point-biserial correlation study of cSBP, cAIx, and Age relationship with demographic, anthropometric, hemodynamic, and vascular parameters of the analyzed population. As can be seen in Table 2, the age and the anthropometric parameters show a positive and significantly association with cSBP and cAIx levels. Moreover, HR shows borderline statistic values of association with cSBP ($p = 0.079$).

Table 3 show a covariance (ANCOVA) study destined to determine if the gender discrimination would be necessary in the RIs of cSBP and cAIx generation using data collected in this research. Also in Table 3, the noncorrected and corrected marginals' means values with standard error and 95% confidence intervals are given for males and females. In the case of cSPB, a first analysis induces to think that adjustments using Models 1, 2, 3, and 4 show no statistically significantly gender differences. However, the comparison of regression lines obtained from males and females showed statistically significant differences; that is to say there are different slopes of the cSBP-age regression lines (see homogeneity of regression slope's test in Table 3(a)). As the ANCOVA analysis and the associated adjusted means values rely on the assumption of the homogeneity of regression slopes in the studied groups. If this assumption is not met ($p < 0.05$) the ANCOVA results are unreliable; consequently, in the analyzed population, it is absolutely necessary to perform different RIs for cSBP for males and females (Table 3(a)). Similar results were obtained when sex-related differences in cAIx were analyzed using Models 3 and 4 (Table 3(b)). Moreover, for all considered models, sex-related differences after Levene's test for equality of variances were also demonstrated (different in terms of the calculated variance). Again, if Levene's test is positive ($p < 0.05$) the variances in the analyzed groups should be considered statistically different (the groups are not homogeneous); so the assumption of homogeneity is not met and the ANCOVA analysis is invalid. As a consequence of the results obtained in cAIx ANCOVA analysis, sex-related RIs should be necessary in this population (Table 3(b)).

TABLE 2: Association between aortic characteristics and anthropometric and haemodynamic parameters.

		Central (aortic) SBP (mmHg)	cAIx (%)	Age (years)
Sex (0: male; 1: female)	R	−.066	.334	−.057
	P	.035	.000	.068
Age (years)	R	.263	−.188	1.000
	P	.000	.000	.000
Body height (cm)	R	.238	−.371	.678
	P	.000	.000	.000
Body weight (Kg)	R	.318	−.362	.617
	P	.000	.000	.000
BMI (Kg/m^2)	R	.320	−.215	.414
	P	.000	.000	.000
Yugulo-symphysis distance (cm)	R	.242	−.378	.656
	P	.000	.000	.000
Heart rate (b.p.m.)	R	.054	.005	−.358
	P	.079	.881	.000
Peripheral SBP (mmHg)	R	.892	−.216	.308
	P	.000	.000	.000
Peripheral MBP (mmHg)	R	.863	−.016	.293
	P	.000	.617	.000
Peripheral DBP (mmHg)	R	.720	.107	.236
	P	.000	.001	.000
Peripheral PP (mmHg)	R	.385	−.336	.131
	P	.000	.000	.000
Central (aortic) SBP (mmHg)	R	1.000	.164	.263
	P	.000	.000	.000
Central (aortic) PP (mmHg)	R	.525	.180	.040
	P	.000	.000	.202
Peripheral (brachial) AIx	R	−.018	.079	−.079
	P	.571	.011	.011
cAIx (%)	R	.164	1.000	−.188
	P	.000	.000	.000
cAIx HR75 (%)	R	.162	.997	−.160
	P	.000	.000	.000
Ejection duration (ms)	R	−.026	.207	.096
	P	.396	.000	.002
Return time (ms)	R	−.118	−.327	.152
	P	.000	.000	.000
Ao-PWV (m/s)	R	.374	.010	.456
	P	.000	.757	.000

BMI: body mass index. SBP, MBP, DBP, and PP: systolic, mean, diastolic, and pulse blood pressure, respectively. AIx: augmentation index. cAIx and cAIx HR75: central (aortic) augmentation index net value and normalized for heart rate equal 75 beats/minute, respectively. Ao-PWV: aortic pulse wave velocity. A $p < 0.05$ was considered statistically significant.

3.3. Reference Intervals (Percentile Analysis) Obtained in the Analyzed Population. As is shown in Table 4, specific percentiles of age-cSBP values for five-year age RIs were generated including the entire population ($n = 1038$), that is, including males and females. Furthermore, a similar analysis was carried out using values corresponding to each year of age (Table A in Supplementary Materials). As seen in Table 5, age-cSBP percentiles corresponding to 5-year age intervals were generated for males ($n = 576$). A similar analysis was done for each year of age, as seen in Table B (see Supplementary Materials). Females ($n = 462$) were analyzed using a similar method, and the obtained RIs can be seen in Table 6 and Table C (see Supplementary Materials). Figures 1(a), 1(b), and 1(c) show specific age-cSBP percentiles for the entire population, males and females, respectively. As expected, there was a positive association between age and cSBP values, representing a gradual and continuous increase in terms of cSBP.

TABLE 3: Sex-related cSBP and cAIx comparison: analysis of covariance (ANCOVA) adjusting by age, heart rate, and/or anthropometric variables (cofactors).

(a)

		cSBP (mMHg): before adjustment			cSBP (mmHg): after adjustment by covariates					Covariates appearing in the model are evaluated at the following values							
		MV	SD	p	MV	SE	95% CI lower bound	95% CI upper bound	p	Age (years)	Body height (cm)	Body weight (Kg)	Yugulo-Symphysis distance (cm)	Heart rate (b.p.m.)	Levene's test	Homogeneity of regression slopes test	Adjusted R^2
Model 1	Male	99.3517	8.39824	<0.001	99.241	.337	98.579	99.903	0.090	15.35	------	------	------	------	0.773	0.002	0.070
	Female	98.2448	8.35555		98.383	.377	97.643	99.122									
Model 2	Male	99.3517	8.39824	<0.001	98.813	.350	98.125	99.500	0.852	15.35	162.67	57.00	47.48	------	0.797	0.011	0.113
	Female	98.2448	8.35555		98.917	.397	98.139	99.696									
Model 3	Male	99.3517	8.39824	<0.001	99.616	.337	98.954	100.278	0.724	15.35	------	------	------	68.43	0.724	0.001	0.101
	Female	98.2448	8.35555		97.916	.378	97.173	98.658									
Model 4	Male	99.3517	8.39824	<0.001	99.061	.345	98.385	99.737	0.415	15.35	162.67	57.00	47.48	68.43	0.859	0.005	0.151
	Female	98.2448	8.35555		98.607	.391	97.841	99.374									

(b)

		cAIx: before adjustment			cAIx: after adjustment by covariates					Covariates appearing in the model are evaluated at the following values							
		MV	SD	p	MV	SE	95% CI lower bound	95% CI upper bound	p	Age (years)	Body Height (cm)	Body weight (Kg)	Yugulo-Symphysis distance (cm)	Heart rate (b.p.m.)	Levene's test	Homogeneity of regression slopes test	Adjusted R^2
Model 1	Male	6.6737	7.40231	<0.001	6.747	.327	6.104	7.389	<0.001	15.35	------	------	------	------	<0.001	0.228	0.138
	Female	12.3474	8.64323		12.257	.366	11.539	12.974									
Model 2	Male	6.6737	7.40231	<0.001	7.72	.337	7.059	8.380	<0.001	15.35	162.67	57.00	47.4846	------	<0.001	0.158	0.193
	Female	12.3474	8.64323		11.043	.381	10.295	11.792									
Model 3	Male	6.6737	7.40231	<0.001	6.411	.328	5.767	7.055	<0.001	15.35	------	------	------	68.43	0.020	0.008	0.163
	Female	12.3474	8.64323		12.675	.368	11.953	13.397									
Model 4	Male	6.6737	7.40231	<0.001	7.447	.329	6.802	8.093	<0.001	15.35	162.67	57.00	47.4846	68.43	0.005	0.006	0.238
	Female	12.3474	8.64323		11.383	.373	10.651	12.115									

cSBP: central (aortic) systolic blood pressure. MV: mean value: SD and SE: standard deviation and error, respectively. CI: confidence interval. cAIx: central (aortic) augmentation index (net value). A $p < 0.05$ was considered statistically significant.

TABLE 4: Age-related reference intervals (RIs) for central (aortic) systolic blood pressure for the entire population (n = 1038).

Age (years)	1th	2.5th	5th	10th	25th	50th	75th	90th	95th	97.5th	99th
5.0	77.6	79.2	80.7	82.3	85.1	88.3	91.6	94.6	96.5	98.1	100.0
6.0	77.5	79.4	81.0	83.0	86.3	90.0	93.9	97.5	99.7	101.7	104.0
7.0	77.5	79.6	81.5	83.6	87.3	91.5	95.9	99.9	102.4	104.6	107.2
8.0	77.7	79.9	81.9	84.2	88.2	92.8	97.5	102.0	104.7	107.1	109.9
9.0	77.9	80.3	82.4	84.8	89.0	93.9	99.0	103.7	106.6	109.1	112.2
10.0	78.2	80.7	82.9	85.4	89.8	94.9	100.2	105.1	108.2	110.8	114.0
11.0	78.6	81.2	83.4	86.0	90.5	95.8	101.3	106.4	109.5	112.3	115.6
12.0	79.0	81.6	83.9	86.6	91.2	96.6	102.2	107.4	110.7	113.5	116.9
13.0	79.5	82.1	84.5	87.2	91.9	97.4	103.1	108.4	111.7	114.6	118.0
14.0	80.0	82.7	85.0	87.8	92.5	98.0	103.8	109.2	112.5	115.4	118.9
15.0	80.5	83.2	85.6	88.3	93.1	98.7	104.5	109.9	113.2	116.2	119.7
16.0	81.1	83.8	86.1	88.9	93.7	99.3	105.1	110.5	113.8	116.7	120.3
17.0	81.7	84.4	86.7	89.5	94.3	99.8	105.6	111.0	114.3	117.2	120.7
18.0	82.3	85.0	87.3	90.1	94.8	100.3	106.0	111.4	114.7	117.6	121.1
19.0	83.0	85.6	87.9	90.6	95.3	100.8	106.5	111.8	115.0	117.9	121.3
20.0	83.6	86.2	88.5	91.2	95.9	101.2	106.8	112.1	115.3	118.1	121.5
21.0	84.3	86.9	89.1	91.8	96.4	101.7	107.2	112.3	115.5	118.2	121.6
21.8	84.8	87.4	89.6	92.3	96.8	102.0	107.4	112.5	115.6	118.3	121.6

TABLE 5: Age-related reference intervals (RIs) for central (aortic) systolic blood pressure for males (n = 576).

Age (years)	1th	2.5th	5th	10th	25th	50th	75th	90th	95th	97.5th	99th
5.0	76.4	78.4	80.1	82.1	85.3	89.0	92.5	95.8	97.7	99.3	101.2
6.0	75.4	77.7	79.7	82.0	85.8	90.0	94.2	98.0	100.2	102.2	104.4
7.0	74.8	77.4	79.6	82.2	86.4	91.1	95.7	99.9	102.4	104.5	107.0
8.0	74.7	77.5	79.8	82.6	87.1	92.1	97.1	101.5	104.2	106.5	109.1
9.0	74.8	77.8	80.3	83.1	87.9	93.1	98.4	103.0	105.8	108.2	111.0
10.0	75.2	78.2	80.8	83.8	88.7	94.1	99.5	104.3	107.2	109.7	112.6
11.0	75.8	78.9	81.5	84.5	89.6	95.1	100.6	105.5	108.5	111.0	113.9
12.0	76.5	79.6	82.3	85.4	90.5	96.1	101.7	106.6	109.6	112.2	115.1
13.0	77.4	80.5	83.2	86.3	91.4	97.0	102.7	107.6	110.6	113.2	116.2
14.0	78.4	81.5	84.2	87.3	92.4	98.0	103.6	108.6	111.6	114.2	117.1
15.0	79.4	82.5	85.2	88.3	93.3	98.9	104.5	109.5	112.4	115.0	118.0
16.0	80.6	83.6	86.3	89.3	94.3	99.9	105.4	110.3	113.2	115.8	118.7
17.0	81.8	84.8	87.4	90.4	95.3	100.8	106.3	111.1	114.0	116.5	119.4
18.0	83.1	86.0	88.6	91.5	96.4	101.7	107.1	111.9	114.7	117.1	120.0
19.0	84.4	87.3	89.8	92.7	97.4	102.7	107.9	112.6	115.3	117.7	120.5
20.0	85.8	88.6	91.0	93.8	98.5	103.6	108.7	113.2	116.0	118.3	121.0
21.0	87.2	90.0	92.3	95.0	99.5	104.5	109.5	113.9	116.5	118.8	121.5
21.6	88.1	90.8	93.1	95.8	100.2	105.1	109.9	114.3	116.9	119.1	121.7

Tables 7, 8, and 9 show specific percentiles of age-cAIx values for five-year age RIs corresponding to the entire population, males and females, respectively. Furthermore, a similar analysis was carried out using values obtained by each year of age (Tables D, E, and F in Supplementary Materials). Figures 2(a), 2(b), and 2(c) show specific age-cAIx percentiles for the entire population, males and females, respectively. As expected, there was a correlation between age and cAIx values.

Specific percentile analysis of cAIx corresponding to each body height level (using 5 cm intervals) of the male cohort is shown in Table 10. Also in Table G, using 1 cm interval is provided in Supplementary Materials. Furthermore, in Table 11 and Table H of the Supplementary Materials, RIs corresponding to the female cohort are showed. Figures 3(a) and 3(b) show body height-cAIx percentiles, corresponding to males and females, respectively.

TABLE 6: Age-related reference intervals (RIs) for central (aortic) systolic blood pressure for females ($n = 462$).

Age (years)	1th	2.5th	5th	10th	25th	50th	75th	90th	95th	97.5th	99th
5.2	79.5	80.8	82.0	83.4	85.7	88.3	91.0	93.5	95.0	96.3	97.9
6.0	79.2	80.9	82.3	84.0	86.8	90.0	93.4	96.4	98.3	100.0	101.9
7.0	79.1	81.0	82.6	84.6	88.0	91.8	95.8	99.5	101.7	103.7	106.0
8.0	79.0	81.1	83.0	85.2	88.9	93.3	97.8	101.9	104.5	106.7	109.4
9.0	79.0	81.3	83.3	85.7	89.8	94.5	99.4	103.9	106.7	109.2	112.1
10.0	79.1	81.5	83.7	86.2	90.5	95.5	100.7	105.5	108.5	111.1	114.3
11.0	79.2	81.7	84.0	86.6	91.1	96.3	101.8	106.8	110.0	112.7	116.0
12.0	79.4	82.0	84.3	87.0	91.6	97.0	102.6	107.9	111.1	114.0	117.4
13.0	79.6	82.3	84.6	87.4	92.1	97.6	103.4	108.7	112.0	115.0	118.5
14.0	79.9	82.5	84.9	87.7	92.5	98.1	103.9	109.4	112.7	115.7	119.2
15.0	80.1	82.8	85.2	88.0	92.9	98.5	104.4	109.8	113.2	116.2	119.8
16.0	80.4	83.1	85.5	88.3	93.2	98.8	104.7	110.2	113.6	116.6	120.1
17.0	80.7	83.4	85.8	88.6	93.5	99.1	104.9	110.4	113.7	116.7	120.3
18.0	81.1	83.8	86.1	88.9	93.7	99.2	105.0	110.4	113.8	116.7	120.3
19.0	81.4	84.1	86.4	89.2	93.9	99.4	105.1	110.4	113.7	116.6	120.1
20.0	81.8	84.4	86.7	89.4	94.1	99.5	105.1	110.3	113.6	116.4	119.8
21.0	82.2	84.8	87.0	89.7	94.2	99.5	105.0	110.1	113.3	116.1	119.4
21.8	82.5	85.1	87.3	89.9	94.3	99.5	104.9	109.9	113.0	115.7	119.0

TABLE 7: Age-related reference intervals (RIs) for central (aortic) augmentation index (cAIx) for the entire population ($n = 1038$).

Age (years)	1th	2.5th	5th	10th	25th	50th	75th	90th	95th	97.5th	99th
5.0	1.8	4.5	7.1	10.2	16.0	23.3	31.4	39.4	44.5	49.1	54.7
6.0	−0.1	2.4	4.7	7.5	12.8	19.3	26.7	34.0	38.6	42.8	48.0
7.0	−1.5	0.8	2.9	5.5	10.3	16.4	23.3	30.0	34.3	38.3	43.0
8.0	−2.6	−0.5	1.5	3.9	8.5	14.2	20.6	27.0	31.1	34.8	39.4
9.0	−3.4	−1.5	0.4	2.7	7.0	12.5	18.7	24.8	28.7	32.3	36.6
10.0	−4.1	−2.3	−0.5	1.7	5.9	11.2	17.1	23.0	26.8	30.3	34.5
11.0	−4.7	−2.9	−1.2	1.0	5.0	10.1	15.9	21.7	25.4	28.8	32.9
12.0	−5.2	−3.4	−1.8	0.3	4.3	9.3	15.0	20.7	24.3	27.7	31.7
13.0	−5.6	−3.8	−2.2	−0.2	3.7	8.7	14.3	19.9	23.6	26.9	30.9
14.0	−5.9	−4.2	−2.6	−0.6	3.3	8.2	13.8	19.4	23.0	26.3	30.4
15.0	−6.1	−4.5	−2.9	−0.9	2.9	7.8	13.4	19.1	22.7	26.0	30.1
16.0	−6.4	−4.7	−3.2	−1.1	2.7	7.6	13.2	18.9	22.5	25.9	30.0
17.0	−6.6	−4.9	−3.4	−1.3	2.5	7.4	13.1	18.8	22.5	25.9	30.0
18.0	−6.7	−5.1	−3.5	−1.5	2.4	7.4	13.1	18.9	22.6	26.1	30.3
19.0	−6.8	−5.2	−3.6	−1.6	2.3	7.4	13.2	19.1	22.9	26.4	30.6
20.0	−6.9	−5.3	−3.7	−1.6	2.3	7.4	13.4	19.3	23.2	26.8	31.1
21.0	−7.0	−5.4	−3.8	−1.7	2.3	7.6	13.6	19.7	23.7	27.3	31.8
21.8	−7.1	−5.4	−3.8	−1.7	2.4	7.7	13.8	20.1	24.1	27.8	32.3

4. Discussion

This research provides the first Latin American database concerning RIs of cSBP and cAIx obtained on a large cohort of healthy children, adolescents, and young adults aged between 5 and 22 years. Moreover, the definition of RIs generated in this study will further improve our ability to identify young populations at high risk and represent a first step toward new approaches in the diagnosis and management of high BP states and/or other altered haemodynamic conditions found in childhood and adolescence. To the best of our knowledge, there are no widely accepted clear cutoff values for central aortic BP levels in pediatric clinical practice, in spite of recent efforts of European researchers [18]. In this context, our study provides percentiles for cSBP and cAIx representing a novel approach to optimize risk stratification in youths.

The cAIx inform about the arterial wave reflection component of the left ventricular afterload. Values of cAIx

TABLE 8: Age-related reference intervals (RIs) for central (aortic) augmentation index (cAIx) for males (n = 576).

Age (years)	1th	2.5th	5th	10th	25th	50th	75th	90th	95th	97.5th	99th
5.0	4.6	6.0	7.2	8.7	11.4	14.6	18.1	21.4	23.4	25.3	27.5
6.0	1.2	2.7	4.1	5.8	8.9	12.7	16.9	21.0	23.6	26.0	28.8
7.0	−1.1	0.4	1.9	3.7	7.0	11.2	15.9	20.6	23.6	26.3	29.6
8.0	−2.6	−1.1	0.3	2.1	5.6	10.0	15.1	20.2	23.4	26.4	30.0
9.0	−3.6	−2.2	−0.8	1.0	4.5	9.0	14.3	19.7	23.1	26.3	30.2
10.0	−4.3	−3.0	−1.6	0.1	3.6	8.2	13.6	19.1	22.7	26.0	30.0
11.0	−4.8	−3.6	−2.3	−0.5	2.9	7.5	13.0	18.6	22.2	25.6	29.7
12.0	−5.2	−4.0	−2.7	−1.0	2.4	7.0	12.4	18.0	21.7	25.1	29.2
13.0	−5.4	−4.3	−3.1	−1.4	1.9	6.5	11.9	17.5	21.1	24.5	28.7
14.0	−5.6	−4.5	−3.3	−1.7	1.6	6.0	11.4	16.9	20.5	23.8	27.9
15.0	−5.6	−4.6	−3.5	−1.9	1.3	5.6	10.9	16.3	19.8	23.1	27.2
16.0	−5.7	−4.7	−3.5	−2.0	1.1	5.3	10.4	15.7	19.2	22.4	26.3
17.0	−5.7	−4.7	−3.6	−2.1	0.9	5.0	10.0	15.1	18.5	21.6	25.4
18.0	−5.6	−4.6	−3.6	−2.1	0.8	4.8	9.6	14.5	17.7	20.7	24.4
19.0	−5.6	−4.6	−3.5	−2.1	0.7	4.6	9.2	13.9	17.0	19.9	23.4
20.0	−5.4	−4.5	−3.4	−2.1	0.7	4.4	8.8	13.3	16.3	19.0	22.3
21.0	−5.3	−4.3	−3.3	−2.0	0.7	4.2	8.4	12.7	15.5	18.1	21.3
21.6	−5.2	−4.2	−3.2	−1.9	0.7	4.1	8.2	12.4	15.1	17.6	20.6

TABLE 9: Age-related reference intervals (RIs) for central (aortic) augmentation index (cAIx) for females (n = 462).

Age (years)	1th	2.5th	5th	10th	25th	50th	75th	90th	95th	97.5th	99th
5.2	3.5	6.8	9.7	13.3	19.8	27.5	35.8	43.7	48.6	53.0	58.2
6.0	1.4	4.4	7.2	10.5	16.5	23.7	31.4	38.8	43.4	47.5	52.4
7.0	−0.5	2.2	4.8	7.8	13.4	20.1	27.3	34.1	38.4	42.3	46.8
8.0	−1.9	0.6	3.0	5.9	11.1	17.4	24.1	30.6	34.7	38.3	42.6
9.0	−2.9	−0.5	1.7	4.4	9.3	15.3	21.8	28.0	31.8	35.3	39.4
10.0	−3.7	−1.4	0.7	3.4	8.1	13.8	20.0	25.9	29.6	33.0	36.9
11.0	−4.2	−2.0	0.1	2.6	7.1	12.7	18.6	24.4	28.0	31.2	35.0
12.0	−4.5	−2.4	−0.4	2.0	6.4	11.8	17.7	23.2	26.7	29.9	33.6
13.0	−4.7	−2.7	−0.7	1.7	6.0	11.3	17.0	22.4	25.9	28.9	32.6
14.0	−4.8	−2.8	−0.9	1.5	5.7	10.9	16.5	21.9	25.2	28.3	31.9
15.0	−4.8	−2.8	−0.9	1.4	5.6	10.7	16.3	21.6	24.9	27.9	31.4
16.0	−4.8	−2.7	−0.8	1.5	5.6	10.7	16.2	21.4	24.7	27.7	31.2
17.0	−4.6	−2.6	−0.7	1.6	5.8	10.8	16.3	21.5	24.8	27.7	31.2
18.0	−4.4	−2.3	−0.5	1.9	6.0	11.0	16.5	21.7	25.0	27.9	31.4
19.0	−4.1	−2.0	−0.1	2.2	6.3	11.4	16.8	22.1	25.3	28.2	31.7
20.0	−3.7	−1.7	0.3	2.6	6.8	11.8	17.3	22.5	25.8	28.7	32.2
21.0	−3.3	−1.2	0.7	3.1	7.3	12.4	17.9	23.1	26.4	29.3	32.8
21.8	−3.0	−0.8	1.1	3.5	7.7	12.9	18.4	23.7	27.0	29.9	33.4

are mainly determined by two factors: (a) aortic stiffness (which in turn determines the "central to peripheral" and "peripheral to central" forward and backward wave components propagation velocities) and (b) distance between aortic root and major wave reflection sites (i.e., aortic bifurcation at the level of pelvic arteries and include small arteries) [30]. Increases in aortic stiffness enhance the speed of wave reflection (resulting in an earlier return of the reflected wave to the ascending aorta) and increase the magnitude of the backward or reflected wave (resulting in an increase in aortic pulse pressure and left ventricle afterload). As a result, frequently when the AS increases the higher the cAIx is [30]. Consequently, the cAIx inform about the vascular wall state as a surrogate index of AS [6, 23]. Additionally, reduced body height is associated with early arrival of reflected waves to the ascending aorta, and consequently is associated with

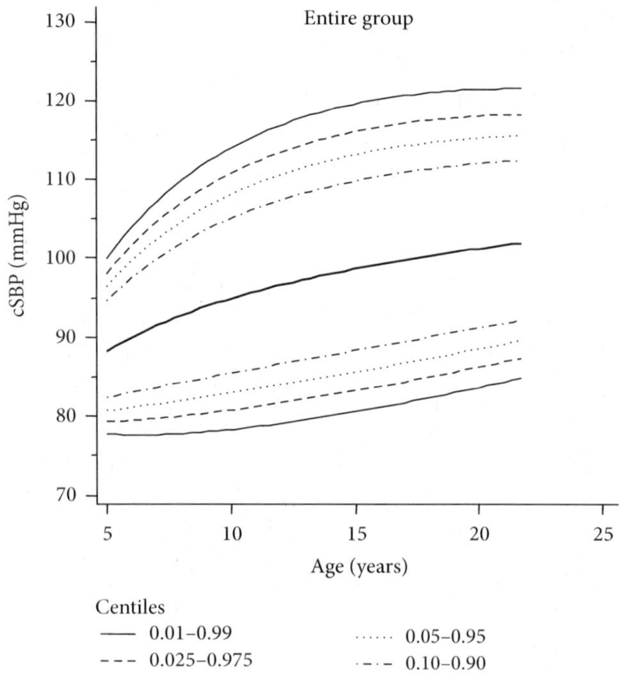

(a) Age specific central (aortic) systolic blood pressure (cSBP) percentiles generated using data of the entire population ($n = 1038$) of children and adolescents

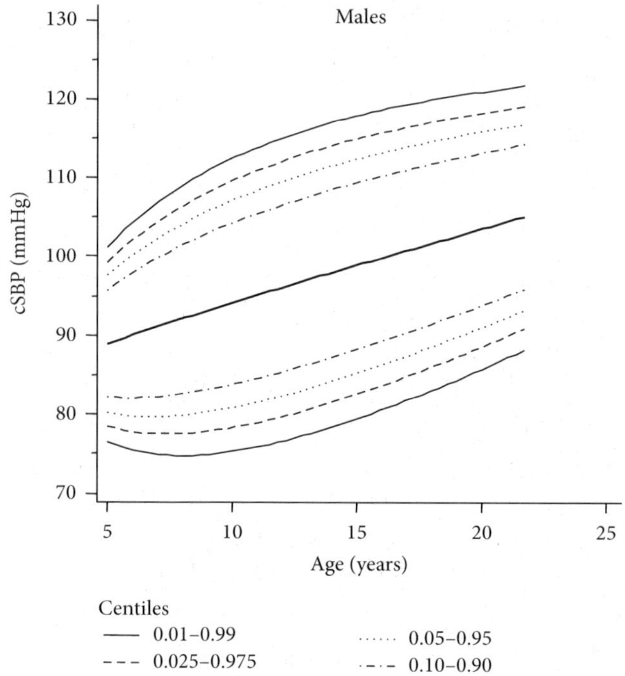

(b) Age specific central (aortic) systolic blood pressure (cSBP) percentiles corresponding to male cohort ($n = 576$) of children and adolescents

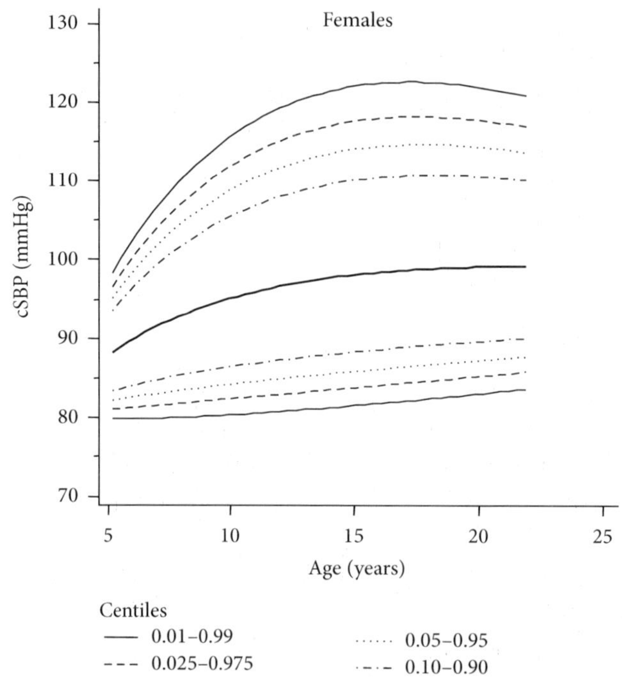

(c) Age specific central (aortic) systolic blood pressure (cSBP) percentiles corresponding to female cohort ($n = 462$) of children and adolescents

FIGURE 1

increased cAIx. Furthermore, high cAIx values implicate that increases of cSBP and/or cPP are determined by early arrival of reflected waves (during left ventricular systolic period). In other words, jointly analyzing the cAIx and cSBP or cPP, it is possible to determine if the levels of cSBP or cPP (i.e., increased) are due (or not) to an increase in the amplitude or early arrival of the reflected waves. Taking into account the determinant of cAIx, subjects with similar

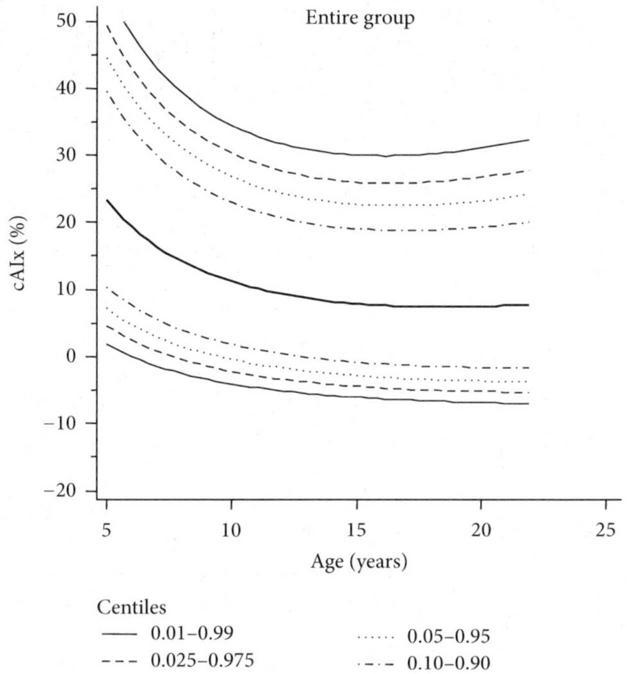

(a) Age specific central (aortic) augmentation index (cAIx) percentiles generated using data of the entire population (n = 1038) of children and adolescents

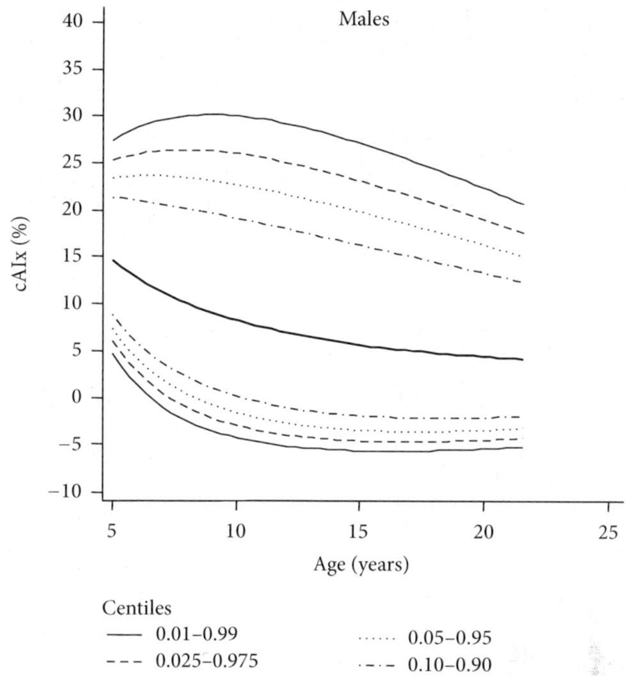

(b) Age specific central (aortic) augmentation index (cAIx) percentiles corresponding to male cohort (n = 576) of children and adolescents

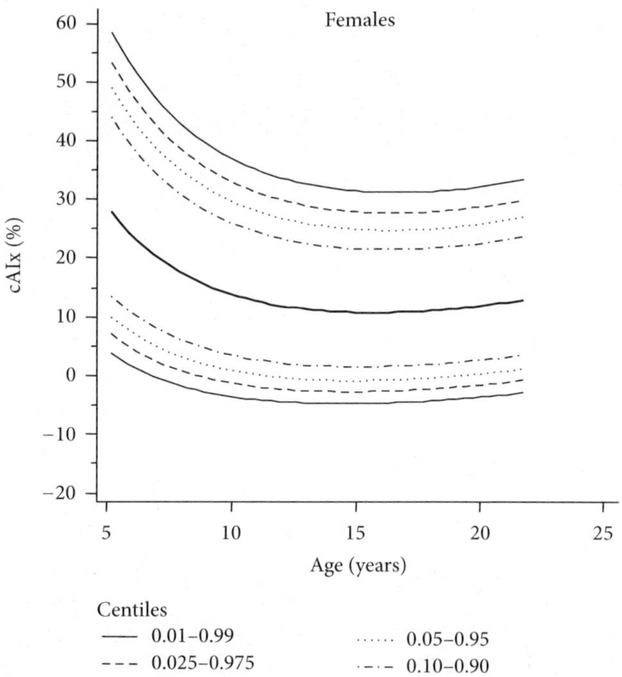

(c) Age specific central (aortic) augmentation index (cAIx) percentiles corresponding to female cohort (n = 462) of children and adolescents

Figure 2

levels of aortic stiffness could exhibit significant differences in cAIx associated with differences in body height. This is particularly important in children and adolescents in which both AS and body height are continuously changing. From this point of view, cAIx would be a very representative index of arterial dynamics and left ventricular afterload, since it evaluates simultaneously AS and changes associated with growth process.

TABLE 10: Body height-related reference intervals (RIs) for central (aortic) augmentation index (cAIx) for males ($n = 576$).

Body height (cm)	1th	2.5th	5th	10th	25th	50th	75th	90th	95th	97.5th	99th
104	5.06	6.36	7.54	8.95	11.43	14.41	17.59	20.62	22.51	24.20	26.23
105	4.79	6.12	7.32	8.76	11.31	14.35	17.62	20.74	22.69	24.44	26.52
110	3.54	4.97	6.26	7.83	10.64	14.03	17.70	21.23	23.45	25.44	27.83
115	2.38	3.87	5.24	6.91	9.93	13.61	17.63	21.52	23.98	26.19	28.85
120	1.31	2.85	4.26	6.01	9.18	13.10	17.41	21.61	24.28	26.69	29.59
125	0.33	1.88	3.33	5.12	8.41	12.52	17.07	21.54	24.39	26.96	30.08
130	−0.58	0.97	2.43	4.25	7.62	11.87	16.62	21.31	24.31	27.03	30.32
135	−1.41	0.11	1.57	3.40	6.82	11.17	16.07	20.93	24.06	26.89	30.33
140	−2.18	−0.69	0.75	2.57	6.01	10.42	15.43	20.43	23.65	26.58	30.14
145	−2.88	−1.44	−0.03	1.76	5.19	9.63	14.71	19.80	23.09	26.09	29.75
150	−3.51	−2.13	−0.77	0.99	4.37	8.81	13.91	19.07	22.41	25.46	29.18
155	−4.09	−2.78	−1.48	0.23	3.56	7.96	13.06	18.24	21.61	24.69	28.46
160	−4.61	−3.38	−2.14	−0.49	2.76	7.09	12.16	17.33	20.70	23.79	27.58
165	−5.07	−3.93	−2.76	−1.18	1.96	6.21	11.21	16.34	19.70	22.79	26.57
170	−5.49	−4.44	−3.34	−1.84	1.19	5.32	10.23	15.30	18.62	21.68	25.44
175	−5.85	−4.90	−3.88	−2.47	0.43	4.43	9.23	14.20	17.47	20.50	24.21
180	−6.16	−5.31	−4.38	−3.06	−0.31	3.54	8.20	13.06	16.27	19.24	22.89
185	−6.42	−5.68	−4.83	−3.61	−1.02	2.66	7.16	11.88	15.02	17.91	21.50
190	−6.63	−6.01	−5.25	−4.13	−1.71	1.80	6.12	10.68	13.72	16.54	20.03
191	−6.67	−6.07	−5.33	−4.23	−1.84	1.62	5.91	10.44	13.46	16.26	19.73

TABLE 11: Body height-related reference intervals (RIs) for central (aortic) augmentation index (cAIx) for females ($n = 462$).

Body height (cm)	1th	2.5th	5th	10th	25th	50th	75th	90th	95th	97.5th	99th
102	−1.63	1.21	3.82	7.03	12.82	19.86	27.47	34.76	39.32	43.40	48.27
105	−1.07	1.71	4.27	7.40	13.02	19.83	27.18	34.20	38.60	42.52	47.20
110	−0.36	2.34	4.80	7.80	13.17	19.65	26.61	33.25	37.40	41.09	45.50
115	0.10	2.71	5.09	7.98	13.12	19.31	25.95	32.26	36.20	39.71	43.89
120	0.32	2.85	5.15	7.93	12.88	18.83	25.19	31.24	35.01	38.37	42.36
125	0.31	2.76	4.99	7.69	12.48	18.22	24.36	30.19	33.82	37.06	40.91
130	0.09	2.48	4.64	7.26	11.92	17.50	23.46	29.12	32.64	35.78	39.52
135	−0.32	2.01	4.12	6.68	11.22	16.67	22.49	28.02	31.47	34.53	38.19
140	−0.90	1.37	3.44	5.95	10.40	15.75	21.47	26.91	30.30	33.32	36.91
145	−1.63	0.60	2.62	5.09	9.47	14.75	20.40	25.78	29.14	32.13	35.69
150	−2.48	−0.30	1.69	4.11	8.45	13.67	19.29	24.64	27.99	30.97	34.52
155	−3.44	−1.31	0.65	3.04	7.34	12.54	18.14	23.49	26.84	29.83	33.40
160	−4.48	−2.40	−0.47	1.89	6.16	11.35	16.96	22.34	25.71	28.72	32.31
165	−5.57	−3.55	−1.66	0.68	4.92	10.11	15.75	21.18	24.58	27.63	31.27
170	−6.70	−4.74	−2.89	−0.58	3.63	8.83	14.52	20.01	23.46	26.56	30.26
175	−7.83	−5.95	−4.15	−1.88	2.31	7.53	13.28	18.84	22.36	25.51	29.29
178	−8.49	−6.67	−4.90	−2.67	1.50	6.74	12.52	18.14	21.70	24.89	28.72

On the other hand, levels of BP are mainly determined by cardiac and vascular factors. Higher (and faster) left ventricular stroke volume is associated with high levels of cSBP and cPP. Otherwise, AS and arrival time and amplitude of wave reflections are the main determinants of cSBP and cPP, while peripheral vascular resistances and cardiac output are the main determinants of MBP and cDBP. In this context, it is important to emphasize that simultaneous measurements of central (aortic) BP and cAIx (using a single device) in children and adolescents allow us not only to know if cSBP and cPP are within physiological levels, but also in case of abnormal values to realize if they were associated or not with increased wave reflection levels (cAIx) [31, 32].

Our data shows that, in agreement with the two largest data bases of cSBP measurement in children and adolescents with oscillometric techniques, males exhibit higher values

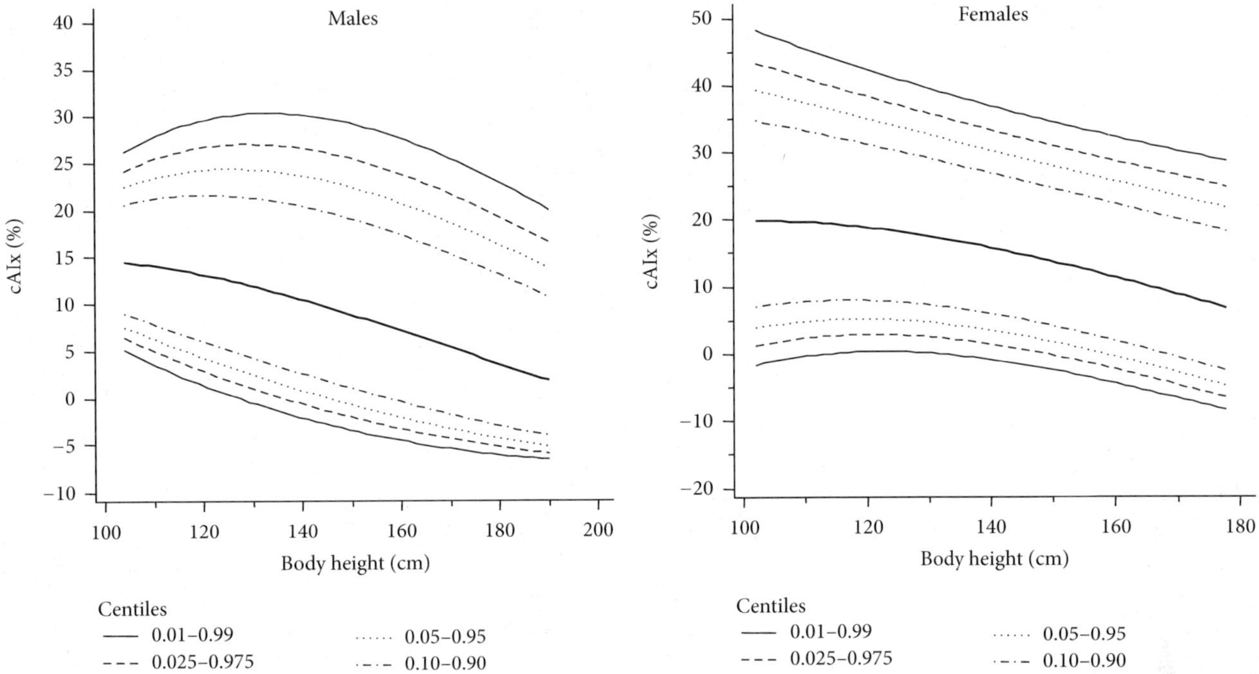

(a) Body height specific central (aortic) augmentation index (cAIx) percentiles corresponding to male cohort ($n = 576$) of children and adolescents

(b) Body height specific central (aortic) augmentation index (cAIx) percentiles corresponding to female cohort ($n = 462$) of children and adolescents

FIGURE 3

of SBP and PP in both central and peripheral arteries [17, 18]. Despite the methodological differences (inclusion and exclusion criteria) in addition to the different devices used between the three studies (see Table 12), it is possible to attempt to compare the cSBP values between our data with the RIs from Hungarian [17] and German pediatric population [18] (Figure 4). In the analyzed population, the 50th percentile corresponding to boys and girls aged between 5 and 22 years shows cSBP values slightly lower than those found by Hidvégi in the Hungarian population using the same technology. Those observations were also valid in boys when 95th percentile was analyzed. However, in girls aged 10 to 17 years, these differences tend to disappear when considering the 95th percentile. On the other hand, in comparison with German database (Mobil-O-Graph System), our data shows that cSBP values in the 50th and the 95th percentiles (both sexes) were slightly higher in children below 10 years, and significantly lower in adolescents over 13 years old than those found by Elmenhorst et al. [18].

On the other hand, values of cAIx show a different behavior with respect to age and gender. As was describe above, our data show that females have higher cAIx values than males (Table 1). These findings are in accordance with the published data of Hidvégi et al. who proved that after 15 years the AIx is higher in females than in males [17]. These authors reported that, in early childhood, the values of AIx are high; however it decreases gradually with age in both genders in ages between 12 and 15 years, increasing afterwards. Moreover, the increased cAIx detected in early childhood cannot be caused by the shorter return time, which is determined by a shorter aortic length [17]. In Figure 5, we compared cAIx percentiles 50th and 75th corresponding ton males and females of the Argentinean population, with those reported by Hidvégi et al. [17]. It is noteworthy that females of both populations exhibit similar cAIx curves, while Argentinean males have lower values than the European cohort before 12 y.o. and higher after ages over 13 y.o.

4.1. Methodological Considerations and Limitations. In this observational study a noninvasive occlusive-oscillometric device to assess arterial function parameters in children and adolescents was used. This validated system provides central aortic BP values that have shown significant correlation with values of cSBP invasively assessed [6, 23]. On the other hand, the use of an arm cuff facilitates epidemiological studies performed in large cohort including children and adolescents [14, 17, 33]. Moreover, the Arteriograph device allows simultaneous quantification of Ao-PWV, AIx, cSBP, and peripheral BP, and the procedure takes only 2-3 min and is well tolerated even in preschool children who experienced only a little discomfort, similar to that observed during noninvasive BP measurement [14].

The lack of standardization in methodologies used to obtain RIs and/or normal values for cAIx, cSBP, and other noninvasive obtained arterial parameters makes difficult to compare different populations. In our research, we used the statistical and methodological approach described by the *Reference Values for Arterial Measurements Collaboration*

Table 12: Subjects characteristics described for Europeans (Germany and Hungary) and our studied populations.

	Elmenhorst et al. 2015	Hidvégi et al. 2015	Díaz et al. (our work)
(1) Characteristics of the sample			
Number of subjects	1445 (females: 715; males: 730)	4619 (females: 2130; males: 2489)	1038 (females: 462; males: 576)
Subjects precedence	Living in Germany (Munich)	Living in Hungary	Living in Argentina (Tandil)
Age interval	8–22 years	3–18 years	5–21 years
Recruitment strategy	Prospective (school-based setting)	Prospective (nursery, elementary, and secondary schools)	Prospective (nursery, elementary, and secondary schools)
Communities	Urban/rural	-------	Urban/rural
Inclusion criteria	Absence of known CV; even if treated	Apparently healthy; Caucasian; without medication	Asymptomatic. (1) None had history of CV, pulmonary, or renal disease; (2) normal brachial BP at the time of examination; (3) none were taking medications, (4) all had normal levels of glycaemia, cholesterol, and triglycerides
Exclusion criteria	Hypertensive BP (<18 years: according to guideline; ≥18 years: 140/90 mmHg); obesity	BMI: 3th–97th percentile; SBP and DBP: 5th–95th percentile	Current and past smokers, diabetic, obese subjects, hypertensive subjects or subjects with averaged high brachial BP levels at the time of the study were excluded
(2) Aortic BP levels and waveform measurement			
Device	Mobil-O-Graph, I.E.M., Stolberg, Germany	Arteriograph, TensioMed Ltd., Budapest, Hungary	Arteriograph, TensioMed Ltd., Budapest, Hungary
Measurement conditions	Supine position after at least 5–10 min of rest	Supine position after 2-3 minutes of rest	Supine position after at least 10 min of rest

Table 12: Continued.

(3) *Characteristics of the subjects*	Elmenhorst et al. 2015 MV	Elmenhorst et al. 2015 SD	Hidvégi et al. 2015 MV	Hidvégi et al. 2015 SD	Díaz et al. (our work) MV	Díaz et al. (our work) SD
Female						
Age (years)	13.8	2.9	10.5	4.8	15.1	3.5
Body height (cm)	157.0	11.6	142.7	22.4	157.1	12.2
Body weight (Kg)	48.8	12.5	37.8	15.6	51.5	11.2
BMI (Kg/m^2)	19.5	3.2	17.4	2.5	20.6	3.0
pSBP (mmHg)	113.5	7.5	110.9	6.0	109.1	8.8
pDBP (mmHg)	66.0	6.8	64.7	3.0	63.6	7.8
pMBP (mmHg)	81.8	6.2	80.2	3.9	78.9	7.3
cSBP (mmHg)	100.5	8.0	100.3	3.3	98.2	8.4
Ao-PWV (m/s)	4.6	0.3	---	---	5.5	0.6
Heart rate (b.p.m.)	---	---	82.6	7.5	72.1	11.6
Yugulo-Symphysis distance (cm)	---	---	42.0	6.6	45.4	4.3
cAIx (%)	---	---	11.9	4.4	12.3	8.6
Male						
Age (years)	13.1	2.6	10.5	4.8	15.5	2.8
Body height (cm)	158.7	15.6	146.3	25.7	167.2	13.7
Body weight (Kg)	49.1	15.2	40.5	18.5	61.4	14.7
BMI (Kg/m^2)	19.0	3.1	17.6	2.4	21.6	3.1
pSBP (mmHg)	114.5	8.3	113.3	8.4	114.0	9.6
pDBP (mmHg)	65.1	6.8	64.7	2.6	62.0	7.2
pMBP (mmHg)	81.6	6.3	81.1	4.3	79.2	7.7
cSBP (mmHg)	100.8	9.7	101.2	4.8	99.4	8.4
Ao-PWV (m/s)	4.7	0.4			5.5	0.6
Heart rate (b.p.m.)	---	---	79.1	8.7	65.5	11.8
Yugulo-Symphysis distance (cm)	---	---	43.9	7.6	49.1	4.9
cAIx (%)	---	---	10.2	4.5	6.7	7.4
All						
Age (years)	13.4	2.8	---	---	15.3	3.1
Body height (cm)	----	----	---	---	162.7	14.0
Body weight (Kg)	----	----	---	---	57.0	14.1
pSBP (mmHg)	114.0	7.9	---	---	111.8	9.6
cSBP (mmHg)	100.7	8.9	---	---	98.9	8.4
Ao-PWV (m/s)	4.7	0.3	---	---	5.5	0.6

BMI: body mass index. pSBP, pMBP, and pDBP: peripheral (brachial) systolic, mean, and diastolic blood pressure, respectively. cAIx: central (aortic) augmentation index. Ao-PWV: aortic pulse wave velocity. CV: cardiovascular. MV: mean value. SD: standard deviation. cSBP: central (aortic) systolic blood pressure, respectively. Data from [18] were directly obtained from average population values published in their manuscript. Data from [17] were obtained from averaging the disaggregated values per year of life (age), for each sex.

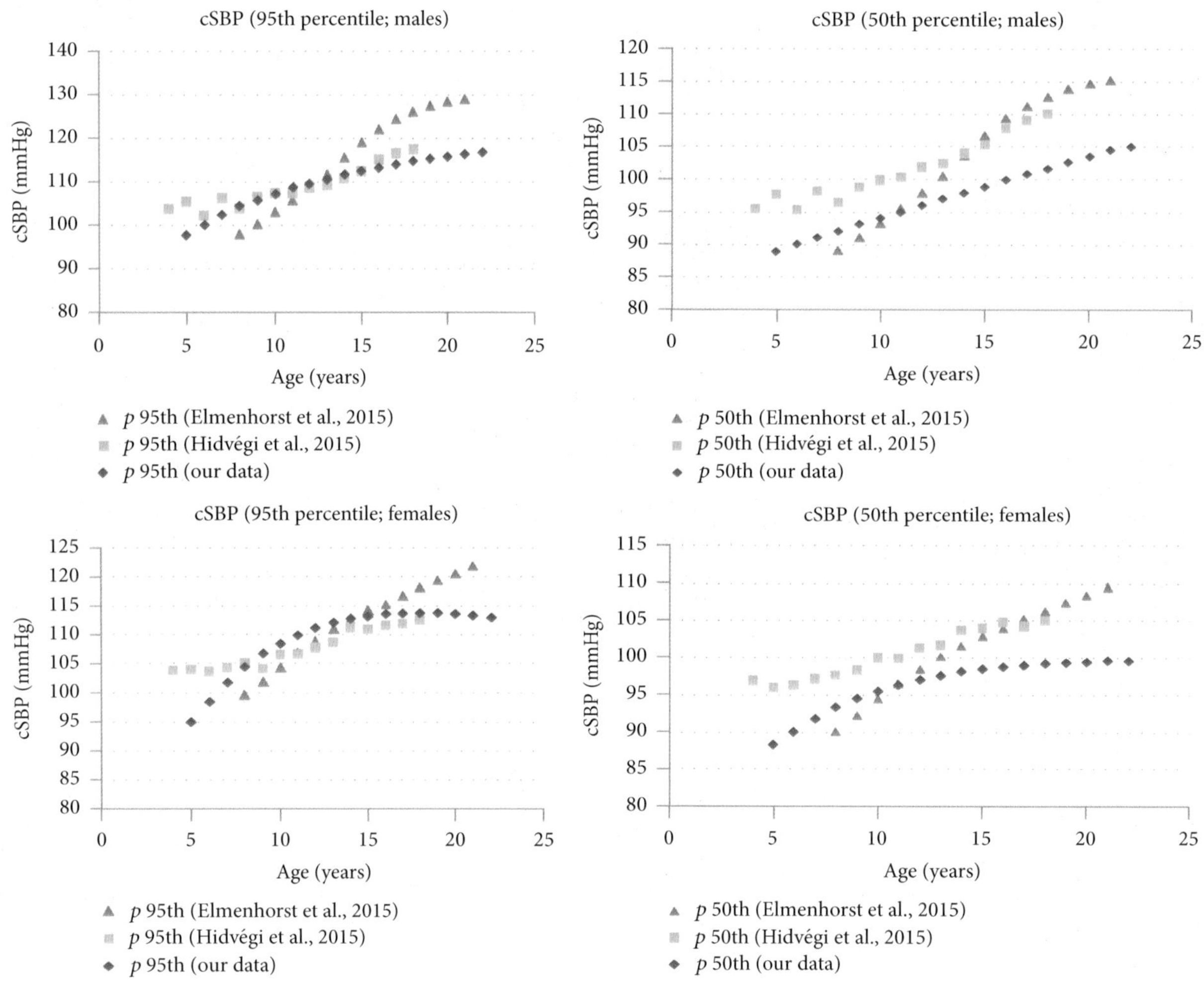

FIGURE 4: Age specific aortic systolic blood pressure (cSBP) percentiles 95th and 50th obtained in males and females of the Argentinean population compared with European date previously reported.

Group [27, 28]. This is not a minor point, since this strategy allows us to compare our data with other databases available around the world.

In this observational study, we used a cross-sectional design; consequently, the relationship between cSBP and cAIx with age should be interpreted with caution. However, generation of these RIs should be generated taking advantage approaches like that used in this research.

5. Conclusion

This study, performed in healthy children, adolescents, and young adults from Argentina with ages 5 to 22 y.o., provides the first RIs and percentile curves of cSBP and cAIx. Additionally, specific body height-related cAIx percentiles are reported for the analyzed population. The RIs and percentiles contribute to the knowledge of arterial dynamic evolution along the normal aging process and the interpretation of data obtained in clinical research and daily clinical practice.

Supplementary Materials

Table A: age-related reference intervals (RIs) for central (aortic) systolic blood pressure for the entire population (n = 1038). Table B: age-related reference intervals (RIs) for central (aortic) systolic blood pressure for males (n = 576). Table C: age-related reference intervals (RIs) for central (aortic) systolic blood pressure for females (n = 462). Table D: age-related reference intervals (RIs) for central (aortic) augmentation index (cAIx) for the entire population (n = 1038). Table E: age-related reference intervals (RIs) for central (aortic) augmentation index (cAIx) for males (n = 576). Table F: age-related reference intervals (RIs) for central (aortic) augmentation index (cAIx) for females (n = 462). Table G: body height-related reference intervals (RIs) for central (aortic) augmentation index (cAIx) for males (n = 576).

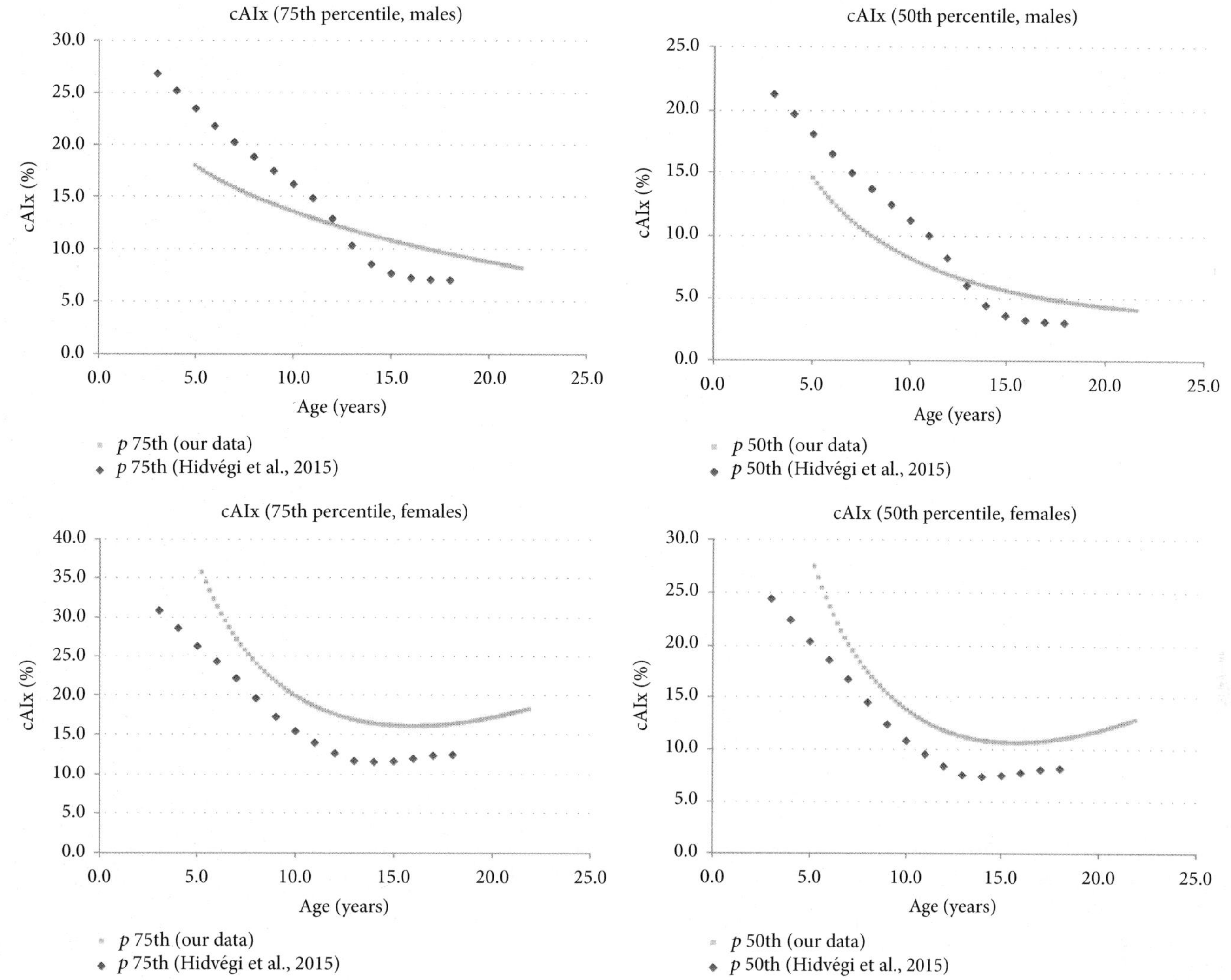

FIGURE 5: Age specific central (aortic) augmentation index (cAIx) percentiles 75th and 50th obtained in males and females of the Argentinean population compared with Hidvégi et al.'s date previously reported.

Table H: body height-related reference intervals (RIs) for central (aortic) augmentation index (cAIx) for females (n = 462). *(Supplementary Materials)*

References

[1] M. Litwin, J. Feber, and M. Ruzicka, "Vascular Aging: Lessons From Pediatric Hypertension," *Canadian Journal of Cardiology*, vol. 32, no. 5, pp. 642–649, 2016.

[2] J. D. Savant, S. L. Furth, and K. E. Meyers, "Arterial Stiffness in Children: Pediatric Measurement and Considerations," *Pulse*, vol. 2, no. 1-4, pp. 69–80, 2014.

[3] E. M. Urbina, L. M. Dolan, C. E. McCoy, P. R. Khoury, S. R. Daniels, and T. R. Kimball, "Relationship between elevated arterial stiffness and increased left ventricular mass in adolescents and young adults," *Journal of Pediatrics*, vol. 158, no. 5, pp. 715–721, 2011.

[4] P. Boutouyrie and S. J. Vermeersch, "Determinants of pulse wave velocity in healthy people and in the presence of cardiovascular risk factors: Establishing normal and reference values," *European Heart Journal*, vol. 31, no. 19, pp. 2338–2350, 2010.

[5] C. M. McEniery, I. R. Hall, A. Qasem, I. B. Wilkinson, and J. R. Cockcroft, "Normal vascular aging: differential effects on wave reflection and aortic pulse wave velocity. The Anglo-Cardiff Collaborative Trial (ACCT)," *Journal of the American College of Cardiology*, vol. 46, no. 9, pp. 1753–1760, 2005.

[6] J. Baulmann, U. Schillings, S. Rickert et al., "A new oscillometric method for assessment of arterial stiffness: comparison with tonometric and piezo-electronic methods," *Journal of Hypertension*, vol. 26, no. 3, pp. 523–528, 2008.

[7] L. M. van Bortel, S. Laurent, P. Boutouyrie et al., "Expert consensus document on the measurement of aortic stiffness in daily practice using carotid-femoral pulse wave velocity," *Journal of Hypertension*, vol. 30, no. 3, pp. 445–448, 2012.

[8] S. Obara, S. Hayashi, A. Hazama, M. Murakawa, and S.-I. Katsuda, "Correlation between augmentation index and pulse wave velocity in rabbits," *Journal of Hypertension*, vol. 27, no. 2, pp. 332–340, 2009.

[9] M. J. Roman, R. B. Devereux, J. R. Kizer et al., "Central pressure more strongly relates to vascular disease and outcome than does brachial pressure: the strong heart study," *Hypertension*, vol. 50, no. 1, pp. 197–203, 2007.

[10] G. Peluso, V. García-Espinosa, S. Curcio et al., "High Central Aortic Rather than Brachial Blood Pressure is Associated with Carotid Wall Remodeling and Increased Arterial Stiffness in Childhood," *High Blood Pressure & Cardiovascular Prevention*, vol. 24, no. 1, pp. 49–60, 2017.

[11] M. Namasivayam, B. J. McDonnell, C. M. McEniery, and M. F. O'Rourke, "Does Wave Reflection Dominate Age-Related Change in Aortic Blood Pressure Across the Human Life Span?" *Hypertension*, vol. 53, no. 6, pp. 979–985, 2009.

[12] P. Skrzypczyk and M. Pańczyk-Tomaszewska, "Methods to evaluate arterial structure and function in children – State-of-the art knowledge," *Advances in Medical Sciences*, vol. 62, no. 2, pp. 280–294, 2017.

[13] E. M. van Leeuwen-Segarceanu, W. F. Tromp, W.-J. W. Bos, O. J. M. Vogels, J. W. Groothoff, and J. H. van der Lee, "Comparison of two instruments measuring carotid-femoral pulse wave velocity: Vicorder versus SphygmoCor," *Journal of Hypertension*, vol. 28, no. 8, pp. 1687–1691, 2010.

[14] M. M. Vanderschuren, C. S. Uiterwaal, C. K. van der Ent, and J. B. Eising, "Feasibility and characteristics of arterial stiffness measurement in preschool children," *European Journal of Preventive Cardiology*, vol. 24, no. 17, pp. 1895–1902, 2017.

[15] E. Lurbe, E. Agabiti-Rosei, J. K. Cruickshank et al., "European Society of Hypertension guidelines for the management of high blood pressure in children and adolescents," *Journal of Hypertension*, vol. 34, no. 10, pp. 1887–1920, 2016.

[16] G. Mancia, R. Fagard, K. Narkiewicz et al., "2013 ESH/ESC Guidelines for the management of arterial hypertension: the Task Force for the management of arterial hypertension of the European Society of Hypertension (ESH) and of the European Society of Cardiology (ESC)," *Journal of Hypertension*, vol. 31, no. 7, pp. 1281–1357, 2013.

[17] E. V. Hidvégi, M. Illyés, F. T. Molnár, and A. Cziráki, "Influence of body height on aortic systolic pressure augmentation and wave reflection in childhood," *Journal of Human Hypertension*, vol. 29, no. 8, pp. 495–501, 2015.

[18] J. Elmenhorst, M. Hulpke-Wette, C. Barta, R. Dalla Pozza, S. Springer, and R. Oberhoffer, "Percentiles for central blood pressure and pulse wave velocity in children and adolescents recorded with an oscillometric device," *Atherosclerosis*, vol. 238, no. 1, pp. 9–16, 2015.

[19] A. Díaz, M. Tringler, J. D. Molina et al., "Blood pressure control and arterial hypertension in children and adolescents from a rural population in Argentina. Preliminary data from Vela Proyect," *Archivos Argentinos de Pediatría*, vol. 108, no. 1, pp. 68–70, 2010.

[20] A. Díaz, C. Galli, M. Tringler, A. Ramírez, and E. I. Cabrera Fischer, "Reference Values of Pulse Wave Velocity in Healthy People from an Urban and Rural Argentinean Population," *International Journal of Hypertension*, vol. 2014, Article ID 653239, 7 pages, 2014.

[21] A. Diaz, M. Tringler, C. Galli, A. Ramirez, and E. I. C. Fischer, "Arterial Stiffness in a Rural Population of Argentina: Pilot Study," *High Blood Pressure & Cardiovascular Prevention*, vol. 22, no. 4, pp. 403–409, 2015.

[22] S. R. Srinivasan, M. G. Frontini, J. Xu, and G. S. Berenson, "Utility of childhood non-high-density lipoprotein cholesterol levels in predicting adult dyslipidemia and other cardiovascular risks: The Bogalusa Heart Study," *Pediatrics*, vol. 118, no. 1, pp. 201–206, 2006.

[23] I. G. Horváth, Á. Németh, Z. Lenkey et al., "Invasive validation of a new oscillometric device (Arteriograph) for measuring augmentation index, central blood pressure and aortic pulse wave velocity," *Journal of Hypertension*, vol. 28, no. 10, pp. 2068–2075, 2010.

[24] J. Sugawara, K. Hayashi, T. Yokoi, and H. Tanaka, "Age-associated elongation of the ascending aorta in adults," *JACC: Cardiovascular Imaging*, vol. 1, no. 6, pp. 739–748, 2008.

[25] L. Stoner, J. Faulkner, A. Lowe et al., "Should the augmentation index be normalized to heart rate?" *Journal of Atherosclerosis and Thrombosis*, vol. 21, no. 1, pp. 11–16, 2014.

[26] P. Royston and E. M. Wright, "A method for estimating age-specific reference intervals ('normal ranges') based on fractional polynomials and exponential transformation," *Journal of the Royal Statistical Society. Series A: Statistics in Society*, vol. 161, no. 1, pp. 79–101, 1998.

[27] L. Engelen, I. Ferreira, C. D. Stehouwer, P. Boutouyrie, and S. Laurent, "Reference intervals for common carotid intima-medi thickness measured with echotracking: relation with risk factors," *European Heart Journal*, vol. 34, no. 30, pp. 2368–2380, 2013.

[28] J. Bossuyt, L. Engelen, I. Ferreira et al., "Reference values for local arterial stiffness. Part B: Femoral artery," *Journal of Hypertension*, vol. 33, no. 10, pp. 1997–2009, 2015.

[29] C. A. Bellera and J. A. Hanley, "A method is presented to plan the required sample size when estimating regression-based reference limits," *Journal of Clinical Epidemiology*, vol. 60, no. 6, pp. 610–615, 2007.

[30] M. Shimizu and K. Kario, "Role of the augmentation index in hypertension," *Therapeutic Advances in Cardiovascular Disease*, vol. 2, no. 1, pp. 25–35, 2008.

[31] J. Castro, V. García-Espinosa, S. Curcio et al., "Childhood obesity associates haemodynamic and vascular changes that result in increased central aortic pressure with augmented incident and reflected wave components, without changes in peripheral amplification," *International Journal of Vascular Medicine*, vol. 2016, Article ID 3129304, 8 pages, 2016.

[32] V. García-Espinosa, S. Curcio, M. Marotta et al., "Changes in Central Aortic Pressure Levels, Wave Components and Determinants Associated with High Peripheral Blood Pressure States in Childhood: Analysis of Hypertensive Phenotype," *Pediatric Cardiology*, vol. 37, no. 7, pp. 1340–1350, 2016.

[33] E. V. Hidvégi, M. Illyés, B. Benczúr et al., "Reference values of aortic pulse wave velocity in a large healthy population aged between 3 and 18 years," *Journal of Hypertension*, vol. 30, no. 12, pp. 2314–2321, 2012.

14

Correlation of Prehypertension with Left Ventricular Mass Assessed by Cardiac Magnetic Resonance Imaging

Tarek M. Mousa,[1] Oluwaseun A. Akinseye,[2] Ketevan Berekashvili,[3] and Olakunle O. Akinboboye[1]

[1]*Queens Heart Institute, 234 36 Merrick Boulevard, Laurelton, NY 11422, USA*
[2]*Department of Medicine, Icahn School of Medicine at Mount Sinai, Queens Hospital Center, 82 68 164th Street, Jamaica, NY 11432, USA*
[3]*Department of Neurology, SUNY Downstate Medical Center, 450 Clarkson Avenue, Brooklyn, NY 11203, USA*

Correspondence should be addressed to Oluwaseun A. Akinseye; oluwaseun.akinseye@mssm.edu

Academic Editor: Tomohiro Katsuya

Introduction. The purpose of this observational cross-sectional study was to assess left ventricular mass (LVM) in prehypertensive individuals in comparison to normotensives and to determine if central blood pressure (BP) correlates better with LVM index (LVMI) than brachial BP. *Methods and Result.* Brachial and central BP measurements were completed at first visit and at 4 weeks in 65 healthy volunteers who were at least 40 years old and not on medication. Subjects were divided into two groups of normotensives and prehypertensives based on JNC-7 criteria and LVM was obtained using cardiac magnetic resonance imaging. Prehypertensives had significantly higher LVMI compared to normotensives ($P < 0.01$). Brachial and central BP also both positively correlate with LVMI ($r = 0.460$, $P < 0.01$; $r = 0.318$, $P = 0.012$, resp.) in both groups and neither method was superior to the other. After multivariate regression analysis and adjusting for cardiovascular risk factors, prehypertension remained an independent determinant of LVM. *Conclusion.* Prehypertension is associated with cardiovascular target organ damage, and central BP was not superior to brachial BP or vice versa for association with LVMI.

1. Introduction

Prehypertension (PHT) was first introduced by the Seventh Joint National Committee on Prevention, Detection, Evaluation, and Treatment of High Blood Pressure (JNC-7) in 2003, replacing former categories of "high-normal" and "above-optimal" blood pressure (BP); and it was defined as systolic BP of 120–139 mmHg or diastolic BP of 80–90 mmHg based on 2 or more properly measured seated BP readings on each of 2 or more office visits [1]. The 2005-2006 National Health and Nutrition Examination Survey estimated 28% of United States adults had PHT [2]. Patients with PHT are at increased risk of developing hypertension and other cardiovascular diseases (CVDs) compared to normotensives [3].

PHT has been associated with significant abnormality of left ventricular (LV) geometry [4]. Although a study done by Zhu et al [5] did not find any statistical difference in the parameters of LV structure between normotensive and prehypertensive subjects, some studies have shown a linear correlation between PHT and increased left ventricular mass (LVM), with target organ damage found in both prehypertensive youths [6, 7] and older population [3, 4] when compared to normotensives. In fact, there has been increased risk of mortality associated with the prehypertensive category of BP [8]. The Prospective Studies Collaboration examined relationship between categories of BP and subsequent mortality by following almost 1 million people with no previous vascular disease prospectively for a total of 12.7 million person-years in 61 observational studies. They concluded that there is a continuous increase in mortality from both stroke and ischemic heart disease from BP of 115/75 mmHg, with a twofold increase in cardiovascular death in those with 20 mmHg higher systolic pressure or a 10 mmHg higher diastolic pressure, a level well within the range of PHT [8].

However, there is currently no indication for pharmacological treatment of this BP category.

Studies have shown that brachial and central BPs may differ, especially the systolic component [9, 10], but debates are still ongoing on which of the two correlates more strongly with left ventricular mass index (LVMI) and other CVD [11–13].

The aim of this study was (1) to assess the strength of association of brachial and central pressure with LVMI and (2) to compare these variables in prehypertensive and normotensive study participants. Cardiac magnetic resonance imaging (MRI) was used to diagnose LVM as it is more precise and reliable compared to other diagnostic modalities [14].

2. Methods

2.1. Study Design. We conducted an observational cross-sectional study of healthy volunteers from September 2008 to September 2009 at Cardiology Division of New York Hospital Medical Center of Queens/Weill Medical College of Cornell University. We recruited our participants using flyers distributed throughout our institution. We enrolled healthy volunteers who were at least 40 years old and not on medication. Exclusion criteria for the study were previous diagnosis of hypertension (HTN), diabetes mellitus (DM), renal disease, CVD, valvular heart disease, and atrial fibrillation.

Detailed history, physical examination, and brachial and central BP measurement were completed at the first visit. Height (m) and weight (kg) were measured and body mass index (BMI) was calculated as weight (kg)/(height (m) × height (m)) and unit was recorded as kg/m^2. The second visit, which was 4 weeks after the first, included the second measurements of brachial and central BP and performing of a cardiac MRI. To ensure a more representative BP value for each patient, the average of the BP measurement at the first and second visit was used for analysis.

Study population was divided into two groups of normotensives and prehypertensives based on their BP measurement, and LVMI was compared in both groups. PHT as defined by JNC-7 criteria is systolic blood pressure (SBP) between 120 and 139 mmHg and diastolic blood pressure (DBP) between 80 and 89 mmHg. Brachial and central BP measurements with their correlation to LVMI were also studied.

The study was approved by Institutional Review Board of New York Hospital Medical Center of Queens.

2.2. Measurements of the Variables

2.2.1. Brachial Blood Pressure. Brachial BP was measured with a BPM-300 noninvasive BP monitor (VSM MedTech Ltd., Vancouver, Canada) after the subject had been in a recumbent position for a minimum of 10 minutes. The device took 6 consecutive BP readings, excluded the first measurement, and derived an average. It uses an oscillometric technique to calculate systolic and diastolic BP. The device meets the Association for the Advancement of Medical Instrumentation Standards.

2.2.2. Central Blood Pressure. SphygmoCor monitor was used to measure central BP. The tonometer, gently pressed against the radial artery pulse, acquires the radial pulse wave and the SphygmoCor's proprietary algorithm derives the pulse wave as it exists in the ascending aorta producing the central BP measurements noninvasively.

2.2.3. Left Ventricular Mass. We used Siemens 1.5T cardiac MRI scanner to obtain LVM. We acquired ECG-gating and breath-holding during contrast-enhanced segmented *k*-space inversion-recovery with steady-state free precession imaging. LVMI was calculated using LV measurements in diastole, divided by height, squared, and expressed as g/m^2.

2.3. Statistical Analysis. Continuous variables were summarized by the mean ± SD. Categorical variables were summarized by frequencies with 95% confidence interval (CI). Pearson r was used for correlations for each variable of interest (i.e., brachial SBP, central SBP, brachial DBP, central DBP, and LVMI). Means of continuous variables were compared with independent t-test statistics.

Multivariate linear regression models were constructed using PHT as the primary risk factor and effect size was adjusted for typical potential confounders (e.g., age, race, gender, BMI, and cardiovascular risk factors); P values ≤ 0.05 were considered statistically significant. Analyses were performed using SPSS statistical software (PASW statistics 18).

3. Results

The study population ($n = 65$) consists of healthy volunteers (Table 1). The average age at the time of enrollment was 54 ± 8 (range from 43 years to 77 years); 65% were female; mean BMI (Kg/m^2) was 27 ± 4 (range of 19–42). 29 (45%) of volunteers were prehypertensive and 36 (55%) were normotensive. 58.5% of volunteers were Caucasian, 27.7% were African Americans, 6.2% were Hispanic, and the rest were Asians. There was no statistically significant difference between prehypertensive and normotensive group in all of the following parameters: age, gender, race, BMI, augmentation pressure, augmentation pressure index, and central SBP.

The main dependent variable we used in our statistical analysis was end diastolic LVMI (using height when calculating the index). Prehypertensives had higher LVMI that was statistically significant as compared to normotensives, $P < 0.01$ (Figure 1). Simple linear regression analysis showed that central SBP has positive statistically significant association with end diastolic LVMI with $P = 0.014$ (standardized beta coefficient = 0.314).

There was no difference between brachial and central DBP (mean brachial DBP = 76 ± 9 mmHg versus central DBP = 77 ± 9 mmHg) (Figure 2); however, there was slightly higher brachial SBP (mean 115.8 ± 12 mmHg) compared with central SBP (mean 106 ± 11 mmHg) (Figure 3).

Pearson's correlation showed statistically significant correlation between central SBP and LVMI ($r = 0.318$, $P = 0.012$) (Figure 4) and brachial SBP and LVMI ($r = 0.460$,

TABLE 1: Patient's characteristics, left ventricular mass index, and blood pressure categories.

	Prehypertensives Yes (n = 29) 45%	Normotensives No (n = 36) 55%	Statistical significance
Age (mean ± SD)	56 ± 9.6	52.8 ± 7.3	0.122
Race (number/%)			
White	17 (58.6)	21 (60)	Not significant
Black	8 (27.6)	10 (28.6)	
Asian	3 (10.4)	1 (2.9)	
Hispanic	1 (3.4)	3 (8.5)	
Gender (number/%)			
Female	18 (62.1)	24 (66.7)	0.796
Male	11 (37.9)	12 (33.3)	
BMI (kg/m^2)	27.5 ± 4.5	26.7 ± 3.8	0.4
BSA (m^2)	1.88 ± 0.26	1.85 ± 0.18	0.57
Augmentation pressure (mmHg)	8.4 ± 5.6	6.3 ± 4.4	0.096
Augmentation pressure index (%)	23.8 ± 13	20.11 ± 14	0.275
LV mass index (g/m^2)	34.45 ± 7.4	29 ± 6	0.002

BMI: body mass index, BSA: body surface area, LV: left ventricle, and LVMI: left ventricular mass index.
Values are presented as mean ± SD.

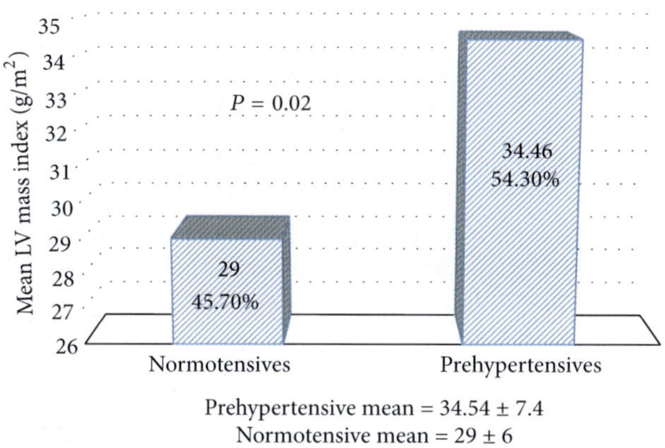

FIGURE 1: LV mass index in prehypertensive versus normotensive volunteers.

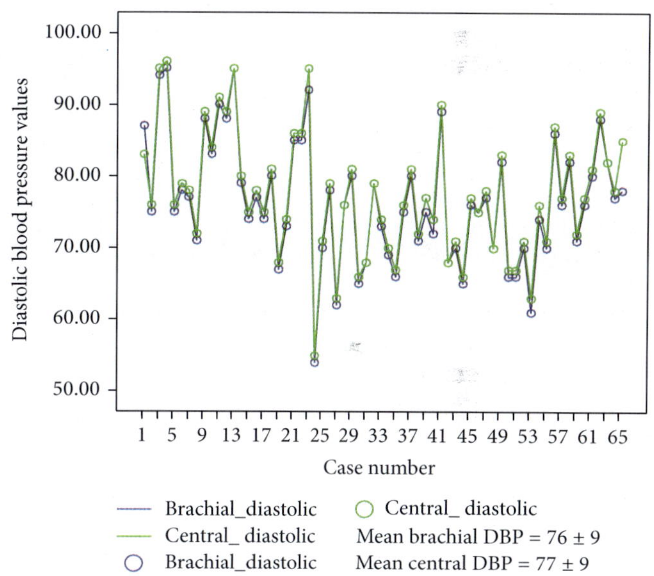

FIGURE 2: Brachial and central diastolic blood pressure measurements.

$P < 0.01$) (Figure 5). The correlation coefficient between brachial DBP and LVMI ($r = 0.521$, $P < 0.01$) and central DBP and LVMI ($r = 0.523$, $P < 0.01$) was similar.

Multivariate linear regression analysis, when adjusted for age, gender, race, and BMI, showed positive statistically significant association between PHT and end diastolic LVMI.

4. Discussion

Prehypertensive individuals have been shown to be at an increased risk of developing hypertension [3]. Although hypertension is a well-documented independent predictor of elevated LVMI [6, 15, 16], few studies have shown the relationship between PHT and structural changes in the LV.

Our study demonstrated a strong relationship between PHT and LVMI when compared to normal BP, even after adjustment for age, gender, race, and BMI. Another principal new finding in present study was that, in both prehypertensives and normotensives, brachial and central BP correlated positively with LVMI, and central BP was not superior to brachial BP or vice versa for association with LVMI.

4.1. Prehypertension and Left Ventricular Mass Index. Manios et al. [17] analyzed the impact of PHT on LVM. They found a statistically significant association between prehypertensives and LVM ($P = 0.03$) compared to normotensive patients after adjustment for baseline characteristics. Our study supports this finding. We were able to establish the importance of PHT category to the increased risk of developing future CVD.

Left ventricular hypertrophy (LVH), measured by LVMI, has been identified as the most powerful risk factor for future cardiovascular events causing morbidity and mortality [15].

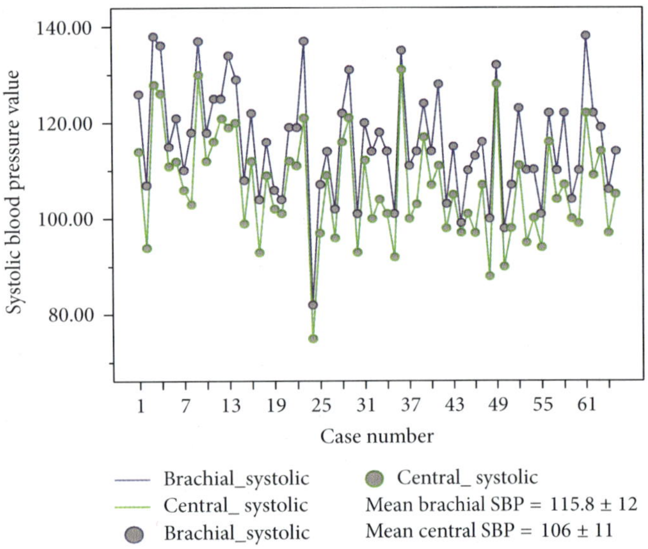

FIGURE 3: Brachial and central systolic blood pressure measurements.

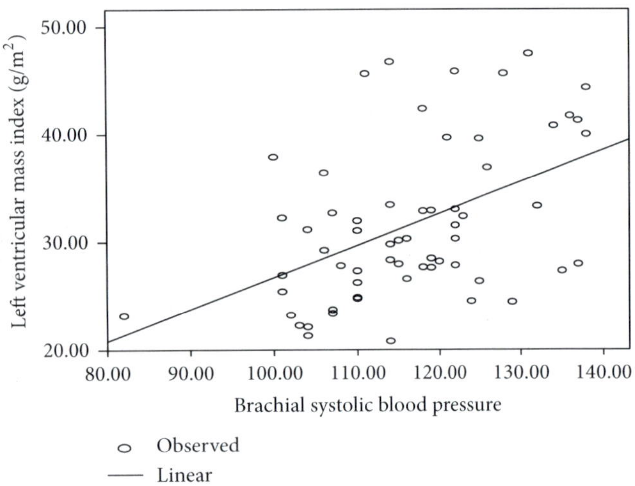

FIGURE 4: Correlation between LV mass index (kg/m^2) and brachial systolic blood pressure.

In fact, Richey et al. [18] studied the relationship between ambulatory BP and increased LVM in children at risk for hypertension and found that the odds ratio (OR) of having elevated LVMI increased by 54% for each incremental increase of standard deviation score (SDS) in 24-hour systolic SDS after controlling for race and BMI (OR = 1.54, unit = 1 SDS, CI = 1.1, 2.15, and $P = 0.011$) and increased by 88% for each increase of 0.1 in BP index (OR = 1.88, CI = 1.03, 3.45, and $P = 0.04$).

PHT is associated with an increased prevalence of LVH [4, 17]. In the Bogalusa Heart Study, Toprak et al. [19], in addition to finding a significantly higher LVMI in prehypertensives compared to normotensives, a finding supported by present study, also found PHT was significantly higher among men than women (35% versus 22%) and among blacks than whites (29% versus 27%). We did not find any significant difference between prehypertensive and normotensive groups

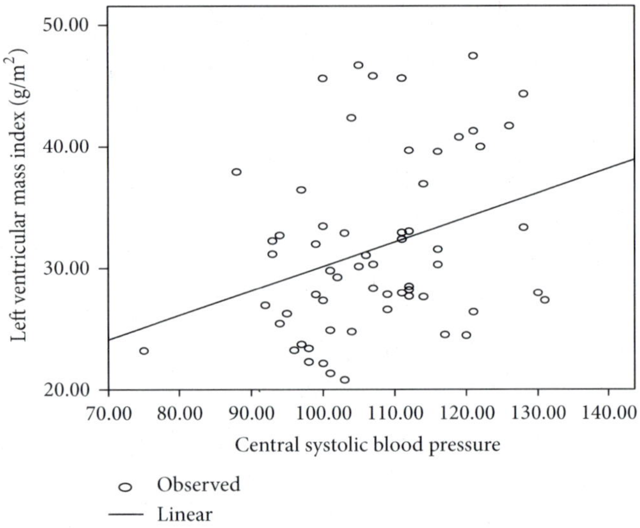

FIGURE 5: Correlation between LV mass index (kg/m^2) and central systolic blood pressure.

by gender or race. The difference between both studies on the significance of race on BP category might be due to the smaller sample size ($n = 65$) of our study compared to the Bogalusa Heart Study ($n = 1379$). The gender differences might be explained by the age difference in both study populations. The average age of present study population was 54 ± 8 (43–77 years) as compared to the Bogalusa Heart Study with age range of 20–44 years. Arterial stiffening increases in both genders with age [20] which may explain why gender was not statistically significant in our prehypertensive group but was in the earlier study which was conducted in a much younger population. However, a recent study that analyzed sex differences in arterial stiffness and ventricular-arterial interactions, done in older population (men 67 ± 9 and women 65 ± 10), showed women had greater aortic stiffening as evidenced by higher aortic characteristic impedance (Zc) which should translate into a greater increase in BP from increased flow during LV ejection [21]. This motivates further research to determine the impact of gender on Zc and its role as a risk for developing PHT and future CVD.

Recent study on 1,940 young participants found higher LVM values in prehypertensives compared to normotensives even after adjustment for covariates [6, 17]. In contrast, Zhu et al. [5] did not find any statistical differences in LVMI between prehypertensives and normotensives. Methodological differences (such as age of study population, inclusion criteria, and ambulatory blood pressure measurement protocol) between these studies may have accounted for the different results.

Elevated LVM is a well-defined independent modifiable risk factor for adverse cardiovascular event [7, 15, 22] and for developing hypertension [7]. In fact, as reported by Urbina et al. [7], the progression of PHT to sustained hypertension was predicted by baseline systolic BP and baseline LVM, with the probability of developing hypertension increasing by 36% for each standard deviation of LVMI. This describes a vicious cycle in which PHT causes elevated LVM which in turn accelerates the progression of PHT to sustained hypertension increasing future risk of CVDs and mortality. Our findings confirmed that subjects with PHT have significantly higher LVMI than normotensives.

4.2. Central versus Brachial Blood Pressure and Left Ventricular Mass Index. Our study showed no difference between the diastolic components of both brachial and central BP but a slightly higher brachial SBP than central SBP (Figures 2 and 3). This supports the finding of a cardiovascular physiology study which showed that, for the same mean arterial pressure, SBP and pulse pressure (PP) are higher in peripheral (brachial) than in central arteries (thoracic aorta, carotid arteries) [23]. The difference, called SBP or PP amplification, is a result of the progressive reduction of the diameter and increase in stiffness from the proximal to the distal arterial vessels and mostly of the modification in the transit of wave reflections [23, 24]. However, even though brachial and centrally measured SBP differ, our observation supports previous evidence that both central and brachial SBP positively correlate with LVMI in normotensive and prehypertensive individuals [11, 12, 25]. The central BP was measured using SphygmoCor monitor which has been shown to have excellent interobserver reproducibility [9] which accords with that reported by other workers using different methodologies [26].

There is an on-going debate on the BP approach that correlates better with LVMI and CVD. Roman et al. [25] reported that LV relative wall thickness and mass index were more strongly related to central than brachial BP, so were the findings in other studies [11, 12]. Na et al. [12] concluded that central BP, measured as central PP, was a stronger predictor of LVMI than peripheral PP (β coefficient = 0.311, P = 0.001 versus β coefficient 0.281, P = 0.003 resp.). Pini et al. [27] also suggested the superior prognostic utility of central BP compared to brachial BP in an unselected geriatric population. In contrast, Dart et al. [13] found that brachial BP but not central BP had a better prognostic impact. A new finding in our study is the nonsuperiority of central BP to brachial BP in correlation with LVMI or vice versa. To the best of our knowledge, this is the first study reporting this finding. Further prospective studies are required to determine whether central BP may be a better predictor of LVMI and future CVD and mortality.

5. Conclusion

In conclusion, this data provides evidence of increased LVMI in prehypertensive patients. An increased LVM has been shown to be an independent modifiable risk factor for adverse cardiovascular events and progression of PHT to sustained hypertension. Current guidelines recommend lifestyle modification for the management of PHT, but this has had no demonstrable effect on public health to date [28]. The Trial of Preventing Hypertension (TROPHY) study demonstrated for the first time that pharmacological treatment of prehypertensives was safe and partially reduced the risk of developing incident hypertension; however, no difference in the occurrence of cardiovascular events was observed between the treatment groups [28]. We recommend further prospective studies to determine whether pharmacological treatment of prehypertensives provides a cost-effective strategy for reducing CVD risks.

In addition, both central and brachial BP positively correlate with LVMI in normotensive and prehypertensive patients and central BP was not superior to brachial BP or vice versa for association with LVMI.

Limitations

Our study population consists of relatively small sample of 65 volunteers which may limit the generalizability of the results. There is need for further studies with larger sample populations to replicate these findings. Furthermore, the average age of our study population was 54 ± 8, with older age individuals underrepresented; however, PHT remained an independent predictor of increased LVMI even in multivariable models where age was entered as covariate.

BMI was indexed to body surface area (BSA) (kg/m^2) in our study; however, there is on-going controversy on the best method to index LVM so as to account for body size. Indexing LVM to BSA is said to underestimate LVM in obese and overweight hypertensive patients when compared to height$^{2.7}$ indexed LVM [29]. Indexing LVM to BSA in present study showed that PHT is associated with LVMI, and this association could have been stronger if LVM was indexed to height$^{2.7}$ as we might have underestimated the prevalence of increased LVM in our study population by using LVM indexed to BSA.

References

[1] A. V. Chobanian, G. L. Bakris, H. R. Black et al., "Seventh report of the joint national committee on prevention, detection, evaluation, and treatment of high blood pressure," *Hypertension*, vol. 42, no. 6, pp. 1206–1252, 2003.

[2] Y. Ostchega, S. S. Yoon, J. Hughes, and T. Louis, "Hypertension awareness, treatment, and control—continued disparities in adults: United States, 2005-2006," *NCHS Data Brief*, vol. 3, no. 3, pp. 1–8, 2008.

[3] P. Kokkinos, A. Pittaras, P. Narayan, C. Faselis, S. Singh, and A. Manolis, "Exercise capacity and blood pressure associations with left ventricular mass in prehypertensive individuals," *Hypertension*, vol. 49, no. 1, pp. 55–61, 2007.

[4] M. B. Lawrence Wright, R. B. Devereux, M. J. Roman et al., "Association of prehypertension by joint national committee 7 criteria with left ventricular structure and function: the strong heart study," *Journal of the American College of Cardiology*, vol. 43, no. 5, supplement 2, p. A513, 2004.

[5] H. Zhu, W. Yan, D. Ge et al., "Cardiovascular characteristics in American youth with prehypertension," *American Journal of Hypertension*, vol. 20, no. 10, pp. 1051–1057, 2007.

[6] J. S. Drukteinis, M. J. Roman, R. R. Fabsitz et al., "Cardiac and systemic hemodynamic characteristics of hypertension and

prehypertension in adolescents and young adults: the Strong Heart Study," *Circulation*, vol. 115, no. 2, pp. 221–227, 2007.

[7] E. M. Urbina, P. R. Khoury, C. McCoy, S. R. Daniels, T. R. Kimball, and L. M. Dolan, "Cardiac and vascular consequences of pre-hypertension in youth," *Journal of Clinical Hypertension*, vol. 13, no. 5, pp. 332–342, 2011.

[8] S. Lewington, R. Clarke, N. Qizilbash, R. Peto, and R. Collins, "Age-specific relevance of usual blood pressure to vascular mortality: a meta-analysis of individual data for one million adults in 61 prospective studies," *The Lancet*, vol. 360, no. 9349, pp. 1903–1913, 2002.

[9] A. Siebenhofer, C. R. W. Kemp, A. J. Sutton, and B. Williams, "The reproducibility of central aortic blood pressure measurements in healthy subjects using applanation tonometry and sphygmocardiography," *Journal of Human Hypertension*, vol. 13, no. 9, pp. 625–629, 1999.

[10] B. Williams, "Central blood pressure: To the heart of the matter," 2010, http://spo.escardio.org/eslides/view.aspx?eevtid=40&fp=5056.

[11] M. J. Roman, R. B. Devereux, J. R. Kizer et al., "Central pressure more strongly relates to vascular disease and outcome than does brachial pressure: the Strong Heart Study," *Hypertension*, vol. 50, no. 1, pp. 197–203, 2007.

[12] J. Na, E. Kim, S. Lim et al., "The relationship between central aortic pressure, brachial blood pressure and left ventricular mass index: in first diagnosed hypertensive patients," *Journal of Hypertension*, vol. 28, p. e498, 2010.

[13] A. M. Dart, C. D. Gatzka, B. A. Kingwell et al., "Brachial blood pressure but not carotid arterial waveforms predict cardiovascular events in elderly female hypertensives," *Hypertension*, vol. 47, no. 4, pp. 785–790, 2006.

[14] P. B. Bottini, A. A. Carr, L. M. Prisant, F. W. Flickinger, J. D. Allison, and J. S. Gottdiener, "Magnetic resonance imaging compared to echocardiography to assess left ventricular mass in the hypertensive patient," *American Journal of Hypertension*, vol. 8, no. 3, pp. 221–228, 1995.

[15] F. H. Messerli and F. C. Aepfelbacher, "Hypertension and left-ventricular hypertrophy," *Cardiology Clinics*, vol. 13, no. 4, pp. 549–557, 1995.

[16] W. B. Kannel, "Left ventricular hypertrophy as a risk factor: the Framingham experience," *Journal of Hypertension*, vol. 9, no. 2, pp. S3–S9, 1991.

[17] E. Manios, G. Tsivgoulis, E. Koroboki et al., "Impact of prehypertension on common carotid artery intima-media thickness and left ventricular mass," *Stroke*, vol. 40, no. 4, pp. 1515–1518, 2009.

[18] P. A. Richey, T. G. DiSessa, M. C. Hastings, G. W. Somes, B. S. Alpert, and D. P. Jones, "Ambulatory blood pressure and increased left ventricular mass in children at risk for hypertension," *Journal of Pediatrics*, vol. 152, no. 3, pp. 343–348, 2008.

[19] A. Toprak, H. Wang, W. Chen et al., "Prehypertension and black-white contrasts in cardiovascular risk in young adults: Bogalusa Heart Study," *Journal of Hypertension*, vol. 27, no. 2, pp. 243–250, 2009.

[20] E. G. Lakatta and D. Levy, "Arterial and cardiac aging: major shareholders in cardiovascular disease enterprises: part I: aging arteries: a 'set up' for vascular disease," *Circulation*, vol. 107, no. 1, pp. 139–146, 2003.

[21] T. Coutinho, B. A. Borlaug, P. A. Pellikka, S. T. Turner, and I. J. Kullo, "Sex differences in arterial stiffness and ventricular-arterial interactions," *Journal of the American College of Cardiology*, vol. 61, no. 1, pp. 96–103, 2013.

[22] A. A. Martinez-Rumayor, J. A. de Lemos, A. K. Rohatgi et al., "Addition of highly sensitive troponin T and N-terminal pro-B-type natriuretic peptide to electrocardiography for detection of left ventricular hypertrophy: results from the Dallas Heart Study," *Hypertension*, vol. 61, no. 1, pp. 105–111, 2013.

[23] W. Nichols and M. O'Rourke, *McDonald's Blood Flow in Arteries. Theoretical, Experimental and Clinical Principles*, Arnold Publishers, London, UK, 5th edition, 2005.

[24] M. E. Safar and J. Blacher, "Carotid versus brachial pulse pressure in elderly persons," *Journal of the American College of Cardiology*, vol. 51, no. 25, pp. 2440–2441, 2008.

[25] M. J. Roman, P. M. Okin, J. R. Kizer, E. T. Lee, B. V. Howard, and R. B. Devereux, "Relations of central and brachial blood pressure to left ventricular hypertrophy and geometry: the Strong Heart Study," *Journal of Hypertension*, vol. 28, no. 2, pp. 384–388, 2010.

[26] I. B. Wilkinson, S. A. Fuchs, I. M. Jansen et al., "Reproducibility of pulse wave velocity and augmentation index measured by pulse wave analysis," *Journal of Hypertension*, vol. 16, no. 12, part 2, pp. 2079–2084, 1998.

[27] R. Pini, M. C. Cavallini, V. Palmieri et al., "Central but not brachial blood pressure predicts cardiovascular events in an unselected geriatric population: the ICARe dicomano study," *Journal of the American College of Cardiology*, vol. 51, no. 25, pp. 2432–2439, 2008.

[28] S. Julius, S. D. Nesbitt, B. M. Egan et al., "Feasibility of treating prehypertension with an angiotensin-receptor blocker," *The New England Journal of Medicine*, vol. 354, no. 16, pp. 1685–1697, 2006.

[29] C. Cuspidi, S. Meani, F. Negri et al., "Indexation of left ventricular mass to body surface area and height to allometric power of 2.7: is the difference limited to obese hypertensives?" *Journal of Human Hypertension*, vol. 23, no. 11, pp. 728–734, 2009.

15

Factors Associated with Outcomes of Percutaneous Transluminal Renal Angioplasty in Patients with Renal Artery Stenosis: A Retrospective Analysis of 50 Consecutive Cases

Tetsutaro Matayoshi,[1,2] Kei Kamide,[1,3] Ryoichi Tanaka,[4,5] Tetsuya Fukuda,[4] Takeshi Horio,[1,6] Yoshio Iwashima,[1] Fumiki Yoshihara,[1] Satoko Nakamura,[1] Hajime Nakahama,[1,7] Yusuke Ohya,[2] and Yuhei Kawano[1,8]

[1] *Division of Hypertension and Nephrology, Department of Medicine, National Cardiovascular Center, Osaka, Japan*
[2] *Department of Cardiovascular Medicine, Nephrology and Neurology, University of the Ryukyus, Okinawa, Japan*
[3] *Division of Health Sciences, Osaka University Graduate School of Medicine, Osaka, Japan*
[4] *Department of Radiology, National Cardiovascular Center, Osaka, Japan*
[5] *Division of Cardiovascular Radiology, Department of Radiology, Iwate Medical University, Iwate, Japan*
[6] *Department of General Internal Medicine 3, Kawasaki Medical School, Okayama, Japan*
[7] *Diage Kobe Clinic, Hyogo, Japan*
[8] *Department of Medical Technology, Teikyo University, Fukuoka Campus, Fukuoka, Japan*

Correspondence should be addressed to Tetsutaro Matayoshi; b987741@med.u-ryukyu.ac.jp

Academic Editor: Masayoshi Soma

Background. The results of recent trials have brought some confusion to the treatment strategy for renal artery stenosis (RAS). To evaluate the applicability of percutaneous transluminal renal angioplasty (PTRA) for RAS, we extracted the factors that may affect the effectiveness of PTRA from cases experienced at a hypertension center. *Methods and Results.* We retrospectively assessed the blood pressure (BP) lowering effects and renoprotective effects in 50 consecutive patients that had hemodynamically significant RAS and had undergone PTRA and stenting during 2001–2005. Subjects were diagnosed with atherosclerotic RAS (42), fibromuscular dysplasia (6), or Takayasu disease (2). After PTRA, BP significantly lowered from 152.3/80.3 mmHg to 132.6/73.2 mmHg ($p < 0.05$), but the estimated glomerular filtration rate (eGFR) did not change significantly. There were no factors associated with the BP lowering effects of PTRA. The baseline resistive index (RI) was negatively correlated with the change in eGFR ($p < 0.05$). After correction for age, sex, BMI, and the dose of contrast medium, the association of RI with change in eGFR remained significant. *Conclusion.* In cases with hemodynamically significant RAS, PTRA lowered BP but was not effective in improving renal function. Higher baseline RI may be a factor for predicting poor clinical course of renal function after PTRA.

1. Introduction

Renal artery stenosis (RAS) is a cause of renovascular hypertension (RVHT) and ischemic nephropathy and has been demonstrated to be a predictor of future cardiovascular events [1]. Percutaneous transluminal renal angioplasty (PTRA) has been one of the common treatments for RAS despite recent developments in therapeutics [2, 3]. Using retrospective data, Bonelli et al. reported that 60–90% of 320 RAS patients who underwent PTRA exhibited some benefits after PTRA [4]. The efficacy of PTRA for the treatment of RVHT differs among causes of RAS, such as atherosclerosis, fibromuscular dysplasia (FMD), and Takayasu arteritis, as well as with or without stent placement. BP lowering effects with a high hypertension cure rate by PTRA are reportedly better in FMD than in atherosclerosis [4]. Cure or improvement rates of RVHT after PTRA are reported to be 8 or 70–76% in atherosclerotic stenosis and 22–24% or 63% in

FMD cases, respectively [4–6]. However, most trials failed to demonstrate significant improvement in renal function after PTRA [5].

Two large-scale randomized controlled clinical trials (RCTs), ASTRAL (Angioplasty and Stent for Renal Artery Lesions) trial [7], and CORAL (Cardiovascular Outcomes in Renal Atherosclerotic Lesions) trial [8] compared PTRA and conventional medication therapy regarding outcomes for BP lowering effects, renal protection (in ASTRAL), and onset of future cardiovascular events (in CORAL). Both studies could not demonstrate any advantages of PTRA compared with conventional medication therapy. STAR (Stent Placement in Patients With Atherosclerotic Renal Artery Stenosis and Impaired Renal Function), an RCT, which enrolled a relatively small number of patients, also could not demonstrate the renoprotective effects of PTRA in patients with RAS and impaired renal function [9]. Consequently, PTRA for RAS has become less recommended [10].

The current guidelines for atherosclerotic RAS recommend PTRA for patients with hemodynamically significant RAS or with the following conditions: flash pulmonary edema, rapidly declining renal function or refractory hypertension [11–15]. Such patients were excluded from ASTRAL and CORAL.

After ASTRAL and CORAL, physicians, such as cardiologists or radiologists, who handle RAS tend to hesitate to perform PTRA. However, recent recommendations and review articles have demonstrated the importance of PTRA [16, 17]. Therefore, therapeutic strategies to treat RAS are confused, and more information about patient selection is needed to perform PTRA. Several reports have clarified the determining factors for PTRA efficacy [18, 19]. Radermacher et al. has reported that a resistive index (RI) > 0.80 evaluated by renal Doppler ultrasonography (RDU) predicted outcomes in BP and renal function after PTRA in patients with RAS whose RA stenosis was over 50% [18]. Therefore, PTRA may be an effective therapy for patients with RAS if it could be performed for patients selected by RI with RDU. As patients with RAS have several features which may affect the prognosis of hypertension and renoprotection, such as the pathogenesis of atherosclerotic RAS, presence of dyslipidemia, diabetes mellitus (DM), renal impairment or renal failure, and their atherosclerotic complications of other arteries [20], such conditions should be considered when making strategies for RAS.

There are few reports on the effectiveness of PTRA, and there are even fewer reports of the Japanese or Asian patients. The aim of this study was to clarify factors associated with outcomes in PTRA for RAS patients with hemodynamically significant stenosis, before ASTRAL and CORAL, to reconsider the effectiveness of PTRA for RAS patients.

2. Subjects and Methods

We retrospectively assessed the influences of several factors on clinical courses of patients who had undergone PTRA. The subjects consisted of 50 consecutive patients who had their first PTRA between January 2001 and September 2005 in the National Cardiovascular Research Center in Osaka, Japan. Patients who had undergone two or more rounds of PTRA for restenosis of the treated lesion or progression of opposite-side RAS were excluded. PTRA was indicated for hemodynamically significant RAS with either of the following: (1) peak systolic velocity $\geq$ 1.8 m/sec by RDU, (2) diameter or area stenosis rate $\geq$ 75% by magnetic resonance imaging angiography, and (3) prolonged vascular, functional, and distribution phases by renogram. Cases without viability of the affected kidneys (RI evaluated by RDU < 0.8 and/or low distribution of the affected kidney evaluated by renogram) were excluded. Renal artery stenting was done in all cases at the ostial and proximal lesion without distal protection or filtration device. The clinical courses after PTRA in our institute were good overall. Major complications, such as cholesterol crystal embolism, dissection of the renal artery, or other vascular disease, were not observed in the present study subjects.

BP was measured on the days before PTRA (w0) and 1-2 weeks after PTRA (w1). Serum creatinine levels (S-Cre: enzymatic method) were obtained at the day before PTRA (W0), 1-2 weeks after (w1), and 1 year (+/−4 weeks) after PTRA (y1).

Primarily, we compared the change in mean blood pressure (MBP), use of antihypertensive drugs, and estimated glomerular filtration rate (eGFR) between before and after PTRA.

MBP was calculated as follows:

$$\text{MBP} = \frac{(\text{Systolic BP} + \text{Diastolic BP} \times 2)}{3}. \quad (1)$$

eGFR was calculated by the following formula:

$$\text{eGFR} = 194 \times \text{S-Cre}^{-1.094} \times \text{age}^{-0.287} \; (\text{if female subjects}, \times 0.739). \quad (2)$$

Successful BP reduction was defined as a 5 mmHg or more reduction in w1 mean BP compared with the measurement at w0 or reduction in the dosage of one or more antihypertensive medicines. Course of renal function (eGFR) was stratified into "not changed or improved" (w0 $\geq$ y1) or "worsened" (w0 < y1).

Additionally, we assessed influences on the BP lowering and renoprotective effects of PTRA by several confounding factors, including age, sex, body mass index (BMI), presence of bilateral stenosis, RI in the affected kidney, impaired glucose tolerance (IGT), DM (DM: expressing DM pattern in oral glycemic tolerance test or currently prescribed hypoglycemic agent), dyslipidemia, RI: (1 – (end diastolic velocity/peak systolic velocity)) [18], plasma renin activity (PRA), MBP (w0) eGFR (<60 mL/min/1.73 m^2), and the dose of contrast medium by univariate and multivariate analysis. We adapted common log conversion of eGFR and PRA for analysis because they did not follow a standard normal distribution.

All data were analyzed using JMP 9 software (SAS Institute Inc., Cary NC US). All continuous values were expressed as the mean +/− SD and categorical variables were reported as percentages. BP and eGFR were examined. The time courses

TABLE 1: Baseline characteristics. Data are described as "mean ± standard deviation," or "number (percentage)." M: male; F: female; BMI: body mass index; IGT: impaired glucose tolerance; DM: diabetes mellitus; PSV: peak systolic velocity; RA: renal arteries; RI: resistive index; SBP: systolic blood pressure; DBP: diastolic BP; S-Cre: serum creatinine; eGFR: estimated glomerular filtration rate; proteinuria: patients who have uric protein ≥ ± or urinary albumin/creatinine ratio ≥ 30; chronic kidney disease: patients who have albuminuria or reduced eGFR (<60 mL/min/1.73 m^2). *Missing data in one of two cases with aortitis. **The volume of iopamidol (300 mg iodine/mL).

	Atherosclerosis	Fibromuscular dysplasia	Aortitis	All subjects
Number (M/F)	42 (34/8)	6 (1/5)	2 (2/0)	50 (37/13)
Age (year)	68.0 ± 7.8	27.0 ± 11.2	28.5 ± 16.3	61.5 ± 17.2
BMI (kg/m^2)	23.3 ± 3.5	22.3 ± 0 2.2	21.4 ± 1.2	23.1 ± 3.3
IGT or DM (%)	21 (50)	0 (0)	0 (0)	21 (42)
Dyslipidemia (%)	27 (64)	1 (17)	0 (0)	28 (56)
Calcium channel blockers (%)	33 (79)	3 (50)	2 (100)	38 (76)
ACE inhibitor (%)	6 (14)	0 (0)	0 (0)	6 (12)
Angiotensin II type 1 receptor blocker (%)	12 (29)	1 (17)	0 (0)	13 (26)
Diuretics (%)	13 (31)	1 (17)	1 (50)	15 (30)
β-Blockers (%)	14 (42)	2 (33)	2 (100)	18 (36)
α-Blockers (%)	4 (10)	0 (0)	0 (0)	4 (8)
Stenosis rate (%)	(82)	(81)	(83)	(82)
Bilateral stenosis (%)	18 (43)	1 (17)	2 (100)	21 (42)
PSV of the affected RA (m/sec)	2.4 ± 0.9	2.3 ± 1.4	5.4 ± 2.4	2.5 ± 1.2
Renal/aorta ratio	2.6 ± 1.0	2.9 ± 1.4	4.1 ± 1.0	2.7 ± 0.9
RI (poststenotic site)	0.66 ± 0.10	0.47 ± 0.1	0.52*	0.63 ± 0.12
PRA (ng/mL/hr)	4.7 ± 6.1	7.3 ± 7.5	4.2 ± 1.4	5.0 ± 6.1
PRA (log converted)	0.41 ± 0.51	0.71 ± 0.37	0.65 ± 0.15	0.45 ± 0.49
PAC (ng/dL)	16.6 ± 10.0	35.5 ± 49.8	14.2 ± 2.1	18.8 ± 19.4
SBP (mmHg)	153 ± 30	151 ± 8	159 ± 27	152 ± 28
DBP (mmHg)	80 ± 14	84 ± 8	86 ± 8	80 ± 13
Pulse Rate (/min)	67 ± 7	68 ± 7	72 ± 3	67 ± 7
S-Cre (mg/dL)	1.39 ± 0.66	0.59 ± 0.13	0.84 ± 0.23	1.28 ± 0.67
eGFR (mL/min/1.73 m^2)	47.2 ± 23.2	113.6 ± 34.7	99.2 ± 45.2	57.2 ± 34.1
eGFR (log converted)	1.63 ± 0.20	2.04 ± 0.13	1.97 ± 0.20	1.69 ± 0.24
Proteinuria (%)	24 (60) $n = 40$	2 (40) $n = 5$	0 (0)	26 (55) $n = 47$
eGFR < 60 mL/min/1.73 m^2 (%)	31 (78) $n = 40$	0 (0) $n = 5$	0 (0)	31 (66) $n = 47$
Chronic Kidney Disease (%)	36 (88) $n = 41$	2 (40) $n = 5$	0 (0)	38 (79) $n = 48$
Dose of Contrast Medium (mL)**	107.6 ± 41.4	102.3 ± 19.4	120*	107.2 ± 38.7

of BP and eGFR were examined using the paired t-test. Between the groups of the BP lowering effects, categorical variables were compared by χ^2 analysis, and continuous variables were compared by unpaired t-test. The influence of each parameter on the regression of eGFR was analyzed by unpaired t-test or linear regression analysis. p values < 0.05 were considered as statistical significant.

3. Results

The characteristics of the 50 patients (male 37, female 13) were as follows. All patients were East Asians. Flash pulmonary edema or rapidly declining renal function was not observed on or before admission. Refractory hypertension and uncontrolled BP (SBP ≥ 140 and/or DBP ≥ 90) despite taking 3 or more antihypertensive drugs, including diuretics, were seen in 8 cases (1 aortitis case and 7 atherosclerotic stenosis cases) among 47 cases (17.0%, 3 of 50 missed BP or drug data from the outpatient clinic before PTRA). Causes of RAS were atherosclerosis (42 cases), FMD (6 cases), and Takayasu aortitis (2 cases), as shown in Table 1. One FMD case was complicated with Moyamoya disease (18-year-old male). The mean age was 61.5 years and mean BMI was 23.1. Twenty-one patients had DM and 8 had IGT. Twenty-seven patients had dyslipidemia. Twenty-one patients (42%) had bilateral RAS, and they were treated with one-step strategy. Mean BP at w0 was 152/80 mmHg, eGFR was 57.2 mL/min/1.73 m^2, and other characteristics and subgroup characteristics divided by causes of RAS are shown in Table 1. Patients with atherosclerotic lesions were older and had a higher rate of coexisting DM and dyslipidemia. Among all patients, 6 were missing w1 BP measurements and 6 were missing y1 S-Cre measurements. The number of patients with an RI of ≥0.80 was only 3. There was no significant relationship between stenosis rate and RI (data not shown).

SBP and DBP were significantly reduced from 152.3/80.3 mmHg to 132.6/73.2 mmHg (Figure 1(a)) after PTRA, and the BP lowering effects continued until 1 year after. The

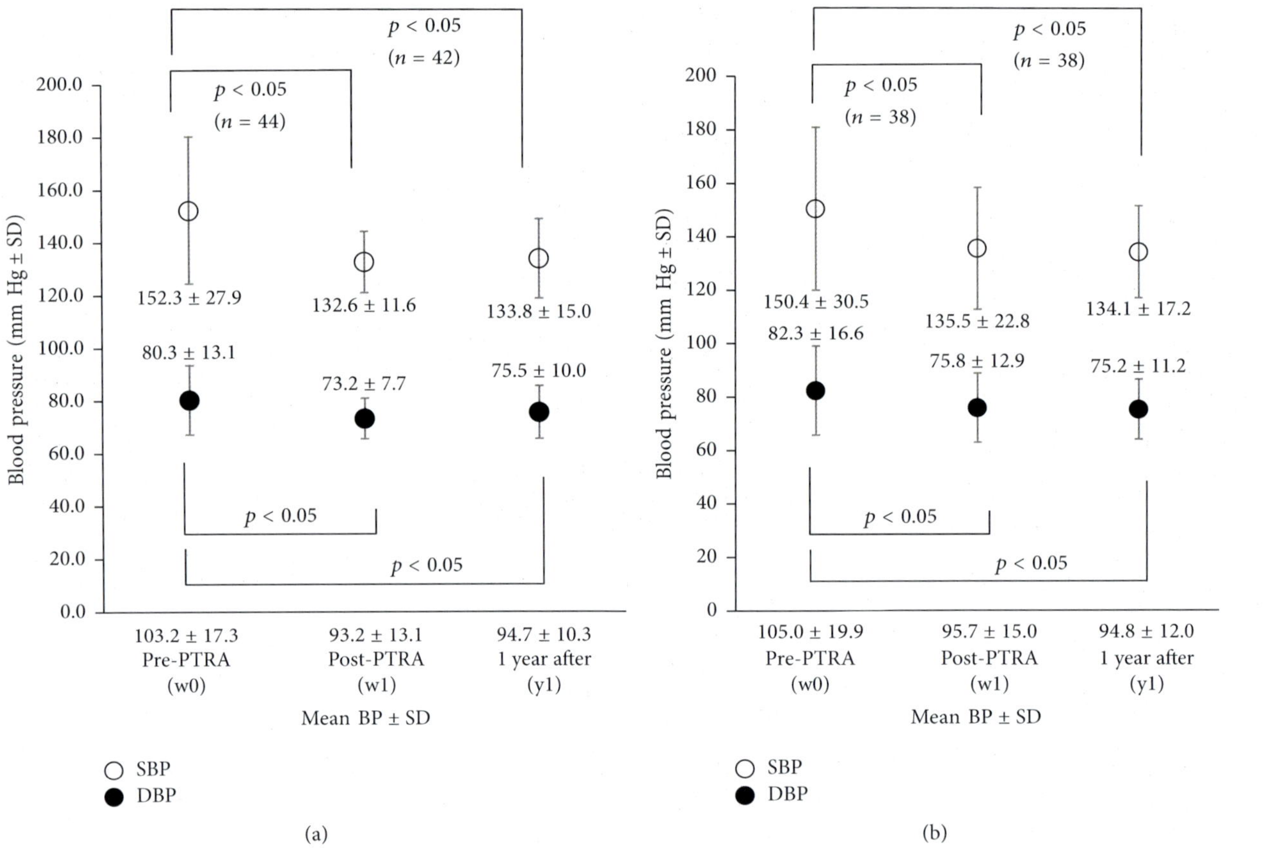

FIGURE 1: Change in blood ressure. (a) All cases. (b) Atherosclerotic RAS only. SBP and DBP were significantly reduced after PTRA, and the BP lowering effects continued until 1 year after. RAS: renal artery stenosis; BP: blood pressure; SBP: systolic BP; DBP: diastolic BP; PTRA: percutaneous transluminal renal angioplasty; SD: standard deviation.

number of drugs patients had taken was significantly reduced from 1.98 to 1.28 ($p < 0.05$, $n = 47$) at the period of 1-2 weeks after PTRA, but the reduction did not last until 1 year after PTRA ($1.95p = 0.39n = 42$). Mean BP reduction of 5 mmHg or more was observed in 29 of 44 patients (66%), and reduced dose of antihypertensive drugs was observed in 23 of 50 (46%). Successful BP reduction was observed in 35 of 48 patients (73%). Limited to cases of atherosclerotic RAS, the reduction in BP remained significant (Figure 1(b)) and the successful BP reduction rate was similar to that of all cases (70% 28/40).

Univariate analysis of predictive and confounding factors for successful BP reduction are shown in Table 2. No items indicated a significant correlation with successful BP reduction.

The changes in average eGFR throughout pre- and post-PTRA and 1 year after are shown in Figure 2. The estimated renal function neither improved nor worsened. Acute renal dysfunction, defined as an S-Cre rise of 0.5 mg/dL or more, was observed in 2 patients with atherosclerotic RAS and type 2 DM. Both patients recovered.

Renal function was "not changed or improved" in 23 of 44 patients (52%) at y1. Univariate analysis of confounding factors for regression of renal function is shown in Table 3(a). Baseline RI was significantly correlated with deterioration of

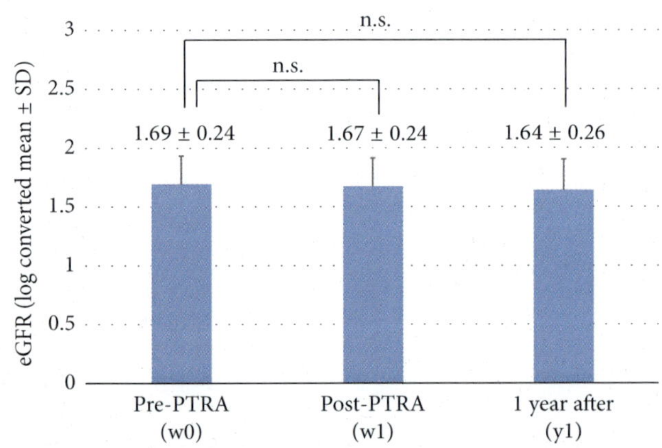

FIGURE 2: Change in eGFR. eGFR was not improved after PTRA. PTRA: percutaneous transluminal renal angioplasty; eGFR: estimated glomerular filtration rate; SD: standard deviation. *Paired t-tests were performed after log conversion of the values.

renal function (Figure 3). Presence of "IGT or DM" tended to correlate with deterioration of renal function at y1 (Student's t-test, $p = 0.05$). There was a significant correlation between presence of "IGT or DM" and baseline RI (without IGT or DM 0.58 +/− 0.09, with IGT or DM 0.71 +/− 0.11,

TABLE 2: Univariate analysis of predictive and confounding factors for successful reduction of blood pressure. Successful reduction of BP was defined as reduction in mean BP of 5 mmHg or more, or reduction of antihypertensive dose. *Logistic regression analysis, other parameters were analyzed with the chi-square test. !Plasma renin activity and eGFR were analyzed after log conversion. BP: blood pressure; BMI: body mass index; IGT: impaired glucose tolerance; DM: diabetes mellitus; eGFR: estimated glomerular filtration rate.

	Number	Odds ratio	p value
Age (years)*	48	5.14	0.25
Sex (female)	48	1.33	0.70
BMI (kg/m^2)*	48	4.61	0.37
IGT or DM	47	0.23	0.09
Dyslipidemia	47	0.59	0.45
Bilateral renal artery stenosis	48	1.08	0.91
Resistive index*	38	0.51	0.30
Plasma renin activity*!	48	0.22	0.29
Mean BP (mmHg)*	47	0.04	0.16
eGFR*!	45	0.20	0.24

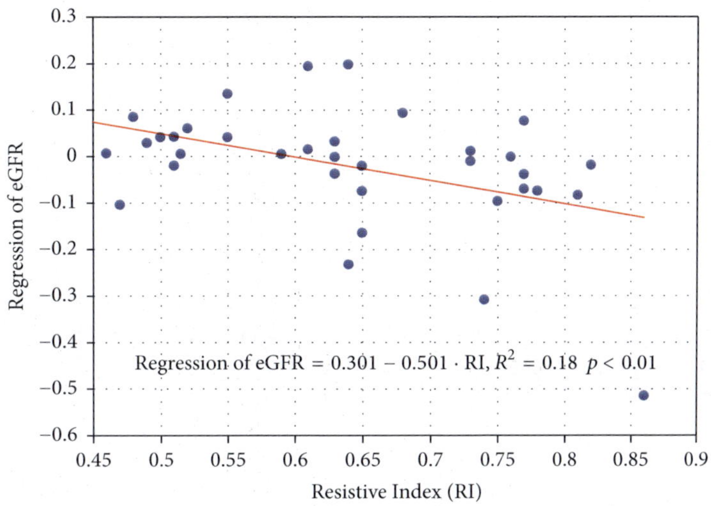

FIGURE 3: RI and regression of eGFR. Baseline RI was significantly correlated with deterioration of renal function. RI: resistive index. eGFR: estimated glomerular filtration rate. Regression of eGFR was calculated as log(eGFR y1) − log(eGFR y0).

$p < 0.01$). We performed multivariate analysis for regression of renal function accounting for age, sex, BMI, baseline RI, and the dose of contrast medium. Baseline RI remained significant for the regression of renal function (Table 4(a)). In the subgroup of atherosclerotic RAS, lower RI showed a significant relationship with regression of renal function after correction for age, sex, BMI, and the dose of contrast medium (Tables 3(b) and 4(b)).

4. Discussion

In the present study, BP was improved in approximately 70% of patients, but the average eGFR remained unchanged from the baseline. We also demonstrated that patients with a higher RI were associated with a poor renal course, as reported by Radermacher et al. [18]. Higher RI is correlated with low eGFR and may be a consequence of finaldprogressed microangiopathy of the kidneys, which causes poorer renal prognosis.

We also demonstrated that patients with glucose intolerance tended to have worsened renal function. Hyperglycemia causes increased glomerular vascular resistance [21]. RI is reported to be higher in patients with DM than in the control [22]. Our data were in accordance with previous reports.

Although prognosis of RAS is known to be different between atherosclerosis and FMD [4], RI demonstrated a significant relationship with regression of renal function in all atherosclerosis patients in the present study. RI seems to be an important prognostic factor.

On the other hand, 12 subjects in the present study lacked RI measurements. The main reasons why the data were unavailable were undetectable blood flow signals in the kidneys due to severe renal damage or marked stenosis of the renal arteries. There were no significant differences in eGFR values between the subjects with available RI measurements and the subjects for which we could not obtain the RI value. Prognostic factors among such patients remain unclear in the present study.

TABLE 3: Univariate analysis of predictive and confounding factors for regression of eGFR. A: all subjects; B: atherosclerotic RAS only; BP: blood pressure; BMI: body mass index; IGT: impaired glucose tolerance; DM: diabetes mellitus; RI: resistive index; eGFR: estimated glomerular filtration rate. Regression of eGFR was calculated as log(eGFR y1) − log(eGFR y0). *Linear regression analysis, other parameters were analyzed with the unpaired t-test. #Plasma renin activity and eGFR were analyzed after log conversion.

(a)

	Number	Mean ± SD		Gradient	R^2	p value
Age (years)*	44			0.00	0.02	0.40
Sex	44	male −0.013 ± 0.118	female −0.058 ± 0.170			0.32
BMI (kg/m^2)*	44			0.01	0.23	0.32
IGT or DM	43	Normal GT 0.01 ± 0.02	IGT or DM −0.07 ± 0.03			0.05
Dyslipidemia	43	Dyslipidemia − −0.06 ± 0.03	Dyslipidemia + 0 ± 0.03			0.15
Bilateral renal artery stenosis	44	Unilateral −0.02 ± 0.03	Bilateral −0.03 ± 0.03			0.66
Baseline RI*	35			−0.50	0.19	<0.05
Plasma renin activity*#	44			0.07	0.05	0.14
Mean blood pressure (mmHg)*	44			0.00	0.07	0.09
eGFR*#	44			−0.08	0.02	0.34
Dose of contrast medium (mL)	47			0.00	0.01	0.55

(b)

	Number	Mean ± SD		Gradient	R^2	p value
Age (years)*	37			0.00	0.00	0.32
Sex	37	male −0.016 ± 0.123	female −0.081 ± 0.204			0.13
BMI (kg/m^2)*	37			0.01	0.01	0.27
IGT or DM	36	Normal GT 0.02 ± 0.13	IGT or DM −0.07 ± 0.15			<0.05
Dyslipidemia	36	Dyslipidemia − −0.08 ± 0.04	Dyslipidemia + 0.00 ± 0.02			0.05
Bilateral renal artery stenosis	37	Unilateral −0.02 ± 0.02	Bilateral −0.03 ± 0.01			0.35
Baseline RI*	30			−0.66	0.23	<0.05
Plasma renin activity*#	37			0.07	0.03	0.16
Mean BP (mmHg)*	34			0.00	0.05	0.10
eGFR*#	37			−0.17	0.03	0.14
Dose of contrast medium (mL)	35			0.00	0.01	0.52

Indication for PTRA in patients with RAS continues to be still controversial because the results of ASTRAL and CORAL failed to demonstrate beneficial effects of PTRA. It is possible that patients who may have benefited from PTRA were excluded and/or patients with mild stenosis were included in these studies.

Although our subjects, who were expected to have better outcomes than the subjects of ASTRAL or CORAL, demonstrated hemodynamically significant RAS, overall regression of renal function was not observed. In the results of ASTRAL, the decline in renal function over time was slightly slower in the revascularization group, but the difference was not significant after 34 months of follow-up [7, 13]. Renal function in our subjects was preserved for 1 year after PTRA. Therefore, a longer follow-up period seems to be needed to demonstrate the renoprotective effects of PTRA. According to the current guidelines [11–15], PTRA is recommended for patients with flash pulmonary edema, rapidly declining renal

TABLE 4: Multivariate linear regression analysis of predictive and confounding factors for regression of eGFR. A: all subjects ($n = 35$); B: atherosclerotic RAS only ($n = 30$); BMI: body mass index; RI: resistive index; eGFR: estimated glomerular filtration rate. eGFR was analyzed after log conversion. Regression of eGFR was calculated as log(eGFR y1) − log(eGFR y0).

(a)

	Parameter estimate	t value	p value
Age (years)	0.00	0.52	0.61
Sex (female)	0.05	2.18	<0.05
BMI (kg/m^2)	0.01	1.81	0.08
Baseline RI	0.72	−3.12	<0.05
Dose of contrast medium	0.00	−1.11	0.28

(b)

	Parameter estimate	t value	P value
Age (years)	0.00	−0.13	0.90
Sex (female)	0.05	1.73	0.10
BMI (kg/m^2)	0.01	1.73	0.09
Baseline RI	0.69	−2.65	<0.05
Dose of contrast medium	0.00	−1.18	0.25

function and refractory hypertension, accelerated hypertension, unexplained unilateral small kidney, or renal arteries affected in the bilateral or single-functioning kidney. Both of the studies were criticized for the low applicability of PTRA for their included subjects.

It has been reported that approximately 20–45% of patients with atherosclerotic RAS are affected in the bilateral or single-functioning kidney [7, 23, 24]. In our study, patients with bilateral RA stenosis were observed in a similar proportion (Table 1). Although the results of the RCTs were negative, PTRA may be effective in limited high-risk cases [11, 12, 14]. However, our study could not demonstrate a correlation between bilateral RAS and improvement of renal function. Our study did not confirm the validity of the current recommendations, mainly due to too few cases and large heterogeneity between cases. On the other hand, the current recommendations for PTRA were mainly based on observational studies or consensus of the specialists [11–15]. Evidence based on the randomized trials is still very limited.

The limitations of our study are that it was a retrospective and single center design, with a limited number of subjects, which could not detect the difference in clinical course between causes of the RAS, and lack of control groups. Although we applied PTRA for patients with hemodynamically significant RAS, our criteria for applicability of PTRA were not strict, and therapeutic methods were at each doctor's discretion in each clinical situation. Furthermore, although the smoking habits of patients seem to be one of the determining factors of clinical outcome [25], we were unable to obtain the data in most cases due to a lack of detailed smoking history records.

5. Conclusion

In cases with hemodynamically significant RAS, PTRA was able to lower BP but was not effective in improving renal function.

Higher baseline RI demonstrated a significant correlation with poor renal outcome after PTRA. The presence of IGT or DM may be associated with poor renal outcome. Caution should be taken when PTRA for RVHT is considered in such patients.

Acknowledgments

The authors thank Mrs. Yoko Saito for her excellent assistance.

References

[1] P. J. Conlon, M. A. Little, K. Pieper, and D. B. Mark, "Severity of renal vascular disease predicts mortality in patients undergoing coronary angiography," *Kidney International*, vol. 60, no. 4, pp. 1490–1497, 2001.

[2] R. V. Tiradentes, C. H. Santuzzi, E. R. G. Claudio et al., "Combined Aliskiren and L-arginine treatment reverses renovascular hypertension in an animal model," *Hypertension Research*, vol. 38, no. 7, pp. 471–477, 2015.

[3] M. Oboshi, Y. Naito, H. Sawada et al., "Attenuation of hypertension and renal damage in renovascular hypertensive rats by iron restriction," *Hypertension Research*, vol. 39, no. 12, pp. 832–839, 2016.

[4] F. S. Bonelli, M. A. McKusick, S. C. Textor et al., "Renal artery angioplasty: Technical results and clinical outcome in 320 patients," *Mayo Clinic Proceedings*, vol. 70, no. 11, pp. 1041–1052, 1995.

[5] T. Zeller, U. Frank, C. Müller et al., "Predictors of improved renal function after percutaneous stent-supported angioplasty of severe atherosclerotic ostial renal artery stenosis," *Circulation*, vol. 108, no. 18, pp. 2244–2249, 2003.

[6] A. Alhadad, I. Mattiasson, K. Ivancev, A. Gottsäter, and B. Lindblad, "Revascularisation of renal artery stenosis caused by

fibromuscular dysplasia: effects on blood pressure during 7-year follow-up are influenced by duration of hypertension and branch artery stenosis," *Journal of Human Hypertension*, vol. 19, no. 10, pp. 761–767, 2005.

[7] The ASTRAL Investigators, "Revascularization versus medical therapy for renal-artery stenosis," *The New England Journal of Medicine*, vol. 361, no. 20, pp. 1953–1962, 2009.

[8] C. J. Cooper, T. P. Murphy, A. Matsumoto et al., "Stent revascularization for the prevention of cardiovascular and renal events among patients with renal artery stenosis and systolic hypertension: rationale and design of the CORAL trial," *American Heart Journal*, vol. 152, no. 1, pp. 59–66, 2006.

[9] L. Bax, A.-J. J. Woittiez, W. P. T. M. Mali et al., "Stent placement in patients with atherosclerotic renal artery stenosis and impaired renal function: a randomized trial," *Annals of Internal Medicine*, vol. 150, no. 12, pp. 840–848, 2009.

[10] I. V. Mohan and V. Bourke, "The management of renal artery stenosis: An alternative interpretation of ASTRAL and CORAL," *European Journal of Vascular and Endovascular Surgery*, vol. 49, no. 4, pp. 465–473, 2015.

[11] A. Levin, S. Linas, F. C. Luft, A. B. Chapman, and S. Textor, "Controversies in renal artery stenosis: a review by the American society of nephrology advisory group on hypertension," *American Journal of Nephrology*, vol. 27, no. 2, pp. 212–220, 2007.

[12] A. T. Hirsch, Z. J. Haskal, N. R. Hertzer et al., "ACC/AHA 2005 Practice Guidelines for the management of patients with peripheral arterial disease (lower extremity, renal, mesenteric, and abdominal aortic): a collaborative report from the American Association for Vascular Surgery/Society for Vascular S urgery, Society for Cardiovascular Angiography and Interventions, Society for Vascular Medicine and Biology, Society of Interventional Radiology, and the ACC/AHA Task Force on Practice Guidelines (Writing Committee to Develop Guidelines for the Management of Patients With Peripheral Arterial Disease): endorsed by the American Association of Cardiovascular and Pulmonary Rehabilitation; National Heart, Lung, and Blood Institute; Society for Vascular Nursing; TransAtlantic Inter-Society Consensus; and Vascular Disease Foundation," *Circulation*, vol. 113, no. 11, pp. e463–e654, 2006.

[13] R. Erbel, V. Aboyans, C. Boileau et al., "The Task Force on the Diagnosis and Treatment of Peripheral Artery Diseases of the European Society of Cardiology (ESC). ESC Guidelines on the diagnosis and treatment of peripheral artery diseases," *European Heart Journal*, vol. 35, no. 41, pp. 2873–2926, 2014.

[14] G. Mancia, R. Fagard, K. Narkiewicz et al., "2013 ESH/ESC Guidelines for the management of arterial hypertension: the Task Force for the management of arterial hypertension of the European Society of Hypertension (ESH) and of the European Society of Cardiology (ESC)," *Journal of Hypertension*, vol. 31, no. 7, pp. 1281–1357, 2013.

[15] K. Shimamoto, K. Ando, T. Fujita et al., "The Japanese Society of Hypertension guidelines for the management of hypertension (JSH 2014)," *Hypertension Research*, vol. 37, no. 4, pp. 253–390, 2014.

[16] C. J. White and S. B. King III, "The 'chicken little' of renal stent trials: The CORAL trial in perspective," *JACC: Cardiovascular Interventions*, vol. 7, no. 1, pp. 111–113, 2014.

[17] S. M. S. Herrmann, A. Saad, and S. C. Textor, "Management of atherosclerotic renovascular disease after Cardiovascular Outcomes in Renal Atherosclerotic Lesions (CORAL)," *Nephrology Dialysis Transplantation* , vol. 30, no. 3, pp. 366–375, 2015.

[18] J. Radermacher, A. Chavan, J. Bleck et al., "Use of Doppler ultrasonography to predict the outcome of therapy for renal-artery stenosis," *The New England Journal of Medicine*, vol. 344, no. 6, pp. 410–417, 2001.

[19] G. Soulez, E. Therasse, S. D. Qanadli et al., "Prediction of clinical response after renal angioplasty: Respective value of renal Doppler sonography and scintigraphy," *American Journal of Roentgenology*, vol. 181, no. 4, pp. 1029–1035, 2003.

[20] S. Nakamura, K. Iihara, T. Matayoshi et al., "The incidence and risk factors of renal artery stenosis in patients with severe carotid artery stenosis," *Hypertension Research*, vol. 30, no. 9, pp. 839–844, 2007.

[21] P. K. Carmines, "The renal vascular response to diabetes," *Current Opinion in Nephrology and Hypertension*, vol. 19, no. 1, pp. 85–90, 2010.

[22] Y. Ohta, K. Fujii, H. Arima et al., "Increased renal resistive index in atherosclerosis and diabetic nephropathy assessed by Doppler sonography," *Journal of Hypertension*, vol. 23, no. 10, pp. 1905–1911, 2005.

[23] C.\ J. Cooper, T. P. Murphy, D. E. Cutlip et al., "Stenting and medical therapy for atherosclerotic renal-artery stenosis," *The New England Journal of Medicine*, vol. 370, no. 1, pp. 13–22, 2014.

[24] J. M. Rimmer and F. J. Gennari, "Atherosclerotic renovascular disease and progressive renal failure," *Annals of Internal Medicine*, vol. 118, no. 9, pp. 712–719, 1993.

[25] U.S. Department of Health and Human Services, *Centers for Disease Control, Office on Smoking and Health. The health consequences of smoking - 50 years of progress*, Rockville, USA, 2014.

16

Brain Angiotensin II Type 1 Receptor Blockade Improves Dairy Blood Pressure Variability via Sympathoinhibition in Hypertensive Rats

Takuya Kishi,[1] Yoshitaka Hirooka,[2] and Kenji Sunagawa[3]

[1] *Department of Advanced Therapeutics for Cardiovascular Diseases, Kyushu University Graduate School of Medical Sciences, 3-1-1 Maidashi, Higashi-ku, Fukuoka 812-8582, Japan*
[2] *Department of Advanced Cardiovascular Regulation and Therapeutics, Kyushu University Graduate School of Medical Sciences, 3-1-1 Maidashi, Higashi-ku, Fukuoka 812-8582, Japan*
[3] *Department of Cardiovascular Medicine, Kyushu University Graduate School of Medical Sciences, 3-1-1 Maidashi, Higashi-ku, Fukuoka 812-8582, Japan*

Correspondence should be addressed to Takuya Kishi; tkishi@cardiol.med.kyushu-u.ac.jp

Academic Editor: Jiguang Wang

Abnormal blood pressure (BP) elevation in early morning is known to cause cardiovascular events. Previous studies have suggested that one of the reasons in abnormal dairy BP variability is sympathoexcitation. We have demonstrated that brain angiotensin II type 1 receptor (AT_1R) causes sympathoexcitation. The aim of the present study was to investigate whether central AT_1R blockade attenuates the excess BP elevation in rest-to-active phase in hypertensive rats or not. Stroke-prone spontaneously hypertensive rats (SHRSP) were treated with intracerebroventricular infusion (ICV) of AT_1R receptor blocker (ARB), oral administration of hydralazine (HYD), or ICV of vehicle (VEH). Telemetric averaged mean BP (MBP) was measured at early morning (EM), after morning (AM), and night (NT). At EM, MBP was significantly lower in ARB to a greater extent than in HYD compared to VEH, though MBP at AM was the same in ARB and HYD. At NT, MBP was also significantly lower in ARB than in HYD. These results in MBP were compatible to those in sympathoexcitation and suggest that central AT_1R blockade attenuates excess BP elevation in early active phase and continuous BP elevation during rest phase independent of depressor response in hypertensive rats.

1. Introduction

Hypertension is established as a major risk factor for cardiovascular disease, and antihypertensive treatments are necessary to prevent the cardiovascular events [1]. We have already various and effective antihypertensive agents. However, it is also true that our antihypertensive treatments could not achieve the optimal blood pressure levels [2, 3]. Among the unmet prevention for hypertensive cardiovascular events, early morning blood pressure elevation is known to be associated with cardiovascular events [4, 5]. Recent several studies have suggested that morning surge should be a crucial target of the treatments for hypertension [6–8]. There are so much various factors to cause morning surge [4, 5], and, among the factors, sympathoexcitation and baroreflex dysfunction are closely associated with blood pressure elevation in the early morning [9].

Sympathetic nerve activity is mediated by brain, especially by rostral ventrolateral medulla (RVLM) known as vasomotor center [10, 11]. In the aspects of sympathoexcitation, we and other investigators have demonstrated that brain oxidative stress in the RVLM causes sympathoexcitation [12–18] and that blockade of angiotensin II type 1 receptor (AT_1R) in the RVLM decreases blood pressure with sympathoinhibition and improvement of baroreflex sensitivity via reduction of oxidative stress [12, 17, 18]. From these backgrounds, the aim of the present study was to investigate whether central AT_1R blockade attenuates the excess blood pressure elevation in early active phase (mimicking early morning surge) with sympathoinhibition and improvement

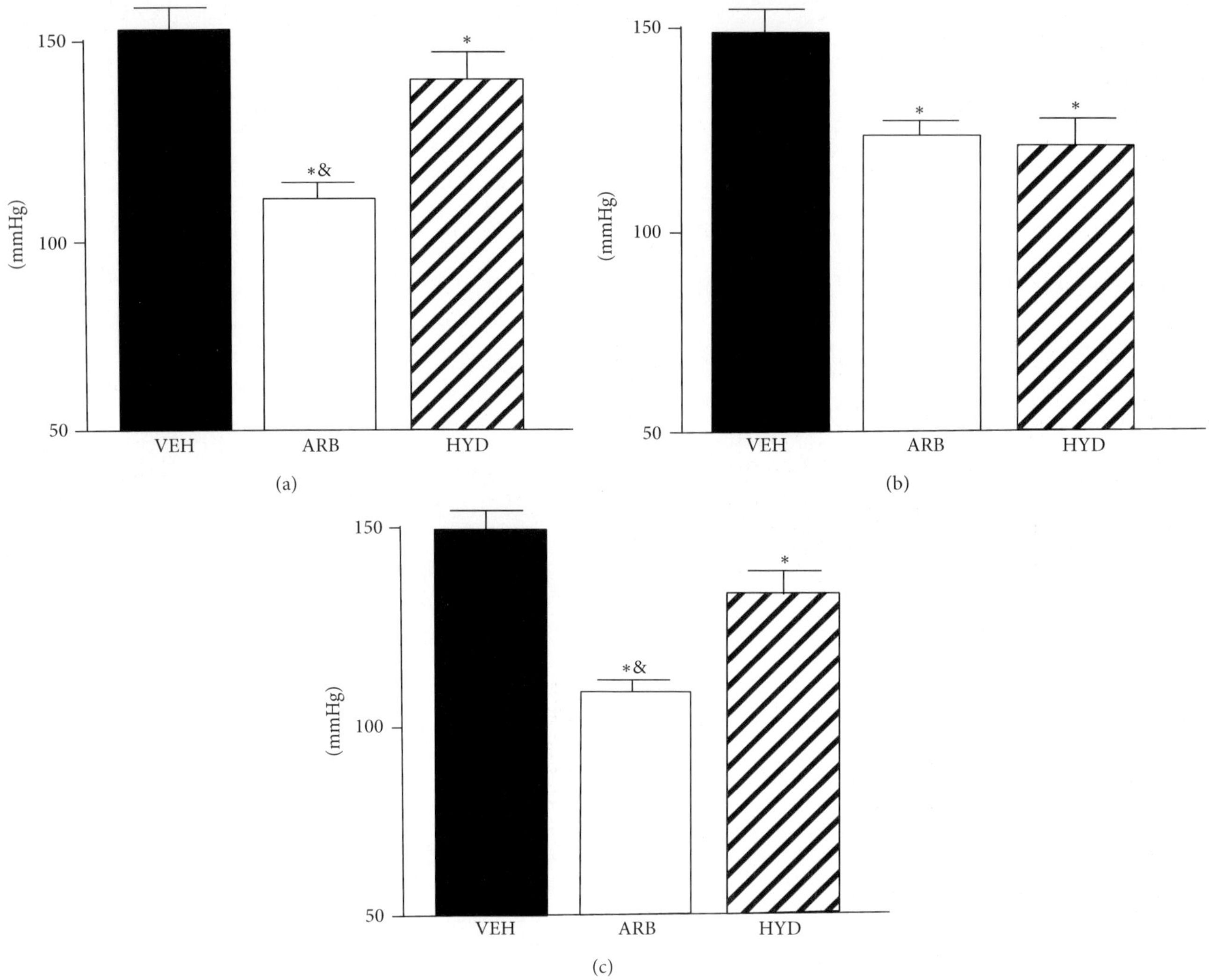

FIGURE 1: Telemetric averaged mean blood pressure in stroke-prone spontaneously hypertensive rats treated with intracerebroventricular infusion of losartan (ARB, $n = 5$), oral-administered hydralazine (HYD, $n = 5$), and intracerebroventricular infusion of vehicle (VEH, $n = 5$) at early morning (a), after morning (b), and night (c). $^{*}P < 0.05$ versus VEH, $^{\&}P < 0.05$ in ARB versus HYD.

of baroreflex in hypertensive rats and if so to determine whether the benefit was independent of depressor response or not.

2. Methods

2.1. Studies and Animals. The study protocol was reviewed and approved by the Committee on the Ethics of Animal Experiments at the Kyushu University Graduate School of Medical Sciences and conducted according to the Guidelines for Animal Experiments of Kyushu University. Experiments were performed on male stroke-prone spontaneously hypertensive rats (SHRSP) as a hypertensive model with sympathoexcitation (14 to 18 weeks old, SLC Japan, Hamamatsu, Japan). SHRSP were divided into 3 groups, treated with intracerebroventricular infusion (ICV) of AT_1R receptor blocker (ARB, $n = 5$), treated with oral administration of hydralazine (HYD, $n = 5$), and treated with ICV of vehicle (VEH, $n = 5$) for 2 weeks.

2.2. Administration of Drugs. In ARB, losartan ($1\,mg{\cdot}kg^{-1}{\cdot}day^{-1}$) in artificial cerebrospinal fluid (aCSF) was infused at 0.5 μL/h for 14 days by using an osmotic minipump (Alzet 2002, DURECT Corporation, Cupertino, CA) into the right lateral cerebral ventricle of the brain, as described previously [17, 19]. In HYD, hydralazine (100 mg/L) was administered in the drinking water. In VEH, only aCSF was infused at 0.5 μL/h for 14 days by using an osmotic minipump.

2.3. Measurements of Mean Blood Pressure and Heart Rate. Mean blood pressure (MBP) and heart rate (HR) were measured using the UA-10 radiotelemetry system (Data Sciences International, Saint Paul, MN, USA) as described previously [12, 17, 18, 20]. Telemetric MBP of 5 minutes three times every

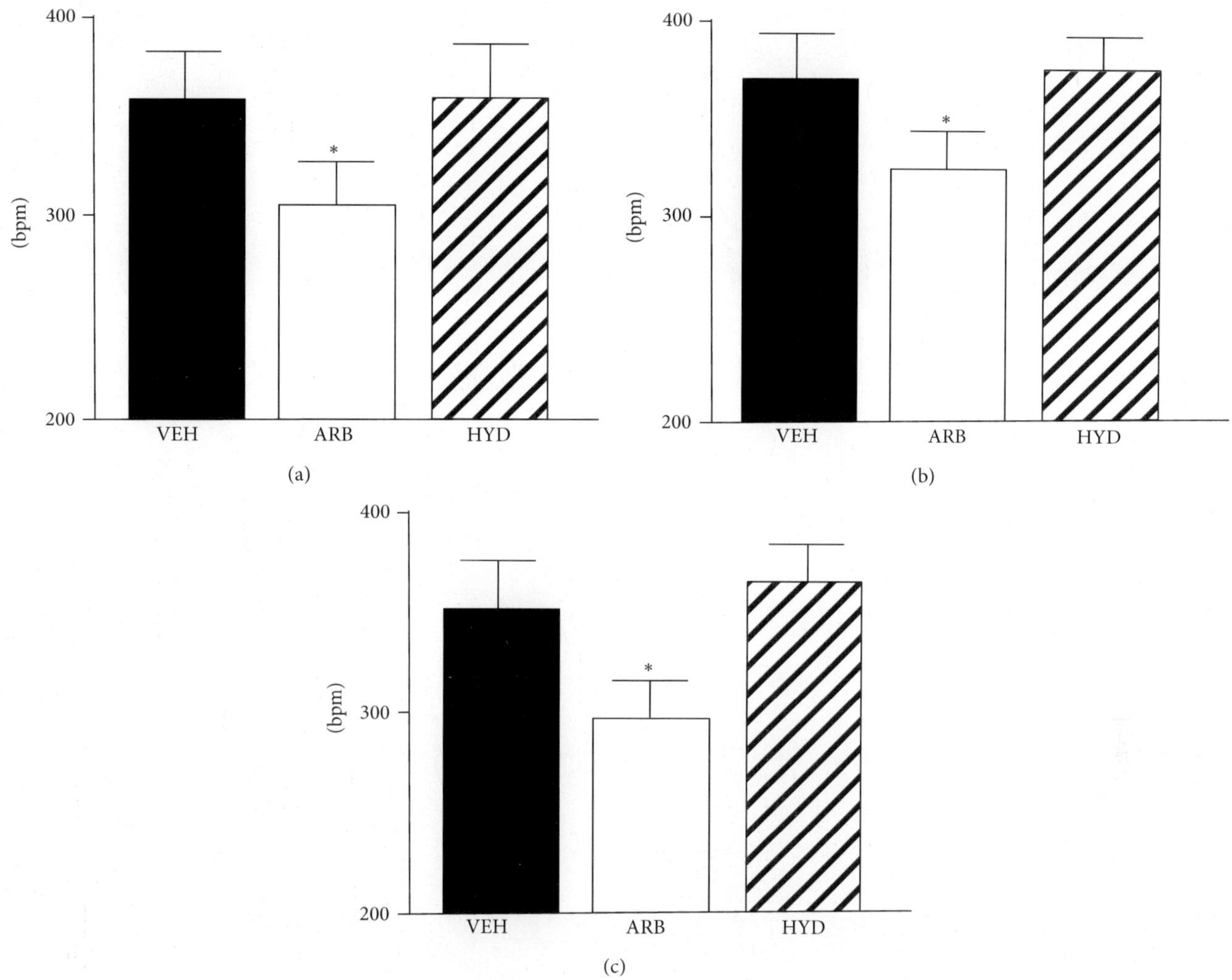

FIGURE 2: Telemetric averaged heart rate in stroke-prone spontaneously hypertensive rats treated with intracerebroventricular infusion of losartan (ARB, $n = 5$), oral-administered hydralazine (HYD, $n = 5$), and intracerebroventricular infusion of vehicle (VEH, $n = 5$) at early morning (a), after morning (b), and night (c). $^*P < 0.05$ versus VEH.

one hour was sampled and averaged at the first 2 hours at dark-active (early morning, EM), mid 2 hours at dark-active (after morning, AM), and mid 2 hours at light-rest phase (night, NT).

2.4. Measurements of Sympathoexcitation. We assessed sympathoexcitation by spectral analysis using an adaptive autoregressive model to provide power spectra for systolic blood pressure (SBP). The low-frequency power of SBP (integrating the spectra between 0.04 and 0.15 Hz) was computed by MATLAB (MathWorks, USA), and sympathoexcitation is presented as the normalized unit of the low-frequency component of SBP (LFnuSBP), as previously done in our and other studies [17, 20–22].

2.5. Assessment of Baroreflex Sensitivity. We assessed baroreflex sensitivity by spontaneous sequence method, as done in our and other previous experiments [17, 20, 23, 24]. In brief, we measured baroreflex sensitivity by using spontaneous sequence method. About 10-minute rest period was obtained in all subjects to allow for stabilization of blood pressure or HR. For analysis of about 5-minute hemodynamic recordings from telemetry system, we selected all sequences of three or more successive heart beats in which there was concordant increase (up sequence) or decrease (down sequence) in arterial systolic blood pressure and peak-to-peak systolic blood pressure interval change. A linear regression was applied to each of the sequences, and an average regression slope was calculated for the sequences. This slope represents the cardiac baroreflex sensitivity. The threshold values for including beat-to-beat systolic blood pressure and its interval changes in a sequence are set at 1 mmHg and 2 milliseconds, respectively.

2.6. Statistical Analysis. All values are expressed as the mean ± SEM. An unpaired t-test was used to compare the parameters in each group. Differences were considered significant when the P value was less than 0.05.

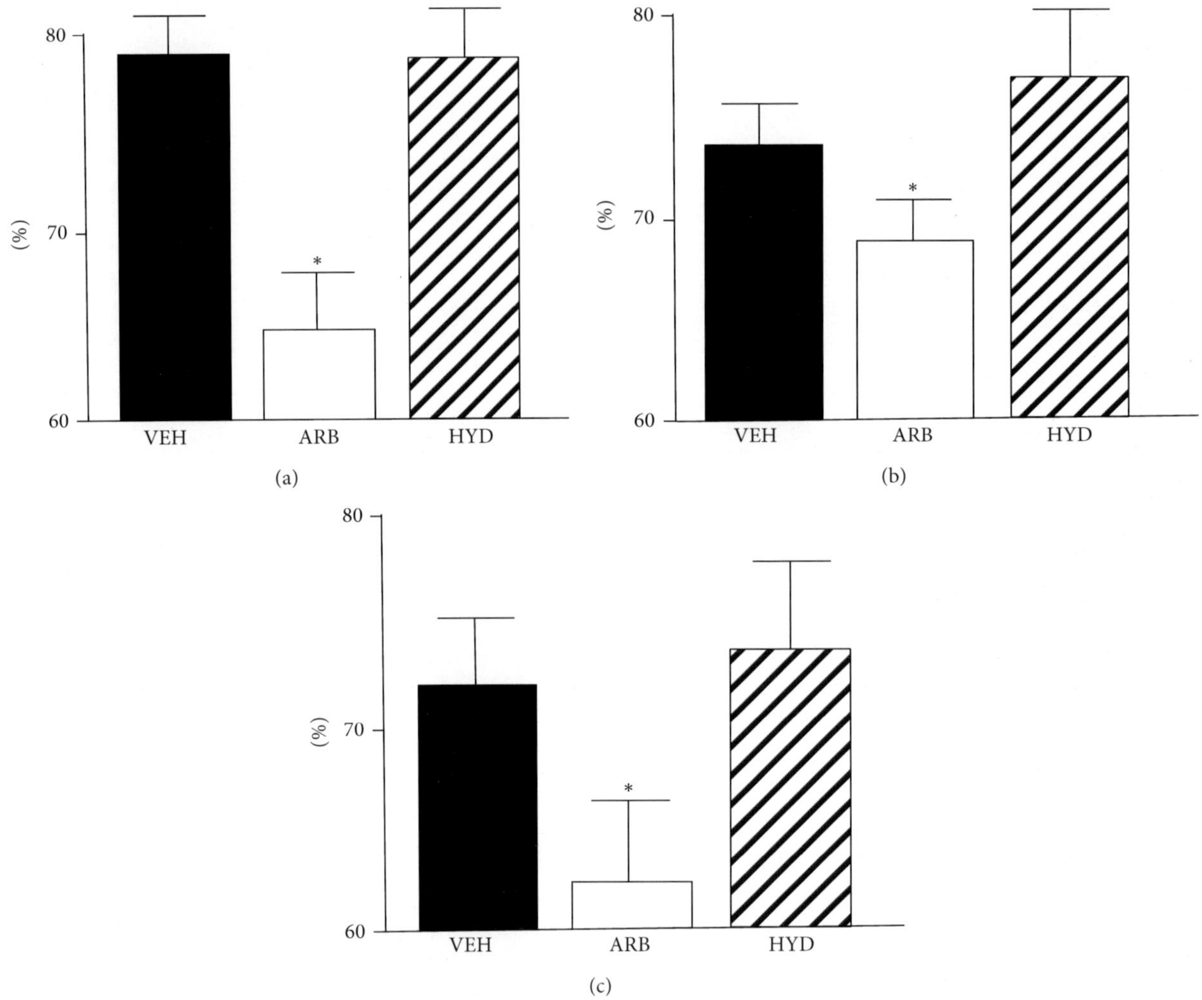

FIGURE 3: Normalized unit of the low-frequency component of systolic blood pressure as parameters f sympathoexcitation in stroke-prone spontaneously hypertensive rats treated with intracerebroventricular infusion of losartan (ARB, $n = 5$), oral-administered hydralazine (HYD, $n = 5$), and intracerebroventricular infusion of vehicle (VEH, $n = 5$) at early morning (a), after morning (b), and night (c). $^{*}P < 0.05$ versus VEH.

3. Results

3.1. Mean Blood Pressure and Heart Rate. At EM, MBP was significantly lower in ARB to a greater extent than in HYD compared to VEH, though MBP at AM was the same in ARB and HYD (Figure 1). At NT, MBP was also significantly lower in ARB than in HYD (Figure 1).

Throughout a day, HR was significantly lower in ARB than in HYD and VEH (Figure 2).

3.2. Sympathoexcitation. LFnuSBP was shown in Figure 3. Throughout EM, AM, and NT, LFnuSBP was significantly lower in ARB than in HYD and VEH. In HYD, LFnuSBP did not differ compared to VEH.

3.3. Baroreflex Sensitivity. Throughout EM, AM, and NT, baroreflex sensitivity was significantly higher in ARB than in HYD and VEH (Figure 4). In HYD, baroreflex sensitivity did not differ compared to VEH (Figure 4).

4. Discussion

Our obtained new findings were as follows. (1) At EM and NT, MBP was decreased in ARB to a greater extent than in HYD. (2) At AM, MBP was the same in ARB and HYD. (3) Throughout EM, AM, and NT, LFnuSBP was significantly lower in ARB than in VEH and HYD, and (4) baroreflex sensitivity was improved in ARB, but not in HYD. These results suggest that central AT_1R blockade would attenuate the excess blood pressure elevation in early active phase and continuous blood pressure elevation during rest phase independent of depressor response in hypertension and that these benefits of central AT_1R blockade on dairy blood pressure variability might be due to sympathoinhibition with baroreflex improvement.

The most impressive results were that central AT_1R blockade attenuates the excess blood pressure elevation in early active phase. Dairy blood pressure variability and/or morning surge is associated with abnormal regulation of sympathetic nerve activity [9], and we have demonstrated that central

[17] T. Kishi, Y. Hirooka, S. Konno, K. Ogawa, and K. Sunagawa, "Angiotensin II type 1 receptor-activated caspase-3 through ras/mitogen-activated protein kinase/extracellular signal-regulated kinase in the rostral ventrolateral medulla is involved in sympathoexcitation in stroke-prone spontaneously hypertensive rats," *Hypertension*, vol. 55, no. 2, pp. 291–297, 2010.

[18] T. Kishi, Y. Hirooka, and K. Sunagawa, "Sympathoinhibition caused by orally administered telmisartan through inhibition of the AT_1 receptor in the rostral ventrolateral medulla of hypertensive rats," *Hypertension Research*, vol. 35, no. 9, pp. 940–946, 2012.

[19] B. S. Huang, M. Ahmad, J. Tan, and F. H. H. Leenen, "Sympathetic hyperactivity and cardiac dysfunction post-MI: different impact of specific CNS versus general AT1 receptor blockade," *Journal of Molecular and Cellular Cardiology*, vol. 43, no. 4, pp. 479–486, 2007.

[20] K. Ogawa, Y. Hirooka, K. Shinohara, T. Kishi, and K. Sunagawa, "Overexpression of manganese superoxide dismutase in rostral ventrolateral medulla of stroke-prone spontaneously hypertensive rats," *International Heart Journal*, vol. 53, pp. 193–198, 2012.

[21] C. Cerutti, M. P. Gustin, C. Z. Paultre et al., "Autonomic nervous system and cardiovascular variability in rats: a spectral analysis approach," *The American Journal of Physiology—Heart and Circulatory Physiology*, vol. 261, no. 4, pp. H1292–H1299, 1991.

[22] M.-L. Tsai, W.-C. Shann, W.-R. Luo, and C.-T. Yen, "Wavelet-based analysis of low-frequency fluctuations of blood pressure and sympathetic nerve activity in rats," *Neuroscience Letters*, vol. 358, no. 3, pp. 165–168, 2004.

[23] M. J. Hilz, H. Marthol, S. Schwab, E. H. Kolodny, M. Brys, and B. Stemper, "Enzyme replacement therapy improves cardiovascular responses to orthostatic challenge in Fabry patients," *Journal of Hypertension*, vol. 28, no. 7, pp. 1438–1448, 2010.

[24] G. Grassi, "Assessment of sympathetic cardiovascular drive in human hypertension: achievements and perspectives," *Hypertension*, vol. 54, no. 4, pp. 690–697, 2009.

[25] Y. Naito, T. Tsujino, M. Matsumoto et al., "The mechanism of distinct diurnal variations of renin-angiotensin system in aorta and heart of spontaneously hypertensive rats," *Clinical and Experimental Hypertension*, vol. 31, no. 8, pp. 625–638, 2009.

[26] Y. Naito, T. Tsujino, Y. Fujioka, M. Ohyanagi, and T. Iwasaki, "Augmented diurnal variations of the cardiac renin-angiotensin system in hypertensive rats," *Hypertension*, vol. 40, no. 6, pp. 827–833, 2002.

[27] Y. Naito, T. Tsujino, D. Kawasaki et al., "Circadian gene expression of clock genes and plasminogen activator inhibitor-1 in heart and aorta of spontaneously hypertensive and Wistar-Kyoto rats," *Journal of Hypertension*, vol. 21, no. 6, pp. 1107–1115, 2003.

[28] H. Li, N.-L. Sun, J. Wang, A.-J. Liu, and D.-F. Su, "Circadian expression of clock genes and angiotensin II type 1 receptors in suprachiasmatic nuclei of sinoaortic-denervated rats," *Acta Pharmacologica Sinica*, vol. 28, no. 4, pp. 484–492, 2007.

A Community-Based Assessment of Hypertension and Some Other Cardiovascular Disease Risk Factors in Ngaoundéré, Cameroon

Olivier Pancha Mbouemboue,[1,2] Diana Derew,[1]
Jacques Olivier Ngoufack Tsougmo,[1,2] and Marcel Tangyi Tamanji[3,4]

[1]*Department of Biomedical Sciences, Faculty of Science, University of Ngaoundéré, P.O. Box 454, Ngaoundéré, Cameroon*
[2]*General Medicine Service, Ngaoundéré Regional Hospital, P.O. Box 45, Ngaoundéré, Cameroon*
[3]*Clinical Laboratory Service, Ngaoundéré Regional Hospital, P.O. Box 45, Ngaoundéré, Cameroon*
[4]*Faculty of Science, University of Buea, P.O. Box 63, Buea, Cameroon*

Correspondence should be addressed to Olivier Pancha Mbouemboue; olivier_pancha@yahoo.fr

Academic Editor: Claudio Borghi

Background and Objective. Cardiovascular diseases are primary causes of death worldwide with well documented risk factors whose varying impacts added to the complexity in CVD management dictate the need for region-specific studies. We aimed at investigating the interactions between CVD risk factors and hypertension in Ngaoundéré. *Methods*. A cross-sectional survey was carried out from March to August 2014. Sociodemographic, fasting blood glucose, blood pressure, and anthropometric data were recorded. Statistical analyses were carried out using SAS software version 9.1. *Results*. 700 adults resident in Ngaoundéré for at least two years consented and were included in the survey. Abdominal obesity, physical inactivity, and hypertension were the dominant risk factors recording 51.1%, 35.4%, and 20.4%, respectively. The prevalence of hyperglycaemia, tobacco consumption, obesity, and alcohol consumption was 5.6%, 8.3%, 9.6%, and 18.1%, respectively. Advanced age, hyperglycaemia, a divorced marital status, and alcohol consumption were independent determinants of high blood pressure. *Conclusion*. Physical inactivity, abdominal obesity, and hypertension were the most prevalent CVD risk factors, and the role of advanced age and hyperglycaemia in the occurrence of high blood pressure was reiterated. Health programs need to focus on effective screening, prevention, and control of CVDs in the Adamawa Region and Cameroon at large.

1. Introduction

Noncommunicable diseases (NCDs) represent an essential public health problem worldwide and their increasing occurrence in Africa simultaneously with infectious diseases is of particular importance [1, 2]. Generally, NCDs account for approximately two-thirds of the global mortality with diabetes and cardiovascular pathologies among other diseases taking the lead [3, 4]. NCDs and cardiovascular diseases (CVDs) contribute, respectively, to 82% and 37% of all the deaths under the age of 70 in developing countries [4]. CVDs represent the first cause of mortality and are responsible for about a third of all deaths worldwide, four-fifths of which occur in developing countries [4, 5]. In Cameroon, CVDs account for 11% of total mortality and central to this problem are associated risk factors defined by WHO as any attribute, characteristic, or exposure of an individual that increases the likelihood of developing the disease [6]. Consequently, CVDs prevention and the reduction of associated mortality will not be effective without direct interventions on these factors including population based investigations on the distribution of and interactions between risk factors, sensitisation, and strengthening awareness of the general population on CVDs prevention needs [7–10]. Although a majority of CVD risk factors are well known and established, the variability of the individual contribution of each risk factor in different communities and ethnic groups, as well as the complexity of the management of CVD patients, necessitates the conduction of specific regional and subregional surveys, worldwide.

Data on the distribution of cardiovascular risk factors in the Adamawa Region of Cameroon is insufficient, forming the basis for this work in investigating and collecting current data on cardiovascular disease risk factors in Ngaoundéré, the principal town of the region, with the aim of contributing to the reduction of cardiovascular risk and prevention of CVDs.

2. Study Area

Our survey was carried out in Ngaoundéré, the headquarter of the Adamawa Region (Figure 1). This region shares boundaries in the south and north with the centre and north regions of Cameroon, respectively, in the west with Nigeria, and in the east with the Central African Republic. It is found in the high altitude guinea savannah ecological zone of Cameroon, possessing a surface area of 62000 km^2, and is characterised by two seasons: a rainy season spanning the period from April to October and a dry season from November to March [11]. The main economic activity in the region is dairy farming and agriculture.

Ngaoundéré town comprises three subdivisions. The main health structure is the Ngaoundéré Regional Hospital which is public, followed by a private protestant hospital. There are also one subdivisional medical centre, one social medical centre at the Ngaoundéré University, four integrated health centres, and many private health centres. The population is made up of several ethnic groups of unequal proportions and distribution among which are the Foulbes, the Bororo, the Haoussas, the Gbaya, the Tikar, the Mboum, and the Dii.

3. Methods

3.1. Study Design, Subjects, and Selection Criteria. We conducted a prospective cross-sectional community-based survey from March to August 2014. We enrolled persons at least 18 years of age who resided in the study area for at least two years and who provided written consent to participate in the survey. Pregnant women and seriously sick persons (bedridden or in terminal phase of chronic disease) were not included in our study.

3.2. Sample Size. The sample size was calculated according to the following Lorenz formula:

$$N = \frac{t^2 \times p(1-p)}{m^2}, \qquad (1)$$

where N is the required sample size, t is Z-score, in our case 1.96 for 95% confidence level, p is the estimated prevalence of the risk factor in the survey zone, and m is the error margin, in our case 0.05 for 5%.

3.3. Sampling Method. We performed a two-stage sampling procedure wherein the quarters within the three subdivisions of the town were initially stratified following socioeconomic characteristics (low, middle, and high class and university area, considering majority of inhabitants). At least one quarter was selected from each subdivision to approximately represent the overall socioeconomic quotas; thus, 7 quarters have been selected. Secondly, households were selected within each quarter using a systematic method where every Kth household was selected beginning with that of the quarter head until the allocated number of participants per quarter attended. The calculated value of K varied depending on the average number of households and inhabitants per household in each quarter. Seven quarters were selected and sensitised with the help of quarter head messengers and community relay workers prior to data collection, after which 100 participants were recruited per quarter.

3.4. Sample and Data Collection Procedure. In the course of our study, all adults per households visited who fulfilled eligibility criteria of the study were enrolled without any discrimination upon their gender or religious, ethnic, or social status. All data were collected and measurements performed in the evenings from 4 p.m. to 6 p.m. at the participant's residence except for fasting blood glucose (FBG) which was measured between 6 a.m. and 9 a.m. the following morning for the same participants from whom data were collected the day before. Participants who could not communicate in French were assisted with translations to the Fulfulde (local) dialect which is widely spoken in the region. We prepared and pretested a semistructured questionnaire with which information on sociodemographics and several epidemiological factors and determinants of cardiovascular disease was collected.

3.5. Measured Variables

3.5.1. Blood Pressure (BP). Arterial blood pressure was measured with the help of a manual mercury sphygmomanometer (ADC Prosphyg model 770) according to the STEPS method described by the WHO [12]. This was performed following a 15-minute rest period, with the individual assuming a sitting position and on both arms, and having an average time lapse of 3 to 5 minutes between paired measurements. Arterial blood pressure measurements of 140/90 mmHg or higher were considered as high blood pressure and results were recorded. Participants with high blood pressure measurements were referred for consultation with a cardiologist for comprehensive examination including other risk factors out of the scope of our study.

3.5.2. Fasting Blood Glucose (FBG). Fasting blood glucose levels were equally measured following WHO recommendations after an 8–12-hour overnight fast, using a glucometer (Accu-Chek® Performa). Hyperglycaemia was defined according to the WHO threshold [12], with measurements being greater than 1.26 g/dL.

3.5.3. Weight. We measured participants' weights using a mechanical balance (mark: SECA), with light weight clothing

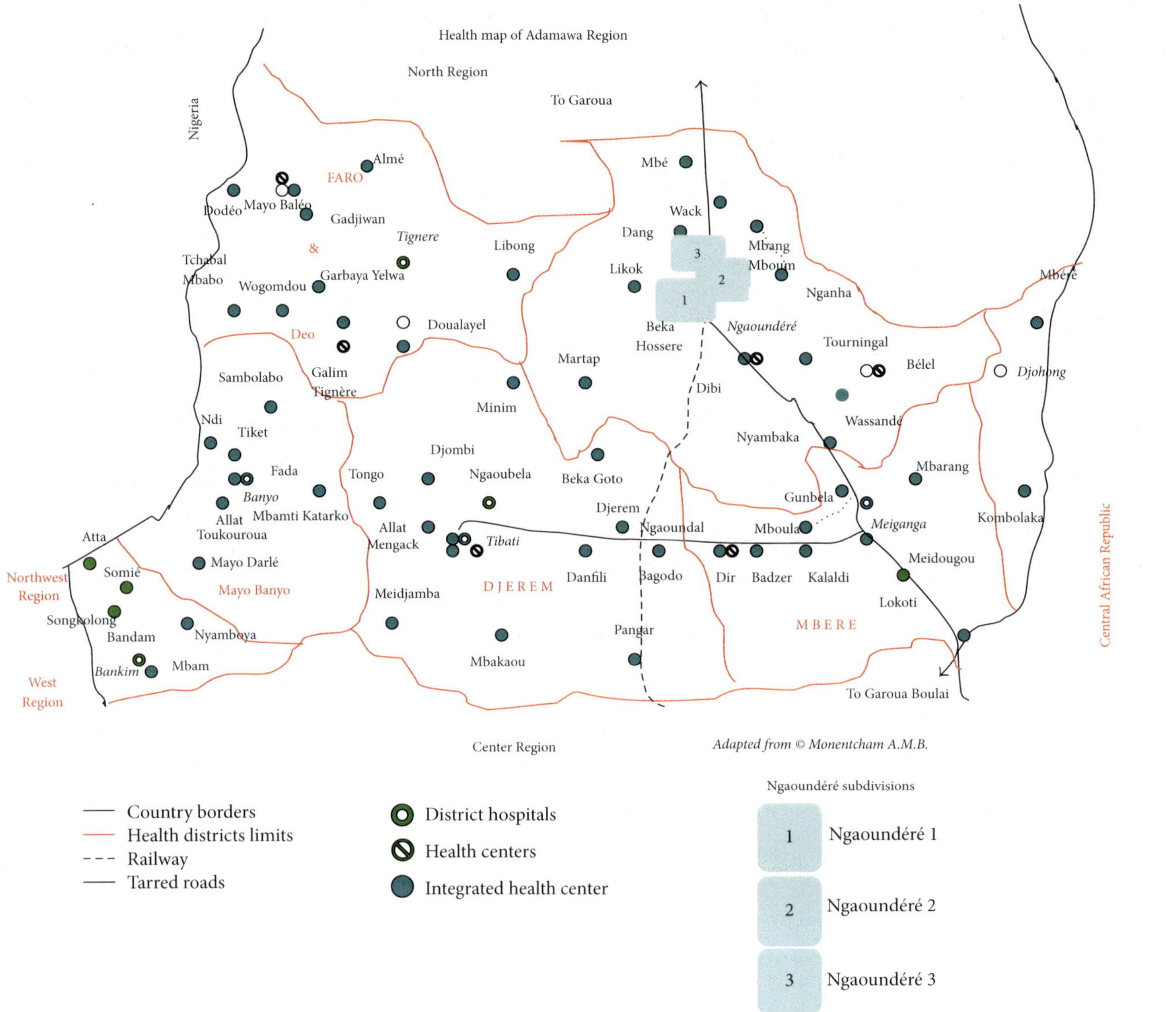

Figure 1: Map of the Adamawa Region of Cameroon, Africa.

and ensuring that the scale was on a flat and stable surface. The measurement of the body weight was done in conformity with the WHO STEPS method [12].

3.5.4. Height. Height measurements were done using a graduated flexible nonextensible ribbon tape (Gulick Measuring Tape©) provided with a spring enabling the adjustment of the tension applied during measurement and having a precision of 0.1 cm. These measurements were done in accordance with the WHO recommendations [12].

3.5.5. Body Mass Index (BMI). Body mass indices were calculated using formula BMI = weight (kg)/height (m^2). WHO thresholds were used to define general obesity, with BMI ≥ 30. Overweight was considered as BMI between 25 and 29 and underweight BMI < 18.5. BMI values between 18.5 and 24.9 were considered normal [13].

3.5.6. Waist Circumference Measurement. Waist circumference as an indicator of abdominal obesity was measured in accordance with the WHO STEPS method using a graduated flexible nonextensible ribbon tape (*see height measurement*)

3.6. Ethical Considerations. The authorisation to carry out this survey was obtained from the Adamawa Regional Delegation of Public Health (ref. N°507/L/HN/DRSPA/SAGE/BPF/NGD) and the Ethical Committee of the Ngaoundéré Regional Hospital (ref. N°1233/L/RC/RA/DSP/HR/NGD/CLE). Participants provided written consent after obtaining information on the nature of the study and its merits and demerits. Specimen collection was performed under aseptic conditions and participant information was handled confidentially. Results per quarter were kept in the corresponding health centres, to be handed to the individual participants by the chief of the centre while ensuring proper referral for those with abnormal values.

3.7. Data Management, Analysis, and Interpretation of Results. All the data collected on the individual record sheet of participants were transferred onto an Excel spreadsheet. The confidentiality of the data was respected by minimising access to the data using a password. The saved data were verified with participants' individual record sheets for conformity and consistency. The data were finally forwarded onto SAS software version 9.1 for analysis with statistical significance stated at $p < 0.05$.

4. Results

4.1. Basic Characteristics of the Study Population. Our survey population was made of 700 adults, with an age range of 18 to 93 years and average age of 36 ± 17 years. Among them were 340 (48.6%) men and 360 (51.4%) women. Two-thirds of this population were made up of Muslims and a third of Christians. The majority of our population were housewives (32%) and were predominantly possessing secondary level education (41.1%). With respect to participants with more than secondary education, women were less educated than men (9.1% against 16.9%).

4.2. Distribution of Cardiovascular Disease (CVD) Risk Factors

4.2.1. High Blood Pressure. A total of 143 (20.43%) of the study participants had BP values above the normal, comprising 9.57% men and 10.86% women. The prevalence of higher-than-normal BP was recorded as 19.71% and 21.1% among male and female participants, respectively. In individuals under the age of 30 years, 9.40% presented higher-than-normal blood pressure and likewise 9.76%, 27.59%, and 45.03% in the age groups 30–39 years, 40–49 years, and >50 years, respectively. Although wide differences were observed between subgroup population weights, divorced persons (53.33%) had the highest frequency of high blood pressure followed by married participants (25.0%). Subpopulation proportions of participants with high BP were the highest among the unemployed (34.29%), followed by household workers (29.91%), and were the least among civil servants (6.19%). Furthermore, frequency distributions of high blood pressure following educational level were performed and it was observed that 87.02% of persons with higher-than-normal blood pressure possessed at most a secondary level of education. The distributions of high blood pressure following sociodemographic characteristics are presented in Table 1.

4.2.2. Obesity and Overweight. Overall, 21.14% of the participants were overweight and 9.57% of the individuals were obese (Figure 2). The distribution of obesity according to gender showed a prevalence of 3.29% among men and 6.28% among women.

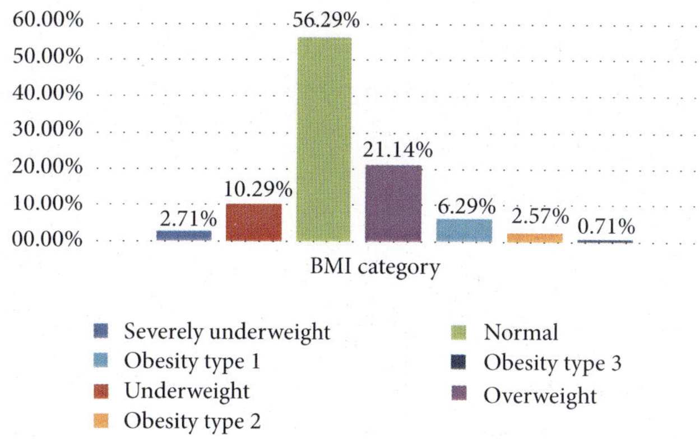

FIGURE 2: Distribution of study participants by BMI categories.

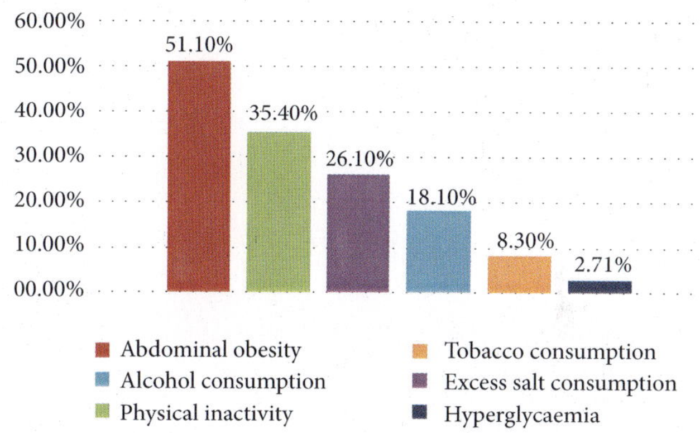

FIGURE 3: Distribution of other CVD risk factors in the study population.

4.2.3. Other CVD Risk Factors. The other CVD risk factors we studied include hyperglycaemia, abdominal obesity, physical inactivity, and excess salt, alcohol, and tobacco consumption. Among these, physical inactivity (35.4%) was highly prevalent, second only to abdominal obesity (51.1%). Hyperglycaemia was the least present in our study population (Figure 3).

Gender based distributions demonstrated high frequencies of abdominal obesity, physical inactivity, and excess salt and alcohol consumption in women relative to men, while higher proportions of the male population were smokers and hyperglycaemic subjects (Figure 4).

4.2.4. Notion of Family History and Hereditary Diabetes, Arterial Hypertension, and Obesity. The possibility for hereditary hypertension, diabetes, and obesity was defined and constituted persons with raised BP (paired), FBG, and BMI measurements, having family history (at least a parent or sibling diagnosed) of hypertension, diabetes, and obesity, respectively. The probability of hereditary (familial) hypertension, diabetes (using hyperglycaemia), and obesity was

Table 1: Distribution of high blood pressure by age, marital status, and gender.

Variable	Total, n	High blood pressure			
		Men, n (%)	Women, n (%)	Total, n (%)	Proportion of the study population (%)
Age (years)					
<30	319	18 (5.64)	12 (3.76)	30 (9.40)	4.29
30–39	123	2 (1.63)	10 (8.13)	12 (9.76)	1.71
40–49	87	13 (14.94)	11 (12.64)	24 (27.59)	3.43
≥50	171	34 (19.88)	43 (25.15)	77 (45.03)	11.00
Marital status					
Unmarried	253	16 (6.32)	10 (3.95)	26 (10.28)	3.71
Married	426	46 (10.80)	59 (13.85)	105 (24.65)	15.00
Widowed	6	3 (50.00)	1 (16.67)	4 (66.67)	0.57
Divorced	15	2 (13.33)	6 (40.00)	8 (53.33)	1.14
Profession					
Farmers	34	2 (5.88)	2 (5.88)	4 (11.76)	0.57
Drivers	26	5 (19.23)	0 (0.00)	5 (19.23)	0.71
Traders	139	19 (13.67)	3 (2.16)	22 (15.83)	0.03
Students	125	9 (7.20)	7 (5.60)	16 (12.80)	2.28
Household workers	224	22 (9.82)	45 (20.09)	67 (29.91)	9.57
Civil servants	117	0 (0.00)	7 (5.98)	7 (6.19)	1.00
Unemployed	35	10 (28.57)	2 (5.71)	12 (34.29)	1.71
Level of education					
Uneducated	92	3 (3.26)	8 (8.70)	11 (11.96)	1.57
Coranic	107	16 (14.95)	18 (16.82)	34 (31.78)	4.86
Primary	121	8 (6.61)	20 (16.53)	28 (23.14)	4.00
Secondary	288	32 (11.11)	26 (9.03)	58 (20.14)	8.29
Higher	92	8 (8.70)	4 (4.35)	12 (13.04)	1.71
Religion					
Atheist	2	0 (0.00)	0 (0.00)	0 (0.00)	0.00
Christian	235	17 (7.23)	18 (7.66)	35 (14.89)	5.00
Muslim	463	50 (10.80)	58 (12.53)	108 (23.33)	15.42

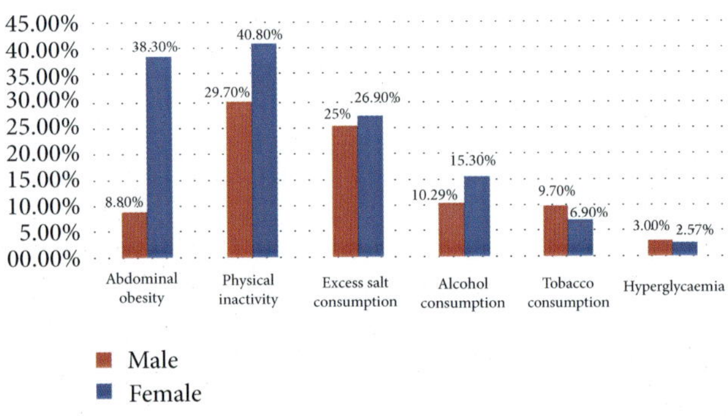

Figure 4: Distribution of other CVD risk factors by gender.

thus estimated at 11.6%, 11.28%, and 4.6%, respectively, in our survey.

4.3. Factors Associated with Hypertension. Based on blood pressure measurements and following JNC-7 recommendations [14], normotensive, prehypertensive, and hypertensive persons were estimated at 67.43%, 12.14%, and 20.43%.

Examining the distribution of high BP between other categories of CVD risk factors, hyperglycaemic persons (46.15%) exhibited the highest prevalence of high BP followed by obese participants (31.34%) and then tobacco consumers (25.86%) as shown in Table 2.

Regression analysis proved that advanced age, alcohol consumption, hyperglycaemia, and a divorced marital status were associated with hypertension. Participants aged 40 to 49 (OR = 3.83; $p = 0.0016$) and 50 years and above (OR = 7.08; $p < 0.0001$) were more likely to have high BP values compared to those under 30 years of age. Likewise, participants with hyperglycaemia compared to normoglycaemia (OR = 4.2; $p = 0.027$) and those divorced compared to unmarried ones (OR = 4.11; $p = 0.0488$) were more prone to high blood pressure values, while alcohol consumers compared to nonconsumers were less likely to have high BP levels (OR = 0.16; $p = 0.0025$) (Table 3).

5. Discussion

Except for some hospital studies involving a reduced number of participants and usually focussed on only one risk factor,

Table 2: Distribution of High BP between other CVD risk factors and gender.

CVD risk factors	Total, n	High blood pressure			
		Men, n (%)	Women, n (%)	Total, n (%)	Proportion of study population (%)
Hyperglycaemia	39	9 (23.08)	9 (23.08)	18 (46.15)	2.57
Obesity	67	15 (22.39)	6 (8.96)	21 (31.34)	3.00
Alcohol consumption	127	8 (6.30)	5 (3.94)	13 (10.24)	1.86
Tobacco consumption	58	7 (12.07)	8 (13.79)	15 (25.86)	2.14
Physical inactivity	248	21 (8.47)	38 (15.32)	59 (23.79)	8.43
Excessive salt consumption	182	12 (6.59)	24 (13.19)	36 (19.78)	5.14

Table 3: Logistic regression for HBP with other CVD risk factors.

Variables	p value	Odds ratio	[95% CI]
Age group			
<30	Reference	1	
30–39	0.8419	0.91	[0.36–2.2]
40–49	0.0016**	3.83	[1.66–8.9]
≥50	<0.0001***	7.08	[3.43–15.2]
Sex			
Male	Reference	1	
Female	0.6820	0.77	[0.35–1.68]
Obesity			
No	Reference	1	
Yes	0.0881	1.04	[0.049–0.22]
Alcohol consumption			
No	Reference	1	
Yes	0.0025**	0.16	[0.046–0.49]
Tobacco consumption			
No	Reference	1	
Yes	0.0561	2.26	[0.95–5.18]
Physical inactivity			
No	Reference	1	
Yes	0.3680	1.03	[0.28–3.70]
Excessive salt consumption			
No	Reference	1	
Yes	0.1450	1.05	[0.52–2.07]
Hyperglycaemia			
No	Reference	1	
Yes	0.0270*	4.20	[1.17–15.2]
Marital status			
Unmarried	Reference	1	
Divorced	0.0488*	4.11	[0.92–18.3]
Married	0.8634	0.80	[0.39–1.62]
Widowed	0.7964	1.2	[0.13–12.5]

***$p < 0.001$; **$p < 0.01$; *$p < 0.05$.

few epidemiological data are available quantifying cardiovascular disease risk factors in northern regions of Cameroon. This community survey carried out in Ngaoundéré town was aimed at studying cardiovascular disease risk factors and their association with hypertension so as to contribute to the improvement of disease prevention, control, and management.

5.1. The Prevalence of Cardiovascular Disease Risk Factors

5.1.1. Arterial Hypertension. Our study showed that approximately one-fifth (20.43%) of the study participants had arterial blood pressure values higher than normal at the time of measurement. Data from a 2004 study by Kengne et al. reported similar rates (20.8%) in Cameroon [15]. Studying a ten-year variation in hypertension in Cameroon, Fezeu et al. (2010) suggested a 2- to 5-fold increase in both urban and rural dwellers of both sexes [16]. The distribution of hypertension in sub-Saharan Africa varies considerably between countries with recent surveys reporting occurrence rates of 27.9% in Ethiopia [17], 31.8% in Nigeria [18], and 47% in Kenya [19], among others. As previously proposed by other authors, we acknowledge the contribution of socioeconomic, environmental, and behavioural determinants to this prevalence, including increasing economic growth and urbanisation, consumption of tobacco and fatty foods, and long periods of risk exposure to these factors due to a long-life experience [20, 21].

5.1.2. Overweight and Obesity. Overweight and obesity were estimated in 21.14% and 9.57% of the study population, respectively, values which are lower than the 23.7% and 11.1% previously reported in Cameroon [15]. Although our results recorded the prevalence of overweight and obesity lower than the 34.5% and 9.5% observed in Kenya [22], 28.2% and 13.8% in Nigeria [18], and 29.6% and 13.0% in Iran [23], respectively, they remain far below the 72.4% recorded in South Africa in 2013 [24]. Gender based distribution of obesity portrayed women (6.28%) to be more affected by obesity than men (3.29%), concurring with previous findings [17, 19, 23]. Our results differ greatly and are much lower than those reported in Western Europe (France: 6.28% in men and 37% in women) and Asia (China: 45% in men and 32% in women) [25]. These differences could be explained by the improved living standards, advanced state of urbanisation, and other inherent sociocultural attributes associated with the latter region.

In addition, we observed that abdominal obesity occurred in about half of our participants (51.1%) in the study. Kengne and coworkers reported 14% and 59.5% prevalence of abdominal obesity in urban dwelling Cameroonian men and women, respectively [15]. Our rate, despite being in line with the reports of Elasmi et al. (2009) in the Grand Tunis population [26], is far higher than the 14.4% observed in Iran [23] and is possibly the result of an increase in the consumption of salts and fatty and energy-rich foods with deprivation in vitamins and mineral salts due to the change in lifestyle habits [27].

5.1.3. Hyperglycaemia. Hyperglycaemia was defined as an increase in blood glucose level above 1.26 g/dL measured after an overnight fast of 8 to 12 hours with or without any associated clinical manifestations. The prevalence of hyperglycaemia was 5.57% in our survey (3% in men and 2.57% in women). Diabetes mellitus has been reported to occur in about 2.9% to 6.2% of Cameroon's rural and urban subpopulations [28], similar to the observed 3.6% in neighbouring Nigeria [18]. This is lower than the results reported in several countries: 11.9% in men and 11.7% in women in South Africa [24], 7.8% in men and 8.5% in women in Congo [29], 7.2% in men and 4.3% in women in France, and 12.6% in men and 9.1% in women in the United States [30]. Probably, our sampling methods could have led to underestimation of the occurrence of hyperglycaemia in our study population as we did not consider diabetic patients on treatment and having normal FBG levels as being hyperglycaemic contrary to the other authors [26, 29].

5.2. Other Cardiovascular Disease Risk Factors

5.2.1. Tobacco and Alcohol. The prevalence of alcohol and tobacco consumption in our survey was 18.1% and 8.3%, respectively, with even much lesser rates reported in rural Kenya [19], findings which are lower than the previously reported 85% and 16% in urban Cameroon [16] and 55.8% and 13% in Nigeria [18]. The prevalence of these two risk factors varies between countries with an unequal distribution between men and women [17, 22]. Inherent sociocultural and economic factors possibly affect these habits in our setting such as the state of reduced urbanisation and the widely practiced Muslim faith.

5.2.2. Excessive Salt Consumption. 26.1% of participants consumed large quantities of salt, which is encouraged by several sociocultural practices. The high consumption of sodium is common in Kenya due to the use of salts to preserve food or render it appetising or to be added to prepared food by consumers [19]. These facts were reflected in our work as several participants from different quarters of the town were observed to consume a large quantity of salts.

5.2.3. Sedentary Lifestyle. Compared to the 35.4% proportion of our participants characterised with a sedentary lifestyle, other African studies have reported relatively higher values of 52.2% [24] and 42.6% [29]. This is likely owing to the fact that animal breeding and farming which are most practiced in this region necessitate important geographical displacement. In our study, however, physical inactivity appeared to be a more dominant risk factor for cardiovascular diseases compared to high blood pressure, thus contradicting reports of other sub-Saharan studies in which arterial hypertension was observed to be the most prevalent CVD risk factor [22, 30].

5.2.4. Hereditary Hypertension, Diabetes, and Obesity. The probability of family heredity of arterial hypertension was found in 11.6% of the study population and likewise 11.28% and 4.6% for diabetes and obesity, respectively. It has been clearly established in previous studies that family history of arterial hypertension is associated with a significant risk of hypertension for both men and women [31]. Our results therefore suggest a relatively high medium- to long-term risk of hypertension in our population.

5.3. Factors Associated with Arterial Hypertension. Previous reports have established the role of advanced age as a risk factor for hypertension [17, 24, 32]. A study carried out in Israel between 2002 and 2007 showed that ten years caused a 1.6-fold rise in the risk of being in a higher JNC-7 category of blood pressure [33]. Regression analysis reiterated the relationship between advanced age and arterial hypertension, as the likelihood of high blood pressure was 3.8-fold ($p = 0.0016$) and 7.1-fold ($p < 0.0001$) the normal for participants aged 40–49 and 50 years and above, respectively, compared to those 30 years of age and below.

Hyperglycaemia is another CVD risk factor which demonstrated an association with hypertension in this study. 46.15% of the participants with raised fasting blood sugar levels had higher-than-normal blood pressure values. These findings are in conformity with the previous literature [34].

Alcohol consumption was inversely associated with arterial blood pressure: consumers of alcohol were less likely to have high BP values compared to nonconsumers ($p = 0.0025$; OR = 0.16). These results are similar to those obtained by Peltzer and Phaswana-Mafuya [24], although other studies hold the notion that the consumption of even very little quantities of alcohol increases the risk of hypertension [35, 36].

5.4. Limitations of This Study. This study was characterised with several limitations with the most significant being the reliability of data analysis based on nonverifiable verbal responses of participants. Also, the evaluation of alcohol and tobacco consumption was incoherent as several participants consumed tobacco in powder form by chewing and others consumed local alcoholic beverages rendering quantification difficult. Lastly, the time frame within which our study was carried out did not permit an elaborate investigation on dietary awareness, patterns, and practice as a function of CVD risk at individual level within the population.

5.5. Conclusion. Our study on cardiovascular diseases risk factors indicates relatively high occurrences of several factors within the Ngaoundéré community with dominant risk factors being abdominal obesity, physical inactivity, excessive salt consumption, arterial hypertension, and alcohol consumption. Furthermore, advanced age, hyperglycaemia, a divorced marital status, and consumption of alcohol were associated with higher-than-normal blood pressure levels.

5.6. Perspectives. This study was carried out in an urban setting within the Adamawa Region where access to health information, services, and promotion programs and socioeconomic and educational levels are relatively higher compared to rural settlements. It is imperative therefore for future studies to be carried in rural communities of the Adamawa Region as well as comparative studies between regions of the Cameroon national territory. This will furnish relevant data necessary for informed decision-making, advocacy, elaboration of health promotion programs, and strengthening the health system in a bid to progressively and sufficiently prevent, control, and manage cardiovascular diseases nationwide.

Competing Interests

The authors declare that they have no competing interests.

Acknowledgments

The authors express immense gratitude to Pr. Elias Nchiwan Nukenine for the supervision of this research work. They also extend their gratitude to all the participants for their enthusiasm and the interest they accorded in this research work. They equally extend gratitude to the Adamawa public health regional delegate, the staff of the corresponding district health services, health centres, community relay workers, and the local community rulers for their monumental collaboration throughout this survey.

References

[1] I. C. Bygbjerg, "Double burden of noncommunicable and infectious diseases in developing countries," *Science*, vol. 337, no. 6101, pp. 1499–1501, 2012.

[2] M. Naghavi, H. Wang, R. Lozano et al., "Global, regional, and national age-sex specific all-cause and cause-specific mortality for 240 causes of death, 1990–2013: a systematic analysis for the Global Burden of Disease Study 2013," *The Lancet*, vol. 385, no. 9963, pp. 117–171, 2015.

[3] M. Ezzati, A. D. Lopez, A. Rodgers, S. V. Hoorn, and C. J. L. Murray, "Selected major risk factors and global and regional burden of disease," *The Lancet*, vol. 360, no. 9343, pp. 1347–1360, 2002.

[4] S. Mendis, T. Armstrong, D. Bettcher et al., *Global Status Report on Noncommunicable Diseases 2014*, WHO Library Cataloguing-in-Publication Data, Geneva, Switzerland, 2014.

[5] WHO, *Global Atlas on Cardiovascular Disease Prevention and Control*, World Health Organization, Geneva, Switzerland, 2011.

[6] World Health Organization, *Noncommunicable Diseases Country Profiles 2014*, WHO Library Cataloguing-in-Publication Data, Geneva, Switzerland, 2014.

[7] H. L. F. Kamga, N. J. C. Assob, D. S. Nsagha, A. L. Njunda, and D. L. Njimoh, "A community survey on the knowledge of neglected tropical diseases in Cameroon," *International Journal of Medicine and Biomedical Research*, vol. 1, no. 2, pp. 131–140, 2012.

[8] M. O. Pancha, A. M. N. Aïdego, M. T. Tamanji, and M. B. Atanga, "Educational needs of hypertensive patients in Buea hospital setting (Cameroon)," *Health Science and Disease*, vol. 16, no. 2, pp. 1–5, 2015.

[9] O. P. Mbouemboue, E. Yiagnigni, A. K. Koona, J. Cacko, and P. Ndobo, "Determinants of hypertension awareness and treatment among patients under cardiology follow-up in A Cameroonian Regional Hospital," *International Journal of Collaborative Research on Internal Medicine & Public Health*, vol. 4, no. 9, pp. 1663–1672, 2012.

[10] P. K. Awah, A. P. Kengne, L. L. K. Fezeu, and J.-C. Mbanya, "Perceived risk factors of cardiovascular diseases and diabetes in Cameroon," *Health Education Research*, vol. 23, no. 4, pp. 612–620, 2008.

[11] F. Tchuenguem Fohouo, S. Tope, A. Mbianda, J. Messi, and D. Bruckner, "Foraging behaviour of *Apis mellifera adansonii* Latreille (Hymenoptera : Apidae) on *Daniellia oliveri*, *Delonix regia*, *Hymenocardia acida* and *Terminalia mantaly* flowers in Ngaoundéré (Cameroon)," *International Journal of Biological and Chemical Sciences*, vol. 4, no. 4, pp. 1180–1190, 2011.

[12] World Health Organization, *The WHO STEPwise Approach to Chronic Disease Risk Factor Surveillance/Non-Communicable Diseases and Mental Health*, WHO, Geneva, Switzerland, 2005.

[13] WHO, *Physical Status: The Use and Interpretation of Anthropometry. Report of a WHO Expert Committee. WHO Technical Report Series 854*, World Health Organization, Geneva, Switzerland, 1995.

[14] A. V. Chobanian, G. L. Bakris, H. R. Black et al., "The Seventh Report of the Joint National Committee on Prevention, Detection, Evaluation, and Treatment of High Blood Pressure: the JNC 7 report," *The Journal of the American Medical Association*, vol. 289, no. 19, pp. 2560–2572, 2003.

[15] A. P. Kengne, P. K. Awah, L. Fezeu, and J. C. Mbanya, "The burden of high blood pressure and related risk factors in urban Sub-Saharan Africa: evidences from Douala in Cameroon," *African Health Sciences*, vol. 7, no. 1, pp. 38–44, 2007.

[16] L. Fezeu, A. P. Kengne, B. Balkau, P. K. Awah, and J. C. Mbanya, "Ten-year change in blood pressure levels and prevalence of hypertension in urban and rural Cameroon," *Journal of Epidemiology and Community Health*, vol. 64, no. 4, pp. 360–365, 2010.

[17] S. M. Abebe, Y. Berhane, A. Worku, and A. Getachew, "Prevalence and associated factors of hypertension: a crossectional community based study in Northwest Ethiopia," *PLOS ONE*, vol. 10, no. 4, Article ID e0125210, 2015.

[18] O. S. Ogah, O. O. Madukwe, U. U. Onyeonoro et al., "Cardiovascular risk factors and non-communicable diseases in Abia state, Nigeria: report of a community-based survey," *International Journal of Medicine & Biomedical Research*, vol. 2, no. 1, pp. 57–68, 2013.

[19] J. Muchira, E. Stuart-Shor, J. Kariuki et al., "Distribution and characteristics of risk factors for cardiovascular-metabolic disease in a rural Kenyan community," *International Journal of Africa Nursing Sciences*, vol. 3, pp. 76–81, 2015.

[20] O. Steichen, "Hypertension artérielle du sujet noir," *la Revue du Praticien*, vol. 60, pp. 654–659, 2010.

[21] J. B. Echouffo-Tcheugui and A. P. Kengne, "Chronic non-communicable diseases in Cameroon—burden, determinants and current policies," *Globalization and Health*, vol. 7, article no. 44, 2011.

[22] M. E. Hendriks, F. W. N. M. Wit, M. T. L. Roos et al., "Hypertension in Sub-Saharan Africa: cross-sectional surveys

in four rural and urban communities," *PLoS ONE*, vol. 7, no. 3, Article ID e32638, 2012.

[23] H. Najafipour, G. Yousefzadeh, A. Forood, M. Karamouzian, M. Shadkam, and A. Mirzazadeh, "Overweight and obesity prevalence and its predictors in a general population: a community-based study in Kerman, Iran (kerman coronary artery diseases risk factors studies)," *ARYA Atherosclerosis*, vol. 12, no. 1, pp. 18–27, 2016.

[24] K. Peltzer and N. Phaswana-Mafuya, "Hypertension and associated factors in older adults in South Africa," *Cardiovascular Journal of Africa*, vol. 24, no. 3, pp. 67–72, 2013.

[25] M. M. Finucane, G. A. Stevens, M. J. Cowan et al., "National, regional, and global trends in body-mass index since 1980: systematic analysis of health examination surveys and epidemiological studies with 960 country-years and 9.1 million participants," *The Lancet*, vol. 377, no. 9765, pp. 557–567, 2011.

[26] M. Elasmi, M. Feki, H. Sanhaji et al., "Prévalence des facteurs de risque cardiovasculaires conventionnels dans la population du Grand Tunis," *Revue d'Épidémiologie et de Santé Publique*, vol. 57, no. 2, pp. 87–92, 2009.

[27] N. Marion and M. N. Berkeley, "Why calories count: from science to politics," *Health Affairs*, vol. 31, no. 9, p. 2150, 2012.

[28] E. Sobngwi, J.-C. N. Mbanya, N. C. Unwin et al., "Physical activity and its relationship with obesity, hypertension and diabetes in urban and rural Cameroon," *International Journal of Obesity*, vol. 26, no. 7, pp. 1009–1016, 2002.

[29] A. Yahia-Berrouiguet, M. Benyoucef, K. Meguenni, and M. Brouri, "Prevalence of cardiovascular risk factors: a survey at Tlemcen (Algeria)," *Medecine des Maladies Metaboliques*, vol. 3, no. 3, pp. 313–319, 2009.

[30] S. Pessinaba, A. Mbaye, G. A. D. Yabeta et al., "Enquete de prévalence des facteurs de risque cardiovasculaire en population générale à Saint-Louis (Sénégal)," *Annales de Cardiologie et d'Angéiologie*, vol. 62, no. 4, pp. 253–258, 2013.

[31] E. Méndez-Chacón, C. Santamaría-Ulloa, and L. Rosero-Bixby, "Factors associated with hypertension prevalence, unawareness and treatment among Costa Rican elderly," *BMC Public Health*, vol. 8, no. 1, article 275, 2008.

[32] J. Kishore, N. Gupta, C. Kohli, and N. Kumar, "Prevalence of hypertension and determination of its risk factors in rural Delhi," *International Journal of Hypertension*, vol. 2016, Article ID 7962595, 6 pages, 2016.

[33] K. Abu-Saad, A. Chetrit, S. Eilat-Adar et al., "Blood pressure level and hypertension awareness and control differ by marital status, sex, and ethnicity: a population-based study," *American Journal of Hypertension*, vol. 27, no. 12, pp. 1511–1520, 2014.

[34] A. Dzudie, A. P. Kengne, W. F. T. Muna et al., "Prevalence, awareness, treatment and control of hypertension in a self-selected sub-Saharan African urban population: a cross-sectional study," *BMJ Open*, vol. 2, no. 4, Article ID e001217, 2012.

[35] I. B. Puddey and L. J. Beilin, "Alcohol is bad for blood pressure," *Clinical and Experimental Pharmacology and Physiology*, vol. 33, no. 9, pp. 847–852, 2006.

[36] A. Briasoulis, V. Agarwal, and F. H. Messerli, "Alcohol consumption and the risk of hypertension in men and women: a systematic review and meta-analysis," *Journal of Clinical Hypertension*, vol. 14, no. 11, pp. 792–798, 2012.

18

Pulse Pressure Relationships with Demographics and Kidney Function in Ashanti, Ghana

Debasish Banerjee,[1] Jacob Plange-Rhule,[1,2] Nihil Chitalia,[1,3] Kwabena Kumi,[2] Frank B. Micah,[2] Francesco P. Cappuccio,[4] and John B. Eastwood[1]

[1]*Department of Renal Medicine and Transplantation, St Georges, University of London, Cranmer Terrace, London SW17 0RE, UK*
[2]*Department of Medicine, Komfo Anokye Teaching Hospital, P. O. Box 134, Kumasi, Ghana*
[3]*Department of Renal Medicine, Darent Valley Hospital, Dartford, Kent DA2 8DA, UK*
[4]*Division of Mental Health & Wellbeing, University of Warwick, Warwick Medical School, Gibbet Hill Road, Coventry CV4 7AL, UK*

Correspondence should be addressed to Debasish Banerjee; debasish.banerjee@stgeorges.nhs.uk

Academic Editor: Claudio Borghi

Introduction. Hypertension, particularly pulse pressure [PP] is a major risk factor for end-stage renal disease. However, the effect of individual components of hypertension namely PP, systolic [SBP] and diastolic blood pressure [DBP] on kidney function, in the general African population is unknown. *Methods.* Data were collected on 944 participants [aged 40-75 y], living in villages in the area around the city of Kumasi, Ghana, on demographics, medications, height, weight, BP and 24-hour creatinine clearance (CrCl). *Results.* The demographic and clinical characteristics were: age 55(11) [mean (SD)] years, females 62%, rural village-dwellers 52%, diabetes 1·5%, BMI 21(4) kg/m^2, 24-hourCrCl as a measure of glomerular filtration rate (GFR) 84(23) ml/min/1.73 m^2. 29% had BP >140/90 mmHg; SBP and DBP were 125/74(26/14) mmHg, PP was 51(17) mmHg. PP increased with age by 0.55(95% CI: 0.46,0.64) mmHg/year. PP was higher (53(17) v 49(15) mmHg; $p < 0.001$) in the semiurban participants. GFR decreased both with increasing PP [-0.19 (-0.27,-0.10 ml/min/1.73 m^2/mmHg; $p < 0.001$] and SBP [-0.09 (-0.14,-0.03) ml/min/1.73 m^2/mmHg; $p < 0.001$] but there was no significant relationship with DBP [-0.04 (-0.15,0.06)]. After adjusting for SBP, the relationship between GFR and PP became steeper [-0.31 (-0.50,-0.12) ml/min/1.73 m^2/mmHg; $p < 0.001$]. Using multivariate regression analysis that included PP, age, gender, BMI, only increasing age [-0.75 (-0.88,-0.62)] and decreasing BMI [0.49 (0.16,0.81)] were associated with decreased kidney function. *Conclusions.* In this homogeneous West-African population, PP increased with age and had a steeper relationship with declining kidney function than SBP or DBP.

1. Introduction

Hypertension is a major risk factor for chronic kidney damage, and while both systolic (SBP) and diastolic blood pressure (DBP) have been implicated as causal factors, it is now clear that SBP is a much stronger predictor of chronic kidney disease than DBP [1–3]. Isolated systolic hypertension (ISH) is becoming particular common especially in elderly, has also been recognised as a risk factor for cardiovascular disease [4–6]. In recent years there has been a growing interest in pulse pressure (PP) [systolic – diastolic pressure] as a marker of target end-organ damage [7]. Elevated PP is mainly due to central arterial stiffness and increases with age. The nature of PP and its association with demographics and kidney function in an African population has not been described.

PP has a stronger relationship than SBP alone with cardiovascular deaths in end-stage renal disease (ESRD) patients [3, 8, 9]. Also, in a predominantly Caucasian population with early and predialysis chronic kidney disease (CKD), we have found a strong relationship between PP and progression of chronic kidney disease, onset of dialysis, and death [2, 10].

Hypertension is common in Ghana, with estimated prevalence of about 29%, and hence a major cause of morbidity and mortality [11, 12]. However the effect of BP, particularly of PP, on kidney disease, in this population, is unknown.

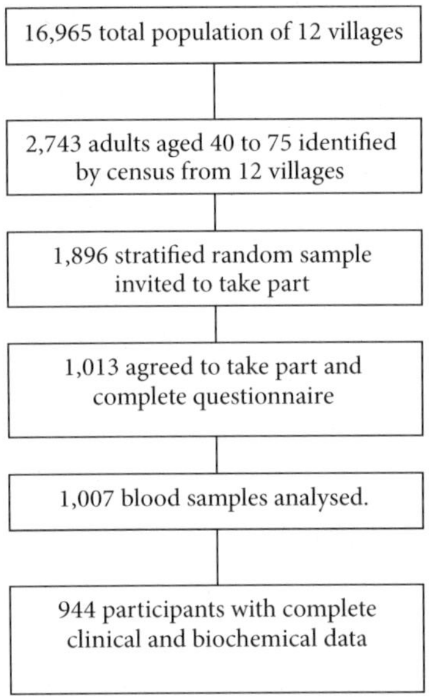

FIGURE 1: Recruitment of participants.

The present study examines the relationships between SBP, DBP, PP, demographic variables, and glomerular filtration rate (GFR), in a community study in villages in Ghana.

2. Methods

2.1. Participants. The present report uses data on 944 individuals [355 men, 589 women] from the 1,103 participants of the baseline survey for a cluster-randomised trial in 12 communities in the Ejisu-Juabeng and Kumasi Districts of the Ashanti Region, clustered around Kumasi, the second largest city in Ghana [11–13]. In this study "rural" refers to villages lacking any real infrastructure; they had no main water supply or sewage and often lacked electricity. These villages were up to 40 km from Kumasi. In contrast, most of the "semiurban" villages had main water and all had electricity; they were within 15 km of Kumasi. From each village, participants aged 40 to 75 were selected using age- and gender-stratified random sampling to ensure that participants from each village matched overall population structure [14]. Individuals with serious mental or physical illness, women pregnant or lactating, and individuals declining to participate were excluded from the study. Individuals with hypertension, diabetes or known renal disease were not excluded (Figure 1).

2.2. Questionnaire. Participants attended a registration centre in their village. After details of the study had been explained in the local language (Twi), individual written consent was obtained. All participants, with the help of a project assistant, completed the questionnaire, which included sections on demographic background, socioeconomic status, health, diet, lifestyle and past and current drug treatment. Ethical approval was granted by the Committee on Human Research Publication and Ethics of the School of Medical Sciences, Kwame Nkrumah University of Science and Technology, Kumasi, and by Wandsworth Research Ethics Committee, London.

2.3. Measurements. Methods are described in detail elsewhere [11–14]. In brief, height was measured to the nearest 0.5 cm using a wooden platform with height rule; footwear was removed. Weight was measured to the nearest 0.5 kg with manual Seca 761 scales (Vogel &Halke, Hamburg, Germany) after participants had removed outer garments and footwear. Blood pressure and pulse rate were measured with an automated sphygmomanometer (OMRON HEM705CP, Omron Matsusaka Co, Matsusaka City, Mie-Ken, Japan), using appropriate cuff size after participants had sat undisturbed for at least 5 minutes. Three readings were taken 1 minute apart. The first was discarded, and the mean of the last two used in the analysis. Hypertension was defined as a systolic BP $\geq$ 140 mm Hg and/or a diastolic BP $\geq$ 90 mm Hg or being on drug therapy for hypertension.

2.4. Blood Samples and 24-Hour Urine Collections. Venous blood samples were taken fasting from each participant. The samples were put into Vacutainer tubes and transported without delay to Komfo Anokye Teaching Hospital. The tubes were centrifuged at 1,500 rpm for 10 minutes at room temperature, and the serum transferred into 5 ml aliquot tubes, which were kept frozen at -20°C until analysed. Serum and urine creatinine were measured using a Jaffe alkaline picrate method (Beckman–Coulter). Our method has been validated against isotope dilution mass spectrometry (IDMS) values for creatinine measurement [11].

Two consecutive timed 24-hour urine collections were obtained from each participant and the excretion of sodium, potassium and creatinine clearance were measured.

2.5. Statistical Analysis. GFR was measured as the mean of two creatinine clearances based on 24-hour urine collections and adjusted for body surface area. 24-hour urinary sodium and potassium were also measured. Body mass index (BMI) was calculated from the equation: BMI = weight/height^2 [kg/m^2]. Data were analysed using SPSS v.17 (Chicago, SPSS Inc). Results are presented as mean $\pm$ SD or median (interquartile range) for continuous variables and relationships between variables using correlation and regression coefficients with 95% confidence intervals. A two-sided p value < 0.05 is taken as statistically significant.

3. Results

3.1. Participants (Table 1). The mean age of the population was 54.6 (11.1) years. 62% were females and 49% rural village dwellers. Only 1.6% of the study population were self-reported diabetics. BMI was 21.1 (4.2) kg/m^2, haemoglobin 12.2 (1.7) g/dl, and creatinine clearance 84 (22) ml/min/1.73 m^2. 24-urine sodium/potassium ratio was 2.3 (1.2) mmol/mmol. The mean BP of the study population was 125/74 (26/14) mmHg with a PP of 51 (17) mmHg. The overall prevalence of hypertension in the population was 28.7%, which higher than in other parts of Africa [12], with 30% of

TABLE 1: Clinical characteristics of the population.

	Females $n = 589$	Males $n = 355$	Total $n = 944$
Age	54.8 (11.5)	54.5 (10.7)	54.6 (11.1)
BMI baseline (kg/m^2)	21.7 (4.7)	20.2 (3.1)**	21.1 (4.1)
Diabetics (%)	1.5%	1.7%	1.6%
Rural dwellers (%)	46.3%	51.5%	48.3%
SBP mean baseline (mmHg)	125.2 (27.1)	125.9 (24.1)	125.4 (26.0)
DBP mean baseline (mmHg)	73.6 (13.5)	75.6 (13.5)*	74.4 (13.4)
Pulse pressure baseline (mmHg)	51.6 (17.5)	50.2 (14.7)	51.1 (16.5)
Serum Haemoglobin (g/dl)	11.7 (1.4)	13.1 (1.9)**	12.2 (1.7)
Serum creatinine (μmol/L)	73 (13)	90 (18)**	79 (17)
Mean 24 hour urinary volume (Litres/day)	1.2 (0.5)	1.1 (0.5)	1.1 (0.5)
Mean 24 hour urinary sodium excretion (mmol/day)	103 (45)	100 (45)	102 (45)
Mean 24 hour urinary potassium excretion (mmol/day)	48 (22)	51 (26)*	49 (23)
Urinary Sodium:potassium ratio (mmol/mmol)	2.4 (1.2)	2.2 (1.2)	2.3 (1.2)
24 hour mean creatinine clearance (ml/min/1.73 m^2)	85 (23)	82 (22)	84 (23)

Mean and (SD) are given for all normally distributed variables.
†: Median and (IQR) for skewed variables (NS).
*for $p < 0.05$.
**for $p < 0.005$.

TABLE 2: Pulse pressure and age relationships in females and males according to age.

	β	95% Confidence interval	P value
Age < 55 years			
Female	0.8	(0.4-1.0)	<0.001
Male	0.5	(0.1-0.8)	0.008
Age > 55 years			
Female	0.44	(0.1-0.7)	0.007
Male	0.36	(-0.5-0.7)	0.84

men and 28% of women diagnosed with hypertension in this study. The prevalence of hypertension was high despite half of the studied population were rural dwellers with a lean body mass. However, only about 8% of men and 4% of women were on any pharmacological treatment for hypertension. PP was higher in the semiurban population than in the rural village dwellers (Table 1). The rural population also had a lower BMI compared to the semiurban population.

3.2. Blood Pressure, Age, and Gender. SBP increased with age by 0.70 [95% CI (0.51 to 0.80); $p < 0.001$] mmHg/year in the overall population. PP also increased with age [0.55 (0.46 to 0.64, $p < 0.001$) mmHg/year]. DBP did not increase significantly with age particularly in subjects 55 years or older [-0.11 to -0.28 to 0.07) mmHg/year; $p = 0.236$]. The increase in blood pressure was seen in both men and women. However, a steeper rise of SBP and PP was noted in women than men at an older age (Figures 2 and 3 and Table 2). The women had a higher mean BMI than men.

3.3. Blood Pressure, Age, Gender, and Kidney Function. Creatinine clearance showed a strong inverse correlation with age; it also correlated inversely with PP and directly with BMI (Figure 4). On univariate analysis, creatinine clearance decreased with increasing PP [$\beta = -0.18$ (95% CI: -0.27 to -0.10) ml/min/1.73 m^2/mmHg, $p < 0.001$] and SBP [$\beta = -0.08$(-0.14 to -0.03) ml/min/1.73 m^2/mmHg, $p = 0.002$], but there was no significant association between creatinine clearance and DBP [$\beta = -0.04$ (-0.14 to 0.06) ml/min/1.73 m^2/mmHg, $p = 0.43$] (Table 3). Creatinine clearance showed a slightly stronger inverse correlation with age in women ($\beta = -0.399$, $p < 0.0001$), compared to men ($\beta = -0.29$, $p < 0.0001$).

Using multivariate analysis, after adjusting for SBP the relationship between creatinine clearance and PP became stronger [-0.25 (-0.53 to -0.14) ml/min/1.73 m^2/mmHg, $p = 0.001$]. In contrast, although creatinine clearance increased with an increase in SBP, the relationship no longer held after adjusting for PP [0.14 (-0.004 to 0.24) ml/min/1.73 m^2/mmHg, $p = 0.06$].

There was no significant difference in creatinine clearance between men and women. [83 ± 21 v 85 ± 23 ml/min/1.73 m^2, $p = 0.16$]. On multivariate regression analysis with creatinine clearance as dependent variable, and age, sex, pulse pressure, BMI and presence of diabetes as independent variables, only age [$\beta = -0.75$ (-0.88 to -0.62), $p < 0.001$] and BMI [$\beta = 0.49$ (0.16 to 0.81), $p = 0.003$] were independent predictors of creatinine clearance.

TABLE 3: Relationship of different blood pressures with kidney function (creatinine clearance).

	β	95% Confidence interval	p value
Univariate analysis			
PP	-0.18	(-0.27 to -0.10)	<0.001
SBP	-0.08	(-0.14 to -0.03)	0.002
DBP	-0.04	(-0.14 to 0.06)	0.43
Bivariate analysis			
PP	-0.31	(-0.50 to -0.12)	<0.001
SBP	0.09	(-0.03 to 0.21)	0.143
PP	-0.22	(-0.32 to -0.12)	<0.001
DBP	0.09	(-0.03 to 0.21)	0.143
SBP	-0.22	(-0.32 to -0.12)	<0.001
DBP	0.31	(0.12 to 0.50)	<0.001

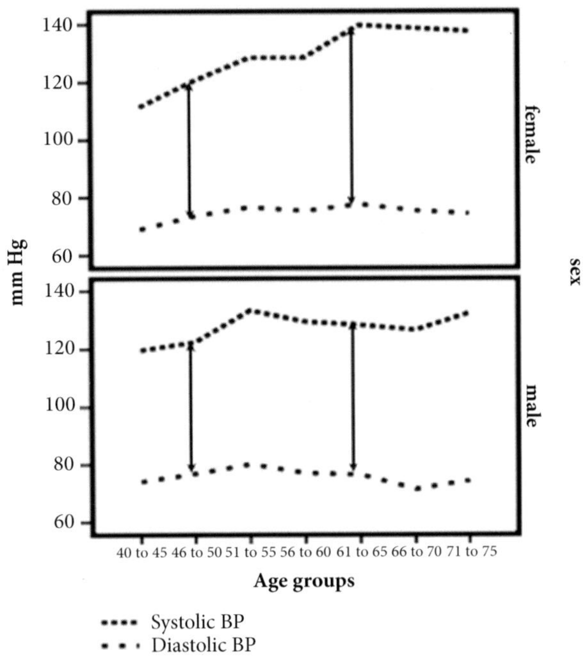

FIGURE 2: The effect of age on systolic and diastolic blood pressure in both genders. The top panel shows the changes in systolic (small dots) and diastolic (large dots) blood pressure variation with different age groups in females; the bottom panel shows the systolic and diastolic blood pressure variation with age in males.

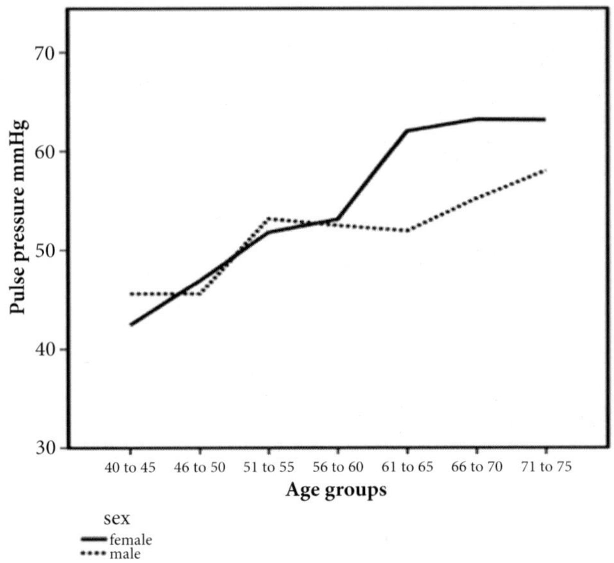

FIGURE 3: Changes of pulse pressure with age in males and females. The bold line shows the change in pulse pressure with different age groups in females; the dotted line shows the change pulse pressure with age in males.

4. Discussion

This is the first study investigating the effects of age, gender, and demographic factors on blood pressure components, along with the effect of blood pressure on kidney function in a rural African population.

Our study shows that hypertension is common in Ghana. We have shown an increase in SBP and PP with age, in both men and women. Both SBP and PP rose with age, the rise being more marked in the women that in the men. Both SBP and PP were higher in the semiurban than in the rural population.

The increase in PP with age is well known, and has been ascribed to increasing central arterial stiffness. The trajectory of rise in PP with age may be gender related and is steeper in women than in men [15]. We have also seen a steeper rise of PP with age in women compared to men in our population, and believe that the higher BMI in women may be a possible explanation.

There is evidence that the higher PP in semiurban populations may be as a consequence of altered dietary habits and sedentary lifestyle leading to an increase in body weight [16]. In our population the higher PP and SBP in the semiurban population may also be explained by the higher BMI in these individuals. Interestingly, this trend of increasing blood pressure with urbanisation was not seen in a study from Tanzania [17].

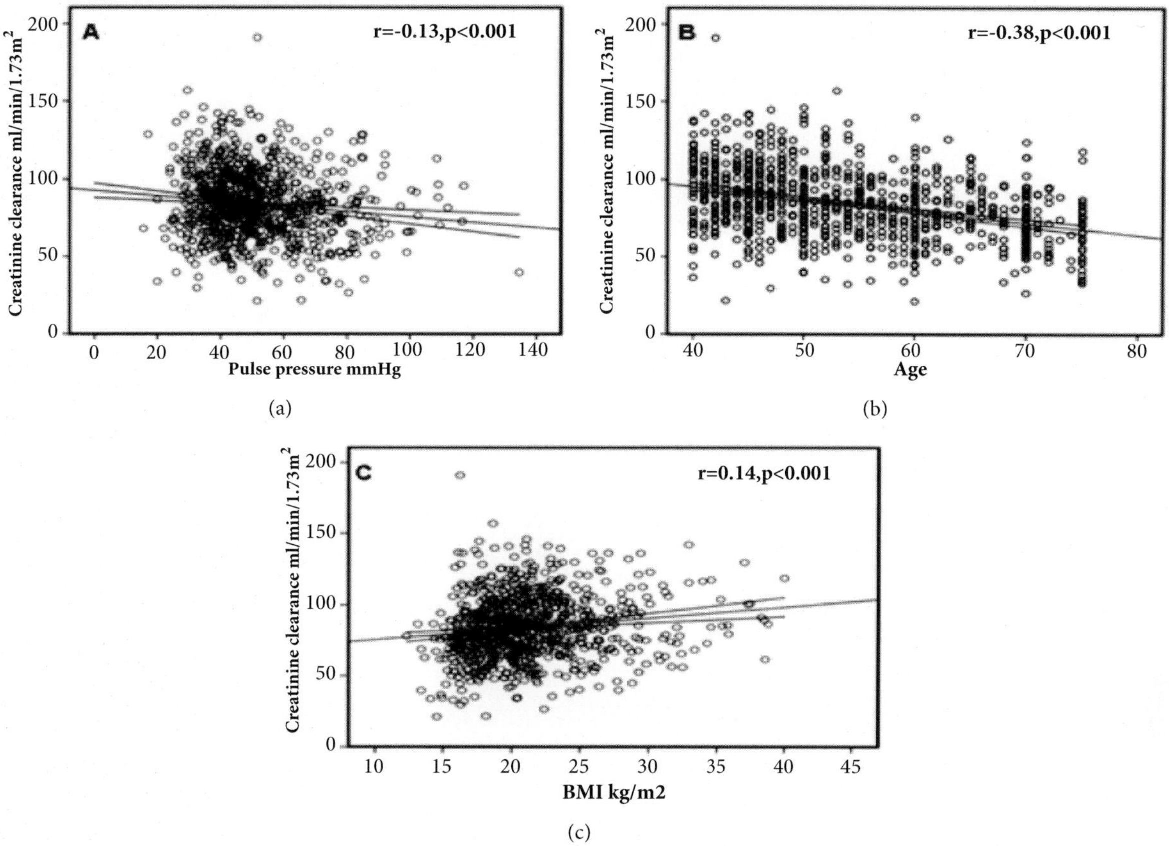

FIGURE 4: Associations of kidney function with pulse pressure, age, and body mass index. (a) demonstrates relationship between pulse pressure and creatinine clearance, (b) demonstrates relationship between age and creatinine clearance, and (c) demonstrates relationship between body mass index and creatinine clearance. The correlation coefficient and p values are shown with individual panels.

PP is a better predictor of CVD than SBP and DBP among middle age Caucasian populations [18, 19]. In our previous studies, in a predominantly Caucasian population, PP was shown to be a good predictor of early chronic kidney disease (CKD) progression, and onset of dialysis, and death in predialysis CKD patients [2, 10]. The study aimed at identifying if pulse pressure is a good marker at predicting CKD, measured with 24 hour urinary creatinine clearance, in West-African rural and semiurban population. Unfortunately none of the accepted gold standard glomerular filtration rate (GFR) measurements were available to us during screening, and as demonstrated in our previous report, none of the current estimated GFR equations accurately predicted the GFR in this population based on 24-hour urinary creatinine clearance adjusted for body surface area. Hence this study measured renal function by the mean of two 24-hour creatinine clearance values.

In summary our study was directed to assessing the role of PP in predicting GFR. PP preformed slightly better than SBP, and both were highly correlated with GFR, unlike DBP, which showed no significant relationship. However, we have found age to be a significant confounder while assessing the impact of blood pressure parameters on GFR. The relationship of pulse pressure with decreasing kidney function was stronger than that with systolic blood pressure. Diastolic blood pressure had no relationship with kidney function.

5. Conclusion

This is the first population study showing gender and demographic differences in blood pressure parameters in a homogeneous West-African population from central Ghana. Sub-Saharan Africans have a higher PP when compared to Caucasians of similar age. We have also demonstrated that PP, a measure of arterial compliance, has a better relationship with declining renal function than measurement of either systolic or diastolic blood pressure. This study does provide support for the notion that in the prevention of cardiovascular disease (including stroke and chronic kidney disease) blood pressure reduction is a vital component of public health policy in Sub-Saharan Africa.

Data Availability

The data used to support the findings of this study are available from the corresponding author upon request.

Disclosure

The data from this study was presented as an abstract in the 12th Congress of African Association of Nephrology, February 2013.

Acknowledgments

The study was supported by grants 060415/Z/00/Z and 069500/Z/02/Z from The Wellcome Trust.

References

[1] M. J. Klag, P. K. Whelton, B. L. Randall et al., "Blood pressure and end-stage renal disease in men," *The New England Journal of Medicine*, vol. 334, no. 1, pp. 13–18, 1996.

[2] D. Banerjee, S. Brincat, H. Gregson et al., "Pulse pressure and inhibition of renin-angiotensin system in chronic kidney disease," *Nephrology Dialysis Transplantation* , vol. 21, no. 4, pp. 975–978, 2006.

[3] M. Tozawa, K. Iseki, C. Iseki, K. Kinjo, Y. Ikemiya, and S. Takishita, "Blood pressure predicts risk of developing end-stage renal disease in men and women," *Hypertension*, vol. 41, no. 6, pp. 1341–1345, 2003.

[4] B. M. Psaty, C. D. Furberg, L. H. Kuller et al., "Isolated Systolic Hypertension and Subclinical Cardiovascular Disease in the Elderly: Initial Findings From the Cardiovascular Health Study," *Journal of the American Medical Association*, vol. 268, no. 10, pp. 1287–1291, 1992.

[5] R. Antikainen, P. Jousilahti, and J. Tuomilehto, "Systolic blood pressure, isolated systolic hypertension and risk of coronary heart disease, strokes, cardiovascular disease and all-cause mortality in the middle-aged population," *Journal of Hypertension* vol. 16, no. 5, pp. 577–583, 1998.

[6] R. C. Grebla, C. J. Rodriguez, L. N. Borrell, and T. G. Pickering, "Prevalence and determinants of isolated systolic hypertension among young adults: the 1999–2004 US National Health and Nutrition Examination Survey," *Journal of Hypertension*, vol. 28, no. 1, pp. 15–23, 2010.

[7] Y.-T. Kao, C.-C. Huang, H.-B. Leu et al., "Ambulatory pulse pressure as a novel predictor for long-term prognosis in essential hypertensive patients," *Journal of Human Hypertension*, vol. 25, no. 7, pp. 444–450, 2011.

[8] D. Banerjee, A. J. Collins, and C. A. Herzog, "Effect of Inflammation on the Relationship of Pulse Pressure and Mortality in Haemodialysis," *Nephron Extra*, vol. 1, no. 1, pp. 292–299, 2011.

[9] P. S. Klassen, E. G. Lowrie, D. N. Reddan et al., "Association Between Pulse Pressure and Mortality in Patients Undergoing Maintenance Hemodialysis," *Journal of the American Medical Association*, vol. 287, no. 12, pp. 1548–1555, 2002.

[10] N. Arulkumaran, R. Diwakar, Z. Tahir, M. Mohamed, J. C. Kaski, and D. Banerjee, "Pulse pressure and progression of chronic kidney disease," *Journal of Nephrology*, vol. 23, no. 2, pp. 189–193, 2010.

[11] J. B. Eastwood, S. M. Kerry, J. Plange-Rhule et al., "Assessment of GFR by four methods in adults in Ashanti, Ghana: the need for an eGFR equation for lean African populations," *Nephrology Dialysis Transplantation* , vol. 25, no. 7, pp. 2178–2187, 2010.

[12] F. P. Cappuccio, F. B. Micah, L. Emmett et al., "Prevalence, detection, management, and control of hypertension in Ashanti, West Africa," *Hypertension*, vol. 43, no. 5, pp. 1017–1022, 2004.

[13] J. Plange-Rhule, F. P. Cappuccio, L. Emmett et al., "A community study of health promotion in rural West Africa: Details of a household survey and population census," *QJM: Monthly Journal of the Association of Physicians*, vol. 95, no. 7, pp. 445–450, 2002.

[14] S. M. Kerry, F. P. Cappuccio, L. Emmett, J. Plange-Rhule, and J. B. Eastwood, "Reducing selection bias in a cluster randomized trial in West African villages," *Clinical Trials*, vol. 2, no. 2, pp. 125–129, 2005.

[15] J. H. Skurnick, M. Aladjem, and A. Aviv, "Sex differences in pulse pressure trends with age are cross-cultural," *Hypertension*, vol. 55, no. 1, pp. 40–47, 2010.

[16] S. Ebrahim, S. Kinra, L. Bowen et al., "The effect of rural-to-urban migration on obesity and diabetes in india: a cross-sectional study," *PLoS Medicine*, vol. 7, no. 4, Article ID e1000268, 2010.

[17] N. Unwin, P. James, D. McLarty et al., "Rural to urban migration and changes in cardiovascular risk factors in Tanzania: A prospective cohort study," *BMC Public Health*, vol. 10, article no. 272, 2010.

[18] A. Benetos, M. Safar, A. Rudnichi et al., "Pulse pressure: a predictor of long-term cardiovascular mortality in a french male population," *Hypertension*, vol. 30, no. 6, pp. 1410–1415, 1997.

[19] S. S. Franklin, S. A. Khan, N. D. Wong, M. G. Larson, and D. Levy, "Is pulse pressure useful in predicting risk for coronary heart disease? The Framingham Heart Study," *Circulation*, vol. 100, no. 4, pp. 354–360, 1999.

19

Herbal and Alternative Medicine Use in Tanzanian Adults Admitted with Hypertension-Related Diseases: A Mixed-Methods Study

Anthony Liwa,[1] Rebecca Roediger,[2] Hyasinta Jaka,[3] Amina Bougaila,[4] Luke Smart,[3,5] Stacey Langwick,[6] and Robert Peck[3,5]

[1]*Department of Clinical Pharmacology, Weill Bugando School of Medicine, Catholic University of Health and Allied Sciences, P.O. Box 1464, Mwanza, Tanzania*
[2]*Department of Internal Medicine, Mount Sinai Hospital, 17 East 102nd St, 7th Floor, New York, NY 10029, USA*
[3]*Department of Internal Medicine, Weill Bugando School of Medicine, Catholic University of Health and Allied Sciences, P.O. Box 1464, Mwanza, Tanzania*
[4]*Weill Cornell Medical College in Qatar, Doha, Qatar*
[5]*Center for Global Health, Department of Medicine, Weill Cornell Medical College, New York, NY, USA*
[6]*Department of Anthropology, Cornell University, 261 McGraw Hall, Ithaca, NY, USA*

Correspondence should be addressed to Anthony Liwa; tonyliwa@gmail.com and Robert Peck; rnp2002@gmail.com

Academic Editor: Markus P. Schlaich

Background. Hypertension is increasingly common in sub-Saharan Africa where traditional medicine use is also common. We conducted a hospital-based, mixed-methods study to determine prevalence, pattern, and correlates of herbal and alternative medicine use in Tanzanian adults hospitalized with hypertension. *Methods.* A standardized questionnaire was administered. In-depth interviews were performed on a subset of participants. Factors associated with herbal medicine use were determined by logistic regression. The association between traditional medicine uses and allopathic medication adherence was determined using ordinal logistic regression. Qualitative data were analyzed according to grounded theory. *Results.* Of 213 adults enrolled, 52 (24.4%) reported using herbs during the previous month and 47 (22.1%) reported concurrent use of herbs and allopathic medicines. Lower educational level, nonprofessional employment, and lack of health insurance were significantly associated with herbal medicine use. Alternative medicines use was not associated with lower medication adherence. Qualitative interviews identified several important themes including reasons for herbal medicine use. *Conclusion.* The use of traditional medicines is very common among patients with hypertension. Adults from low socioeconomic status, those with misunderstandings about hypertension, and those without health insurance were more likely to take herbs. Open, nonjudgmental communication between healthcare workers and patients regarding use of traditional medicines must be encouraged in Africa.

1. Background

The burden of hypertension is increasing in sub-Saharan Africa (SSA) [1], with an age-standardized prevalence of ~40% in adults over 25 years of age [2]. Of adults with hypertension in Tanzania, only ~35% are aware of their diagnosis, ~5% are on treatment, and ~1% are controlled [3]. At our own hospital in Tanzania, hypertension is the second most common diagnosis on the medical wards accounting for >15% of all admissions, hospital days, and deaths [4].

WHO has defined "traditional medicine" as sum total of the knowledge, skills, and practices based on the theories, beliefs, and experiences indigenous to different cultures, whether explicable or not, used in the maintenance of health, as well as in the prevention, diagnosis, improvement, or treatment of illnesses. "Herbal medicines," on the other hand, in a more specific term include herbs, herbal materials, herbal preparations, and finished herbal products that contain active ingredients parts of plants. In the current study we used terms "herbal" to describe traditional medicine that is derived from plants and "alternative medicine" to describe other traditional medicines.

Traditional medicine use in hypertension and its related diseases can lead to adverse outcome, related to delay in seeking proper treatment, leading to increased severity or complications of the disease, drug interactions, and poor adherence to allopathic medicines that are known to control the disease [5]. Although traditional medicine use is common in sub-Saharan Africa (SSA) [5–9], little is known about its overlap with hypertension. In our own, recent meta-analysis, we found only 4 published studies reporting data regarding herbal and alternative medicine use in adults with hypertension in Africa. These 4 studies indicated that 25–65% of adults with hypertension reported use of herbal and alternative medicines [10].

To the best of our knowledge, no published data exists regarding the pattern of herbal and alternative medicine use among adult inpatients or the association between herbal and alternative medicine use and antihypertensive medications adherence. Specifically, it determined (1) the prevalence and pattern of herbal and alternative medicine utilization, (2) factors associated with herbal medicine use, and (3) whether herbal or alternative medicine use was associated with medication nonadherence. We hypothesized that herbal and other alternative medicine use is common among Tanzanians hospitalized with hypertension-related diseases and is associated with nonadherence to allopathic medicines.

2. Methods

2.1. Study Setting. This study was conducted in the adult medical wards of Bugando Medical Centre (BMC). BMC is a tertiary and teaching hospital that serves the Lake region in the northwestern part of mainland Tanzania.

2.2. Study Design and Recruitment of Participants. To provide better understanding of the problem of herbal and other alternative medicines use, the current study was conducted prospectively by a hospital-based mixed quantitative and qualitative research design and was conducted concurrently between April and October 2014. The subjects for this study were selected from patients hospitalized at the medical wards of BMC. All adults (>18 years of age) admitted with hypertension-related diagnoses were approached within 24 hours of admission and invited to participate in our study.

Blood pressure measurement was done at least twice (once on each arm) after 5 minutes of sitting using a mercury sphygmomanometer. If either or both first 2 blood pressure measurements are elevated, a 3rd blood pressure measurement was taken and the average of the 2nd and 3rd measurements was considered for the diagnosis of hypertension.

Diagnoses of hypertensive diseases, that is, hypertensive stroke, hypertensive heart failure, or hypertensive renal failure, were made per WHO International Statistical Classification of Diseases and Related Health Problems 10th Revision (ICD-10) version for 2010. Adults with altered mental status were excluded since they could not provide adequate or reliable information.

2.3. Data Collection and Analysis. A structured researcher-administered questionnaire with both closed ended and open-ended questions was used to collect quantitative data from eligible patients. The questionnaire consisted of sections that assessed patient information such as age, gender, marital status, education level, and duration of disease. Responses on patients' knowledge about hypertension, use of herbal and other alternative medicines, reasons for herbs use, sources of herbs, and adherence to antihypertensive medications were obtained.

Adherence to antihypertensive medications was measured using a Morisky Medication Adherence Scale, the 4-item scale (MMAS-4). MMAS-4 is a self-reported commonly used adherence-screening tool. It is composed of 4 yes/no questions about past medication use patterns and is validated in antihypertensive patients in several countries [11, 12].

Data were coded and entered into Microsoft Excel 2010 software (Microsoft Corporation, Redmond, WA, USA) and analyzed using STATA version 12 (StataCorp, Collage Station, Texas). Categorical variables were described as proportions (percentiles) and continuous variables were described as medians [interquartile ranges]. Differences between patient groups were calculated along with 95% confidence intervals (CI). To examine potential factors associated with the current use of herbal and alternative medicines, univariate and multivariate logistic regression were conducted. Factors associated with adherence to allopathic antihypertensive medications were explored using ordinal logistic regression. The Brant test was used to assess the proportional odds assumption. A two-sided p value < 0.05 was considered significant. Since this was an exploratory analysis, we did not make any adjustment for multiple comparisons.

12 study subjects who used herbal or other alternative medicines were selectively chosen and underwent in-person, semi-structured interviews. The primary investigator conducted these interviews in a private space on the medical wards and they were ~20 minutes long. Interviews were conducted in Kiswahili, recorded, transcribed, and then translated into English by a professional translation service.

The analysis process had two levels. We started collecting qualitative data through open-ended questions. As we reviewed the data collected, repeated ideas, concepts, or elements become apparent and were eventually tagged with inductive and deductive *codes*, which were extracted from the data. The second level involved collection of data, and as data were rereviewed, codes were grouped into themes and then into categories. These categories were the basis for new theory. Two independent researchers (AL and RP) identified themes and supporting quotations were selected.

In-depth interviews were performed on 12 adults admitted with hypertension. After breaking data into conceptual components, these concepts were theorized, integrated, and refined, and four themes/theories emerged: (i) lack of understanding about hypertension, (ii) the exact identity of herbal remedies being often unknown, (iii) contradictory opinions on risks of concurrent use of allopathic and herbal medications, and (iv) 3 common reasons for herbal medicine use.

2.4. Ethical Approval. Ethical approval for the study was obtained from the Bugando Research Ethics Committee in Tanzania and the Institutional Review Board of Weill Cornell Medical College. Each participating patient provided written informed consent. Consent to participate in this study did not affect the clinical care of the patients.

3. Results

3.1. Enrollment. Between April 1 and October 1, 377 adults were hospitalized to the medical wards of Bugando Medical Centre with hypertension-related diseases. Of these, 164 were excluded for the following reasons: 147 were unable to give a reliable history due to altered mental status (mostly due to stroke or hypertensive encephalopathy), 9 declined to participate in the study, and 8 were discharged within 24 hours (before enrollment could occur). The remaining 213 adults consented and were enrolled.

3.2. Demographic Characteristics. Among the 213 adult inpatients enrolled in our study, 112/213 (52.6%) were female, the median age was 56 years [45–67], and only 34/213 (16.0%) had completed secondary school education. Most study subjects (162/213 (76.1%)) were aware of their hypertension before admission but 51/213 (23.9%) were newly diagnosed to have hypertension during the current hospital admission. Most (159/213 (74.7%)) had a previous history of using antihypertensive medications but only 103/213 (48.4%) was taking medications before hospitalization. Of the 159 study subjects who reported prior use of antihypertensive medications, 35/159 (22.0%) reported high adherence, 38/159 (23.9%) reported medium adherence, and 86/159 (54.1%) reported low adherence to antihypertensive medications. The average years of patient illness were 5 years [2–5, 10–14]. Most (173/213 (81.2%)) had at least 1 comorbid condition: 54/173 (24.5%) had heart failure, 39/173 (18.4%) had diabetes mellitus, 24/173 (11.3%) had kidney disease, and 20/173 (9.4%) reported a history of stroke. The characteristics of the study population are presented in Table 1.

3.3. Outcomes. Of the 213 Tanzanian adults in patients with hypertension that participated in the study, 161/213 (75.6%) reported using herbal and alternative medicines at some point in their life. 69/213 (32.4%) used herbal and alternative medicines specifically to manage hypertension at some point in their life and 52/213 (24.4%) used herbal and alternative medicines in the past month before admission to the hospital. 38/213 (17.8%) of the respondents admitted to having stopped allopathic medications for herbal and alternative medicines and 47/213 (22.1%) reported to the concurrent use of herbal and alternative medicines and allopathic medications. Only 20/213 (9.4%) reported having been asked about traditional medicine use by their admitting doctor. Herbal and other alternative medicines use did not differ significantly by gender. The other outcomes related to the utilization of

TABLE 1: Sociodemographic and clinical characteristics of 213 consecutive adults hospitalized at Bugando Medical Centre with hypertension-related diseases.

Variable Proportion (%) Median [IQR]	Value (n = 213)
Female gender	112 (52.6)
Age (years)	56 [45–67]
Education level	
Not completed primary school	58 (27.2)
Completed primary school	121 (56.8)
Completed secondary school	34 (16.0)
Occupation	
Farmer	78 (36.6)
Small scale business	54 (25.4)
Professional, business, or student	81 (38.0)
Health insurance	70 (32.9)
Hypertension diagnosis	
New diagnosis	51 (23.9)
Previously diagnosed	162 (76.1)
Medication adherence (MMAS-4 score)*	
High (0)	35 (22.0)
Medium (1-2)	38 (23.9)
Low (3-4)	86 (54.1)
Systolic blood pressure	160 [150–180]
Diastolic blood pressure	100 [90–120]
Is hypertension curable (or is it a lifelong condition)?	
No (hypertension is a lifelong condition)	95 (44.6)
Yes (hypertension is curable)	118 (55.4)
Is there anything that can be done to prevent hypertension?	
Yes	54 (25.4)
No	159 (74.7)
Years since hypertension diagnosis	5 [2–10]
Place of diagnosis	
Hospital	194 (91.1)
Other	19 (8.9)
History of hypertensive medication	159 (74.7)
Currently on hypertensive medication	103 (48.4)
Prevalence of comorbid conditions	173 (81.2)
Heart failure	54 (24.5)
Diabetes mellitus	39 (18.4)
Kidney disease	24 (11.3)
Stroke	20 (9.4)

*MMAS-4, Morisky Medication Adherence Scale, the 4-item scale; IQR, interquartile range.

Table 2: Herbal medicine utilization patterns in 213 consecutive adults hospitalized to Bugando Medical Centre with hypertension-related diseases.

Outcome Proportion (%) Median [IQR]	Total ($n = 213$)	Female ($n = 112$)	Male ($n = 101$)	p value
Used herbal medicine in last month*	52 (24.4)	26 (23.2)	26 (25.7)	0.67
Ever attended a traditional healer for any reason	144 (67.6)	77 (68.8)	67 (66.3)	0.71
Ever attended traditional healer for hypertension	59 (27.7)	29 (25.9)	30 (29.7)	0.54
Ever used herbal medicine for any reason	161 (75.6)	35 (31.3)	74 (73.3)	0.46
Ever used herbs for hypertension	69 (32.4)	38 (33.9)	31 (30.7)	0.61
Practiced religious healing for hypertension	30 (14.1)	17 (15.2)	13 (12.9)	0.63
Using herbal medicine in hospital	10 (4.7)	5 (5.0)	5 (4.5)	0.87
Stopped allopathic medicines for herbal medicine	38 (17.8)	17 (15.2)	21 (20.8)	0.29
Used herbal medicine with allopathic medicines	47 (22.1)	28 (25.0)	19 (18.8)	0.28
Believes it is okay to use herbal medicine with allopathic medicines	152 (71.4)	76 (67.9)	76 (75.3)	0.24
Traditional healer has asked about allopathic medicines	20 (9.4)	8 (7.1)	12 (11.9)	0.24
Doctors have asked about herbal medicines	20 (9.4)	11 (9.8)	9 (8.9)	0.82

*Primary study outcome; IQR, interquartile range.

herbal and alternative medicine are presented in detail in Table 2.

3.4. Factors Associated with Herbal Medicine Use. Table 3 displays the results of our logistic regression analysis to determine factors associated with herbal medicine use for hypertension in the past month before admission. Patients with higher categories of education (secondary education to college education) were less likely to consume herbal medicine compared to their counterparts ($p < 0.007$; OR = 0.49; CI 0.29–0.82). Professionals (salaried workers), businessmen (business owners), and government employees were also less likely to consume herbal medicine compared to farmers ($p = 0.002$; OR = 0.27; CI 0.11–0.61). Study subjects with medical insurance were also less likely to use herbal medicines ($p = 0.001$; OR = 0.24; CI 0.10–0.57). Stroke was the only comorbid condition that was significantly associated with herbal medicine use ($p = 0.008$; OR = 3.60; CI 1.40–9.21).

3.5. Factors Associated with Allopathic Medication Adherence. Table 4 displays our ordinal logistic regression analysis of factors associated with poor medication adherence. Higher education level (secondary school and above) was associated with better medication adherence ($p = 0.04$; OR = 0.63; CI 0.40–0.99 for lower adherence). Study subjects who believed that hypertension could not be cured with a short course of traditional or allopathic medicines also had better medication adherence ($p = 0.001$; OR = 0.34; CI 0.18–0.63 for low adherence). In addition, study subjects who were diagnosed with hypertension in places other than a health facility were less likely to be adherent to the antihypertensive medications ($p = 0.02$; OR = 3.80; CI 1.21–11.85). Of note, neither herbal and alternative medicine use nor attendance to traditional healers was significantly associated with nonadherence. In fact, none of the variables for herbal and alternative medicine utilization were significantly associated with nonadherence.

3.6. Herbal Remedies and Other Alternative Therapies. Among the 161 patients who reported to use herbal and alternative medicine, 134/161 (83.2%) did not know the names of the herbs that they were consuming. Of the 27/161 (16.8%) patients who knew the names of the herbs that they were taking, 21/161 (13.0%) patients mentioned taking more than one herbal preparation. The most frequent remedies that were mentioned include *garlic* (11), *ginger* (3) *honey* (2), *carrots (2), avocado seeds* (2), *bit roots* (1), *wood charcoal* (1), *papaya seeds* (1), *lemons* (1), *onions* (1), and *aloe vera* (1). Other patients mentioned plant derived remedies known by tribal names including Mronge seeds *(Moringa oleifera)* (2), Kuwarumbizo (Ikizu tribe) (1), Engeni tree (1), and Nyabururu (Sukuma tribal name) (1). Four (4) study subjects reported using "Chinese medicines" but were not able to give specific names. Some patients also mentioned commercially available remedies/products including "Herbal Works" (1) and "Forever Living" health products (1).

3.7. Reasons for Herbal Medicine Use. The 69 study subjects who had used herbal medicines specifically for the treatment of hypertension were asked to provide reasons for herbal medicine use: 22/69 (31.9%) reported using herbal medicines because they still believed in traditional ways of treatment and customs of healthcare; 12/69 (17.4%) were convinced by friends or people who have claimed to have been cured by herbs; 11/69 (15.9%) were looking for other options for treatment; 7/69 (10.2%) reported pressure from a spouse or family member; 5/69 (7.3%) reported that they did not want to go to hospital because of uncaring attitude of hospital staff; 3/69 (4.4%) patients used herbal medicines because they did not have funds to go to hospital; 3/69 (4.4%) patients wanted

TABLE 3: Characteristics and factors associated with the current use of herbal medicine in the month prior to hospital admission.

Variable Proportion (%) Median [IQR]	Herbal users ($n = 52$)	Herbal nonusers ($n = 161$)	Odds ratio [95% CI]	p value
Female gender	26 (23.2)	86 (76.8)	0.87 [0.47–1.63]	0.67
Age category (years)				
≤45	13 (21.7)	47 (78.3)	1	
46–55	12 (30.0)	28 (7.0)	1.55 [0.62–3.86]	
56–65	11 (20.1)	43 (79.6)	0.93 [0.37–2.28]	
>65	16 (27.1)	43 (72.9)	1.35 [0.58–3.12]	0.65
Education level				
Not completed primary school	21 (36.2)	37 (63.8)		
Completed primary school	27 (22.3)	94 (77.7)		
Completed secondary school	4 (11.8)	30 (88.2)	0.49 [0.29–0.82]	0.007
Occupation				
Farmer	25 (32.1)	53 (68.0)	1	
Small scale business	18 (33.3)	36 (66.7)	1.06 [0.51–2.21]	
Professional, business, or student	9 (11.1)	72 (88.9)	0.27 [0.11–0.61]	0.002
Health insurance				
No insurance	45 (31.5)	98 (68.5)	1	
Insurance	7 (10.0)	63 (90.0)	0.24 [0.10–0.57]	0.001
Hypertension diagnosis				
New diagnosis	13 (25.5)	38 (74.5)	1	
Previously diagnosed	39 (24.1)	123 (75.9)	0.93 [0.45–1.92]	0.84
Years of diagnosis				
≤1	16 (32.0)	34 (38.0)		
2–4	7 (16.7)	35 (83.3)	0.43 [0.16–1.16]	
5–9	8 (28.6)	20 (71.4)	0.85 [0.31–2.34]	
≥10	21 (24.4)	72 (77.4)	0.62 [0.29–1.34]	0.34
Systolic blood pressure				
≤140	8 (18.2)	36 (81.8)		
141–160	17 (27.9)	44 (72.1)	1.74 [0.67–4.50]	
161–180	16 (29.6)	38 (70.4)	1.89 [0.72–4.97]	
>180	11 (20.4)	43 (79.6)	1.15 [0.42–3.17]	0.45
Currently on hypertensive medication	38 (23.9)	121 (76.1)	1.53 [0.81–2.89]	0.77
Is hypertension curable (or is it a lifelong condition)?				
No (hypertension is a lifelong condition)	34 (28.8)	84 (71.2)		
Yes (hypertension is curable)	18 (19.0)	77 (81.1)	0.58 [0.30–1.11]	0.098
Is there anything that can be done to prevent hypertension?				
Yes	8 (14.8)	46 (85.2)		
No	44 (27.7)	115 (72.3)	0.46 [0.19–1.04]	0.06
Place of diagnosis				
Hospital	47 (24.2)	147 (75.8)		
Other	5 (26.3)	14 (73.7)	1.12 [0.38–3.27]	0.34
MMAS Question 1 (ever forget to take medicines)	5 (12.5)	35 (87.5)	0.42 [0.14–1.26]	0.12
MMAS Question 2 (have problems remembering to take medicines)	5 (14.3)	30 (85.7)	0.54 [0.18–1.63]	0.28
MMAS Question 3 (when feel better stops taking medicines)	12 (21.8)	43 (78.2)	1.21 [0.46–3.18]	0.70
MMAS Question 4 (stop taking medicines when feeling worse with medicines)	1 (11.1)	8 (88.9)	0.46 [0.55–3.92]	0.44

TABLE 3: Continued.

Variable Proportion (%) Median [IQR]	Herbal users ($n = 52$)	Herbal nonusers ($n = 161$)	Odds ratio [95% CI]	p value
Medication adherence (MMAS-4)[#] score				
High adherence (0)	8 (22.9)	27 (77.1)		
Medium adherence (1-2)	9 (23.7)	29 (76.3)		
Low adherence (3-4)	21 (24.4)	65 (75.6)	1.64 [0.66–1.64]	0.85
Prevalence of comorbid condition	44 (25.4)	129 (74.6)	1.36 [0.59–3.18]	0.47
Individual comorbid conditions				
Diabetes mellitus	9 (23.1)	30 (76.9)	0.9 [0.40–2.10]	0.82
Kidney disease	7 (29.2)	17 (70.8)	1.32 [0.51–3.38]	0.57
Stroke	10 (50)	10 (50)	3.60 [1.40–9.21]	0.008
Heart failure	10 (18.5)	44 (81.5)	0.63 [0.29–1.36]	0.24

[#] MMAS-4, Morisky Medication Adherence Scale, the 4-item scale; IQR, interquartile range; CI, confidence interval.

to lose weight; 2/69 (2.9%) patients were convinced by radio advertisement; 2/69 (2.9%) reported to have been bewitched to think traditional ways were the better option; 1/69 (1.5%) reported that he was previously cured of hypertension with herbs; and 1/69 (1.5%) was advised by a local healer who knew the herbs.

3.8. Qualitative Analysis. In-depth interviews and the following themes emerged: (i) lack of understanding about hypertension, (ii) the exact identity of herbal remedies being often unknown, (iii) contradictory opinions on risks of concurrent use of allopathic and herbal medications, and (iv) 3 common reasons for herbal medicine use.

3.8.1. Lack of Understanding about Hypertension. Participants in this study consistently expressed a limited understanding of hypertension and reported having received very little education about this condition:

> *I do not know what it is, except that they have tested me and they said I have high blood pressure. (Male, 42 years)*

3.8.2. Exact Identity of Herbal Remedies Being Often Unknown. There are many forms in which herbal medicines were prepared, the most common of which were extracts from plants which were either diluted or boiled to obtain its liquid form through steam. Whole herb consumption was also practiced either fresh or in dried form.

> *What I know it is a tree, but I do not know what kind of a tree... I found that the stuff has already been pounded... you just mix it with water and drink it... they put one, two or even five kinds of those trees. (Female, 48 years)*

3.8.3. Contradictory Opinions on Risks of Concurrent Use of Allopathic and Herbal Medications. Participants expressed differing opinions regarding whether it is acceptable to take both allopathic and herbal medications at the same time:

> *There is a problem... you cannot mix medications because if you mix you will not know what is making you feel better. (Male, 55 years)*

> *Yes you take them [herbs] as well except that you must know your time. (Male, 42 years)*

3.8.4. 3 Common Reasons for Herbal Medicines Use. Interest in herbal medicines was commonly attributed to 3 main reasons: (i) lack of funds to go to hospital, (ii) pressure from relatives and friends, and (iii) the desire for a complete cure:

> *Sometimes you do not have money.... now someone comes and say that I was helped by avocado seeds and you see it's free you prepare it to obtain good health. (Female, 50 years)*

> *If you are sick, the advice come from any human being... because you are sick, you do not have a choice... if someone come and tell you that I have been helped by this certain tree, you go and dig it up. (Female, 49 years)*

> *They said that they treat diseases that cannot be cured in hospitals by using traditional medicines. (Male, 65 years)*

4. Discussion

Herbal and other alternative medicines use is highly prevalent among Tanzanian adults admitted with hypertension-related conditions and many of those adults were using herbs specifically for hypertension. More than 75% of the adults in our study reported using herbal medicines in the past and nearly 70% had attended a traditional healer. Approximately 25% of adults were currently using herb specifically for management of hypertension. This study is the first to describe the pattern of herbal and alternative medicine in African inpatients. This pattern is broadly similar to findings from hypertension clinics in South and West Africa [6, 7, 13, 14], as well as

TABLE 4: Factors associated with medication nonadherence by ordered logistic regression in 213 consecutive adults hospitalized to Bugando Medical Centre with hypertension-related diseases.

Variable Proportion (%) Median [IQR]	High adherence (MMAS; 0) $n = 35$ (%)	Medium adherence (MMAS; 1-2) $n = 38$ (%)	Low adherence (MMAS; 3-4) $n = 86$ (%)	Odds ratio [95% CI]	p value
Female gender	23 (28.1)	16 (19.5)	43 (52.4)	0.74 [0.41–1.34]	0.31
Age category					
≤45	12 (33.3)	9 (25.0)	15 (41.7)		
46–55	4 (12.9)	10 (32.3)	17 (54.8)		
56–65	11 (25.0)	7 (15.9)	26 (59.1)		
>65	8 (16.7)	12 (25.0)	28 (58.3)	1.24 [0.95–1.62]	0.12
Education level					
Not completed primary school	5 (11.9)	9 (21.4)	28 (66.7)		
Completed primary school	25 (27.5)	18 (19.8)	48 (52.8)		
Completed secondary school	5 (19.2)	11 (42.3)	10 (38.5)	0.63 [0.40–0.99]	0.04
Occupation					
Farmer	14 (25.9)	9 (16.7)	31 (57.4)		
Small scale business	5 (14.3)	10 (28.6)	20 (57.1)		
Professional, business, or student	16 (22.9)	19 (27.1)	35 (50.0)	1.20 [0.53–2.74]	0.68
No insurance	21 (21.2)	22 (22.2)	56 (56.6)	0.80 [0.44–1.48]	0.47
Systolic blood pressure					
≤140	8 (20.5)	14 (35.9)	17 (43.6)		
141–160	9 (20.5)	7 (15.9)	28 (63.6)	1.78 [0.78–4.08]	
161–180	7 (20.0)	8 (22.9)	20 (57.1)	1.45 [0.62–3.42]	
>180	11 (26.8)	9 (22.0)	21 (51.2)	1.09 [0.48–2.45]	0.51
Is hypertension curable (or is it a lifelong condition)?					
No (hypertension is a lifelong condition)	23 (28.8)	25 (31.3)	32 (40.0)		
Yes (hypertension is curable)	12 (15.2)	13 (16.5)	54 (68.4)	0.34 [0.18–0.63]	0.001
Is there anything that can be done to prevent hypertension?					
Yes	6 (12.8)	15 (31.9)	26 (55.3)		
No	29 (25.9)	23 (20.5)	60 (53.6)	1.30 [0.68–2.49]	0.43
Years of diagnosis					
1	12 (24.0)	10 (20)	28 (56.0)		
≥2	8 (19.1)	12 (28.6)	22 (52.4)		
≥5	8 (28.6)	4 (14.3)	16 (57.1)		
≥10	7 (18.0)	12 (30.8)	20 (51.3)	0.99 [0.77–1.28]	0.93
Place of diagnosis					
Hospital	35 (24.8)	34 (24.1)	72 (51.1)		
Other	0	4 (22.2)	14 (77.8)	3.80 [1.21–11.85]	0.02
Ever used herbs for hypertension	14 (20.6)	19 (27.9)	35 (51.5)	0.92 [0.50–1.67]	0.77
Ever used herbs for any reason	24 (20.7)	33 (28.5)	59 (50.9)	1.32 [0.72–2.67]	0.44
Ever attended traditional healer	24 (22.6)	28 (26.4)	54 (50.9)	1.36 [0.72–2.60]	0.35
Stopped allopathic medications for herbal medicine	7 (20.6)	6 (17.7)	21 (61.8)	0.72 [0.34–1.54]	0.40
Concurrent use of allopathic medications and herbal medicine	8 (21.1)	8 (21.1)	22 (57.9)	0.85 [0.42–1.72]	0.64
Believes it is okay to use herbal medicines with allopathic medicines	26 (2.6)	27 (23.5)	62 (53.9)	1.06 [0.54–2.05]	0.87
Prevalence of comorbid conditions	30 (22.2)	34 (25.2)	71 (52.6)	−0.33 [−1.20–0.55]	0.46
Individual comorbid conditions					
Diabetes mellitus	5 (15.2)	13 (39.4)	15 (45.5)	−0.14 [−0.4–0.56]	0.67
Kidney disease	6 (33.3)	1 (5.6)	11 (61.1)	0.01 [−0.1–1.02]	0.98
Stroke	2 (10.5)	5 (26.3)	12 (63.16)	0.52 [−0.43–0.47]	0.29
Heart failure	10 (21.3)	10 (21.3)	27 (57.5)	0.17 [−0.49–0.83]	0.61

MMAS-4 refers to Morisky Medication Adherence Scale, the 4-item scale; IQR, interquartile range; CI, confidence interval.

community-based studies in Eastern and Western African countries [8, 9]. In all of these settings, approximately one-quarter of African adults with hypertension reported the use of traditional medicines and most of these were using herbal medicines. Because herbal medicines in particular are such an important part of hypertension self-management throughout Africa, collaboration with traditional healers should be explored as a possible route for improving hypertension care [9].

In the current study, nearly 20% of adults reported stopping their allopathic medicines for herbal medicine and >20% were concurrently using both herbal and allopathic medications. More than 70% of patients believed that there is no problem to use herb together with allopathic medications. These findings are concerning. Although some of the herbs used by our study subjects are likely harmless, most patients did not know what they were taking, and concurrent use of some herbs could hamper the effectiveness of allopathic antihypertensive drugs such as the interaction between St. John's Wart and calcium channel blockers or the interaction between garlic and thiazide diuretics [15, 16]. Interactions between herbs and cardiovascular drugs could also increase the toxicological effects of cardiovascular drugs such as the interaction between garlic and warfarin or the interaction between *Ginseng* and Digoxin [5, 17, 18]. Sodium-sparing herbal aquaretics such as dandelions, for example, may offset antihypertensive effects of thiazide diuretics [16]. The use of *ginseng* with digoxin is associated with increased digoxin concentration in the blood and hence digoxin toxicity [19]. African adults with hypertension who are using herbs clearly require counseling not to stop their allopathic medicines for herbs as well as counseling as to possible interactions between the herbs they are using and their cardiovascular medications.

Factors that were significantly associated with the use of herbal medicines for hypertension included lower education level, nonprofessional occupation, lack of medical insurance, and history of comorbid stroke. The lower education level was also found to be associated with the use of herbal medicines in Nigeria [14]. Occupation has also been shown to be associated with herbal medicine use in another study from West Africa [9]. It is possible, though, that individuals of higher education level and occupation status are simply less willing to report herbal medicine use and this deserves further investigation. Inability to afford allopathic medicines was associated with herbal medicine use in Ghana [6]. The association between herbal medicine use and stroke may be related to the cultural perception in Tanzania that stroke may have an extra-biological (i.e., "magical") origin, a perception that has been associated with herbal medicine use in other studies [9]. These data indicate populations for whom more intensive counseling should be provided regarding herbal medicines. Providing insurance may have a beneficial effect.

Among patients who were aware of the herbal preparations that they are taking, garlic was the most frequently used herb. Garlic *(Allium sativum)* has been closely studied. Garlic has demonstrated multiple cardiovascular benefits that include lowering blood pressure, inhibiting platelet aggregation, enhancing fibrinolytic activity, and reducing cholesterol and triglyceride levels. However, despite all this evidence the routine use has not been advised because of methodological shortcomings of the published literature [20] and extreme caution is advised if garlic is taken concomitantly with CYP2E1 substrates [15] or in patients taking warfarin [16]. Studies are needed to determine possible benefits and harms of native African herbs that are used by traditional healers for hypertension.

Over 90% of study subjects reported that their doctors did not ask them about the use of either herbs or other alternative therapies for hypertension. These findings are consistent with other studies from West Africa which indicate (1) that the overwhelming majority of healthcare workers are not aware of the herbal medicine use of the hypertensive adults in their care [6, 14] and (2) that a leading reason for this is fear and lack of inquiry of the part of the healthcare worker [6].

In our study, current use of traditional medicines for hypertension was not associated with lower compliance to allopathic medicines, as it has been in prior studies [6, 13]. It is therefore important that doctors not only ask about herbs and other alternative therapies among adults admitted with hypertension but also provide careful, specific, and nonjudgmental recommendations. The authors suspect that more patients will be willing to listen and follow advice if clinicians apply this careful, discerning approach. Further studies are needed to determine the best way to ask and educate about herbal medicine use in the African context.

5. Conclusion

The use of herbs and other alternative therapies are very common among patients with hypertension. Nearly a quarter of the hypertensive adults in our study reported recently taking herbs specifically for the treatment of hypertension. Adults from low socioeconomic status, those with misunderstandings about hypertension, and those without insurance were more likely to take herbs. Study subjects often chose to take herbs due to poverty, family pressure, and a desire for a complete cure. Use of herbal or alternative therapies was not associated with noncompliance. Their doctors had asked very few patients about herbal medicine use. Open, nonjudgmental communication between healthcare workers and patients regarding use of herbs and other alternative medicines must be encouraged in Africa. Future investigations should focus on identifying the magnitude of the problem in the community level, traditional healer's knowledge about hypertension, and the timing of initiation of herbal use and alternative therapies.

Additional Points

See http://apps.who.int/classifications/icd10/browse/2010/en#/I10-I15.

Conflicts of Interest

Anthony Liwa was supported by United States Agency for International Development (USAID) leadership training program. Luke Smart and Robert Peck have each received grants from the National Institutes of Health Fogarty International Center (Grant nos. R25TW009337 and K01TW010281, resp.). Other authors report no specific funding in relation to this research and have no conflicts of interest to disclose.

Authors' Contributions

Anthony Liwa and Robert Peck were involved with research concept, data collection, data analysis, interpretation of results, and writing of manuscript. Rebecca Roediger, Amina Bougaila, and Hyasinta Jaka were involved in data collection. Luke Smart and Stacey Langwick contributed to the research concept and review of manuscript. All authors reviewed and approved the final manuscript.

Acknowledgments

The authors acknowledge the tremendous assistance provided by ward staff (nurses, doctors, and medical students) in the identification of patients with hypertension.

References

[1] S. Ramirez, D. Enquobahrie, G. Nyadzi et al., "Prevalence and correlates of hypertension in rural Africa," *Journal of Human Hypertension*, vol. 24, pp. 786–795, 2010.

[2] M. E. Hendriks, F. W. N. M. Wit, T. M. Akande et al., "Effect of health insurance and facility quality improvement on blood pressure in adults with hypertension in nigeria a population-based study," *JAMA Internal Medicine*, vol. 174, no. 4, pp. 555–563, 2014.

[3] M. J. Dewhurst, F. Dewhurst, W. K. Gray, P. Chaote, G. P. Orega, and R. W. Walker, "The high prevalence of hypertension in rural-dwelling Tanzanian older adults and the disparity between detection, treatment and control: a rule of sixths?" *Journal of Human Hypertension*, vol. 27, no. 6, pp. 374–380, 2013.

[4] R. N. Peck, E. Green, J. Mtabaji et al., "Hypertension-related diseases as a common cause of hospital mortality in Tanzania: a 3-year prospective study," *Journal of Hypertension*, vol. 31, no. 9, pp. 1806–1811, 2013.

[5] G. A. Mansoor, "Herbs and alternative therapies in the hypertension clinic," *American Journal of Hypertension*, vol. 14, no. 9 I, pp. 971–975, 2001.

[6] I. A. Kretchy, F. Owusu-Daaku, and S. Danquah, "Patterns and determinants of the use of complementary and alternative medicine: a cross-sectional study of hypertensive patients in Ghana," *BMC Complementary and Alternative Medicine*, vol. 14, article 44, 2014.

[7] O. C. Amira and N. U. Okubadejo, "Frequency of complementary and alternative medicine utilization in hypertensive patients attending an urban tertiary care centre in Nigeria," *BMC Complementary and Alternative Medicine*, vol. 7, article 30, 2007.

[8] F. Nuwaha and G. Musinguzi, "Use of alternative medicine for hypertension in Buikwe and Mukono districts of Uganda: A cross sectional study," *BMC Complementary and Alternative Medicine*, vol. 13, article no. 301, 2013.

[9] P. E. Osamor and B. E. Owumi, "Complementary and alternative medicine in the management of hypertension in an urban Nigerian community," *BMC Complementary & Alternative Medicine*, vol. 10, article 36, 2010.

[10] A. C. Liwa, L. R. Smart, A. Frumkin, H.-A. B. Epstein, D. W. Fitzgerald, and R. N. Peck, "Traditional herbal medicine use among hypertensive patients in sub-Saharan Africa: A systematic review," *Current Hypertension Reports*, vol. 16, no. 6, article no. 437, 2014.

[11] D. E. Morisky, L. W. Green, and D. M. Levine, "Concurrent and predictive validity of a self-reported measure of medication adherence," *Medical Care*, vol. 24, no. 1, pp. 67–74, 1986.

[12] X. Tan, I. Patel, and J. Chang, "Review of the four item morisky medication adherence scale (MMAS-4) and eight item morisky medication adherence scale (MMAS-8)," *Innovations in Pharmacy*, vol. 5, pp. 1–8, 2014.

[13] K. Peltzer, "Health beliefs and prescription medication compliance among diagnosed hypertension clinic attenders in a rural South African Hospital," *Curationis*, vol. 27, no. 3, pp. 15–23, 2004.

[14] N. S. Olisa and F. T. Oyelola, "Evaluation of use of herbal medicines among ambulatory hypertensive patients attending a secondary health care facility in Nigeria," *International Journal of Pharmacy Practice*, vol. 17, no. 2, pp. 101–105, 2009.

[15] A. A. Izzo and E. Ernst, "Interactions between herbal medicines and prescribed drugs: An updated systematic review," *Drugs*, vol. 69, no. 13, pp. 1777–1798, 2009.

[16] L. G. Miller, "Herbal medicinals: selected clinical considerations focusing on known or potential drug-herb interactions," *Archives of Internal Medicine*, vol. 158, no. 20, pp. 2200–2211, 1998.

[17] A. Fugh-Berman, "Herb-drug interactions," *The Lancet*, vol. 355, no. 9198, pp. 134–138, 2000.

[18] T. Kupiec and V. Raj, "Fatal seizures due to potential herb-drug interactions with Ginkgo biloba," *Journal of Analytical Toxicology*, vol. 29, no. 7, pp. 755–758, 2005.

[19] S. McRae, "Elevated serum digoxin levels in a patient taking digoxin and Siberian ginseng," *Canadian Medical Association Journal*, vol. 155, no. 3, pp. 293–295, 1996.

[20] N. H. Mashour, G. I. Lin, and W. H. Frishman, "Herbal medicine for the treatment of cardiovascular disease: clinical considerations," *Archives of Internal Medicine*, vol. 158, no. 20, pp. 2225–2234, 1998.

20

An Analysis of Anthropometric Indicators and Modifiable Lifestyle Parameters Associated with Hypertensive Nephropathy

Christiana Aryee,[1,2] William K. B. A. Owiredu,[1,3] James Osei-Yeboah,[1,4] Ellis Owusu-Dabo,[5,6] Edwin F. Laing,[1,3] and Isaac K. Owusu[7]

[1] *Department of Molecular Medicine, School of Medical Sciences, Kwame Nkrumah University of Science and Technology, Kumasi, Ghana*
[2] *Becton Dickinson Biosciences Technical Services, West Africa, Accra, Ghana*
[3] *Department of Clinical Biochemistry, Diagnostic Directorate, Komfo Anokye Teaching Hospital, Kumasi, Ghana*
[4] *Department of Medical Laboratory Sciences, School of Allied Health Sciences, University of Health and Allied Sciences, Ho, Ghana*
[5] *School of Public Health, Kwame Nkrumah University of Science and Technology, Kumasi, Ghana*
[6] *Kumasi Centre for Collaborative Research in Tropical Medicine, Kwame Nkrumah University of Science and Technology, Kumasi, Ghana*
[7] *Department of Medicine, School of Medical Sciences, Kwame Nkrumah University of Science and Technology and Komfo Anokye Teaching Hospital, Kumasi, Ghana*

Correspondence should be addressed to William K. B. A. Owiredu; wkbaowiredu@yahoo.com

Academic Editor: Tomohiro Katsuya

The surge in prevalence of chronic noncommunicable diseases like hypertension and chronic kidney disease has been linked with modifiable lifestyle practices and increased body fat. This study sought to compare the association between different modifiable lifestyle practices, adiposity indices, renal function parameters, and hypertension as well as the predictive implications for levels of these parameters in target cardiac organ damage among an urban Ghanaian hypertensive population. Using a hospital-based case-control study design, 241 Ghanaian indigenes from the Kumasi metropolis were recruited for this study. The case group was made up of 180 hypertensives and 61 normotensives served as controls. In addition to sociodemographic data, standard haemodynamic, anthropometric, renal function, and cardiac organ damage assessments were done. The prevalence of chronic kidney disease (CKD) ranged from 13.3% to 16.6% depending on the equation used in estimating the glomerular filtration rate (eGFR). Percentage cluster distribution by chronic kidney disease was observed to be significantly tilted toward the upper quartiles (3rd and 4th) of the haemodynamic parameters measured. Chronic kidney disease was significantly higher among self-reported smokers and alcoholic hypertensives. In this urban population, adiposity was associated with hypertension and renal insufficiency. Chronic kidney disease was associated with hypertension and cardiac abnormalities.

1. Background

High blood pressure is a major health problem all over the world [1]. Ghana and other countries in Sub-Saharan Africa (SSA) are experiencing an epidemic of cardiovascular diseases propelled by rapidly increasing rates of hypertension [2]. A reciprocal or bidirectional relationship has been postulated for hypertension and end-stage chronic kidney disease (ESCKD) [3]. Hypertension is a key pathogenic factor linked to deterioration of kidney function, whilst the most common forms of secondary hypertension are attributable to chronic kidney disease [4–6]. According to Commodore-Mensah et al. [7], hypertension is the leading cause of renal failure in Ghana, whilst Owiredu et al. [8] estimated a 20-fold higher increased risk of death through cardiovascular complications among chronic kidney disease (CKD) patients than any other cause in the general population.

The upsurge in chronic noncommunicable diseases has been attributed to modifiable lifestyle practices characterized by sedentary lifestyle and a resultant obesity [9–13]. Evidence that hypertension is related to increases in body fat is well established in the literature [14–22]. Epidemiological studies of the impact of obesity on outcome in chronic kidney disease (CKD) remain conflicting, with several well-designed studies even suggesting a survival advantage for obese end-stage renal disease (ESRD) patients [23–25].

This study sought to compare the association between different modifiable lifestyle practices, adiposity indices, renal function parameters, and hypertension as well as the predictive implications for levels of these parameters in target cardiac organ damage among an urban Ghanaian hypertensive population.

2. Material and Methods

2.1. Study Participants. A hospital-based case-control study was conducted between November 2012 and September 2013. Two hundred and forty-one participants were involved in this study. One hundred and eighty (108) nondiabetic hypertensive patients were attending clinic at the Komfo Anokye Teaching Hospital (KATH) and the Precise Specialist Clinic, all in Kumasi, Ghana, and sixty-one (61) age-matched normotensive controls were from the Kumasi metropolis. The study participants were recruited from a population of adult individuals between the ages of 22 and 87 years. Criteria for the case group were patients diagnosed with hypertension who were not suffering from diabetes and were of consent age. The control group were normotensive age-matched healthy individuals with no past history of diabetes, cardiac, renal, and hepatic dysfunction, or dyslipidaemia, living in the Kumasi metropolis, who consented to participate in this study. The detailed characteristics of study participants have been published in an earlier work [26].

2.2. Sociodemographic Data Capture (Questionnaire). Self-reported structured questionnaire was administered to determine duration of hypertension and treatment status, smoking status, alcohol intake, educational level, physical activity levels, occupation, the usage of nonprescribed orthodox and herbal medications, family history of hypertension, current and past symptoms of cerebrovascular disease, and peripheral vascular and coronary heart diseases.

2.3. Blood Pressure (BP) Measurement. Blood pressure (BP) and pulse rate measurements were done using the Omron M5-I digital fully automatic blood pressure monitor (OMRON Healthcare Europe BV Wegalaan 57 NL-2132 JD Hoofddorp). After participants had sat quietly for at least ten minutes, three measurements were taken at one-minute intervals on the right arm in a seated position, with arm supported at heart level and feet flat on the floor using an appropriate sized cuff. Hypertension was diagnosed when the mean of the second and third blood pressure (BP) measurements was equal or above 140/90 mmHg or when participants reported use of antihypertensive medication which was verified from their hospital files [27, 28].

2.4. Anthropometric Variables. Anthropometric measurements included height to the nearest millimeter without shoes and weight to the nearest 0.1 kg in light clothing. Subjects were weighed on a bathroom scale (Zhongshan Camry Electronic Co. Ltd., Guangdong, China) and their height was measured with a Seca stadiometer with the participant standing erect with back straight, heels together, and feet slightly apart at a 60-degree angle. Waist circumference (to the nearest centimeter) was measured with a Gulick II spring-loaded measuring tape (Gay Mills, WI) midway between the inferior angles of the ribs and the suprailiac crests. The hip circumference was measured as the maximal circumference over the hip circumference (HC) at the level of the widest diameter around the gluteal protuberance in centimeters. Body mass index (BMI) was calculated by dividing weight (kg) by height squared (m^2). The waist-to-hip ratio (WHR) was calculated by dividing the waist circumference (cm) by the hip circumference (cm). Waist-to-height ratio was calculated by dividing the waist circumference (cm) by the height circumference (cm). Other calculated adiposity indices were as follows:

(1) Conicity index (CI) [29]:

$$\mathrm{CI} = \frac{\text{Waist Circumference (m)}}{\left[0.109 \times \sqrt{\text{Weight (Kg)}/\text{Height (m)}}\right]} \tag{1}$$

(2) Abdominal volume index (AVI) [30]:

$$\mathrm{AVI} = \frac{\left[2\left(\text{Waist C (cm)}\right)^2 + 0.7\left\{\text{Waist C (cm)} - \text{Hip C (cm)}\right\}^2\right]}{1000} \tag{2}$$

(3) Body Adiposity Index (BAI) [31]:

$$\mathrm{BAI} = \frac{\text{Hip Circumference (cm)}}{\left[\text{Height (m)}\right]^{1.5}} - 18. \tag{3}$$

2.5. Biochemical Assays. Venous blood samples were collected after an overnight fast (12–16 hours) between 7 am and 10 am. About 5 mL of venous blood was drawn from the antecubital vein of which four mL was dispensed into vacutainer® plain tubes and one mL was dispensed into fluoride oxalate tubes. After centrifugation at 500 ×g for 15 minutes, the serum and plasma were stored at −80°C until assayed. Parameters that were determined include fasting blood glucose (FBG) to exclude participants with diabetes, urea, creatinine, uric acid, potassium, sodium, and chloride. The methods adopted for the determination of the urea, creatinine, and uric acid were predetermined by the reagent manufacturer (Dialab GmbH, IZ-NÖ Süd, Hondastrasse, A-2351 Wiener Neudorf,

Austria). Ion Selective Electrode (ISE) method was used to assay electrolytes (AVL 9180 Electrolyte Analyzer, Roche Diagnostics, Switzerland, http://www.roche.com/index.htm) at the Komfo Anokye Teaching Hospital in Kumasi. All other biochemical analytical investigations were carried out at the Kumasi Centre for Collaborative Research in Tropical Medicine (KCCR) located at the Kwame Nkrumah University of Science and Technology, Kumasi.

2.6. Clinical Assessment. All the 241 participants underwent clinical assessment to determine target organ damage. Detailed history, physical examination, chest X-ray, 12-lead resting electrocardiogram (ECG), and transthoracic echocardiogram (ECHO) were done. All diagnoses and interpretation were performed by consultant radiologists and cardiologists.

2.7. Diagnosis of Chronic Kidney Disease. Estimate glomerular filtration rate (GFR) was calculated from serum creatinine according to Cockcroft-Gault (CG) equation as follows:

$$\text{eGFR} = \frac{(140 - \text{Age}) \times \text{Weight}}{72 \times \text{Serum Creatinine}} (\times\ 0.85 \text{ if female}). \quad \text{(CG)}$$

2.8. Four-Variable Modification of Diet in Renal Disease.

$$\text{eGFR} = 186 \times \text{SCr}^{-1.154} \times \text{Age}^{-0.203} \times (1.212) \times (0.742 \text{ if female}). \quad \text{(4v-MDRD)}$$

The eGFR results from the various renal function equations were used to stratify the study population into five categories corresponding to the five stages of CKD in the K/DOQI CKD classification [32]. Chronic kidney disease was classified as eGFR $< 60\ \text{mL/min/1.73 m}^2$ (stages 3, 4 and 5; see Table 5) [33].

2.9. Diagnosis of Heart Failure. Heart failure was diagnosed, using the modified Framingham criteria for diagnosis of heart failure [34]. Major criteria included paroxysmal nocturnal dyspnea, raised jugular venous pressure, cardiomegaly, basal crepitation, S3 gallop, and acute pulmonary oedema. Minor criteria included tachycardia, orthopnea, exertional dyspnea, nocturnal cough, hepatomegaly, and diuretic use. Heart failure was diagnosed if the participant had two major and one minor or one major and two minor criteria. Other complications of hypertension included cardiomegaly (without heart failure), stroke or transient ischaemic attack, and chronic kidney disease.

2.10. Statistical Analysis. Normality of all continuous variables was tested. All nonparametric variables were normalized by log transformation before analysis. Results obtained after analysis of log transformed variables were converted by antilog. Continuous variables were expressed as their mean ± SEM, whereas categorical variables were presented as count and proportion. Comparisons of the general characteristics of the hypertensive group against the normotensive group were performed using unpaired t-tests, chi square (χ^2) tests, or Fisher exact tests where appropriate. Analysis of variance (ANOVA) and Bonferroni post hoc test were used to compare more than two means, whilst a post hoc linear contrast test was used for trend analysis of continuous variables. A level of $p < 0.05$ was considered as statistically significant for all analyses. IBM Statistical Package for the Social Sciences (SPSS Inc., Chicago, USA (http://www.spss.com) version 20.00) and GraphPad Prism version 6.00 GraphPad software, San Diego, California, USA (http://www.graphpad.com/), for windows were used for statistical analysis where appropriate.

3. Results

Two hundred and forty-one (241) adult Ghanaians were recruited for the study. The sociodemographic characteristics of the participants, as shown in Table 2, involved 61 (25.3%) normotensives and 180 (74.7%) hypertensives, of which 40 patients representing 16.6% of the study population were newly diagnosed hypertensives who were not on any hypertensive drugs and were classified as drug-naive. Female participation was higher in each of the three categories of subjects. The informal sector employees dominated the case group. Significantly self-reported alcohol intake and smoking were both found to be more prevalent among the hypertensives, peaking in each case in the drug-naive group. No significant differences were recorded in the rest of the sociodemographic parameters assessed between the three different groups of participants evaluated in this study (see Table 2).

Among all the parameters evaluated as shown in Table 3, no statistically significant variation was recorded between the newly diagnosed hypertensives and their counterparts on treatment. Higher anthropometric indices were recorded among both hypertension groups compared with the normotensives; however, in the case of body mass index (BMI) and waist-to-hip ratio (WHR) the difference was not statistically significant. The hypertensives presented with significantly higher mean serum biochemical indices of renal dysfunction and electrolytes levels than their normotensive counterparts. The average concentration of microalbumin excreted in the urine as well as the glomerular filtration rate estimated by both (4v-MDRD) and (CG) equations was comparable among the treatment-naïve hypertensives and the normotensives (see Table 3).

Among the general study population after adjusting for age and gender, positive additive changes in waist-to-height ratio (WHtR) as well as both the abdominal body frame factors (waist circumference (WC); hip circumference (HC)), the abdominal body region volumetric models for central obesity (conicity index (CI); abdominal volume index (AVI)) and body fat deposition (body adiposity index (BAI)) were associated with corresponding incremental changes in the haemodynamic measures (hypertension), the serum biochemical kidney profile measures, and renal insufficiency (decreasing eGFR). Among the hypertensive subpopulation, positive association was observed between the anthropometric measures and the serum biochemical kidney profile (K^+, Na^+, Cl^-, urea, creatinine, and UA) as well as renal

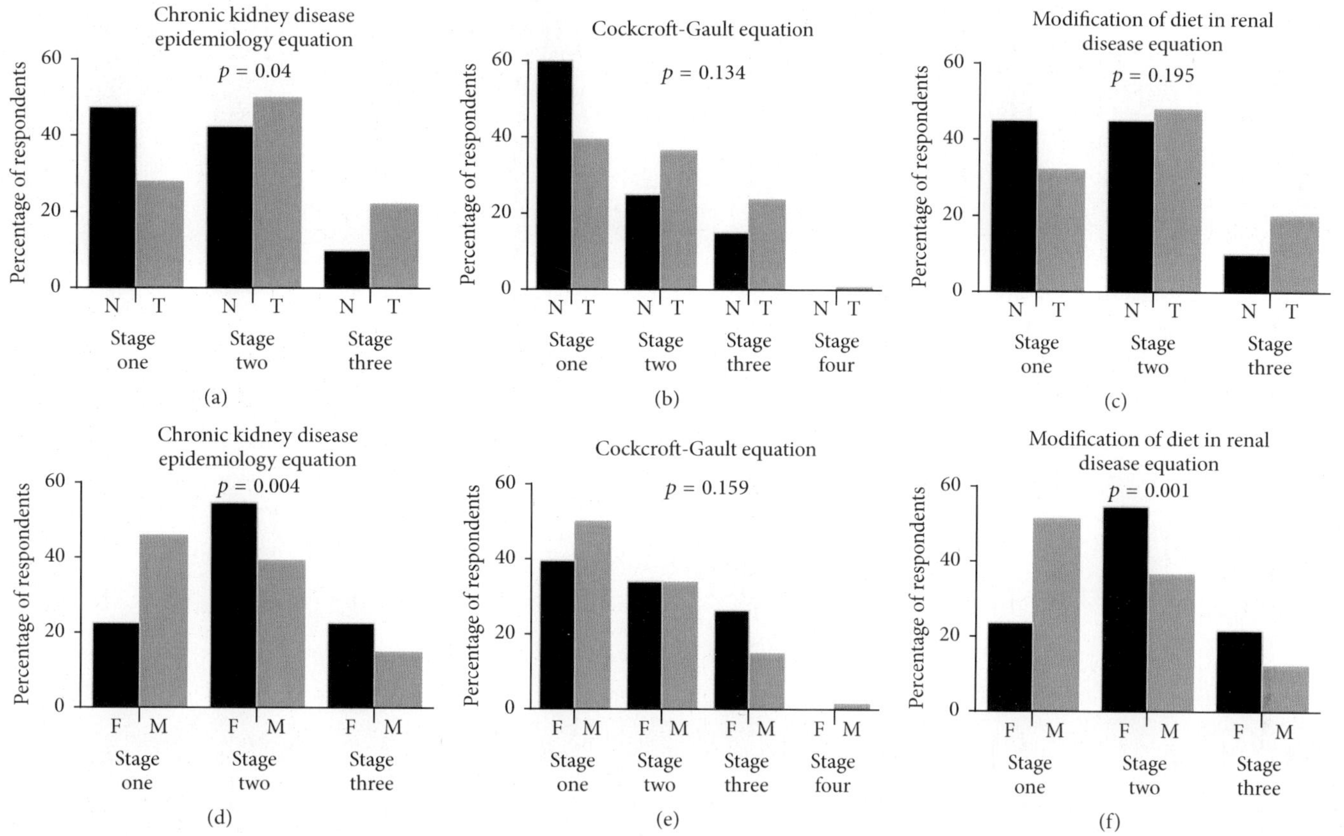

FIGURE 1: Estimates of the prevalence of CKD in the study population using the renal function equations stratified by therapy and gender. N: drug naïve, T: therapy, F: female, and M: male.

insufficiency. With the exception of pulse, no significant correlation was observed between the anthropometric measures and the haemodynamic measures among the hypertensive subpopulation.

Among both the general study population and the hypertension subgroup increasing levels of serum potassium, urea, creatinine, and uric acid were associated with increasing renal insufficiency. Significant association between the haemodynamic measures and the serum biochemical kidney profile was more profound in the general study population than the hypertension subgroup (see Table 4).

Among the total population of 241 participants, 13.3% presented with chronic kidney disease (CKD) when assessed by the four-variable modification of diet in renal disease (4v-MDRD) equation. The Cockcroft-Gault (CG) recorded 16.6% and the chronic kidney disease epidemiology collaboration (CKD-EPI) equation recorded 14.5%. All patients presenting with CKD belong to the hypertension group. With the exception of one study participant who was observed to be in stage four by the Cockcroft-Gault (CG) equation, all CKD patients observed were in the third stage (see Table 5).

Among the hypertensive patients who were newly diagnosed and thus treatment-naïve and those who were on therapy irrespective of the equation used in assessing glomerular filtration rate, the group on therapy recorded a greater percentage of end-stage chronic kidney disease (CKD) than their naïve counterparts; however, with the exception of the chronic kidney disease epidemiology collaboration (CKD-EPI) equation (see Figure 1(a)), this difference was not statistically significant (see Figures 1(a) and 1(c)). With the exception of the Cockcroft-Gault (CG) equation (see Figure 1(e)), significant gender differences in the incidence of CKD were observed. Using the CKD-EPI equation, 22.6% of hypertensive females presented with CKD compared to 14.9% of hypertensive males (see Figure 1(d)). Twenty-one and seven percent (21.7%) of females compared to 12.2% of males presented with CKD as per the four-variable modification of diet in renal disease (4v-MDRD) equation (see Figure 1(f)).

Irrespective of the equation used in estimating the glomerular filtration rate (GFR), self-reported nonalcoholics presented with significantly higher percentage of chronic kidney disease (CKD) than the alcoholics (23.6% versus 16.7%; 30.6% versus 16.7%; and 20.8% versus 15.7) for chronic kidney disease epidemiology collaboration (CKD-EPI), Cockcroft-Gault (CG), and four-variable modification of diet in renal disease (4v-MDRD) equations, respectively.

From Figure 2(d), significantly higher percentage of smokers (37.9%) were observed with CKD, compared to their counterparts who did not smoke (15.9%), a similar outcome was observed with the use of (4v-MDRD) where (37.9%) of smokers presented with CKD compared to (13.9%) of nonsmokers (see Figure 2).

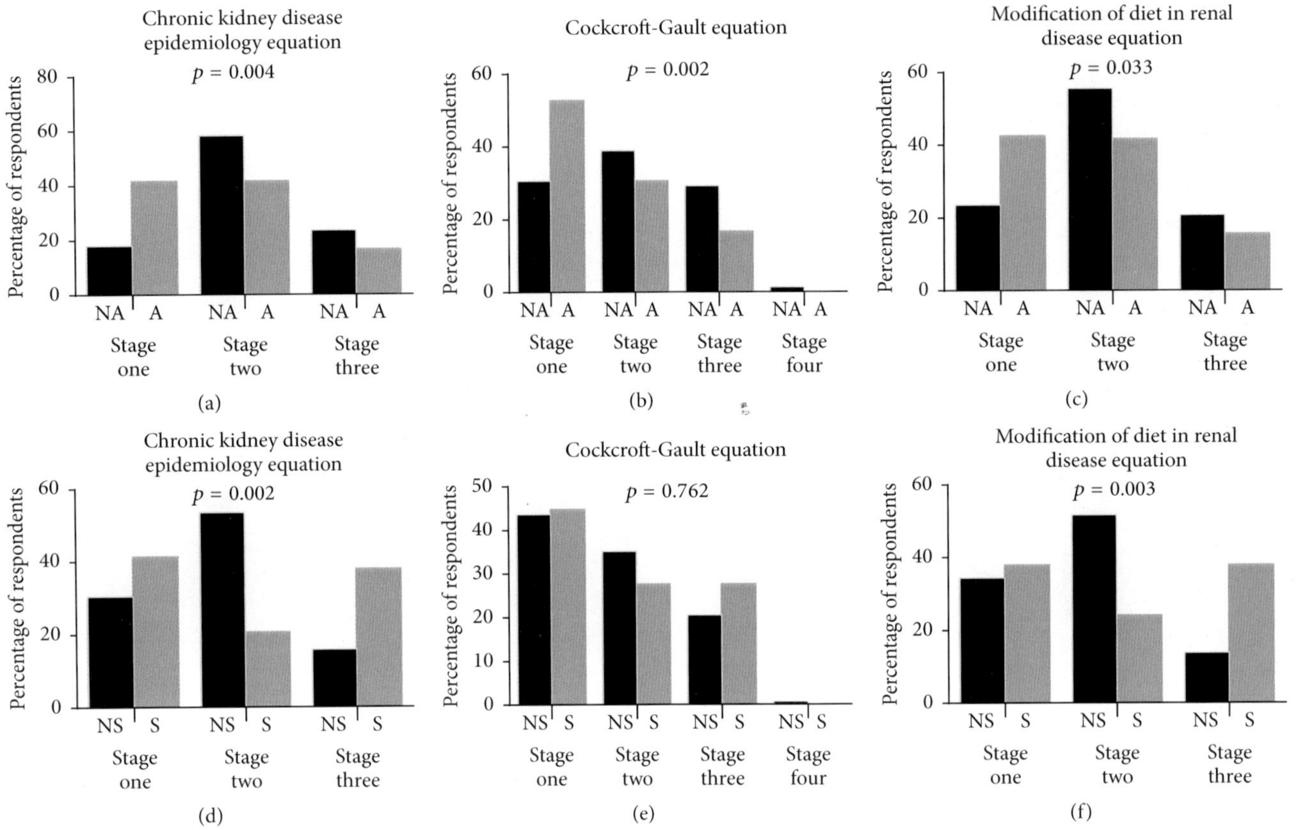

FIGURE 2: Estimates of the prevalence of CKD in the study population using the renal function equations stratified by alcohol consumption and smoking status. NA: nonalcoholic, A: alcoholic, S: smoker, and NS: nonsmoker.

Almost all participants presenting with chronic kidney disease (CKD) clustered at the upper quartiles (3rd and 4th) of systolic blood pressure. The exception included 10% of CKD subjects who clustered at the lower quartiles (7.5% and 2.5% for 1st and 2nd quartiles, resp.) of systolic blood pressure when Cockcroft-Gault (CG) equation was used to estimate the glomerular filtration rate. Percentage cluster distribution by CKD was observed to be significantly tilted toward the upper quartiles of diastolic blood pressure. Though not statistically significant, the majority of CKD participants clustered in the third and fourth quartiles of pulse, irrespective of the renal function equation used. The majority of participants presenting with microalbuminuria clustered in the upper quartiles of the haemodynamic parameters evaluated (see Figure 3).

The prevalence of microalbuminuria among the alcoholic subjects was 32.4% compared to 27.8% among the nonalcoholics. Study participants who smoked recorded a higher percentage of microalbuminuria compared to nonsmokers and also a higher number of smokers were found to cluster at increasing levels of microalbuminuria compared to nonsmokers. Patients using herbal medicine had higher microalbuminuria (32.7%) than those who were not using herbal medications (27.6%). Even though higher microalbuminuria was observed among the physically active group, severity of microalbuminuria was more profound in their nonactive counterparts (see Figure 4).

In general, significant additive linear relationship was observed for all serum renal biochemical parameters assayed with progressive quartile increment of haemodynamic indices. The exception was observed with the average levels of uric acid among the diastolic quartile cluster distribution, where no significant linearity was observed.

Irrespective of the renal function equation used in the estimation of the glomerular filtration rate among the study population, participants presenting with cardiac abnormalities (left ventricular hypertrophy-electrocardiograph, left ventricular hypertrophy-echocardiograph, and cardiomegaly-X-ray) recorded significant prevalence of chronic kidney disease compared to their counterparts who were without the specific abnormal heart condition (see Table 6).

4. Discussion

Earlier reports by Addo et al. [35] and Osafo et al. [36] put the calculated incidence of renal insufficiency (eGFR < 60 mL/min/1.73 m^2; stages 3, 4, and 5) among different hypertensive populations in Accra Ghana at 4.1% and 27.8%, respectively. The estimates of hypertensive kidney target organ damage burden for the present study (17.80%–22.22%) compared to the earlier records in the previous studies but were higher than the former and lower than the latter. The difference in CKD burden for the hypertensive cohort

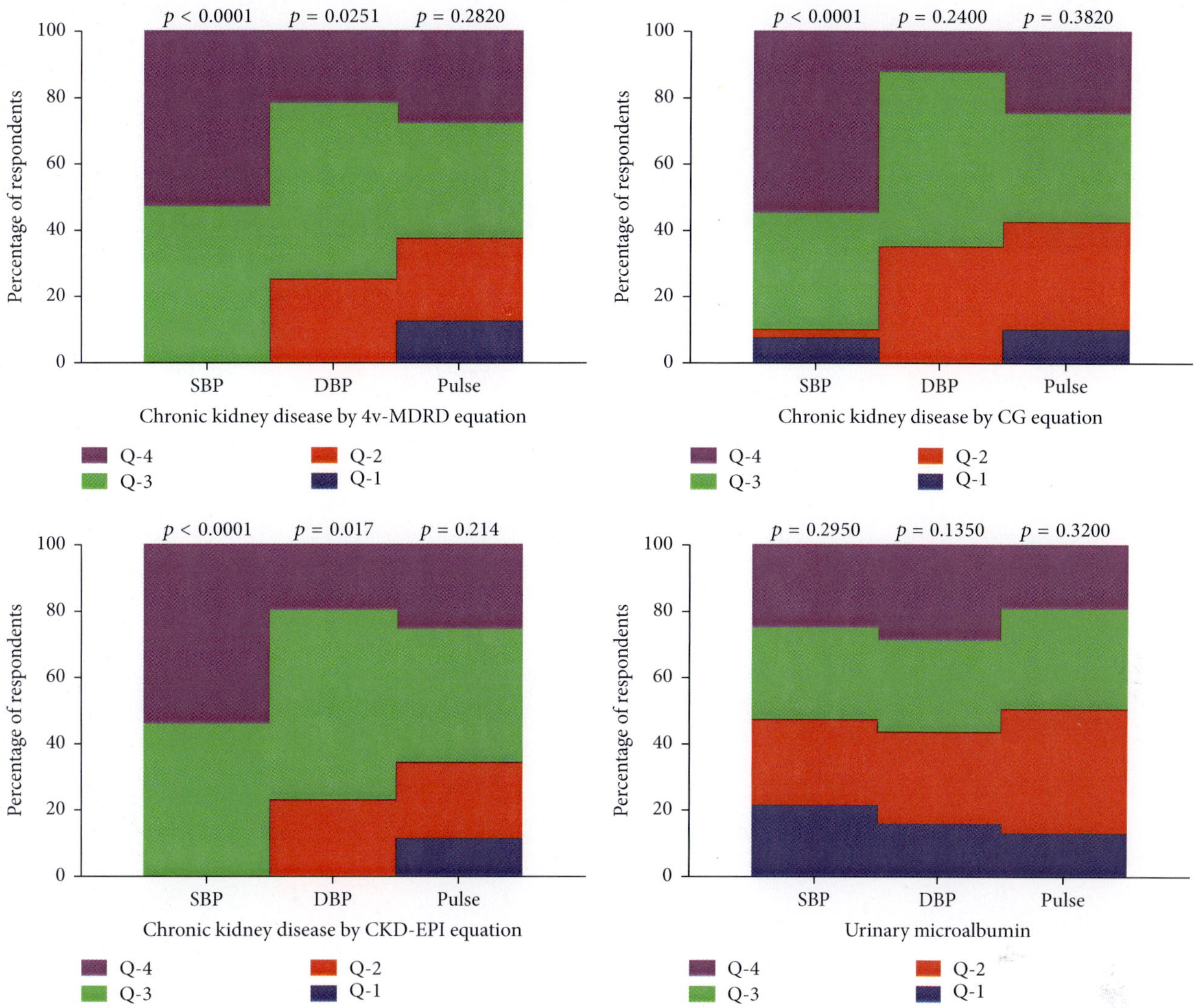

FIGURE 3: Renal insufficiency quartile cluster distributions with haemodynamic parameters. SBP: systolic blood pressure, DBP: diastolic blood pressure, Q-1: first quartile, Q-2: second quartile, Q-3: third quartile, and Q-4: fourth quartile. p value for linear by linear association is significant at 0.05 for two tail.

was perhaps due to differences in study population characteristics; thus, the work of Addo et al. [35] involved a population survey whilst that of Osafo et al. [36] and the present study were hospital-based studies. Again the fact that the study of Osafo et al. [36] included 14.7% of subjects with preexisting diabetes mellitus whereas the present study involved only nondiabetic hypertensives may account for the higher CKD incidence recorded in the previous report. Adu [37] in an editorial in the Ghana Medical Journal estimated the prevalence of hypertension in the African population at 10% and posited that hypertension accounts for 38.8% of the aetiology of CKD and is possibly the leading cause of target kidney organ damage among this population.

The incidence of CKD was higher among the hypertensive study participants on treatment than the treatment-naïve group. The increased duration of chronic diseases like hypertension has usually been linked with deterioration of sequelae and survival. Also the institution of drug therapy in the management of hypertension is usually associated with advancing disease state and this may account for the higher target kidney organ damage observed among the hypertensives on treatment.

Gender differences in health vary according to differential vulnerabilities in males and females, which may be as a result of biological or sociodemographic differences [38, 39]. In the case of chronic kidney disease among hypertensives, vulnerability seems to be more tilted toward the female gender than the male gender [4, 40]. This finding is in agreement with observations made in this study (see Figure 1). Wang et al. [40] have suggested that the stronger association between obesity and chronic kidney disease in women than in men could account for this phenomenon. In Ghana, obesity is reported to be significantly higher among females than in males [13, 41]. Among hypertensives, obesity was found to be significantly higher ($p = 0.0337$) among females (57.5%) compared to the males (40.5%).

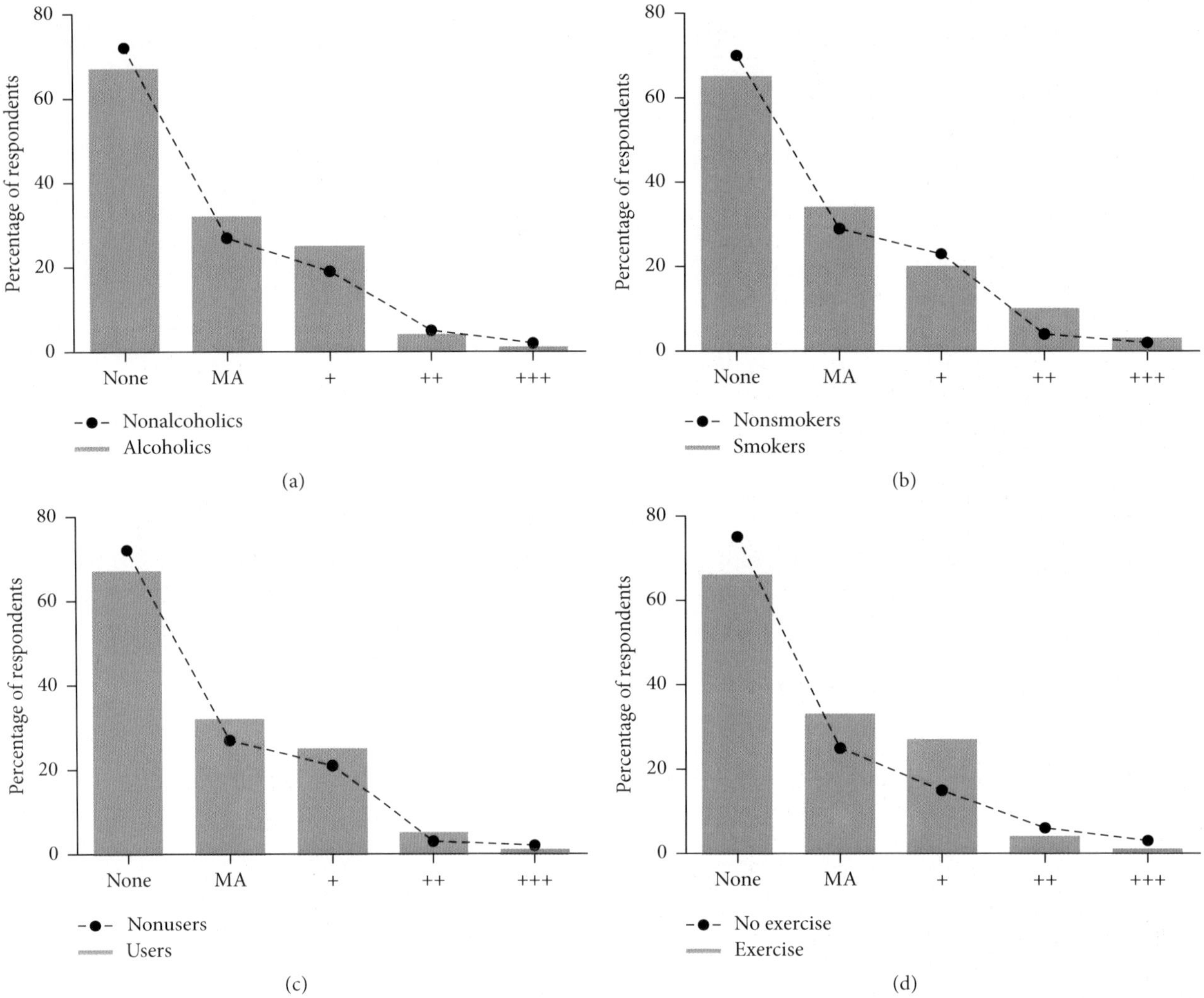

FIGURE 4: Prevalence of microalbuminuria among hypertension subjects stratified by sociodemographic characteristics. MA: microalbuminuria. (a) Alcohol intake, (b) smoking status, (c) herbal medicine intake, and (d) physical activity level.

The raging debate of alcohol consumption as a modifiable lifestyle trait influencing both hypertension and kidney outcomes in the scientific literature has become even more intense in recent times because of the great importance it confers due to the seemingly large numbers of the population any prognostic outcome may affect. In the current study, self-reported alcohol consumption was recorded among more than half of the study population (130 (53.9%)) with a significantly higher presence among the hypertensives than the normotensives (see Table 1). Deleterious association of alcohol consumption with hypertension is available in the Ghanaian literature [10, 42, 43]. Plausible mechanisms elucidated for such adverse effects include stimulation of corticosteroid, catecholamine, vasopressin production, and drug interaction causing resistance to drug therapy and direct pressor effect due to alcohol induced arteriolar vasoconstriction [44–46].

The findings of the current study are consistent with those of Renaud et al. [47] and Reynolds et al. [48] both of whom reported an inverse association between alcohol consumption and chronic kidney disease among hypertensives (see Figure 2). However, due to our inability to determine the threshold dose level of alcohol intake among the study population, drawing inferences for causality of alcohol dose response was not possible [46, 49]. It is therefore appropriate to concur with Reynolds et al. [48] who called for caution in the interpretation of similar results, since epidemiologically a suggested J- or U-shaped relationship exists between alcohol consumption and coronary heart diseases. Thus, the apparent benefits of moderate drinking on kidney and coronary heart disease mortality are offset at higher drinking levels by increasing risk of death from other types of heart diseases (cardiomyopathy, arrhythmia, etc.), neurological disorders, cancer, liver cirrhosis, and traffic accidents [46, 50].

Despite the recent report from the HUNT study suggesting smoking is not a major determinant of adverse blood pressure and other component cardiovascular disease risk factors [51] and the report from the population-based Malmö-Diet-and-Cancer-Cohort which found that the associated risk of cardiovascular disease and cardiovascular disease mortality conferred by genetic variation on chromosome

TABLE 1: Equations for chronic kidney disease epidemiology collaboration (CKD-EPI).

Gender	Serum creatinine μmol/L (mg/dL)	Estimated glomerular equation
Female	≤62 (≤0.7)	$\text{eGFR} = 166 \times \left(\frac{\text{Serum Creatinine}}{0.7^{-0.329}}\right) \times (0.993)^{\text{Age}}$
Female	>62 (>0.7)	$\text{eGFR} = 166 \times \left(\frac{\text{Serum Creatinine}}{0.7^{-1.209}}\right) \times (0.993)^{\text{Age}}$
Male	≤80 (≤0.9)	$\text{eGFR} = 163 \times \left(\frac{\text{Serum Creatinine}}{0.9^{-0.411}}\right) \times (0.993)^{\text{Age}}$
Male	>80 (>0.9)	$\text{eGFR} = 163 \times \left(\frac{\text{Serum Creatinine}}{0.9^{-1.209}}\right) \times (0.993)^{\text{Age}}$

TABLE 2: Sociodemographic characteristics of the population under study stratified by hypertension and treatment status.

Parameter	Control	HPT-naïve	HPT-therapy	p value
Respondents	61 (25.3)	40 (16.6)	140 (58.1)	*nd*
Female	45 (73.8)	22 (55.0)	84 (60.0)	0.0980
Male	16 (26.2)	18 (45.0)	56 (40.0)	
Formal sector	45 (74.2)	10 (24.4)	44 (31.7)	<0.0001
Informal sector	16 (25.8)	30 (75.6)	96 (68.3)	
Alcoholics	22 (36.1)	32 (80.0)	76 (54.3)	<0.0001
Smokers	3 (4.9)	9 (22.5)	20 (14.3)	0.0340
Exercise	36 (59.0)	27 (67.5)	89 (63.6)	0.6760
Positive family history	40 (65.6)	31 (77.5)	104 (74.3)	0.3330
Herbal medicine intake	33 (54.1)	24 (60.0)	79 (56.4)	0.8430
Nonprescribed drug intake	36 (59.0)	22 (55.0)	82 (58.6)	0.9090

Data is presented as figure with corresponding percentage in parenthesis. HPT-naïve: newly diagnosed hypertensive not on antihypertensive drugs; HPT-therapy: hypertensives on antihypertensives. p is significant at 0.005.

9p21 may be attenuated by smoking [52], there is consensus on the association of smoking with adverse cardiovascular and renal outcome [53–59].

In the present study, self-reported smoking was 13.3% among the total study population and significantly higher among the hypertensives compared to normotensives (16.1% versus 4.9%). In agreement with the findings of adverse renal events associated with cigarette smoking among various study populations [53, 60–63], current smoking status was associated with chronic kidney disease among hypertensives (see Figure 2). Plausible mechanisms of smoking attributed renal injury include increased blood pressure and heart rate; altered diurnal blood pressure rhythm; increased sympathetic nerve activity; nicotine induced mesangial cell proliferation and increased production of fibronectin; arteriosclerosis of renal and intrarenal arteries and arterioles; growth factor activation (angiotensin II, endothelin-1, and TGF-1); oxidative stress; impaired lipoprotein and glycosaminoglycan metabolism; tubulotoxicity; direct endothelial cell toxicity; increased aggregation of platelet; modulation of immune mechanisms; vasopressin-mediated antidiuresis and insulin resistance [4, 64].

Excess weight gain is a major risk factor for essential hypertension and end-stage renal disease (ESRD) [65, 66]. In the present study, higher anthropometric indices were recorded among the hypertensive groups compared to the normotensives and, after adjusting for age and gender, positive additive changes in anthropometric indices were associated with corresponding incremental changes in the haemodynamic measurements (hypertension), the serum kidney profile estimates, and renal insufficiency (decreasing eGFR). According to the Guyton hypothesis, sustained hypertension can occur only when there is a derangement of pressure natriuresis [6, 67, 68]. Obesity related resetting of the kidney-fluid apparatus to a hypertensive level is consistent with the model of hypertension by volume overload [69]. Documented pathogenic mechanisms include enhanced sympathetic nervous system activity, increased activity of the systemic renin-angiotensin system, low atrial natriuretic peptide levels, and physical compression of the kidneys by fat deposits within and around the kidneys, coupled with increased abdominal pressure due to accumulation of excess visceral fat, all of which can cause sodium retention [65, 70–72]. This enhanced sodium avidity shifts the pressure natriuresis curve to the right, thereby necessitating higher arterial pressure to excrete the day's salt intake and maintain sodium balance and volume homeostasis [67, 73].

There is an accumulating body of clinical and experimental data implicating obesity as an important causative factor in renal disease [74–76]. Several alterations in renal structure and function have been associated with obesity [77]. The compensatory mechanisms to maintain sodium balance in obesity in the long term lead to increased systemic arterial pressure, creating a haemodynamic burden on the kidneys which causes glomerular injury [65]. Deposition of extracellular matrix throughout the renal medulla and the ducts of Bellini compresses the renal parenchyma toward the pole of the kidney resulting in the formation of round-shaped, enlarged kidneys in obese subjects [69].

There is intense debate as to whether hypertension causes kidney disease or vice versa [4]. High blood pressure is a key pathogenic factor that contributes to the deterioration of kidney function [78]. Conversely, chronic kidney disease (CKD) is the most common form of secondary hypertension

TABLE 3: Haemodynamic, anthropometric, serum biochemical kidney profile and estimated glomerular filtration rate of the study population stratified by hypertension status.

Parameter	Control	HPT-naïve	HPT-therapy	p value
SBP (mmHg)	117.38 ± 0.96	152.00 ± 3.27	155.46 ± 1.82	<0.0001
DBP (mmHg)	73.28 ± 0.77	100.50 ± 1.34	101.46 ± 0.94	<0.0001
Pulse (BPM)	51.41 ± 0.91	76.85 ± 2.20	81.74 ± 1.77	<0.0001
MAP (mmHg)	87.98 ± 0.63	117.67 ± 1.81	119.46 ± 1.01	<0.0001
WC (cm)	69.10 ± 1.57	97.65 ± 2.80	95.69 ± 1.58	<0.0001
HC (cm)	71.82 ± 1.56	102.20 ± 3.20	101.42 ± 2.12	<0.0001
BMI (Kg/m^2)	29.36 ± 0.65	29.80 ± 0.71[a]	29.52 ± 0.39[a]	0.9018
WHR	0.96 ± 0.01	0.97 ± 0.01[a]	0.97 ± 0.0[a]	0.9356
WHtR	0.45 ± 0.01	0.60 ± 0.11	0.59 ± 0.13	<0.0001
AVI	9.86 ± 0.45	19.74 ± 1.16	19.09 ± 0.66	<0.0001
Conicity index	0.929 ± 0.11	1.28 ± 0.04	1.25 ± 0.02	<0.0001
BAI	19.49 ± 0.90	31.14 ± 1.60	31.40 ± 1.17	<0.0001
Potassium (mmol/L)	3.20 ± 1.03	3.76 ± 1.05	3.82 ± 1.03	0.0001
Sodium (mmol/L)	134.89 ± 1.35	139.43 ± 3.20	146.86 ± 2.39	<0.0001
Chloride (mmol/L)	94.89 ± 1.35	106.13 ± 1.12	112.73 ± 1.03	<0.0001
Urea (mmol/L)	3.71 ± 0.09	5.66 ± 0.31	5.77 ± 0.14	<0.0001
Creatinine (μmol/L)	69.08 ± 1.48	86.81 ± 4.29	91.71 ± 2.38	<0.0001
Uric acid (μmol/L)	125.68 ± 1.02	157.19 ± 1.07	176.66 ± 1.05	<0.0001
Microalbuminuria (mg)	4.52 ± 1.14	5.60 ± 1.21[a]	7.38 ± 1.12	0.0336
4v-MDRD (mL/min/1.73 m^2)	127.63 ± 1.03	101.78 ± 1.13[a]	87.05 ± 1.06	0.0002
CG (mL/min/1.73 m^2)	130.24 ± 1.03	103.26 ± 1.12[a]	82.61 ± 1.05	<0.0001
CKD-EPI (mL/min/1.73 m^2)	131.23 ± 1.03	90.33 ± 1.06	81.49 ± 1.05	<0.0001

Data is presented as mean ± standard error of the mean. HPT-naïve: newly diagnosed hypertensive not on antihypertensive drugs, HPT-therapy: hypertensives on antihypertensives, SBP: systolic blood pressure, DBP: diastolic blood pressure, MAP: mean arterial pressure, WC: waist circumference, HC: hip circumference, BMI: body mass index, WHR: waist-to-hip ratio, WHtR: waist-to-height ratio, AVI: abdominal volume index, BAI: body adiposity index, 4v-MDRD: four-variable modification of diet in renal disease, CG: Cockcroft-Gault, CKD-EPI: chronic kidney disease epidemiology collaboration. Bonferroni post hoc[a]: no statistically significant difference compared with control.

[6], thus making the kidney both a cause and a victim of hypertension [5]. In the current study, chronic kidney disease was observed only among the participants presenting with hypertension, irrespective of the predictive equation used in estimating the glomerular filtration rate. The association between hypertension and CKD was also evident as percentage cluster distribution of participants presenting with chronic kidney disease predominantly segregated with the upper quartiles (3rd and 4th quartiles) of the haemodynamic indices (SBP, DBP, and pulse; see Figure 3). The strength of association was found to be more pronounced with systolic blood pressure rather than diastolic blood pressure, posing a greater risk for cardiovascular events and kidney disease progression.

Serum elevation of kidney excretory products like electrolytes and metabolites of purine and amino acid catabolism (uric acid and urea) in hypertensives has traditionally been attributed to decreased glomerular filtration rate (GFR) as a result of the effect of hypertension on renal function. A reduction in renal blood flow as a consequence of increasing renal vascular resistance leads to decreased distal tubular flow rate which leads to increased reabsorption and decreased excretion [68, 79, 80]. Significantly higher levels of serum electrolytes as well as urea and uric acid were observed among the hypertensive subgroup compared to their normotensive counterparts (see Table 2). The assertion that serum kidney excretory products are only secondary to residual confounding factors that have a pathogenically inert relationship with hypertension and renal disease is giving way. Serum kidney excretory products are now viewed as pathophysiologically active independent attribution factors for the cause and progression of hypertension and renal disease [81–85].

Linear additive relationship was observed for all serum electrolytes as well as urea and uric acid with progressive quartile increment of haemodynamic indices measured in this study. After adjusting for age and gender in the present study, surfeit urea and uric acid were significantly associated with renal insufficiency (see Table 3). Often considered a beneficial antioxidant, recent epidemiologic and experimental studies have demonstrated that hyperuricaemia is a major and an independent risk factor for the development of renal disease, hypertension, and adverse cardiovascular outcome [79, 83, 84, 86, 87]. Possible adverse effects of uric acid on the vasculature have been linked to increased chemokine and cytokine expression [88], induction of renal vasoconstriction mediated by endothelial dysfunction, activation of the renin-angiotensin system [87], and stimulation of oxidative stress in vascular smooth muscle cell (VSMC) proliferation, mediated

TABLE 4: Partial correlation coefficients of haemodynamic parameters, anthropometric variables, and biochemical kidney markers of study population (upper right sided) and indices of hypertension group (lower left sided), adjusted for age and gender.

Index	SBP	DBP	Pulse	MAP	WC	HC	BMI	WHR	WHtR	CI	AVI	BAI	K^+	Na^+	CL^-	Urea	Creat	UA	MA	MDRD	CG	EPI
SBP		.51**	.20**	.85**	.20**	.16*	−0.03	0.04	.19**	.24**	.18**	.30**	0.07	.23**	.39**	.21**	.15*	0.10	−0.09	−0.03	−0.01	−0.06
DBP	.39**		.25**	.89**	.19**	.19**	0.05	0.00	0.12	.17**	.16*	.28**	0.01	.35**	.52**	0.11	.13*	0.01	0.01	0.00	0.08	−0.02
Pulse	0.02	0.01		.26**	.64**	.69**	.17**	0.07	.58**	.57**	.68**	.66**	.22**	.20**	.40**	.22**	0.05	.29**	0.01	−0.01	0.11	−0.01
MAP	.83**	.83**	0.02		.22**	.20**	0.01	0.02	.18**	.24**	.19**	.31**	0.04	.33**	.53**	.18**	.16*	0.06	−0.04	−0.01	0.04	−0.05
WC	0.04	−0.07	.60**	−0.02		.95**	.37**	0.1	.93**	.89**	.99**	.86**	.19**	.14*	.40**	.29**	.21**	.44**	0.08	−.18**	0.03	−.20**
HC	0.02	−0.04	.66**	−0.01	.94**		.33**	−0.12	.88**	.84**	.96**	.90**	.23**	.13*	.35**	.26**	.21**	.47**	0.06	−.21**	−0.01	−.21**
BMI	−0.06	0.01	.18*	−0.03	.37**	.32**		0.03	.47**	−0.03	.33**	.43**	0.02	0.00	0.09	0.01	0.06	−0.03	0.12	−0.11	.19**	−0.10
WHR	0.04	−0.02	0.08	0.01	0.07	−.16*	0.00		0.10	0.10	0.09	−0.10	−0.04	0.00	0.03	0.07	−0.08	−0.09	0.01	.17**	.18**	0.09
WHtR	0.07	−0.09	.55**	−0.01	.93**	.86**	.42**	0.07		.80**	.92**	.95**	.16*	0.12	.33**	.29**	.20**	.43**	0.1	−.21**	−0.04	−.22**
CI	0.10	−0.08	.51**	0.01	.87**	.81**	−0.09	0.08	.80**		.89**	.75**	.16*	.15*	.37**	.29**	.19**	.49**	0.05	−.16*	−0.1	−.18**
AVI	0.04	−0.07	.65**	−0.02	.99**	.96**	.33**	0.07	.92**	.87**		.88**	.21**	0.11	.36**	.29**	.20**	.46**	0.07	−.18**	0.01	−.20**
BAI	0.05	−0.07	.60**	−0.01	.86**	.89**	.39**	−0.13	.95**	.73**	.87**		.24**	.25**	.40**	.35**	.27**	.52**	0.11	−.30**	−.14*	−.32**
K^+	0.02	−0.10	.21**	−0.05	.20**	.24**	0.09	−0.05	.19*	.15*	.22**	.21**		.21**	0.11	.20**	.16*	.19**	−0.03	−.14*	−0.1	−0.11
Na^+	0.06	.16*	0.04	0.14	−0.06	−0.04	−0.04	−0.02	−0.04	0.04*	0.06	−0.02	.20**		.35**	.16*	0.10	−0.03	−0.02	0.08	0.11	0.02
CL^-	0.12	0.10	0.09	0.13	0.14	0.11	0.04	0.06	0.10	0.12	.16*	0.06	0.03	0.03		.31**	.18**	.21**	0.08	−0.04	0.08	−0.08
Urea	0.09	−0.12	0.08	−0.02	.20**	.17*	0.00	0.09	.22**	.19*	.21**	.20**	.18*	0.04	0.02		.38**	.29**	−0.05	−.23**	−.18**	−.27**
Creat	0.09	0.04	−0.03	0.08	.17*	.17*	0.07	−0.11	.17*	0.14*	.16*	.17*	0.15	0.05	0.06	.36**		.30**	0.02	−.80**	−.73**	−.79**
UA	0.02	−0.14	.24**	−0.07	.45**	.46**	−0.06	−0.13	.43**	.49**	.45**	.42**	.18*	−0.12	0.11	.24**	.27**		0.02	−.29**	−.27**	−.27**
MA	−0.13	−0.06	−0.04	−0.11	0.02	0.00	0.10	0.04	0.05	0.00	0.02	0.03	−0.04	−0.08	0.09	−0.09	0.03	0.03		−0.05	−0.03	−0.05
MDRD	−0.02	0.04	0.01	0.01	−.20**	−.22**	−0.13	0.21	−.22**	−.16*	−.19*	−.24**	−.15*	0.10	0.00	−.23**	−.81**	−.29**	−0.06		.92**	.90**
CG	−0.05	0.05	0.08	−0.01	−0.06	−0.09	.15*	0.20	−0.12	−.19*	−0.06	−.16*	−0.12	0.07	0.04	−.23**	−.77**	−.29**	−0.07	.94**		.81**
EPI	−0.03	0.05	0.04	0.01	−.20**	−.21**	−0.13	0.11	−.22**	−.17*	−.19*	−.22**	−0.12	0.05	−0.01	−.26**	−.80**	−.26**	−0.06	.90**	.83**	

SBP: systolic blood pressure, DBP: diastolic blood pressure, MAP: mean arterial pressure, WC: waist circumference, HC: hip circumference, BMI: body mass index, WHR: waist-to-hip ratio, WHtR: waist-to-height ratio, CI: conicity index, AVI: abdominal volume index, K^+: potassium, Na^+: sodium, CL^-: chloride, creat: creatinine, UA: uric acid, MA: microalbumin, MDRD: four-variable modification of diet in renal disease, CG: Cockcroft-Gault, and EPI: chronic kidney disease epidemiology collaboration. *Correlation is significant at 0.05 and **correlation is significant at 0.01.

TABLE 5: Estimates of the prevalence of CKD in the study population using the renal function equations.

Parameter	4v-MDRD			CG			CKD-EPI		
eGFR (mL/min/1.73 m^2)	Total	Control	Case	Total	Control	Case	Total	Control	Case
Stage 1 (≥90)	120 (49.80)	57 (93.40)	63 (35.00)	136 (56.40)	57 (93.40)	79 (43.90)	117 (48.50)	59 (96.70)	58 (32.20)
Stage 2 (60 to 89)	89 (36.90)	4 (6.60)	85 (47.20)	65 (27.00)	4 (6.60)	61 (33.90)	89 (36.90)	2 (3.30)	87 (48.30)
Stage 3 (30 to 59)	32 (13.30)	0 (0.00)	32 (17.80)	39 (16.20)	0 (0.00)	39 (21.70)	35 (14.50)	0 (0.00)	35 (14.50)
Stage 4 (15 to 29)	0 (0.00)	0 (0.00)	0 (0.00)	1 (0.40)	0 (0.00)	1 (0.60)	0 (0.00)	0 (0.00)	0 (0.00)
Stage 5 (<15)	0 (0.00)	0 (0.00)	0 (0.00)	0 (0.00)	0 (0.00)	0 (0.00)	0 (0.00)	0 (0.00)	0 (0.00)
CKD (Stages 3 + 4 + 5)	32 (13.30)	0 (0.00)	32 (17.80)	40 (16.60)	0 (0.00)	40 (22.22)	35 (14.50)	0 (0.00)	35 (19.40)

Data is presented as absolute values with corresponding percentage in parenthesis. 4v-MDRD: four variable modification of diet in renal disease, CG: Cockcroft-Gault, CKD-EPI: chronic kidney disease epidemiology collaboration, eGFR: estimated glomerular filtration rate, and CKD: chronic kidney disease.

TABLE 6: Staged renal insufficiency stratified by the presence of clinical manifestation of cardiac disorder (nonspecific sinuses, left ventricular hypertrophy, and heart enlargement).

Parameter	Equation	Condition	Stage 1	Stage 2	Stage 3	Stage 4	p value
Left ventricular hypertrophy (electrocardiograph)	4v-MDRD	*Absent*	66 (74.12)	17 (19.10)	6 (6.74)	0 (0.00)	$p < 0.0001$
		Present	54 (35.53)	72 (47.37)	26 (17.11)	0 (0.00)	
	CG	*Absent*	68 (76.40)	12 (13.48)	9 (10.11)	0 (0.00)	$p < 0.0001$
		Present	68 (44.74)	53 (34.87)	30 (19.74)	1 (0.67)	
	CKD-EPI	*Absent*	66 (74.16)	17 (19.10)	6 (6.74)	0 (0.00)	$p < 0.0001$
		Present	51 (33.55)	72 (47.37)	29 (19.08)	0 (0.00)	
Left ventricular hypertrophy (echocardiograph)	4v-MDRD	*Absent*	62 (76.54)	16 (19.75)	3 (3.70)	0 (0.00)	$p < 0.0001$
		Present	58 (36.25)	73 (45.63)	29 (18.13)	0 (0.00)	
	CG	*Absent*	65 (80.25)	12 (14.83)	4 (4.94)	0 (0.00)	$p < 0.0001$
		Present	71 (44.38)	53 (33.13)	35 (21.88)	1 (0.63)	
	CKD-EPI	*Absent*	64 (79.00)	14 (17.30)	3 (3.70)	0 (0.00)	$p < 0.0001$
		Present	53 (33.10)	75 (46.90)	32 (20.00)	0 (0.00)	
Cardiomegaly (X-ray)	4v-MDRD	*Absent*	74 (71.80)	21 (20.40)	8 (7.80)	0 (0.00)	$p < 0.0001$
		Present	46 (33.30)	68 (49.30)	24 (17.40)	0 (0.00)	
	CG	*Absent*	79 (76.70)	18 (17.48)	6 (5.83)	0 (0.00)	$p < 0.0001$
		Present	57 (41.30)	47 (34.06)	33 (23.91)	1 (0.73)	
	CKD-EPI	*Absent*	64 (79.00)	14 (17.30)	3 (3.70)	0 (0.00)	$p < 0.0001$
		Present	53 (33.10)	75 (46.90)	32 (20.00)	0 (0.00)	

Data is presented as figure with percentage in parenthesis. 4v-MDRD: four-variable modification of diet in renal disease, CG: Cockcroft-Gault, and CKD-EPI: chronic kidney disease epidemiology collaboration equation.

by the mitogen-activated protein (MAP) kinase pathway [89] and increased vascular C-reactive protein (CRP) expression [88].

5. Conclusion

In this urban population, chronic kidney disease was associated with hypertension and cardiac abnormalities. Adiposity was associated with hypertension and renal insufficiency. Modifiable lifestyle practices (smoking and alcoholism) increased the risk of hypertension, whilst smoking increased kidney target organ damage among hypertensives.

Additional Points

Limitation of Study. The threshold dose level of alcohol intake could not be established from this study; thus, inferences for causality of alcohol dose response were not feasible. Further studies will be required to help determine the threshold dose of alcohol intake.

Ethical Approval

The participation of the respondents who are all indigenes of Ghana was voluntary and informed consent was obtained from each of them after thorough explanation of what the study entailed. This study was approved by the School of Medical Sciences and KATH Committee on Human Research Publications and Ethics (CHRPE/08/11).

Competing Interests

The authors have declared that no competing interests exist.

Authors' Contributions

This work was carried out in collaboration between all authors. Authors William K. B. A. Owiredu, Isaac K. Owusu, Edwin F. Laing, Ellis Owusu-Dabo, and James Osei-Yeboah conceptualized and designed the study. Authors Isaac K. Owusu, Christiana Aryee, and Ellis Owusu-Dabo recruited the study participants. Authors Isaac K. Owusu, Christiana Aryee, James Osei-Yeboah, William K. B. A. Owiredu, and Ellis Owusu-Dabo generated the data. Authors Christiana Aryee, James Osei-Yeboah, William K. B. A. Owiredu, and Isaac K. Owusu analyzed the data. Authors Isaac K. Owusu, Christiana Aryee, William K. B. A. Owiredu, and James Osei-Yeboah drafted the manuscript. Authors Isaac K. Owusu, Christiana Aryee, William K. B. A. Owiredu, James Osei-Yeboah, Ellis Owusu-Dabo, and Edwin F. Laing reviewed the manuscript for intellectual content and each author approved the final manuscript.

Acknowledgments

The authors' gratitude goes to the doctors, nurses, and ancillary staff of the cardiac clinic of Komfo Anokye Teaching Hospital for their assistance during the study period. The authors are also most grateful to the nurses of the Precise Specialist Clinic for their dedicated service during the segment of the study at their clinic. The authors are most indebted to the Biomedical Scientists at the Kumasi Centre for Collaborative Research in Tropical Medicine especially Mr. Michael Frimpong and Miss Esimebia Agbodidi for their assistance in the assays. The authors are thankful for the insightful suggestions of Dr. Christian Obirikorang, Department of Molecular Medicine.

References

[1] D. B. Munaretti, A. R. Barbosa, M. D. F. N. Marucci, and M. L. Lebrão, "Self-rated hypertension and anthropometric indicators of body fat in elderly," *Revista da Associacao Medica Brasileira*, vol. 57, no. 1, pp. 25–30, 2011.

[2] G. Ogedegbe, J. Plange-Rhule, J. Gyamfi et al., "A cluster-randomized trial of task shifting and blood pressure control in Ghana: study protocol," *Implementation Science*, vol. 9, no. 1, article 73, 2014.

[3] P. Stenvinkel, J. J. Carrero, J. Axelsson, B. Lindholm, O. Heimbürger, and Z. Massy, "Emerging biomarkers for evaluating cardiovascular risk in the chronic kidney disease patient: how do new pieces fit into the uremic puzzle?" *Clinical Journal of the American Society of Nephrology*, vol. 3, no. 2, pp. 505–521, 2008.

[4] M. K. Haroun, B. G. Jaar, S. C. Hoffman, G. W. Comstock, M. J. Klag, and J. Coresh, "Risk factors for chronic kidney disease: a prospective study of 23,534 men and women in Washington County, Maryland," *Journal of the American Society of Nephrology*, vol. 14, no. 11, pp. 2934–2941, 2003.

[5] E. Morgado and P. L. Neves, "Hypertension and chronic kidney disease: cause and consequence-therapeutic considerations," in *Antihypertensive Drugs*, 2012.

[6] F. M. Tedla, A. Brar, R. Browne, and C. Brown, "Hypertension in chronic kidney disease: navigating the evidence," *International Journal of Hypertension*, vol. 2011, Article ID 132405, 9 pages, 2011.

[7] Y. Commodore-Mensah, L. J. Samuel, C. R. Dennison-Himmelfarb, and C. Agyemang, "Hypertension and overweight/obesity in Ghanaians and Nigerians living in West Africa and industrialized countries: a systematic review," *Journal of Hypertension*, vol. 32, no. 3, pp. 464–472, 2014.

[8] W. Owiredu, R. Ephraim, N. Amidu, B. E. Jnr, and E. Laing, "Oxidative stress among ghanaian patients presenting with chronic kidney disease," *Journal of Medical and Biomedical Sciences*, vol. 1, no. 1, pp. 28–37, 2012.

[9] K. Entsua-Mensah, A. Doku, and I. Adzamli, "The National cardiothoracic centre, Accra Ghana: proceedings of the second International update course in cardiology—improving the coverage of cardiology services," *Pan African Medical Journal*, vol. 11, no. 1, 2012.

[10] J. Addo, C. Agyemang, L. Smeeth, A. D. G. Aikins, A. K. Edusei, and O. Ogedegbe, "A review of population-based studies on hypertension in Ghana," *Ghana Medical Journal*, vol. 46, no. 2, pp. 4–11, 2012.

[11] S. Agyei-Mensah and A. de-Graft Aikins, "Epidemiological transition and the double burden of disease in Accra, Ghana," *Journal of Urban Health*, vol. 87, no. 5, pp. 879–897, 2010.

[12] G. Santulli, M. Ciccarelli, B. Trimarco, and G. Iaccarino, "Physical activity ameliorates cardiovascular health in elderly subjects: the functional role of the β adrenergic system," *Frontiers in Physiology*, vol. 4, article 209, 2013.

[13] R. Biritwum, J. Gyapong, and G. Mensah, "The epidemiology of obesity in Ghana," *Ghana Medical Journal*, vol. 39, no. 3, p. 82, 2005.

[14] E.-M. Backé, A. Seidler, U. Latza, K. Rossnagel, and B. Schumann, "The role of psychosocial stress at work for the development of cardiovascular diseases—a systematic review," *International Archives of Occupational and Environmental Health*, vol. 85, no. 1, pp. 67–79, 2012.

[15] R. Gillum, M. Mussolino, and J. Madans, "Body fat distribution and hypertension incidence in women and men. The NHANES I epidemiologic follow-up study," *International Journal of Obesity and Related Metabolic Disorders*, vol. 22, no. 2, pp. 127–134, 1998.

[16] D. Blair, J.-P. Habicht, E. A. Sims, D. Sylwester, and S. Abraham, "Evidence for an increased risk for hypertension with centrally located body fat and the effect of race and sex on this risk," *American Journal of Epidemiology*, vol. 119, no. 4, pp. 526–540, 1984.

[17] P. Parab-Waingankar and S. Rao, "Obesity and hypertension among urban affluent adult males from Pune, India," *The Indian Journal of Nutrition and Dietetics*, vol. 52, no. 1, pp. 32–44, 2015.

[18] A. Chandra and A. T. Turer, "Reply: does body adiposity better predict obesity-associated cardiometabolic risk than body mass index?" *Journal of the American College of Cardiology*, vol. 65, no. 6, pp. 633–633, 2015.

[19] S. Anoop, A. Misra, S. Bhardwaj, and S. Gulati, "High body fat and low muscle mass are associated with increased arterial stiffness in Asian Indians in North India," *Journal of Diabetes and Its Complications*, vol. 29, no. 1, pp. 38–43, 2015.

[20] S. Wang, Y. Liu, F. Li, H. Jia, L. Liu, and F. Xue, "A novel quantitative body shape score for detecting association between obesity and hypertension in China," *BMC Public Health*, vol. 15, no. 1, article 7, 2015.

[21] Y.-X. Zhang and S.-R. Wang, "Distribution of subcutaneous fat and the relationship with blood pressure in obese children

and adolescents in Shandong, China," *Paediatric and Perinatal Epidemiology*, vol. 29, no. 2, pp. 156–161, 2015.

[22] N. C. Sundgren, W. Vongpatanasin, B.-M. D. Boggan et al., "IgG receptor FcγRIIB plays a key role in obesity-induced hypertension," *Hypertension*, vol. 65, no. 2, pp. 456–462, 2015.

[23] J. Axelsson, "The emerging biology of adipose tissue in chronic kidney disease: from fat to facts," *Nephrology Dialysis Transplantation*, vol. 23, no. 10, pp. 3041–3046, 2008.

[24] P. Iglesias and J. J. Díez, "Adipose tissue in renal disease: clinical significance and prognostic implications," *Nephrology Dialysis Transplantation*, vol. 25, no. 7, pp. 2066–2077, 2010.

[25] R. Agarwal, J. E. Bills, and R. P. Light, "Diagnosing obesity by body mass index in chronic kidney disease: an explanation for the 'obesity paradox?'," *Hypertension*, vol. 56, no. 5, pp. 893–900, 2010.

[26] I. K. Owusu, C. Aryee, W. K. Owiredu, J. Osei-Yeboah, E. Owusu-Dabo, and E. Laing, "Analysis of atherogenic and anthropometric profiles of normotensive and hypertensive ghanaians in the kumasi metropolis," *British Journal of Medicine and Medical Research*, vol. 7, no. 5, pp. 378–397, 2015.

[27] D. Lemogoum, Y. K. Seedat, A. F. B. Mabadeje et al., "Recommendations for prevention, diagnosis and management of hypertension and cardiovascular risk factors in sub-Saharan Africa," *Journal of Hypertension*, vol. 21, no. 11, pp. 1993–2000, 2003.

[28] I. K. Owusu, "Causes of heart failure as seen in Kumasi Ghana," *Internet Journal of Third World Medicine*, vol. 4, no. 3, 2007.

[29] M. Ruperto, G. Barril, and F. J. Sánchez-Muniz, "Conicity index as a contributor marker of inflammation in haemodialysis patients," *Nutricion Hospitalaria*, vol. 28, no. 5, pp. 1688–1695, 2013.

[30] M. Vuga, "Conceptual review of issues with practical abdominal obesity measures," in *Section on Statistics in Epidemiology-JSM*, 2009.

[31] R. Lategan, V. L. Van den Berg, and C. M. Walsh, "Body adiposity indices are associated with hypertension in a black, urban Free State community: original research," *African Primary Health Care and Family Medicine*, vol. 6, no. 1, pp. 1–7, 2014.

[32] KDOQI, "Clinical practice guidelines and clinical practice recommendations for anemia in chronic kidney disease," *American Journal of Kidney Diseases*, vol. 47, pp. S11–S145, 2006.

[33] A. S. Levey, K.-U. Eckardt, Y. Tsukamoto et al., "Definition and classification of chronic kidney disease: a position statement from Kidney Disease: Improving Global Outcomes (KDIGO)," *Kidney International*, vol. 67, no. 6, pp. 2089–2100, 2005.

[34] P. A. McKee, W. P. Castelli, P. M. McNamara, and W. B. Kannel, "The natural history of congestive heart failure: the Framingham study," *The New England Journal of Medicine*, vol. 285, no. 26, pp. 1441–1446, 1971.

[35] J. Addo, L. Smeeth, and D. A. Leon, "Hypertensive target organ damage in Ghanaian civil servants with hypertension," *PLoS ONE*, vol. 4, no. 8, Article ID e6672, 2009.

[36] C. Osafo, M. Mate-Kole, K. Affram, and D. Adu, "Prevalence of chronic kidney disease in hypertensive patients in ghana," *Renal Failure*, vol. 33, no. 4, pp. 388–392, 2011.

[37] D. Adu, "Haemodialysis treatment for end stage chronic kidney disease and acute kidney injury in Africa," *Ghana Medical Journal*, vol. 47, no. 1, pp. 1–2, 2013.

[38] H.-Y. Shin, M.-H. Shin, and J.-A. Rhee, "Gender differences in the association between self-rated health and hypertension in a Korean adult population," *BMC Public Health*, vol. 12, article 135, 2012.

[39] A. A. Saeed, N. A. Al-Hamdan, A. A. Bahnassy, A. M. Abdalla, M. A. F. Abbas, and L. Z. Abuzaid, "Prevalence, awareness, treatment, and control of hypertension among Saudi adult population: a national survey," *International Journal of Hypertension*, vol. 2011, Article ID 174135, 8 pages, 2011.

[40] Y. Wang, X. Chen, Y. Song, B. Caballero, and L. J. Cheskin, "Association between obesity and kidney disease: a systematic review and meta-analysis," *Kidney International*, vol. 73, no. 1, pp. 19–33, 2008.

[41] A. G. B. Amoah, "Sociodemographic variations in obesity among Ghanaian adults," *Public Health Nutrition*, vol. 6, no. 8, pp. 751–757, 2003.

[42] W. K. Bosu, "Epidemic of hypertension in Ghana: a systematic review," *BMC Public Health*, vol. 10, no. 1, article 418, 2010.

[43] A. A. Newlove, W. B. Owusu, and A. Charles, "The relationship between lifestyle variables, blood pressure and dietary habits of male adult miners in Ghana," *Asian Journal of Clinical Nutrition*, vol. 4, no. 3, pp. 98–106, 2012.

[44] L. J. Beilin and I. B. Puddey, "Alcohol and hypertension," *Clinical and Experimental Hypertension—Part A: Theory and Practice*, vol. 14, no. 1-2, pp. 119–138, 1992.

[45] J. F. Potter, L. T. Bannan, and D. G. Beevers, "Alcohol and hypertension," *British Journal of Addiction*, vol. 79, no. 4, pp. 365–372, 1984.

[46] A. L. Klatsky, "Alcohol-associated hypertension: when one drinks makes a difference," *Hypertension*, vol. 44, no. 6, pp. 805–806, 2004.

[47] S. C. Renaud, R. Guéguen, P. Conard, D. Lanzmann-Petithory, J.-M. Orgogozo, and O. Henry, "Moderate wine drinkers have lower hypertension-related mortality: a prospective cohort study in French men," *American Journal of Clinical Nutrition*, vol. 80, no. 3, pp. 621–625, 2004.

[48] K. Reynolds, D. Gu, J. Chen et al., "Alcohol consumption and the risk of end-stage renal disease among Chinese men," *Kidney International*, vol. 73, no. 7, pp. 870–876, 2008.

[49] M. C. Dufour, "What is moderate drinking," *Alcohol Research & Health*, vol. 23, no. 1, pp. 5–14, 1999.

[50] D. P. Agarwal, "Cardioprotective effects of light-moderate consumption of alcohol: a review of putative mechanisms," *Alcohol and Alcoholism*, vol. 37, no. 5, pp. 409–415, 2002.

[51] B. O. Åsvold, J. H. Bjørngaard, D. Carslake et al., "Causal associations of tobacco smoking with cardiovascular risk factors: a Mendelian randomization analysis of the HUNT study in Norway," *International Journal of Epidemiology*, vol. 43, no. 5, pp. 1458–1470, 2014.

[52] V. Hamrefors, B. Hedblad, G. Hindy et al., "Smoking modifies the associated increased risk of future cardiovascular disease by genetic variation on chromosome 9p21," *PLoS ONE*, vol. 9, no. 1, Article ID e85893, 2014.

[53] N. Ishizaka, Y. Ishizaka, E.-I. Toda et al., "Association between cigarette smoking and chronic kidney disease in Japanese men," *Hypertension Research*, vol. 31, no. 3, pp. 485–492, 2008.

[54] S. R. Orth, H. Ogata, and E. Ritz, "Smoking and the kidney," *Nephrology Dialysis Transplantation*, vol. 15, no. 10, pp. 1509–1511, 2000.

[55] W. C. Willett, A. Green, M. J. Stampfer et al., "Relative and absolute excess risks of coronary heart disease among women who smoke cigarettes," *The New England Journal of Medicine*, vol. 317, no. 21, pp. 1303–1309, 1987.

[56] F. Doyle, D. Rohde, A. Rutkowska, K. Morgan, G. Cousins, and H. McGee, "Systematic review and meta-analysis of the impact

of depression on subsequent smoking cessation in patients with coronary heart disease: 1990 to 2013," *Psychosomatic Medicine*, vol. 76, no. 1, pp. 44–57, 2014.

[57] A. S. Go, D. Mozaffarian, V. L. Roger et al., "Heart disease and stroke statistics 2014 update: a report from the American Heart Association," *Circulation*, vol. 129, no. 3, pp. e28–e292, 2014.

[58] R. M. Nance, J. A. Delaney, M. Blaha et al., "Abstract P133: modeling smoking in relation to cardiovascular disease risk in the multi-ethnic study of atherosclerosis (MESA)," *Circulation*, vol. 129, supplement 1, Article ID AP133, 2014.

[59] J. S. Tolstrup, U. A. Hvidtfeldt, E. M. Flachs et al., "Smoking and risk of coronary heart disease in younger, middle-aged, and older adults," *American Journal of Public Health*, vol. 104, no. 1, pp. 96–102, 2014.

[60] I. Maeda, T. Hayashi, K. K. Sato et al., "Cigarette smoking and the association with glomerular hyperfiltration and proteinuria in healthy middle-aged men," *Clinical Journal of the American Society of Nephrology*, vol. 6, no. 10, pp. 2462–2469, 2011.

[61] L. Ryom, A. Mocroft, O. Kirk et al., "Predictors of advanced chronic kidney disease and end-stage renal disease in HIV-positive persons," *AIDS*, vol. 28, no. 2, pp. 187–199, 2014.

[62] K. Yamagata, K. Ishida, T. Sairenchi et al., "Risk factors for chronic kidney disease in a community-based population: a 10-year follow-up study," *Kidney International*, vol. 71, no. 2, pp. 159–166, 2007.

[63] B. Stengel, M. E. Tarver-Carr, N. R. Powe, M. S. Eberhardt, and F. L. Brancati, "Lifestyle factors, obesity and the risk of chronic kidney disease," *Epidemiology*, vol. 14, no. 4, pp. 479–487, 2003.

[64] S. R. Orth and S. I. Hallan, "Smoking: a risk factor for progression of chronic kidney disease and for cardiovascular morbidity and mortality in renal patients—absence of evidence or evidence of absence?" *Clinical Journal of the American Society of Nephrology*, vol. 3, no. 1, pp. 226–236, 2008.

[65] J. E. Hall, J. R. Henegar, T. M. Dwyer et al., "Is obesity a major cause of chronic kidney disease?" *Advances in Renal Replacement Therapy*, vol. 11, no. 1, pp. 41–54, 2004.

[66] P. Mathieu, P. Poirier, P. Pibarot, I. Lemieux, and J.-P. Després, "Visceral obesity the link among inflammation, hypertension, and cardiovascular disease," *Hypertension*, vol. 53, no. 4, pp. 577–584, 2009.

[67] R. N. Re, "Obesity-related hypertension," *Journal Information*, vol. 9, no. 3, 2009.

[68] I. A. H. AL-Hamdani, "Estimation of serum uric acid, urea and creatinine in essential hypertensive patients," *Tikrit Medical Journal*, vol. 16, no. 1, 2010.

[69] V. Kotsis, S. Stabouli, S. Papakatsika, Z. Rizos, and G. Parati, "Mechanisms of obesity-induced hypertension," *Hypertension Research*, vol. 33, no. 5, pp. 386–393, 2010.

[70] A. H. A. Mazairac and J. A. Joles, "Renal sinus adiposity and hypertension," *Hypertension*, vol. 56, no. 5, pp. 814–815, 2010.

[71] A. M. Sharma, S. Engeli, and T. Pischon, "New developments in mechanisms of obesity-induced hypertension: role of adipose tissue," *Current Hypertension Reports*, vol. 3, no. 2, pp. 152–156, 2001.

[72] J. E. Hall, A. A. da Silva, J. M. do Carmo et al., "Obesity-induced hypertension: role of sympathetic nervous system, leptin, and melanocortins," *The Journal of Biological Chemistry*, vol. 285, no. 23, pp. 17271–17276, 2010.

[73] L. Landsberg, L. J. Aronne, L. J. Beilin et al., "Obesity-related hypertension: pathogenesis, cardiovascular risk, and treatment," *The Journal of Clinical Hypertension*, vol. 15, no. 1, pp. 14–33, 2013.

[74] S. D. Navaneethan, J. P. Kirwan, S. Arrigain, M. J. Schreiber, M. J. Sarnak, and J. D. Schold, "Obesity, anthropometric measures and chronic kidney disease complications," *American Journal of Nephrology*, vol. 36, no. 3, pp. 219–227, 2012.

[75] E. Ejerblad, C. M. Fored, P. Lindblad, J. Fryzek, J. K. McLaughlin, and O. Nyrén, "Obesity and risk for chronic renal failure," *Journal of the American Society of Nephrology*, vol. 17, no. 6, pp. 1695–1702, 2006.

[76] J. E. Hall, "The kidney, hypertension, and obesity," *Hypertension*, vol. 41, no. 3, pp. 625–633, 2003.

[77] K. Rahmouni, M. L. G. Correia, W. G. Haynes, and A. L. Mark, "Obesity-associated hypertension: new insights into mechanisms," *Hypertension*, vol. 45, no. 1, pp. 9–14, 2005.

[78] G. L. Bakris and E. Ritz, "The message for World Kidney Day 2009: hypertension and kidney disease: a marriage that should be prevented," *Kidney International*, vol. 75, no. 5, pp. 449–452, 2009.

[79] R. J. Johnson, D.-H. Kang, D. Feig et al., "Is there a pathogenetic role for uric acid in hypertension and cardiovascular and renal disease?" *Hypertension*, vol. 41, no. 6, pp. 1183–1190, 2003.

[80] P. Habbu, M. Sugoor, and B. Kale, "Serum inorganic phosphorus Level along with serum potassium as a best marker in the diagnosis and prognosis of Chronic Kidney Disease (CKD)," *Journal of Chemical, Biological and Physical Sciences A*, vol. 4, no. 2, pp. 1922–1926, 2014.

[81] H. J. Adrogué and N. E. Madias, "Sodium and potassium in the pathogenesis of hypertension," *The New England Journal of Medicine*, vol. 356, no. 19, pp. 1966–1978, 2007.

[82] I. Drenjančević-Perić, B. Jelaković, J. H. Lombard, M. P. Kunert, A. Kibel, and M. Gros, "High-salt diet and hypertension: focus on the renin-angiotensin system," *Kidney and Blood Pressure Research*, vol. 34, no. 1, pp. 1–11, 2011.

[83] J. F. Baker, E. Krishnan, L. Chen, and H. R. Schumacher, "Serum uric acid and cardiovascular disease: recent developments, and where do they leave us?" *The American Journal of Medicine*, vol. 118, no. 8, pp. 816–826, 2005.

[84] P. B. Mellen, A. J. Bleyer, T. P. Erlinger et al., "Serum uric acid predicts incident hypertension in a biethnic cohort: the Atherosclerosis Risk in Communities study," *Hypertension*, vol. 48, no. 6, pp. 1037–1042, 2006.

[85] X. Zhou, L. Matavelli, and E. D. Frohlich, "Uric acid: its relationship to renal hemodynamics and the renal renin-angiotensin system," *Current Hypertension Reports*, vol. 8, no. 2, pp. 120–124, 2006.

[86] T. S. Perlstein, O. Gumieniak, G. H. Williams et al., "Uric acid and the development of hypertension: the Normative Aging Study," *Hypertension*, vol. 48, no. 6, pp. 1031–1036, 2006.

[87] R. J. Johnson, M. S. Segal, T. Srinivas et al., "Essential hypertension, progressive renal disease, and uric acid: a pathogenetic link?" *Journal of the American Society of Nephrology*, vol. 16, no. 7, pp. 1909–1919, 2005.

[88] J. Kanellis and D. H. Kang, "Uric acid as a mediator of endothelial dysfunction, inflammation, and vascular disease," *Seminars in Nephrology*, vol. 25, no. 1, pp. 39–42, 2005.

[89] D. B. Corry, P. Eslami, K. Yamamoto, M. D. Nyby, H. Makino, and M. L. Tuck, "Uric acid stimulates vascular smooth muscle cell proliferation and oxidative stress via the vascular renin-angiotensin system," *Journal of Hypertension*, vol. 26, no. 2, pp. 269–275, 2008.

Designing a Cocreated Intervention with African American Older Adults for Hypertension Self-Management

Kathy D. Wright,[1] Carolyn H. Still,[2] Lenette M. Jones,[3] and Karen O. Moss[2]

[1] *College of Nursing, Discovery Themes-Chronic Brain Injury, The Ohio State University, Columbus, OH 43210, USA*
[2] *Frances Payne Bolton School of Nursing, Case Western Reserve University, Cleveland, OH 44106-4904, USA*
[3] *School of Nursing, University of Michigan, Ann Arbor, MI 48109, USA*

Correspondence should be addressed to Kathy D. Wright; wright.2104@osu.edu

Academic Editor: Omotayo O. Erejuwa

Hypertension is a lifelong disease that requires self-management. Additionally, there are disparities in hypertension self-management that disproportionately affect African Americans. Interventions designed in collaboration with older adults have the potential to improve hypertension self-management. The purpose of this design paper is to describe the process in which African American older adults and nurse researchers cocreated an intervention to address stress in the self-management of hypertension. A semistructured interview guide was used to elicit feedback on self-management behaviors to cocreate an intervention with the participants. Participants provided constant iterative feedback on the design used for the intervention. Participants prioritized the content and mode of delivery. African American older adults with hypertension ($N = 31$; 87% women) participated in two focus group sessions. The primary stressors identified by the group that influenced their blood pressure self-management were as follows: (a) measuring blood pressure and using home blood pressure monitors; (b) difficulty communicating with family and friends; (c) sleep management and pain at night; and (d) healthy eating. Based on the participants' feedback, we created four biweekly (2-hour) group sessions that incorporated their suggestions and addressed their concerns. Health care providers can use this technique to engage African American older adults in participant-centered hypertension self-management.

1. Introduction

Hypertension self-management is complex, particularly among older African American individuals who are affected by additional factors. These factors that are thought to contribute to disparities in hypertension include low self-efficacy, limited social support, increased stress due to racism or discrimination, and perceived lack of control over whether or not one will develop hypertension [1–3]. In addition, socioeconomic disadvantages (i.e., low income, low education, and neighborhood safety) [3, 4] increase the cumulative stressors that African Americans experience and contribute to acute and chronic stress responses that interfere with self-management and produce poor health outcomes [3, 5].

Hypertension self-management includes taking prescribed medications as directed, managing daily stress, eating a balanced diet, and performing regular physical activity, each of these is associated with improved outcomes [6]. The frequency with which these activities are performed differs by race [4], with the poorest self-management and clinical outcomes being reported in African Americans [4, 5]. Because hypertension is a lifelong disease that requires self-management, there is a need to better understand the hypertension self-management strategies employed by African American older adults to improve blood pressure control [7, 8].

Studies of hypertension self-management, however, frequently do not account for the full range of contextual factors that influence African American older adults' decisions to engage in self-management behaviors. For example, African Americans who perceive stress as the cause of their hypertension are less likely to engage in self-management behaviors [9]. In addition, interventions designed on behalf of these older adults do not take into consideration personal preferences. Increasing attention is being focused on how to design an appealing and effectively tailored program for African American older adults with hypertension. Yet, little is known about the needs and preferences of African American older adults who could benefit from hypertension self-management. This insight is critical to designing and testing patient-centered interventions that are feasible and acceptable to African American older adults.

An innovative approach to gaining critical insights into designing patient-centered interventions is cocreation. *Cocreation* is a collaborative approach to engaging stakeholders in solving complex problems. Unlike community-based participatory research, cocreation can be used with smaller groups in situations when involving an entire community may not be feasible [10, 11]. In cocreation, a stakeholder is defined as an individual that can contribute to resolution of a problem and benefit from the new solution. [11]. The stakeholders are invited to collaborate with others, asked to identify the problem, and work toward an acceptable solution. Cocreation as a methodology comes from the business management literature and has been recently used in health services research to connect those in academia with clinicians, patients, and other consumers [10, 11]. Advantages of cocreation include that it engages stakeholders early and in a "real-world setting," which has the potential of increasing dissemination [11]. Successful cocreation includes creativity and shared governance with stakeholders in developing an intervention [10].

As an example, pharmacists used cocreation between physicians and patients to reduce inappropriate polypharmacy in the primary care setting [12]. *Deprescribing*, the process of stopping medications where the risks outweigh the benefits, was the focus of the cocreated intervention. The researchers identified providers as primary stakeholders and cocreation partners. Anderson et al. [12] conducted a literature review and held focus groups with 20 general practitioners to create a deprescribing program. The general practitioners wanted to have interactive training workshops, as mechanism for identifying at-risk patients. The workshops also allowed the option of referring the patient to an expert. After integrating the literature and focus group feedback, the researchers worked with a general practitioners and a computer programmer to design a software query. The query was designed to be used with the existing electronic medical record software [12]. The intervention cocreated by the researchers and general practitioners was designed to be practical and protocol-driven, to ease the burden of use during the patient encounter. The outcomes they expected to improve were a reduction of unnecessary medications and increased patient and general practitioner satisfaction.

Based on the previous evidence supporting cocreation, we decided to cocreate a hypertension self-management intervention with community-dwelling African American older adults. The purpose of this paper is to describe the process of cocreation to develop a hypertension self-management intervention in our sample.

2. Materials and Methods

We used the cocreation approach to conduct focus groups to develop an intervention for hypertension self-management with African American older adults. In our study, the older adult is the stakeholder who engages in self-management of health. The focus group design was used to gather participants' perspectives on engaging in self-management activities such as sleep hygiene, exercise, diet, meditation, prayer, smartphones, healthy self-management behaviors, and other participant-generated stress reduction activities. The focus group study was approved by the University Hospitals of Cleveland Institutional Review Board.

2.1. Participants. A sample of community-dwelling African American adults aged 60 and older with a self-reported diagnosis of hypertension were recruited. Potential participants were assessed from the general community and using an established research participant registry maintained by the principal investigator (PI) from previous research conducted in the community. Participants were screened by phone to ensure that enrollment criteria were met. Inclusion criteria were as follows: (1) self-identified as African American, (2) a diagnosis of hypertension, and (3) a reported age of 60 years or older. Exclusion criteria were as follows: (1) non-English speaking or (2) a diagnosis of severe cognitive impairment. Based on their availability to attend the focus group sessions, participants self-selected into two groups (a Wednesday group and a Saturday group). Each of the groups met twice for session that lasted two hours.

2.2. Materials. A demographic data sheet was developed for age, gender, and race. A digital voice recorder and paper for writing field notes were used for the focus group sessions. A graphic recorder was present during one of the focus groups and systematically graphed (using pictures and words) the thoughts expressed by the participants. REDCap data management and survey program was used to store the data on a secure server.

2.3. Procedure. The focus group and the cocreated intervention sessions were held in a private meeting room at a local older adult community center. Additional details related to the convenience and comfort of participants (e.g., free parking and venue near participants' homes) were used in selecting the location for the focus groups and subsequent participant cocreated intervention. To mitigate issues related to transportation, bus passes ($5.00 each), taxi cabs (average cost $30.00 round trip), or gas cards ($5.00 each) were provided to each participant to defray the cost of travel. The participants were surveyed as to the best dates and times to meet. The schedule was created and adapted so that the maximum number of participants could attend.

At the beginning of each session, the PI made introductory comments and asked each participant to speak one at a time without the use of personal identifiers to maintain privacy. Three graduate student-nurse research assistants (two African American women and one Native American man) were present to assist with notetaking and facilitation of the discussion. Participants were reminded at the beginning of each meeting, as indicated in the consent form, that the session would be audio-recorded. Cocreated ground rules were initially established and maintained for each session.

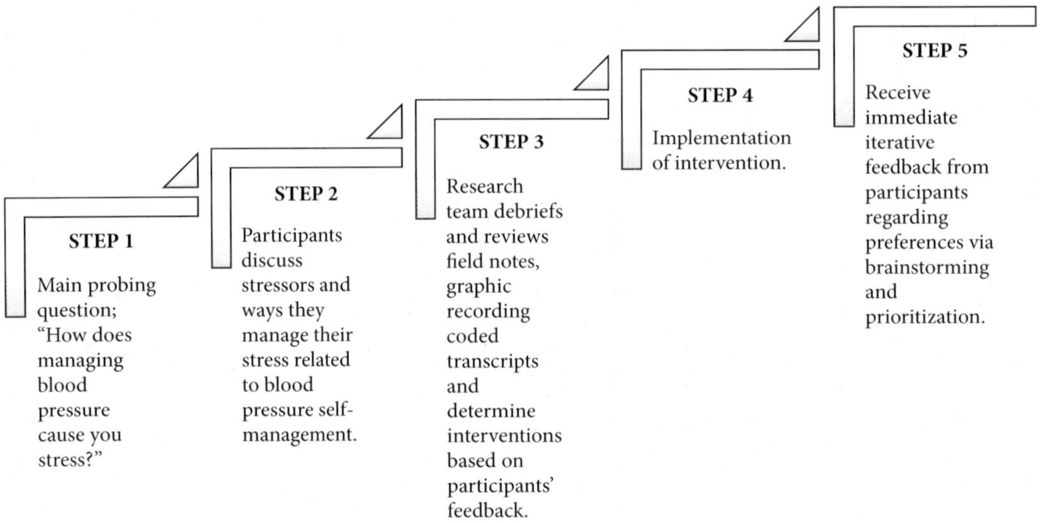

FIGURE 1: Steps to develop the cocreated intervention from focus group sessions.

The session began with focus group questions to elicit their preferences for hypertension self-management.

To determine the types of activities participants might want and suggestions for adaptation, the PI demonstrated proposed activities. The PI demonstrated a 15-minute mindfulness exercise, a strategy to reduce stress and promote relaxation [13]. Participants then completed the mindfulness exercise while in a seated position. In addition, a single content component of a kindness-based meditation was demonstrated, delivered by using the free Stop, Breathe & Think™ application. Finally, we discussed the Dietary Approaches to Stop Hypertension (DASH) diet [14], commonly recommended to people with hypertension, and each participant was provided a copy of the diet [15]. Participants were free to opt out of any of the activities. We elicited feedback on each of the activities to develop the cocreated intervention.

Investigators collected field notes during the focus group sessions in addition to audio recordings. Debriefings were held after each focus group session among with principal investigator and research assistants to review field notes to identify the preferred content for an intervention. During the debriefing session, we listed out the common themes that arose from our field notes and direct observation. Using an iterative process and member fact checking [16], the content of the intervention was verified. In the follow-up session with participants, we used fact checking to test the components of the intervention. We used brainstorming with the participants to prioritize the list of preferred interventions.

Participants returned 14–21 days later for a second focus group. The PI provided a sample presentation of the cocreated intervention based on the feedback and preferences from the previous focus group sessions. Brainstorming was used to design the content of the cocreated intervention [17]. The top 3–5 recommendations from the group were included in the intervention design. A detailed report of the content analysis that led to the intervention development that included three rounds of coding is under review in [17]. Figure 1 illustrates an example of the decision process that was used to provide content for the intervention.

At the end of each focus group, participants received an honorarium in the form of a $50 gift card. Participants that participated in both groups received a total of $100. If a participant was unable to attend the second focus group session, we offered a one-on-one appointment with a research staff member, to ensure that their preferences for the intervention content would be included in the cocreated intervention.

2.4. Analytical Approach. Data analysis began after data were collected from the first focus group. The research team met between focus groups to begin designing a prototype of the intervention that was reviewed with participants at each focus group session (two cohorts met twice each). Data processing focused on identifying salient themes that informed the subsequent focus groups. Each transcript was checked for accuracy against the audio recordings. All transcribed data were deidentified, and audio files were destroyed once the transcripts were verified. A beginning list of themes was reviewed and verified by participants during each focus group session, which led the discussion for the cocreated intervention. This manuscript presents information on the design process used for the cocreated intervention. The results from the qualitative analyses are presented in a separate paper [17].

Investigator generated satisfaction surveys adapted from Bowen et al. [18] were distributed to gather data regarding overall satisfaction with the intervention, intent to use the intervention in the future, appropriateness of the intervention, and cultural relevance. The questions were on a visual analog scale with responses ranging from 1 (very poor) to 10 (excellent).

3. Results

Table 1 displays the demographic characteristics of the sample. Of the 49 African American older adults that were

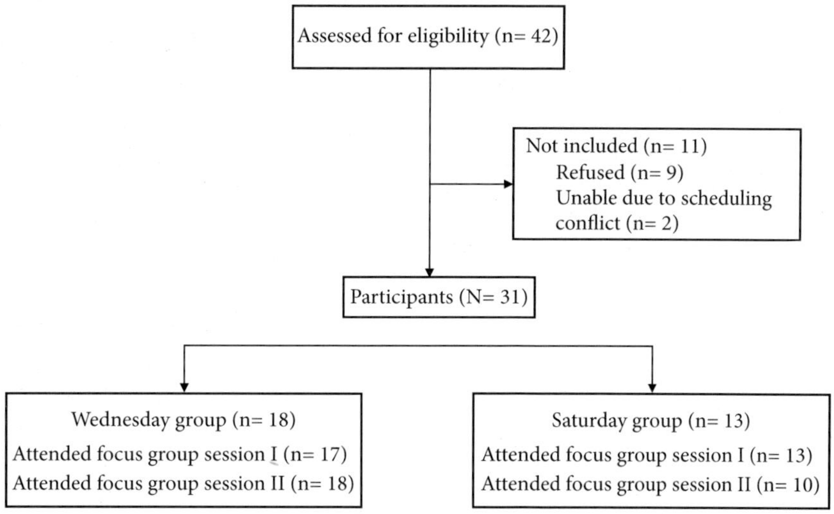

FIGURE 2: Recruitment, enrollment, and participation in focus group sessions.

TABLE 1: Demographic characteristics of community dwelling older adults with hypertension.

Variable participants (N = 31)	n	Percentage
Gender		
Female	27	87%
Male	4	13%
Age (years)		
60–69	13	42%
70–79	12	39%
80–89	5	16%
90–99	1	3%
Ethnicity		
Not Hispanic or Latino	23	74%
Hispanic or Latino	8	26%
Race		
White/Caucasian	0	0%
Black/African-American	31	100%

screened by phone, 31 were enrolled and 87% were women (n = 27). Figure 2 lists the number of participants who were screened, enrolled, and attended the Saturday or Wednesday session. Eighteen participants were assigned to Focus Group 1 (Wednesday group) and thirteen belonged to Focus Group 2 (Saturday group). Thirty participants participated in Session I and 28 participated in Session II. The Saturday group and the Wednesday group met two times and had an average attendance of 15 participants. One participant attended both Saturday and Wednesday. One participant switched after the first Saturday session to the Wednesday group due to work conflict.

Mode of Delivery of the Cocreated Intervention. The participants unanimously agreed that they wanted a group delivered intervention as opposed to an one-on-one intervention. The participants guided intervention delivery by deciding on the topics to be covered, number of sessions, type of experts they wanted to deliver the education session (e.g., requested a dietitian), how long the sessions should last (2 hours), and number of sessions that they wanted. They also selected the time of day and venue for delivery of the interventions. They told us the type of homework that they wanted to do between sessions (e.g., completing a sleep diary and food diary and logging their blood pressure at home). Participants did not want the presenter of the sessions to dominate the conversation. They wanted time for suggestions and answers. They wanted time also to provide peer support to each other in the form of recipe exchanges and cooking appliance recommendations (e.g., one person recommended using the participant compensation to purchase a vegetable steamer).

Prioritized Topics for the Cocreated Intervention. The primary stressors identified by the group that influenced their blood pressure self-management were as follows: (a) measuring their blood pressure and using home blood pressure monitors; (b) difficulty communicating with family and friends; (c) organizing sleep management and pain at night; and (d) determining ways to engage in healthy eating. Based on participants' feedback, we created four biweekly (2-hour) group sessions that incorporated their suggestions and concerns. One health provider (either a registered nurse or licensed dietitian) led each session. Exercise as a way to self-manage hypertension was not brought up by participants in the focus groups.

At the request of the focus group members who helped to cocreate the intervention, the researchers successfully sought permission from the IRB to retain the participants in order for them to "try out" the cocreated intervention. An addendum to the original protocol and consent form were approved by the University Hospitals of Cleveland IRB. The series was titled "Team Learning to Take Control (TLC)," and the individual sessions were named "TLC-Monitoring Your Blood Pressure," "TLC-Communication," "TLC-Sleep and Pain," and "TLC-Healthy Eating and Learning Portions (HELP)."

Satisfaction with the Cocreated Intervention. In order to assess the participants' satisfaction with the cocreated intervention, we asked each participant to complete a four-item survey. Twenty-six surveys were completed and five were missing at random. Concerning satisfaction with the intervention, 100% responded with a score of eight or higher. Ninety-nine percent stated they would continue using what they learned from the intervention. The appropriateness of the intervention was rated 8–10 by (n = 24, 92.3%) and rated 6 by (n = 2, 7.7%) of the respondents. The cultural relevance of the intervention was rated 8–10 (n = 22, 84.6%) and rated 7 by (n = 4, 15.4%) of the respondents.

4. Discussion

This purpose of this paper was to describe the process of cocreating an intervention for hypertension self-management. Using cocreation in our study between the nurse researcher and the older adult allowed the participant (rather than the academic) to drive the design of the intervention. Participants guided intervention content by telling us what they wanted kept or removed. Participants shared their concerns around communicating with family, understanding blood pressure, and coping with the challenges of following a healthy diet. The majority of participants in the study highly rated the intervention. This may be due to their investment in the design of the intervention.

The use of a cocreated hypertension self-management intervention with a group of community-dwelling African American older adults is novel. The literature is scant on the development, use, and effectiveness of cocreated interventions. Previous studies have shown that cocreation has been effective in developing interventions [12]. The benefits of bringing together a group of individuals who share some commonalities toward a common goal are not novel [10, 11]. Using the cocreation technique in health education has the potential to have far-reaching benefits to populations at high risk of facing chronic or even co- or multimorbidities.

Although there are inconsistencies about the effects of ethnicity and gender on research participation, the group and researcher ethnic background can potentially influence participation in the focus groups [19]. Having facilitators and interventionists of a similar ethnic background may have led participants to feel more comfortable about disclosing information. We did not collect any additional data that could have led support to this assumption.

A commonly recommended intervention by nurses to patients with hypertension is exercise. However, the participants did not mention exercise as a way to self-manage hypertension. Although it was discussed in brief in the intervention delivery as appropriate, we did not push the idea of adopting an exercise routine nor make it the sole focus of an intervention session because that would have taken the power and control away from the participants.

The cocreation method is not without its challenges. One major benefit and challenge to cocreation is shared governance over the process. Interference with this process could lead to misguided results. This allowed us to demonstrate how the community-based participatory tenet of trust building over time may work in this sample of older adults with hypertension from conception of the cocreated idea to implementation. Accommodations are often needed to promote participation. For example, in a polypharmacy study, the researchers indicated that it was difficult to schedule meeting times due to the busy nature of the clinic environment [12]. This was not a challenge for our study because our participants were mostly retired or had part-time jobs. They did, however, have transportation challenges and care responsibilities for grandchildren that we took into consideration to schedule meetings. There were a couple of occasions where a participant who was a grandparent needed to bring a grandchild to a focus group meeting. As a group, the members were willing to be flexible.

While our study provides insight into working with community-dwelling African American older adults with hypertension, additional studies are needed to examine cocreated interventions in diverse samples and across chronic illnesses. Cocreated interventions allow further examination of specific self-management strategies and specific skill sets of patients. The next steps of the cocreated intervention will include (1) analyzing our data to determine what the participants found most useful and (2) using assistive technology to manage medication routines.

5. Limitations

Due to the positive responses to participation in the focus groups, each group was larger in size than typically recommended. This may have further reduced the likelihood that individuals who are already less likely to speak up in a group setting to do so. Additionally, the male to female ratio in the groups may have reduced the likelihood of the male perspective being included in the discussion. In a mixed gender sample, there could be less to bring up sexually related topics. As a universal limitation of focus groups, the generalizability of results is limited.

6. Implications for Nursing Practice

Nurses lead development of educational interventions. Cocreation helps reduce the power imbalance in research settings. Cocreation helps establish the nurse researcher and participant as equal partners [20]. The methodology used in this study to promote health education can be incorporated into around other common topics to promote health education in a nonthreatening setting with the use of peer support. Cocreation can be applied in community-based settings, such as faith-based and civic organizations. There are potential benefits to transforming this process into other homogenous groups (i.e., other disease states or age groups).

Changes will be made to the cocreated intervention based upon the feedback of the participants such as increasing the number of sessions from four to six and providing more examples of healthy ethnic recipes. Because of the age of the focus group participants in this study, there is a potential for changes made to their self-management practices to influence their social support system across the lifespan. If the participants were caring for their grandkids, they would be able to lead by example through grocery shopping practices and cooking habits. Future adaptations might include a family component and a group for men.

7. Conclusions

We present our experience cocreating an intervention through focus groups. Other researchers can use cocreation techniques to develop interventions. The benefits of interventions developed in this manner may be heightened by virtue of addressing what the participants indicate would most help them.

Disclosure

The content is solely the responsibility of the authors and does not necessarily represent the official views of the NIH.

Acknowledgments

This publication was made possible by the Clinical and Translational Science Collaborative of Cleveland (KL2TR000440) from the National Center for Advancing Translational Sciences (NCATS) component of the National Institutes of Health and NIH Roadmap for Medical Research and the National Institutes of Nursing Research of the National Institutes of under Awards nos. P30NR015326-02S and T32 NR014213. The Additionally, the Discovery Themes-Chronic Brain Injury supported Dr. Wright (https://discovery.osu.edu/chronic-brain-injury).

References

[1] L. M. Lewis, C. Ogedegbe, and G. Ogedegbe, "Enhancing adherence of antihypertensive regimens in hypertensive African-Americans: current and future prospects," *Expert Review of Cardiovascular Therapy*, vol. 10, no. 11, pp. 1375–1380, 2012.

[2] D. R. Williams, "Race, socioeconomic status, and health the added effects of racism and discrimination," *Annals of the New York Academy of Sciences*, vol. 896, pp. 173–188, 1999.

[3] D. R. Williams and P. B. Jackson, "Social sources of racial disparities in health," *Health Affairs (Millwood)*, vol. 24, no. 2, pp. 325–334, 2005.

[4] P. Herd, B. Goesling, and J. S. House, "Socioeconomic position and health: the differential effects of education versus income on the onset versus progression of health problems," *Journal of Health and Social Behavior*, vol. 48, no. 3, pp. 223–238, 2007.

[5] K. J. August and D. H. Sorkin, "Racial and ethnic disparities in indicators of physical health status: do they still exist throughout late life?" *Journal of the American Geriatrics Society*, vol. 58, no. 10, pp. 2009–2015, 2010.

[6] A. V. Chobanian, G. L. Bakris, and H. R. Black, "Seventh report of the Joint National Committee on prevention, detection, evaluation, and treatment of high blood pressure," *Hypertension*, vol. 42, no. 6, pp. 1206–1252, 2003.

[7] L. N. Borrell, N. D. Crawford, D. S. Barrington, and K. N. Maglo, "Black/white disparity in self-reported hypertension: the role of nativity status," *Journal of Health Care for the Poor and Underserved*, vol. 19, no. 4, pp. 1148–1162, 2008.

[8] A. P. Carson, G. Howard, G. L. Burke, S. Shea, E. B. Levitan, and P. Muntner, "Ethnic differences in hypertension incidence among middle-aged and older adults: the multi-ethnic study of atherosclerosis," *Hypertension*, vol. 57, no. 6, pp. 1101–1107, 2011.

[9] P. A. James, S. Oparil, B. L. Carter et al., "2014 Evidence-based guideline for the management of high blood pressure in adults: report from the panel members appointed to the Eighth Joint National Committee (JNC 8)," *Journal of the American Medical Association*, vol. 311, no. 5, pp. 507–520, 2014.

[10] T. Greenhalgh, C. Jackson, S. Shaw, and T. Janamian, "Achieving Research Impact Through Co-creation in Community-Based Health Services: Literature Review and Case Study," *Milbank Q*, vol. 94, no. 2, pp. 392–429, 2016.

[11] C. L. Jackson and T. Greenhalgh, "Co-creation: a new approach to optimising research impact?" *The Medical Journal of Australia*, vol. 203, no. 7, pp. 283-284, 2015.

[12] K. Anderson, M. M. Foster, C. R. Freeman, and I. A. Scott, "A multifaceted intervention to reduce inappropriate polypharmacy in primary care: research co-creation opportunities in a pilot study," *Medical Journal of Australia*, suppl. 7, pp. S41–S44, 2016.

[13] J. M. Sorrell, "Meditation for Older Adults: A New Look at an Ancient Intervention for Mental Health," *Journal of Psychosocial Nursing and Mental Health Services*, vol. 53, no. 5, pp. 15–19, 2015.

[14] D. E. Epstein, A. Sherwood, P. J. Smith et al., "Determinants and consequences of adherence to the dietary approaches to stop hypertension diet in African-American and white adults with high blood pressure: results from the ENCORE trial," *Journal of the Academy of Nutrition and Dietetics*, vol. 112, no. 11, pp. 1763–1773, 2012.

[15] L. J. Appel, C. M. Champagne, and D. W. Harsha, "Effects of comprehensive lifestyle modification on blood pressure control: main results of the PREMIER clinical trial," *Journal of the American Medical Association*, vol. 289, no. 16, pp. 2083–2093, 2003.

[16] Y. S. Lincoln and E. G. Guba, *Naturalistic Inquiry*, Sage Publications, Newbury Park, CA, USA, 1985.

[17] K. Moss, C. Still, L. Jones, and K. D. Wright, "Hypertension self-management perspectives from African American older adults," *Western Journal of Nursing Research*, 2018, In press.

[18] D. J. Bowen, M. Kreuter, and B. Spring, "How we design feasibility studies," *American Journal of Preventive Medicine*, vol. 36, no. 5, pp. 452–457, 2009.

[19] R. Luebbert and A. Perez, "Barriers to Clinical Research Participation Among African Americans," *Journal of Transcultural Nursing*, vol. 27, no. 5, pp. 456–463, 2016.

[20] K. J. August, A. Haas, A. Ommaya, and L. W. Green, *Exploring challenges, progress, and new models for engaging the public in the clinical research enterprise: Clinical research roundtable workshop summary*, National Academies Press: The National Academies of Sciences, Engineering and Medicine, 2003.

The Prevalence and Social Determinants of Hypertension among Adults in Indonesia: A Cross-Sectional Population-Based National Survey

Karl Peltzer [1,2] **and Supa Pengpid** [2,3]

[1] *HIV/AIDS/STIs and TB (HAST), Human Sciences Research Council, Pretoria 0001, South Africa*
[2] *Department of Research and Innovation, University of Limpopo, Sovenga 0727, South Africa*
[3] *ASEAN Institute for Health Development, Mahidol University, Salaya, Thailand*

Correspondence should be addressed to Karl Peltzer; karl.peltzer@tdt.edu.vn

Academic Editor: Claudio Borghi

Background. Hypertension is the most significant avoidable cause of morbidity and mortality, yet nationally representative adult data on Indonesia have not been available. The study aimed at assessing the prevalence and determinants of hypertension, including sociodemographic variables, weight status, health behaviour, and psychosocial stress and support risk factors. *Methods.* The Indonesia Family Life Survey (IFLS-5) interviewed and examined in a national population-based cross-sectional study 29965 individuals aged 18 years and older, mean age 43.3 years (SD=15.3). Blood pressure, body height and weight, dietary behaviour, physical activity, tobacco use, and psychosocial variables were measured. Logistic regression analyses were used to estimate determinants of hypertension by gender. *Results.* The prevalence of hypertension among study participants was 33.4 % (95 % CI: 32.7-34.0), among males 31.0% (95% CI: 30.2, 31.9), and among females 35.4% (95% CI: 34.6, 36.3). Among hypertensives, 42.9% were aware, 11.5% were treated, and 14.3% were controlled. In fully adjusted analyses, in both men and women, older age, no or elementary education, being overweight or obese, and having visited an outpatients health facility in the past 4 weeks were positively associated hypertension. Significant linear relationships of hypertension were found with age (P for trend <0.001) and body mass index (BMI) (P for trend < 0.001). In addition, among men having quit tobacco use and depressive symptoms were positively associated with hypertension, while current tobacco use was negatively associated with hypertension. Moreover, among women lower subjective economic status was associated with hypertension. *Conclusions.* The prevalence of hypertension was high and awareness was low, and treatment and control were very low. Significant multilevel public health interventions are urgently needed to improve the diagnosis, treatment, and control of hypertension in Indonesia.

1. Introduction

Chronic noncommunicable diseases (NCDs) have become an enormous health burden in low- and middle-income countries [1]. The scale of the increase of NCDs can be particularly observed in Southeast Asia, such as in Indonesia, where a limited budget has been allocated to combat the growing NCD epidemic [2]. The three top causes of death in Indonesia are stroke (21.2%), ischaemic heart disease (8.9%), and diabetes mellitus (6.5%) [3]. Major adult NCD risk factors in Indonesia include current tobacco smoking (in 2011) 35% (67% in men and 3% in women), high blood pressure or hypertension (in 2008) 27.8% (29.1% in men and 26.5% in women), and obesity (in 2008) 4.8% (2.6% in men and 6.0% in women) [4].

Hypertension is a preventable illness condition and has been found to be associated with an unhealthy lifestyle, including tobacco smoking, a lack of physical activity, and alcohol consumption [1]. Increasing trends in the prevalence of hypertension have been shown in high- and low- and middle-income countries [5, 6]. Comparable with the global trend, "the single most attributable cause for mortality in South-East Asia" is hypertension with an increasing trend [7]. Hussain et al. [8] found in the "2007 Indonesian Family Life Survey (IFLS-4)" a prevalence of 47.8% with hypertension in individuals 40 years and older. In other national population-based surveys in Southeast Asia the prevalence of hypertension was in Malaysia 43.5% (≥30 years in 2011) [9], in Myanmar 30.1% (15-64-year-olds in 2009) [10], in Sri Lanka 23.7% (≥18 years in 2005-2006) [11], and in Vietnam 25.1% (≥25 years in 2002-2008) [12], while in two other Asian countries the national prevalence of hypertension was in China 29.6% (≥18 years in 2010) [13] and in Iran 25% (25-64-year-olds in 2005) [14]. There is a lack of data on the adult (15 years and older) hypertension prevalence in Indonesia.

Hypertension is a preventable disease but recent studies found a low prevalence of antihypertensive medication treatment. In the 2007 IFLS4 survey (40-65 years) in Indonesia, 37% of individuals with hypertension were diagnosed or aware and 25% were treated with prescribed antihypertensive medication [8]. In the previously reported national population-based surveys in China (≥18 years and older), 42.6% were aware of their hypertension status and 34.1% received antihypertensive treatment [13], in Iran (25-64 year-olds) 34% were aware and 24.8% treated [14], and in Vietnam [≥25 years] 48.4% were aware and 29.5% received treatment [12]. In a community study with participants (35-70 years) from 17 mainly low- and middle-income countries, 46.5% were aware of their hypertension diagnosis and 32.5% were treated [15]. These studies indicate the very important need for the improvement of the diagnosis and treatment of hypertension [15].

Various risk factors have been found to be linked with hypertension, including sociodemographics (older age, female or male gender, lower education level, and lower household income) [8, 10–12, 14–17], geolocality (urban residence) [10, 12, 18], and other risk factors, including body weight status and health behaviour and psychosocial stress and support. Higher body mass index (BMI) has been found to be positively [8, 10, 13, 15–17] and underweight status negatively [10] associated with hypertension. Various dietary behaviours were also associated with hypertension, including insufficient fruit and vegetable intake [19–21], consumption of fatty foods [22, 23] and fast foods [24, 25], and sugar and soft drink consumption [26]. A number of studies found an association between physical inactivity [10, 13, 27–29], smoking [29, 30], and hypertension. Some studies, e.g., [31], found that a higher frequency of doctor visits was associated with having hypertension in addition to psychosocial stress [32, 33], including depression [34], low life satisfaction [35, 36], and less social cohesion [37] and lack of social support [32].

The aim of this study was to assess the prevalence of hypertension and to identify sociodemographic, weight status, health behaviour, psychosocial stress, and support risk factors for hypertension based on a cross-sectional survey of the IFLS-5 in 2014-15 in Indonesia.

2. Materials and Methods

2.1. Study Design and Participants. Data were analysed from the "Indonesia Family Life Survey (IFLS-5)", a continuing demographic and health survey that began in 1993 and had since four rounds of data collection, with the fifth wave (IFLS-5) having been completed in 2015 [38]. The community surveys collected data on household, individual, and community level using a multistage stratified sampling [38]. The sampling frame of the first survey in 1993 was based on households from 321 enumeration areas (EAs) (20 households were randomly selected from each urban EA, and 30 households were selected from each rural EA) in 13 out of 27 Indonesian provinces that were selected representing 83% of the Indonesian population in 1993; more details are available in [38]. At household level, several randomly selected household members were asked to provide detailed individual information. In the IFLS-5, 16,204 households and 29965 18 years and older individuals were interviewed and had complete blood pressure measurements. In the IFLS-5, "the dynasty recontact rate was 92% and for the individual target households (including split off households as separate) the re-contact rate was 90.5%." [39]. Although the survey is longitudinal, we restricted our analysis to the IFLS-5 because it was the only survey to include complete hypertension information for persons 18 years and older.

2.2. Measures. Measures included blood pressure measurements, anthropometric measurements, and questionnaire items on sociodemographic factors, dietary behaviour, physical activity, tobacco use, health care utilization, psychosocial stress, and support.

2.2.1. Blood Pressure (BP) Measurements and Classification. Three successive measurements of systolic and diastolic blood pressure (BP) were recorded with an Omron meter, HEM-7203, by regular trained interviewers on household members 18 years and older at home in a seated position [38]. Mostly a normal sized cuff was used, while large cuffs were available when needed [38]. The first BP measurement was conducted at the onset of the research interview, with two subsequent assessments during the course of the interview [38]. Information was collected on awareness (having been diagnosed of hypertension by a doctor, nurse, paramedic, and trained mid-wife) and treatment of hypertension (currently taking prescribed medication on a weekly basis to manage your hypertension). The current analysis is restricted to individuals who had information on hypertension measurement, awareness, and treatment. For the three measurements of each systolic and diastolic blood pressure average blood pressure was calculated arithmetically.

Blood pressure was classified using JNC 7 algorithm [39]. "Hypertension was defined as systolic BP ≥140 mm Hg and/or DBP ≥90 mm Hg and/or current use of antihypertensive medication. Normotension was defined as BP values <120/80 mm Hg in individuals who were not taking antihypertensive medication" [39].

Sociodemographic factors were assessed with questions on age, gender, education, residential status, subjective socioeconomic background, and country region. Subjective economic status was assessed by the question "Please imagine a six-step ladder where on the bottom (the first step), stand the poorest people, and on the highest step (the sixth step), stand the richest people. On which [economic] step are you today?" The answers ranged from (1) poorest to (6) richest [38].

2.2.2. Weight Status and Health Behaviour

Anthropometric Measurements. Heights were measured to the nearest millimetre using a Seca plastic height board (model 213) [38]. Weights were taken to the nearest tenth of a kilogram using a Camry model EB1003 scale [38]. Body mass index (BMI) was calculated as weight in kg divided by height in metre squared and classified according to Asian criteria: normal weight (18.5 to <23.0 kg/m^2), overweight (23.0 to <25.0 kg/m^2) and obese (25+ kg/m^2) [40].

Vegetable consumption was measured with two items, "How many days in the past week, (1) Green leafy vegetables and (2) carrots had been eaten?" [38].

Fruit consumption was assessed with three questions on, "How many days in the past week, (1) Banana, (2) Mango and (3) Papaya had been eaten?" [38].

Additional dietary variables included "on how many days in the past week, (1) Fast food, (2) Fried snacks (tempe, tahu, bakwan, etc.), and (3) Soft drinks (Coca cola, sprite, etc.) had been consumed?" [38].

Physical Activity. Physical activity was assessed using a modified version of the International Physical Activity Questionnaire (IPAQ) short version, for the last 7 days (IPAQ-S7S). We used the instructions given in the IPAQ manual [41] and categorized physical activity according to the official IPAQ scoring protocol [42] as low, moderate, and high.

Tobacco use was assessed with two questions: (1) "Have you ever chewed tobacco, smoked a pipe, smoked self-enrolled cigarettes, or smoked cigarettes/cigars?" (Yes, No) and (2) "Do you still have the habit or have you totally quit?"(Still have, Quit) [38]. Responses were grouped into never, quitters, and current tobacco users.

Health care utilization was assessed with the question, "Whether visited any outpatient health care clinic in one month prior to survey or not?" (Yes, No) [38].

2.2.3. Psychosocial Stress and Support. The *Centres for Epidemiologic Studies Depression Scale (CES-D:* 10 items) was used to assess depressive symptoms, and scores 10 or more were classified as having depressive symptoms [43] (Cronbach's alpha = 0.71).

Life satisfaction was assessed with one item, "Please, think about your life as a whole. How satisfied are you with it?" Response option ranged from 1: completely satisfied to 5: not at all satisfied [38].

Social support or capital was assessed with 4 items (selected from 11 items through factor analysis), "During the last 12 months did you participate or use?..." (1) Community meeting, (2) Voluntary labour, (3), Programme to improve the village/neighbourhood, and (4) Religious activities. Response options were "yes" or "no" [38] (Cronbach's alpha 0.60).

2.3. Data Analysis. Descriptive statistics were used to describe the study variables of the study population and Chi-square test to calculate difference in proportions. Nonparametric tests were used for trend analyses across ordered groups. Logistic regression (forced entry) analyses were used to test significant determinants of hypertension status, with hypertension serving as the dichotomous outcome variable and in Model 1 age served as independent predictor variable and in Model 2 sociodemographics, health, nutrition, psychosocial stress, and social capital served as the independent predictor variables. We also examined linear associations by exposure categories in each model (p for trend) in the assessment of hypertension prevalence. "Cross-section analysis weights were applied to correct both for sample attrition from 1993 to 2014, and then to correct for the fact that the IFLS1 sample design included over-sampling in urban areas and off Java. The cross-section weights are matched to the 2014 Indonesian population, again in the 13 IFLS provinces, in order to make the attrition-adjusted IFLS sample representative of the 2014 Indonesian population in those provinces"[38]. Both the 95% confidence intervals and P values were adjusted considering the survey design of the study. All analyses were conducted with STATA software version 13.0 (Stata Corporation, College Station, TX, USA).

3. Results

3.1. Sample Characteristics. The total sample included 29965 individuals 18 years and older, with complete hypertension measures (females: 52.7%; mean age 43.3 years, SD: 15.3, age range of 18–109 years) from Indonesia. Overall, 33.4% of the population had hypertension, 31.0% among men and 35.4% among women. Among hypertensives 42.9% were aware that they had hypertension, which was significantly higher in women (50.1%) than men (33.7%) and in urban (44.5%) than rural areas (41.1%). Of the population with hypertension, 11.5% were currently using prescribed antihypertensive medication, and 14.3% had controlled their blood pressure (<140 mm Hg and diastolic blood pressure <90 mm Hg). Women (14.0%) were more often than men (8.4%) and urban dwellers (13.0%) more often than rural dwellers (9.9%) using currently prescribed antihypertensive medication. Of those participants with hypertension, only 14.3% controlled their blood pressure. Mean systolic blood pressure was 1.1 mmHg higher for men than for women, while mean diastolic blood pressure was 0.2 mmHg higher for women than for men. The prevalence of BMI obesity was higher in women (42.0%) than in men (23.0%), while the current tobacco use prevalence was significantly higher in men (67.2%) than in women (3.0%) (see Table 1).

The prevalence of hypertension increases overall and for both sexes by age group from 18 to 29 years to 70 years and above (*P* for trend <0.001). The prevalence of hypertension is higher among males than females at the age 18 to 29 years, while from 40 years and older the prevalence of hypertension is higher among women than men. Further the prevalence of hypertension decreases overall and for both sexes (and stronger for females) by education from having no education to having higher education (*P* for trend <0.001) (see Table 2).

4. Association between Psychosocial Risk Factors and Hypertension

Table 3 shows associations (odds ratios) between independent variables and the prevalence of hypertension, in Model 1

TABLE 1: Sample characteristics.

Variable name	Variable specification	Total	Male	Female	P value
Sample	N (%)	29965	13997 (47.3)	15969 (52.7)	
Mean age in years (SD)	Range 18-109, mean (SD)	43.3 (15.3)	42.0 (15.3)	42.6 (15.2)	0.056
Systolic blood pressure	mmHg, mean (SD)	130.9 (21.9)	131.8 (19.2)	130.1 (24.1)	<0.001
Diastolic blood pressure	mmHg, mean (SD)	80.1 (11.9)	80.0 (11.7)	80.2 (12.1)	0.004
Hypertension	%	33.4	31.0	35.4	<0.001
Of hypertensives	Aware, %	42.9	33.7	50.1	<0.001
Of hypertensives	Treated, %	11.5	8.4	14.0	<0.001
Of hypertensives	Controlled, %	14.3	12.4	15.7	<0.001
Education	None/elementary, %	44.0	39.1	48.4	<0.001
Subjective economic background	Poor, % Medium, % Rich, %	25.5 46.6 27.9	27.4 48.9 23.7	23.8 44.6 31.6	<0.001
Residence	Urban, %	58.6	58.6	58.7	0.198
Region	Sumatra, % Java, % Main islands[1], %	22.7 54.6 22.7	23.4 54.2 22.4	22.1 54.9 23.0	0.027
Body weight status and health behaviour					
Body Mass Index (BMI)	Normal, % Underweight, % Overweight, % Obese, %	40.2 11.2 16.0 32.4	48.3 13.5 15.2 23.0	33.2 9.0 16.8 42.0	<0.001
Vegetable consumption[2]	<7 days/week, %	57.6	58.3	56.7	<0.001
Fruit consumption[3]	<3 days/week, %	58.1	59.6	56.8	<0.001
Fast food	≥once week, %	10.6	9.8	11.2	0.033
Fried snacks	4-7 times/week, %	25.6	26.3	25.3	0.147
Soft drinks	≥once week, %	18.5	24.9	12.8	<0.001
Physical activity	Low, % Moderate, % High, %	48.3 26.6 25.1	43.1 22.9 34.0	49.7 30.0 20.3	<0.001
Tobacco use	Never, % Quit, % Current, %	62.2 5.0 32.8	23.2 9.6 67.2	95.9 1.1 3.0	<0.001
Health care utilization	Past 4 weeks, %	18.8	14.6	23.9	<0.001
Psychosocial stress and support					
Depression symptoms	Scores ≥10, %	22.8	22.2	23.4	0.177
Life satisfaction	High-yes, %	42.7	40.2	44.9	<0.001
Social support/capital	High-yes, %	37.9	50.6	26.4	<0.001

[1]Major island groups: Bali, West Nusa Tenggara, South Kalimantan, and South Sulawesi; [2]vegetable: green leafy vegetables and/or carrots; [3]fruits: banana and/or mango and/or papaya.

adjusted for age, and in Model 2 adjusted for all covariates in the table. In fully adjusted models in both men and women, older age, no or elementary education, being overweight or obese, and having visited an outpatients health facility in the past 4 weeks were positively associated with hypertension. Both among men and among women being underweight was negatively associated with hypertension. In addition, among men having quit tobacco use and depressive symptoms were positively associated with hypertension, while current tobacco use was negatively associated with hypertension. Moreover, among women lower subjective economic status was associated with hypertension. In Model 1, the prevalence of hypertension was higher among men in urban than rural areas, while this became insignificant in Model 2, the fully adjusted model. Significant positive linear relationships of hypertension were found among both men and women with

TABLE 2: Prevalence of hypertension among individuals 18 years and older in Indonesia.

Variable	Total sample	Male		Female		Total	
	N	n	% (95% CI)	N	% (95% CI)	N	% (95% CI)
All	29965	4040	31.0 (30.2, 31.9)	4925	35.4 (34.6, 36.3)	8965	33.4 (32.7, 34.0)
Age group							
18-29	8488	535	13.9 (12.8, 15.2)	433	9.3 (8.4, 10.2)	968	11.6 (10.9, 12.4)
30-39	8444	804	19.2 (17.8, 20.5)	834	19.5 (18.2, 20.9)	1638	19.3 (18.4, 20.3)
40-49	5586	874	31.3 (29.5, 33.2)	1093	39.1 (37.2, 41.1)	1967	35.6 (34.3, 37.0)
50-59	3834	809	45.6 (43.1, 48.2)	1167	56.7 (54.4, 59.0)	1967	51.3 (49.5, 53.0)
60-69	2105	582	58.1 (54.7, 61.4)	730	66.0 (62.8, 69.0)	1312	62.1 (59.8, 64.4)
70 or more	1508	436	67.1 (63.1, 70.9)	668	79.3 (76.0, 82.3)	1104	74.1 (71.5, 76.4)
			P- trend <0.001		*P*- trend <0.001		*P*- trend <0.001
Education							
None	1568	200	47.2 (41.8, 52.6)	699	59.3 (56.0, 62.5)	899	56.1 (53.2, 58.8)
Elementary	9741	1525	36.8 (35.2, 38.4)	2292	45.2 (43.8, 46.7)	3817	41.5 (40.4, 42.6)
High school	14305	1736	25.7 (24.6, 26.9)	1537	24.6 (23.5, 25.8)	3273	25.2 (24.4, 26.0)
Higher education	4294	567	30.1 (27.9, 32.5)	365	20.0 (18.1, 22.1)	932	25.1 (23.4, 26.6)
			P- trend <0.001		*P*- trend <0.001		*P*- trend <0.001

age (P<0.001) and BMI (P<0.001), and negative relationships among men with tobacco use (P=0.006) and among women with economic background (P=0.015) (see Table 3).

5. Discussion

In this first nationally representative population-based survey on hypertension in Indonesia, the age-adjusted prevalence in all adults (18 years and older) was 33.4% (48.6% in 40 years and older) in 2014-15, which is similar to the prevalence among 40 years and older in the 2007 survey in Indonesia (47.8%) [8], the Myanmar survey in 2009 of 30.1% in 15-64-year-olds [10], and the China survey in 2010 of 29.6% in individuals 18 years and older [13], and similar to the global adult (≥20 years) prevalence in low- and middle-income countries (31.5%) [44], but higher than in Iran [14, 45], Sri Lanka [11], and Vietnam [12].

Of those who had hypertension only 42.9% were aware (44.9% among 40 years and older) and 11.5% were using prescribed antihypertensive medication (13.8% among 40 years and older) in this 2014-15 survey. This seems to show an increase in the awareness (from 37% in 2007 to 44.9% in 2014-15) but a decrease in the proportion of treatment (from 25% in 2007 to 11.5% in 2014-15) [8]. The proportion of awareness in this study was also similar to figures reported from China [13], Vietnam [12], and globally in low- and middle-income countries [15, 45]; however, the proportion of reported treatment was in this study significantly lower than in other countries, including China [13], Iran [14], Vietnam [12], and globally in low- and middle-income countries studies [15, 45]. The awareness and treatment of hypertension was in this study greater among women than men, as also found previously [8]. The awareness and treatment of hypertension was higher in urban than rural areas. This may be because of lack of access to health care services in rural areas [8]. The increase in the awareness of hypertension may be attributed to community-based integrated coaching posts that enable community participation in the early detection of hypertension [46]. These findings seem to suggest that despite some improvement in the awareness of hypertension more should be achieved, in particular among men, and appropriate treatment needs to be seriously improved, especially also among men and in rural areas.

This study found, in agreement with various studies [8, 10–12, 14–17], that older age and lower educational level were among both men and women associated with hypertension. Lower subjective economic status was among women but not among men associated with hypertension. Although the prevalence of hypertension increased overall and for both sexes by age group from 18 to 29 years to 70 years and above, the prevalence of hypertension was higher among males than females at the age 18 to 29 years, while from 40 years and older the prevalence of hypertension was higher among women than men. One possible reason for this age differential among the sexes can be because the prevalence rates of obesity, as one important risk factor for hypertension, are higher in boys than girls among children, adolescents, and young adults [47–49] but higher in females in the adult age groups [49]. The high prevalence of hypertension in the group with low or no education in this study may be related to having a higher number of risk factors such as stress, poor dietary habits, poor working conditions, and lack of access to health services [50]. Urban residence increased the odds for hypertension in previous studies [10, 12, 18] but in this study it was only significant in bivariate analysis among men and nonsignificant for women. It seems that the urban-rural differences in the prevalence of hypertension, as found in the 2007 IFLS [8], no longer exist in the 2013-14 IFLS in Indonesia.

Regarding weight variables, being underweight was protective and being overweight or obese increased the odds

TABLE 3: Predictors of hypertension by gender.

Variable	Male		Female	
	Age-adjusted (95% CI)[a]	AOR (95% CI)[b]	Age-adjusted (95% CI)[a]	AOR (95% CI)[b]
Sociodemographics				
Education				
High school or Higher education	1 (Reference)	1 (Reference)	1 (Reference)	1 (Reference)
None or elementary	1.13 (1.03, 1.25)**	1.15 (1.02, 1.28)*	1.34 (1.22, 1.47)***	1.39 (1.25, 1.54)***
Subjective economic background				
Poor	1 (Reference)	1 (Reference)	1 (Reference)	1 (Reference)
Medium	1.06 (0.95, 1.18)	0.94 (0.84, 1.05)	0.87 (0.78, 0.97)*	0.89 (0.79, 0.99)*
Rich	1.18 (1.04, 1.34)**	0.98 (0.85, 1.12)	0.82 (0.73, 0.93)**	0.85 (0.75, 0.96)*
P for trend	0.011	0.842	0.002	0.015
Residence				
Rural	1 (Reference)	1 (Reference)	1 (Reference)	1 (Reference)
Urban	1.17 (1.07, 1.28)***	1.02 (0.92, 1.12)	1.07 (0.98, 1.16)	1.08 (0.98, 1.18)
Region				
Sumatra	1 (Reference)	1 (Reference)	1 (Reference)	1 (Reference)
Java	0.97 (0.88, 1.08)	0.96 (0.86, 1.07)	1.04 (0.94, 1.15)	0.98 (0.88, 1.10)
Main islands	1.06 (0.94, 1.20)	1.03 (0.90, 1.17)	1.06 (0.94, 1.20)	1.11 (0.97, 1.26)
Body weight status and health behaviour				
Body Mass Index (BMI)				
Underweight	0.66 (0.56, 0.78)***	0.63 (0.53, 0.74)***	0.72 (0.60, 0.86)***	0.69 (0.57, 0.84)***
Normal	1 (Reference)	1 (Reference)	1 (Reference)	1 (Reference)
Overweight	1.93 (1.70, 2.20)***	1.99 (1.74, 2.26)***	1.29 (1.13, 1.48)***	1.32 (1.15, 1.51)***
Obese	3.01 (2.70, 3.36)***	3.02 (2.69, 3.39)***	2.18 (1.96, 2.43)***	2.24 (2.01, 2.50)***
P for trend	<0.001	<0.001	<0.001	<0.001
Vegetable consumption less than daily (base=daily)	0.92 (0.84, 1.01)	0.94 (0.86, 1.04)	1.07 (0.98, 1.16)	1.03 (0.93, 1.12)
Fruit consumption <trice/week (base=trice or more)	0.90 (0.82, 0.99)*	0.99 (0.90, 1.09)	1.02 (0.93, 1.11)	1.04 (0.94, 1.14)
Fast food (once or more/week) (base= <once)	1.12 (0.96, 1.31)	0.96 (0.81, 1.14)	0.99 (0.85, 1.14)	1.00 (0.86, 1.17)
Fried snacks (4-7 times/week) (base=0-3 times)	1.06 (0.96, 1.18)	1.04 (0.93, 1.15)	1.12 (1.02, 1.24)*	1.10 (0.99, 1.21)
Soft drinks (once or more/week) (base= <once)	1.12 (1.00, 1.25)*	1.05 (0.94, 1.18)	0.97 (0.84, 1.11)	0.97 (0.84, 1.12)
Physical activity				
Low	1 (Reference)	1 (Reference)	1 (Reference)	1 (Reference)
Moderate	1.18 (1.05, 1.32)**	1.20 (1.07, 1.40)**	1.02 (0.92, 1.13)	1.01 (0.91, 1.11)
High	0.86 (0.78, 0.96)**	0.95 (0.85, 1.06)	1.00 (0.89, 1.12)	1.00 (0.88, 1.12)
P for trend	0.011	0.487	0.945	0.951
Tobacco use				
Never	1 (Reference)	1 (Reference)	1 (Reference)	1 (Reference)
Quit	1.22 (1.04, 1.43)*	1.19 (1.00, 1.40)*	1.43 (0.94, 2.16)	1.56 (0.98, 2.48)
Current	0.74 (0.66, 0.82)***	0.88 (0.79, 0.99)*	0.92 (0.73, 1.17)	1.00 (0.78, 1.29)
Health care utilization	1.25 (1.11, 1.41)***	1.16 (1.02, 1.32)*	1.23 (1.12, 1.36)***	1.22 (1.10, 1.35)***
Psychosocial stress and support				
Depression symptoms	1.12 (1.01, 1.24)*	1.17 (1.04, 1.31)**	1.12 (1.01, 1.24)*	1.09 (0.98, 1.21)
Life satisfaction (high) (base=low)	0.96 (0.88, 1.06)	0.91 (0.83, 1.01)	0.97 (0.89, 1.06)	0.97 (0.89, 1.06)
Social support/capital (high) (base=low)	0.97 (0.88, 1.06)	0.95 (0.87, 1.05)	0.92 (0.83, 1.01)	0.93 (0.83, 1.02)

AOR: Adjusted Odds Ratio; CI: Confidence Interval; [a]adjusted for age; [b]adjusted for all covariates; *** represents P<.001; ** represents P<.01; * represents P<.05.

of having hypertension. The association between overweight/obesity and hypertension has been confirmed in a number of studies [8, 10, 13, 15–17]. Overweight or obesity may be associated with hypertension independently but it could also be mediated through unhealthy diet and inadequate physical activity [14]. The negative association between being underweight and hypertension was also found in a study in Myanmar [10]. Some studies [e.g., [51]] suggest that about two-thirds of the prevalence of hypertension may be attributed to obesity.

As found in a number of previous studies [10, 13, 27–29], moderate physical activity was in this study among men but not among women negatively associated with hypertension. The elevated blood pressure among the female participants of the study may not be attributable to physical inactivity but linked to other factors such as obesity [52]. In agreement with some previous studies [22, 23], this study found that consumption of fatty foods (fried snacks) was among women associated with hypertension.

Unlike previous studies [19–21, 24–26], this study did not find an association between fruit and vegetable, soft drink, fatty foods (fried snacks), fast food consumption, and hypertension. Current smoking is a significant risk factor for hypertension [29, 30]. However, in this study among men only former tobacco use was positively associated with hypertension, while current tobacco use was negatively associated with hypertension. Among smokers in this study the number of cigarettes smoked per day (Mean=11.7) did not differ between hypertensives and nonhypertensives (Mean: 11.9) (P=0.150). It is possible that the impact of current tobacco use on hypertension is delayed, and, thus, current tobacco use may not be closely correlated with hypertension [53]. In a life-course impact of smoking on hypertension study, Gao et al. [53] found that current number of cigarettes smoked per day was negatively associated with the risk of hypertension; however, the increase of life-course-adjusted number of cigarettes smoked per day was associated with higher risks of hypertension.

The burden of having hypertension may also be expressed in the association between past 4 weeks outpatient health care utilization and hypertension, as also found in a previous study [31] of hypertension. In terms of psychosocial stress and support, this study found, in agreement with previous studies [32–34], that depression was among men (and in bivariate analysis among women) positively related to hypertension. Hyperreactivity of the sympathetic nervous system and genetic influences seem to be influencing mechanisms in the relationship between depression and hypertension [54]. Unlike previous studies [32, 35–37], this study did not find an association between low life satisfaction and lack of social support or capital and hypertension.

6. Study Limitations

Apart from anthropometric and blood pressure measurements, a study limitation was that all the other information assessed in this analysis was based on self-reporting. It is possible that certain behaviours were over- or underreported. Several essential determinants for hypertension such as serum fasting blood surge, Low-Density Lipoprotein (LDL), and total cholesterol (TC) were not assessed in this study and should be included in future studies. Further, it was a cross-sectional study and causal relationships between risk factors and the development of hypertension can be established. Another limitation was that salt intake and heavy alcohol use, which are determinants of hypertension, were not assessed in this study.

7. Conclusion

The study found a high prevalence of hypertension in a representative sample of the general adult population in Indonesia. Less than half of hypertensives were aware and a minority were treated and controlled. Several risk factors, including sociodemographic variables (older age, lower education, being female, and lower socioeconomic status), body weight status (overweight or obese), health behaviour (physical inactivity), and psychosocial stress (depression), have been identified, which can help in guiding intervention programmes. Interventions programmes operating at multiple levels are urgently needed that can increase awareness of hypertension, access to high blood pressure treatment, and community wide health behaviour interventions that were identified and known to be effective in reducing high blood pressure levels. Future studies may want to include additional measures such as salt intake and alcohol consumption.

Abbreviations

BMI: Body mass index
DBP: Diastolic blood pressure
CES-D: Centres for Epidemiologic Studies Depression Scale
EA: Enumeration area
IFLS: Indonesian Family Life Survey
IPAQ: International Physical Activity Questionnaire
LDL: Low-density lipoprotein
NCD: Noncommunicable disease
SBP: Systolic blood pressure.

Data Availability

The data underlying this study belong to the Indonesia Family Life Survey and are accessible via the RAND website: http://www.rand.org/labor/FLS/IFLS.html.

Ethical Approval

The IFLS has been approved by ethics review boards of RAND and University of Gadjah Mada in Indonesia [38].

Authors' Contributions

Karl Peltzer and Supa Pengpid conceived and designed the analysis. Karl Peltzer drafted the manuscript and Supa Pengpid made critical revision of the manuscript for key intellectual content. All authors read and approved the final version of the manuscript. All authors have agreed to authorship and order of authorship for this manuscript.

Acknowledgments

The research was conducted based on the IFLS-5 conducted by RAND (http://www.rand.org/labor/FLS/IFLS.html). We thank RAND for providing the access to the survey data and the study participants who provided the survey data.

References

[1] World Health Organization (WHO). Global status report on noncommunicable diseases 2014. Geneva, Switzerland: WHO, 2014.

[2] J. Schröders, S. Wall, M. Hakimi et al., "How is Indonesia coping with its epidemic of chronic noncommunicable diseases? A systematic review with meta-analysis," *PLoS ONE*, vol. 12, no. 6, p. e0179186, 2017.

[3] World Health Organization (WHO). Indonesia: WHO statistical profile, 2012. http://www.who.int/gho/countries/idn.pdf?ua=1.

[4] World Health Organization (WHO). Noncommunicable diseases country profiles 2014. http://apps.who.int/iris/bitstream/10665/128038/1/9789241507509_eng.pdf.

[5] M. M. Ibrahim and A. Damasceno, "Hypertension in developing countries," *The Lancet*, vol. 380, no. 9841, pp. 611–619, 2012.

[6] B. M. Egan, Y. Zhao, and R. N. Axon, "US trends in prevalence, awareness, treatment, and control of hypertension, 1988–2008," *The Journal of the American Medical Association*, vol. 303, no. 20, pp. 2043–2050, 2010.

[7] R. Castillo, "Prevalence and management of hypertension in Southeast Asia," *J Hypertens*, supplement 1, p. e4, 2016.

[8] M. A. Hussain, A. A. Mamun, C. Reid, R. R. Huxley, and Y. Li, "Prevalence, Awareness, Treatment and Control of Hypertension in Indonesian Adults Aged ≥40 Years: Findings from the Indonesia Family Life Survey (IFLS)," *PLoS ONE*, vol. 11, no. 8, p. e0160922, 2016.

[9] C. Naing, P. N. Yeoh, V. N. Wai, N. N. Win, L. P. Kuan, and K. Aung, "Hypertension in Malaysia: An Analysis of Trends From the National Surveys 1996 to 2011," *Medicine*, vol. 95, no. 2, p. e2417, 2016.

[10] M. B. Bjertness, A. S. Htet, H. E. Meyer et al., "Prevalence and determinants of hypertension in Myanmar - a nationwide cross-sectional study," *BMC Public Health*, vol. 16, no. 1, 2016.

[11] P. Katulanda, P. Ranasinghe, R. Jayawardena, G. R. Constantine, M. H. Rezvi Sheriff, and D. R. Matthews, "The prevalence, predictors and associations of hypertension in Sri Lanka: A cross-sectional population based national survey," *Clinical and Experimental Hypertension*, vol. 36, no. 7, pp. 484–491, 2014.

[12] P. T. Son, N. N. Quang, N. L. Viet et al., "Prevalence, awareness, treatment and control of hypertension in Vietnam—results from a national survey," *Journal of Human Hypertension*, vol. 26, no. 4, pp. 268–280, 2012.

[13] J. Wang, L. Zhang, F. Wang, L. Liu, and H. Wang, "Prevalence, awareness, treatment, and control of hypertension in China: results from a national survey," *American Journal of Hypertension*, vol. 27, no. 11, pp. 1355–1361, 2014.

[14] A. Esteghamati, M. Abbasi, S. Alikhani et al., "Prevalence, awareness, treatment, and risk factors associated with hypertension in the Iranian population: The national survey of risk factors for noncommunicable diseases of Iran," *American Journal of Hypertension*, vol. 21, no. 6, pp. 620–626, 2008.

[15] C. K. Chow, K. K. Teo, S. Rangarajan et al., "Prevalence, awareness, treatment, and control of hypertension in rural and urban communities in high-, middle-, and low-income countries," *Journal of the American Medical Association*, vol. 310, no. 9, pp. 959–968, 2013.

[16] S. Cuschieri, J. Vassallo, N. Calleja, N. Pace, and J. Mamo, "The Effects of Socioeconomic Determinants on Hypertension in a Cardiometabolic At-Risk European Country," *International Journal of Hypertension*, vol. 2017, Article ID 7107385, 7 pages, 2017.

[17] M. E. Hendriks, F. W. N. M. Wit, M. T. L. Roos et al., "Hypertension in Sub-Saharan Africa: cross-sectional surveys in four rural and urban communities," *PLoS ONE*, vol. 7, no. 3, Article ID e32638, 2012.

[18] C. Agyemang, "Rural and urban differences in blood pressure and hypertension in Ghana, West Africa," *Public Health*, vol. 120, no. 6, pp. 525–533, 2006.

[19] B. Li, F. Li, L. Wang, and D. Zhang, "Fruit and Vegetables Consumption and Risk of Hypertension: A Meta-Analysis," *The Journal of Clinical Hypertension*, vol. 18, no. 5, pp. 468–476, 2016.

[20] L. Wang, J. E. Manson, J. M. Gaziano, J. E. Buring, and H. D. Sesso, "Fruit and vegetable intake and the risk of hypertension in middle-aged and older women," *American Journal of Hypertension*, vol. 25, no. 2, pp. 180–189, 2012.

[21] D. Zhao, Y. Qi, Z. Zheng et al., "Dietary factors associated with hypertension," *Nature Reviews Cardiology*, vol. 8, no. 8, pp. 456–465, 2011.

[22] C. Ezekwesili, C. Ononamadu, O. Onyeukwu, and N. Mefoh, "Epidemiological survey of hypertension in Anambra state, Nigeria," *Nigerian Journal of Clinical Practice*, vol. 19, no. 5, pp. 659–667, 2016.

[23] A. M. El-Badawy, H. M. Al-Kharusi, and S. A. Al-Ghanemy, "Health habits and risk factors among Omanis with hypertension," *Saudi Medical Journal*, vol. 26, no. 4, pp. 623–629, 2005.

[24] X. Xu, J. Byles, Z. Shi, P. McElduff, and J. Hall, "Dietary pattern transitions, and the associations with BMI, waist circumference, weight and hypertension in a 7-year follow-up among the older Chinese population: A longitudinal study," *BMC Public Health*, vol. 16, no. 1, article no. 743, 2016.

[25] S. Kar and B. Khandelwal, "Fast foods and physical inactivity are risk factors for obesity and hypertension among adolescent school children in east district of Sikkim, India," *Journal of Natural Science, Biology and Medicine*, vol. 6, no. 2, pp. 356–359, 2015.

[26] W. Cheungpasitporn, C. Thongprayoon, P. J. Edmonds et al., "Sugar and artificially sweetened soda consumption linked to hypertension: A systematic review and meta-analysis," *Clinical and Experimental Hypertension*, vol. 37, no. 7, pp. 587–593, 2015.

[27] M. Borjesson, A. Onerup, S. Lundqvist, and B. Dahlof, "Physical activity and exercise lower blood pressure in individuals with hypertension: Narrative review of 27 RCTs," *British Journal of Sports Medicine*, vol. 50, no. 6, pp. 356–361, 2016.

[28] A. Giday and B. Tadesse, "Prevalence and determinants of hypertension in rural and urban areas of southern Ethiopia," *Ethiop Med J*, vol. 49, pp. 139–147, 2011.

[29] S. S. De Ramirez, D. A. Enquobahrie, G. Nyadzi et al., "Prevalence and correlates of hypertension: A cross-sectional study among rural populations in sub-Saharan Africa," *Journal of Human Hypertension*, vol. 24, no. 12, pp. 786–795, 2010.

[30] A. Leone, "Smoking and hypertension: independent or additive effects to determining vascular damage?" *Current Vascular Pharmacology*, vol. 9, no. 5, pp. 585–593, 2011.

[31] E. Macia, P. Duboz, and L. Gueye, "Prevalence, awareness, treatment and control of hypertension among adults 50 years and older in Dakar, Senegal," *Cardiovascular Journal of Africa*, vol. 23, no. 5, pp. 265–269, 2012.

[32] Y. Cuffee, C. Ogedegbe, N. J. Williams, G. Ogedegbe, and A. Schoenthaler, "Psychosocial risk factors for hypertension: an update of the literature," *Current Hypertension Reports*, vol. 16, no. 10, p. 483, 2014.

[33] M.-Y. Liu, N. Li, W. A. Li, and H. Khan, "Association between psychosocial stress and hypertension: a systematic review and meta-analysis," *Neurological Research*, vol. 39, no. 6, pp. 573–580, 2017.

[34] A. T. Ginty, D. Carroll, T. J. Roseboom, A. C. Phillips, and S. R. De Rooij, "Depression and anxiety are associated with a diagnosis of hypertension 5 years later in a cohort of late middle-aged men and women," *Journal of Human Hypertension*, vol. 27, no. 3, pp. 187–190, 2013.

[35] V. Romero Martinez, E. Silva, and J. Villasmil, "Relationship between life satisfaction levels and high blood pressure in adolescents: PP.14.43," *Journal of Hypertension*, vol. 28, p. e260, 2010.

[36] S. Mojon-Azzi and A. Sousa-Poza, "Hypertension and life satisfaction: An analysis using data from the Survey of Health, Ageing and retirement in Europe," *Applied Economics Letters*, vol. 18, no. 2, pp. 183–187, 2011.

[37] M. S. Mujahid, A. V. D. Roux, and J. D. Morenoff, "Neighborhood characteristics and hypertension," *Epidemiology*, vol. 19, no. 4, pp. 590–598, 2008.

[38] J. Strauss, F. Witoelar, and B. Sikoki, *The Fifth Wave of the Indonesia Family Life Survey (IFLS5): Overview and Field Report*, vol. 1, RAND Corporation, 2016.

[39] A. V. Chobanian, G. L. Bakris, and H. R. Black, "Seventh report of the Joint National Committee on prevention, detection, evaluation, and treatment of high blood pressure," *Hypertension*, vol. 42, no. 6, pp. 1206–1252, 2003.

[40] C. P. Wen, T. Y. David Cheng, S. P. Tsai et al., "Are Asians at greater mortality risks for being overweight than Caucasians? Redefining obesity for Asians," *Public Health Nutrition*, vol. 12, no. 4, pp. 497–506, 2009.

[41] C. L. Craig, A. L. Marshall, and M. Sjöström, "International physical activity questionnaire: 12-country reliability and validity," *Medicine & Science in Sports & Exercise*, vol. 35, no. 8, pp. 1381–1395, 2003.

[42] International Physical Activity Questionnaire (IPAQ). IPAQ Scoring Protocol. https://sites.google.com/site/theipaq/.

[43] E. M. Andresen, J. A. Malmgren, W. B. Carter, and D. L. Patrick, "Screening for depression in well older adults: evaluation of a short form of the CES-D (Center for Epidemiologic Studies Depression Scale)," *American Journal of Preventive Medicine*, vol. 10, no. 2, pp. 77–84, 1994.

[44] K. T. Mills, J. D. Bundy, T. N. Kelly et al., "Global disparities of hypertension prevalence and control: A systematic analysis of population-based studies from 90 countries," *Circulation*, vol. 134, no. 6, pp. 441–450, 2016.

[45] M. Hosseini, M. Yousefifard, M. Baikpour et al., "Twenty-year dynamics of hypertension in Iranian adults: age, period, and cohort analysis," *Journal of the American Society of Hypertension*, vol. 9, no. 12, pp. 925–934, 2015.

[46] World Health Organization (WHO). The Republic of Indonesia health system review. Health systems in transition. Vol-7, Number -1. New Dehli: WHO Regional Office for South-East Asia.

[47] S. Pengpid and K. Peltzer, "Overweight, obesity and associated factors among 13-15 years old students in the association of Southeast Asian Nations member countries, 2007-2014," *Southeast Asian Journal of Tropical Medicine and Public Health*, vol. 47, no. 2, pp. 250–261, 2016.

[48] K. Peltzer and S. Pengpid, "The Association of Dietary Behaviors and Physical Activity Levels with General and Central Obesity among ASEAN University Students," *AIMS Public Health*, vol. 4, no. 3, pp. 301–303, 2017.

[49] C. N. Rachmi, M. Li, and L. Alison Baur, "Overweight and obesity in Indonesia: prevalence and risk factors—a literature review," *Public Health*, vol. 147, pp. 20–29, 2017.

[50] C. Erem, A. Hacihasanoglu, M. Kocak, O. Deger, and M. Topbas, "Prevalence of prehypertension and hypertension and associated risk factors among Turkish adults: trabzon hypertension study," *Journal of Public Health*, vol. 31, no. 1, pp. 47–58, 2009.

[51] E. Afrifa-Anane, C. Agyemang, S. N. A. Codjoe, G. Ogedegbe, and A. De-Graft Aikins, "The association of physical activity, body mass index and the blood pressure levels among urban poor youth in Accra, Ghana," *BMC Public Health*, vol. 15, no. 1, 2015.

[52] R. M. Krauss, M. Winston, B. J. Fletcher, and S. M. Grundy, "Obesity: Impact on cardiovascular disease," *Circulation*, vol. 98, no. 14, pp. 1472–1476, 1998.

[53] K. Gao, X. Shi, and W. Wang, "The life-course impact of smoking on hypertension, myocardial infarction and respiratory diseases," *Scientific Reports*, vol. 7, no. 1, 2017.

[54] A. Z. Scalco, M. Z. Scalco, J. B. S. Azul, and F. Lotufo Neto, "Hypertension and depression.," *Clinics (São Paulo, Brazil)*, vol. 60, no. 3, pp. 241–250, 2005.

23

Comparative Evaluation of Adiposity Indices as Predictors of Hypertension among Brazilian Adults

Maurílio T. Dutra,[1,2] Diego B. V. Reis,[1] Karla G. Martins,[1] and André B. Gadelha[3]

[1] *Technical School of Health, State Department of Education of the Federal District, Brasília, Brazil*
[2] *Federal Institute of Education, Science and Technology of Brasília, Brasília, Brazil*
[3] *Mauá Institute of Research and Education, Vicente Pires, Federal District, Brazil*

Correspondence should be addressed to Maurílio T. Dutra; mauriliotiradentes@gmail.com

Academic Editor: Markus P. Schlaich

Purpose. To compare several anthropometric indices in the prediction of hypertension among adults. *Methods.* This is a cross-sectional study. Five hundred and eighteen adult men and women (40.9 ± 10.5 years; 1.62 ± .09 m; 72.3 ± 15.6 kg) volunteered to participate and underwent blood pressure and anthropometric measures. Anthropometric assessments were used to calculate body mass index (BMI), waist circumference (WC), waist-to-hip ratio (WHR), waist-to-stature ratio (WSR), body adiposity index (BAI), and conicity index (C). Comparisons between men and women were carried out by independent t-test and chi-square test. Cut-off points for each adiposity index to predict hypertension were obtained using Receiver Operating Characteristic (ROC) curve analyses. The significance level was set at $P \leq .05$. *Results.* All adiposity indices regarding both genders showed significant odds ratios, except BAI (odds ratio: 1.534; CI: 0.916–2.571) for women. In men, WHR and WSR were considered as more balanced indices regarding their sensitivity (AUC: 73.8 and 71.4, respectively) and specificity (AUC: 77.6 and 73.1, respectively). In women, WHR and WSR presented areas under the ROC curves higher than C index ($P = .007$) and BAI ($P = .03$), respectively. *Conclusion.* Indices that consider abdominal adiposity such as WC, WHR, and WSR have a stronger relationship with hypertension compared to others.

1. Introduction

Hypertension is characterized by high and sustained values of blood pressure (BP). It is a chronic multifactorial condition often associated with functional and structural alterations in several organs. Also, hypertension is related to metabolic alterations with a consequent increase in the risk of fatal and nonfatal cardiovascular events [1]. As it is highly prevalent both in developed [2] and low-to-middle-income countries [3], hypertension has been considered a major public health issue worldwide [4]. Particularly, Brazil is a middle-income country that presents a high prevalence of hypertension, reaching 25% of the population [5].

Risk factors for hypertension include age, gender, ethnicity, socioeconomic status, and lifestyle-related factors, such as sodium intake and sedentary lifestyle [1]. Moreover, excess body weight caused by genetic and/or sedentarism and bad nutrition is commonly associated with the incidence of hypertension [1]. Noteworthy, several adiposity indices, such as body mass index (BMI), waist circumference (WC), conicity index (C), and waist-to-hip-ratio (WHR), have been extensively applied to assess cardiovascular risk factors among adults and elderly people [6–8]. In fact, studies have shown that those indices, particularly when WC is accounted for, are good predictors of hypertension [7, 8].

In addition, other adiposity indices that may be useful for predicting cardiovascular diseases have been proposed in the literature, such as the body adiposity index (BAI) [9] and the waist-to-stature ratio (WSR) [10]. Previous results indicate that BAI is a good and valid index for estimating body fat [9]. Meanwhile, WSR was found to be more strongly associated with cardiovascular risk factors (i.e., lipid profile and blood pressure) than BMI, WHR, and WC in a representative sample of Chinese people [10].

As anthropometric derived indices are cost-effective strategies to assess and manage health outcomes, it would be useful to analyze which of those indices has the best sensitivity and specificity to predict hypertension. Of note, middle-income countries like Brazil have been facing a growing incidence of obesity and hypertension [1, 11]. Thus, a comparative evaluation of traditional and newer adiposity indices in the prediction of hypertension among Brazilian people is warranted. Therefore, the aim of the present investigation was to analyze and compare several anthropometric indices in the prediction of hypertension among Brazilian adults.

2. Materials and Methods

2.1. Study Design. The present cross-sectional study was designed to analyze and compare several anthropometric indices in the prediction of hypertension among Brazilian adults. To reach this aim, adults of both genders underwent anthropometric evaluations in several locations of an urban community of the Federal District, Brazil. People were invited as they walked through the evaluation sites that had previously been set up by the researchers in distinct locations of the community. Participants answered a questionnaire addressing medical history, hypertension diagnosis, tobacco use, alcohol consumption, and physical activity habits. Body mass and height, as well as waist and hip circumferences, were measured to analyze adiposity indices. Also, blood pressure was measured twice, after a 10-minute seated rest. Adiposity indices were compared as to their sensitivity and specificity to predict hypertension. This study complies with the Helsinki Declaration and the procedures were approved by the Institution Review Board.

2.2. Sample. A total of six hundred and seventy-six people volunteered to participate. Eligibility criteria for the present analysis were as follows: to be aged between 20 and 60 years old and to live in the community for at least one year. All subjects who did not meet these two eligibility criteria were excluded from the present analysis. Thus, this study reports data from the five hundred and eighteen adult men and women (40.9 ± 10.5 years; 1.62 ± .09 m; 72.3 ± 15.6 kg) who were eligible and completed blood pressure and anthropometric measures. All participants were informed about the study procedures and voluntarily signed an informed consent form.

2.3. Blood Pressure and Hypertension. It is known that office measurements of blood pressure (BP) do not reflect diurnal variation and nocturnal BP levels [12]. Thus, hypertension was determined in the present study by analyzing participant's answers in the medical history questionnaire. All subjects were oriented to answer the questionnaire based on clinical examination performed prior to the present investigation. Therefore, it was assumed that all subjects that reported hypertension did so based on previous diagnostic made by a cardiologist through accurate method, such as 24 h ambulatory BP monitoring. Nevertheless, BP of each volunteer was measured twice by trained technicians after a 10-minute seated rest. Measurements were taken by auscultation using a mercury sphygmomanometer. Systolic BP and diastolic BP were defined as the points of the appearance and disappearance of Korotkoff sounds, respectively. Mean of the two measurements was calculated and recorded as the BP value. These values were used as secondary data to assess hypertension adopting systolic and diastolic BP cutoffs of 140 mmHg and 90 mmHg, respectively [13]. In addition, prevalence of diabetes *mellitus*, smoking status, alcohol consumption, and physical activity status were also assessed by questionnaire.

2.4. Anthropometry. Total body mass was measured in a digital scale to the nearest 0.50 g (OMROM HBF 510, OMRON Healthcare Inc., Lake Forest, IL). Height was measure to the nearest 0.1 cm using a portable stadiometer (Sanny®, São Bernardo do Campo, SP, Brazil). Waist circumference was assessed at the level of umbilicus, and hip circumference was determined at the level of the maximum extension of the buttocks posteriorly in a horizontal plane. Thus, WHR and WSR ratios were calculated as waist divided by hip and height (in centimeters), respectively. BMI was calculated as weight divided by height squared (kg/m^2) and BAI was calculated according to the following equation [9]:

$$\text{BAI} = \left[\frac{(\text{hip circumference})}{\left((\text{height})^{1.5}\right)} - 18 \right]. \qquad (1)$$

Finally, the conicity index was determined according to the following equation [14]:

$$\text{Conicity index} = \frac{\text{waist circumference (m)}}{0.109\sqrt{(\text{total body mass (kg)}/\text{height (m)})}}. \qquad (2)$$

2.5. Statistical Analysis. Descriptive data are expressed as mean and standard deviation unless otherwise noted. The normal distribution of data was examined using the Kolmogorov-Smirnov test. Comparisons between men and women were carried out by independent t-test and chi-square test for continuous and categorical variables, respectively. The cut-off points for each adiposity index to predict hypertension were obtained using Receiver Operating Characteristic (ROC) curve analyses. Thus, areas under the ROC curves and the confidence intervals (CI: 95%) were used to compare the ability of each adiposity index to predict hypertension. Therefore, odds ratios (CI: 95%) for the presence of hypertension considering the identified cut-off points for each adiposity index were calculated. Moreover, Mantel-Haenszel provided common odds ratios adjustments for age, smoking, physical activity, diabetes, and alcohol consumption. The significance level was set at $P \leq .05$, and all analyses were conducted using the Statistical Package for Social Sciences (SPSS 20.0).

3. Results

The overall prevalence of hypertension was 24.3% (95% CI: 20.3–28.0). Rates by gender were 23.9% (95% CI: 17.6–30.1)

TABLE 1: Descriptive values and comparison between genders (mean ± SD).

	Men	Women	P
n	176	342	
Age (years)	41.3 ± 10.5	40.7 ± 10.5	.514
Height (m)	1.71 ± 0.1	1.6 ± 0.1	**.001**
Body weight (kg)	81.0 ± 14.7	67.8 ± 14.2	**.001**
Body mass index (kg/m^2)	27.7 ± 4.3	27.2 ± 5.1	.222
Waist circumference (cm)	93.2 ± 11.9	85.0 ± 11.5	**.001**
Hip circumference (cm)	101.0 ± 8.3	102.1 ± 10.4	.203
Waist-to-hip ratio	0.92 ± 0.1	0.83 ± 0.1	**.001**
Waist-to-stature ratio	0.55 ± 0.1	0.54 ± 0.1	.287
Body adiposity index (%)	27.3 ± 3.7	33.6 ± 5.3	**.001**
Conicity index (AU)	1.2 ± 0.1	1.2 ± 0.1	**.001**
Systolic BP (mmHg)	124.1 ± 13.2	120.3 ± 13.7	**.003**
Diastolic BP (mmHg)	79.9 ± 10.4	77.7 ± 9.8	**.016**

Note. AU: Arbitrary units. BP: blood pressure.

and 24.6% (95% CI: 19.9–29.2) for men and women, respectively, with no differences between groups (X^2 = .031; P = .861). Based on BP values, overall prevalence was slightly lower (20.8%; 95% CI: 17.2–24.5) with no differences between genders (23.3% and 19.6% for men and women, respectively; X^2 = .966 P = .326). Overall prevalence of diabetes *mellitus* was 4.4% (95% CI: 2.9–6.2). Rates by gender were 4.5% and 4.4% for men and women, respectively, with no difference between groups (X^2 = .007; P = .933). In addition, there was no difference between genders with regard to smoking status (8.0% and 6.4% for men and women, respectively; X^2 = .416; P = .519). However, chi-square test showed a significant difference between gender groups regarding the prevalence of alcohol consumption (42.0% and 24.3% for men and women, respectively; X^2 = 17.384; $P < .001$) and physically active status (74.4% and 52.9% for men and women, respectively; X^2 = 22.441; $P < .001$). None of the participants reported heart disease.

Table 1 shows descriptive values regarding genders and its comparisons. Of note, no differences were observed for age, BMI, hip circumference, and WSR ratio between gender groups.

ROC curves for each adiposity index according to sensitivity and specificity in the diagnosis of hypertension for men and women are presented in Figures 1 and 2, respectively. Regarding men's difference between areas under the ROC curves, pairwise comparisons highlighted C index, WHR, and WSR as higher than BMI ($P < .001$), WC ($P < .05$), and BAI ($P < .001$). Furthermore, BAI showed highest sensitivity (97.6) to predict HAS, meanwhile C index presented highest specificity (83.6). Moreover, both WHR and WSR were considered as more balanced indices regarding their sensitivity (73.8 and 71.4, respectively) and specificity (77.6 and 73.1, respectively). In women, WHR and WSR presented areas under the ROC curves higher than C index (P = .007) and BAI (P = .03), respectively.

Table 2 shows the odds ratios and confidence intervals for the presence of hypertension regarding each adiposity index above the proposed cut-off values. All adiposity indices regarding both genders showed significant odds ratios, except the BAI (odds ratio: 1.534; CI: 0.916–2.571) for women. Moreover, after adjustments for age, smoking, physical activity, diabetes, and alcohol consumption, the odds ratios for BAI in men was no longer statistically significant (odds ratio: 10.489; CI: 0.788–139.597). Interestingly, in women, there was no significant odds ratio after the adjustments.

4. Discussion

The purpose of this cross-sectional investigation was to analyze and compare several anthropometric indices in the prediction of hypertension among Brazilian adults. In general, the adiposity indices were more sensitive to predict hypertension in men. Of note, both WC and WSR presented values with the highest balance of sensitivity and specificity in the prediction of hypertension in men. Moreover, WC and WSR presented the highest sensitivity, while WHR presented the highest specificity to predict hypertension in women. Also, the prevalence of hypertension was 24.3%, without differences between genders. Finally, after adjustments for age, smoking, physical activity, diabetes, and alcohol consumption, all adiposity indices, except for BAI, showed significant odds ratios in men. On the other hand, there was no significant odds ratio in women after the adjustments.

Worldwide cut-off recommendations for BMI, WC, and WHR are 30 kg/m^2 (both genders), 102 and 88 cm (men and women), and 0.90 and 0.85 cm (men and women), respectively [15]. Using these recommended cut-off points of BMI and WC to define obesity, a previous study [7] in a Brazilian sample (n = 592, both genders) observed hazard ratios adjusted for age and blood pressure of 1.08 (0.52–2.24, P = .82) and 1.74 (0.93–3.26, P = .08) for BMI in men and women, respectively. Regarding WC, hazard ratios were 1.78 (0.76–4.09, P = .18) for men and 1.72 (1.09–2.73, P = .02) for women. As only WC for women presented a significant ability to predict hypertension, the authors of that study concluded that the risk for hypertension may be better defined by higher WC than higher BMI. In general, the results of the present study presented lower cut-off values when compared to the aforementioned. For instance, WC cut-off points to predict hypertension were 9.0 cm lower in men and 9.5 cm lower in women than the general cut-off recommended by the World Health Organization. This is an important finding that highlights the need for continuously educating people about hypertension risk factors in the sample of this study.

Moreover, there is a gap for the cut-off points of WSR, BAI, and C index. Despite this gap, a recent investigation observed that WSR is more strongly associated with hypertension than BMI, WC, and WHR in men and women from India and Pakistan [8]. In line with this, a previous research analyzing a large sample of Chinese men and women (n = 2895; 25–74 years old) observed that WSR was the best index in predicting elevated systolic and diastolic BP in women when compared to BMI, WC, and WHR (WSR likelihood ratios in that study were 3.05 and 3.38 for systolic

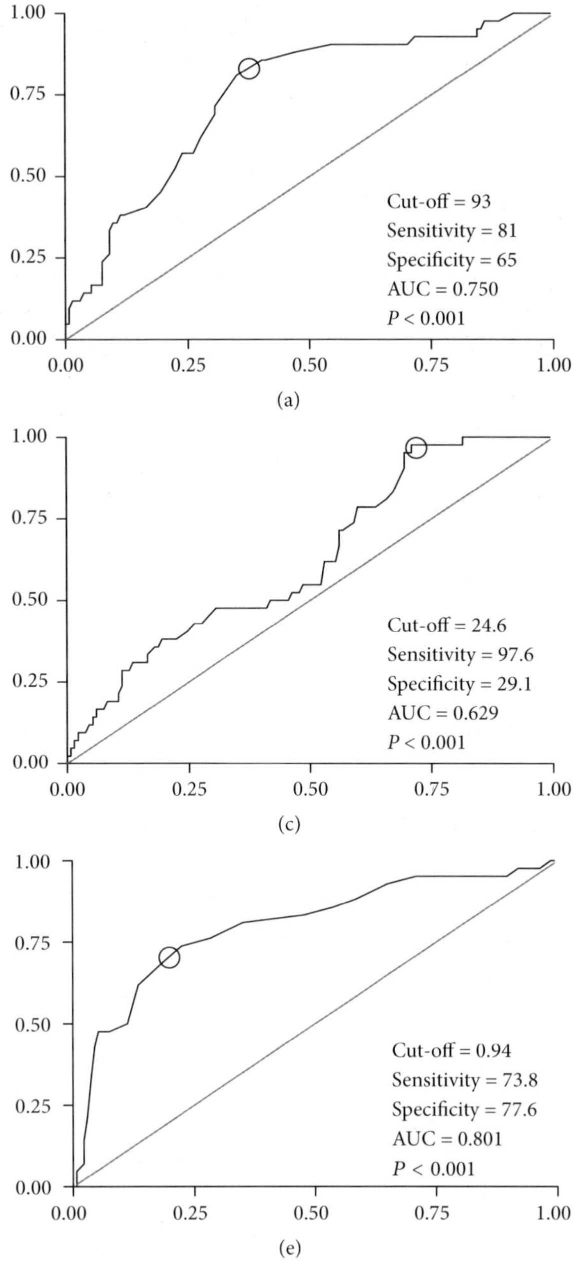

FIGURE 1: Receiver Operating Characteristic curve according to sensitivity (x-axis) and specificity (y-axis) of (a) waist circumference; (b) body mass index; (c) body adiposity index; (d) conicity index; (e) waist-to-hip ratio; (f) waist-to-stature ratio, in men. AUC: area under the curve.

TABLE 2: Odds ratios (OR, confidence interval: 95%) for hypertension.

	Men (n = 176)		Women (n = 342)	
Indices	OR (CI = 95%)	Adjusted OR	OR (CI = 95%)	Adjusted OR
WC	7.87 (3.37–18.37)	4.29 (1.51–12.22)	2.20 (1.21–4.02)	1.40 (0.67–2.96)
BMI	5.17 (2.04–13.08)	6.33 (1.61–24.84)	2.07 (1.21–3.54)	1.84 (0.94–3.61)
BAI	16.22 (2.16–122.22)	10.49 (0.79–139.60)	1.53 (0.92–2.57)	1.50 (0.89–2.56)
C Index	10.18 (4.63–22.38)	6.60 (1.90–22.95)	1.76 (1.03–3.03)	1.35 (0.68–2.68)
WHR	7.97 (3.62–17.54)	3.34 (1.30–8.58)	2.51 (1.48–4.26)	1.95 (0.99–3.84)
WSR	6.66 (3.04–14.14)	4.20 (1.57–11.21)	2.20 (1.21–4.02)	1.48 (0.69–3.18)

Note. Odds ratio adjusted for age, smoking, physical activity, diabetes, and alcohol consumption.

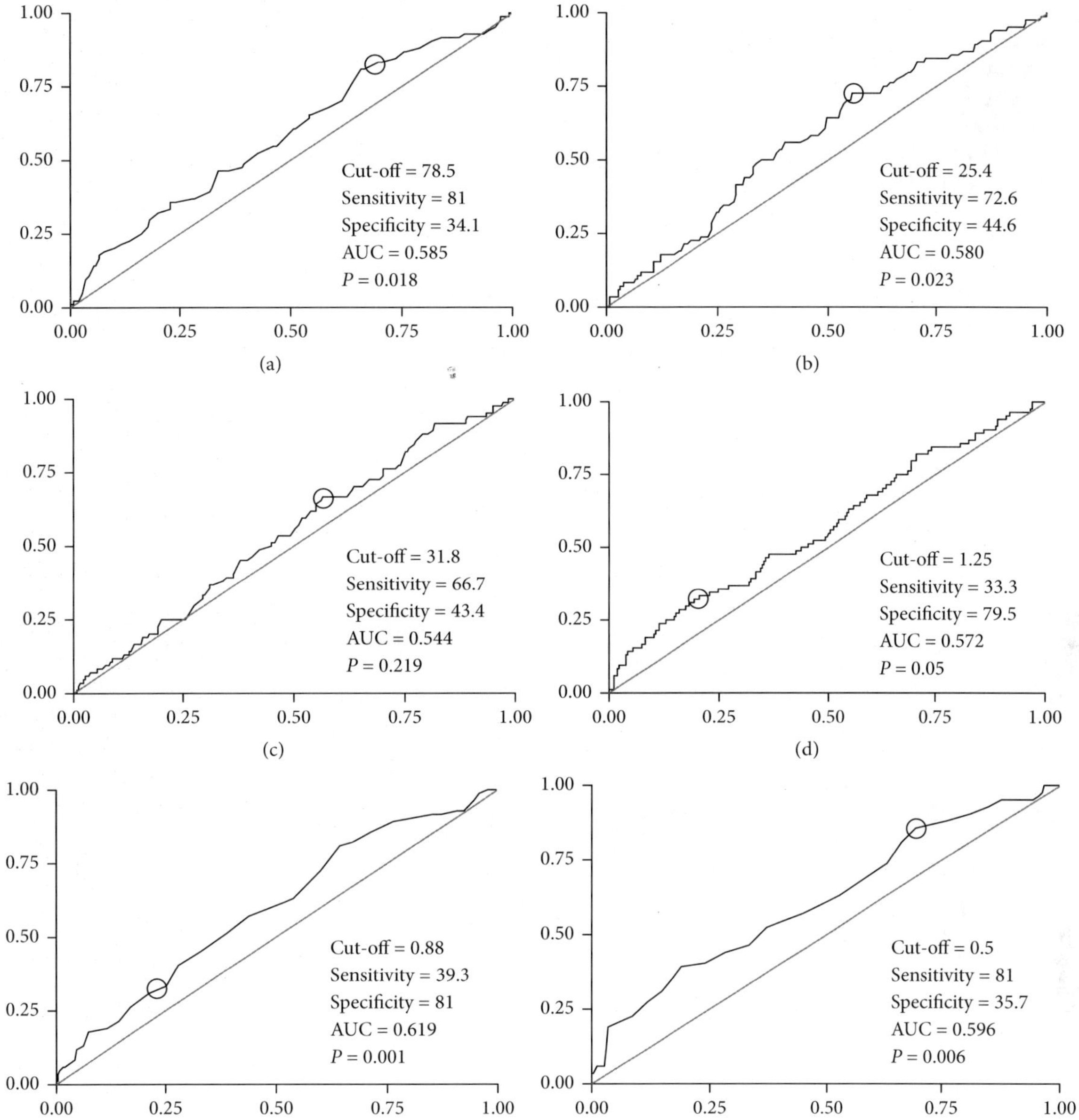

FIGURE 2: Receiver Operating Characteristic curve according to sensitivity (x-axis) and specificity (y-axis) of (a) waist circumference; (b) body mass index; (c) body adiposity index; (d) conicity index; (e) waist-to-hip ratio; (f) waist-to-stature ratio, in women. AUC: area under the curve.

and diastolic BP, respectively) [10]. In addition, in a large sample (n = 3971, both genders) of Arab adults, Al-Daghri and colleagues [16] found that WSR was the most sensitive index, but rather modest, in determining hypertension (AUC 0.66, $P < .001$). In the present research, these values were even higher (see Figures 1 and 2). However, as Al-Daghri et al. did not present sensitivity and specificity for genders separately, further comparison with the present study is limited. In general, the present investigation does not totally corroborate those previous data, once none of the indices presented significant odds ratios to predict hypertension in women after the adjustments, while all of them (except BAI) presented significant odds ratio to predict hypertension in men.

Regarding newer adiposity indices such as BAI, further investigations are clearly warranted, as previous research came up with conflicting results. For instance, a recent report identified BAI to be a useful index to predict hypertension in adult obese women from India (n = 131; odds ratio = 3.28, CI: 1.95–5.51, P = .001) [17]. In the present study, BAI did not present significant odds ratio in women, nor in men, after adjusting for age, smoking, physical activity, diabetes, and alcohol consumption. Indeed, there is evidence that BAI may be an inferior index to predict body fatness and cardiovascular risk factors (i.e., including systolic and diastolic blood pressure) compared to BMI and WC [18, 19]. In the Bogalusa Heart Study [19], for example, the authors showed that the correlation between BAI and a sum of cardiovascular risk factors (lipids, fasting insulin and glucose, and blood pressure) in 2367 men and women (18–49 years old) is significantly weaker when compared with BMI and WC ($r = .49$, .58, and .61, respectively).

Interestingly, in the present study, adiposity indices were more sensitive to predict hypertension in men. Moreover, indices that consider abdominal obesity (i.e., WC and WSR) presented high balance of sensitivity and specificity to predict hypertension in men, but not in women. This finding can be explained by the differences of fat distribution between genders. Indeed, men usually present more fat in the central region of the body, and abdominal fat accumulation (i.e., android pattern) is associated with higher risk for cardiovascular diseases, independent of total body mass or BMI; otherwise, fat accumulation in the subcutaneous or appendicular skeleton (i.e., usually presented by women) is considered to be less harmful [20, 21]. These findings corroborate previous findings and the guidelines of the World Health Organization which states that measures of abdominal obesity are better than BMI as predictors of hypertension and other cardiovascular risk factors [15, 22]. In light of the present results allied with previous investigations regarding differences in gender, the "need to develop sex specific cut-off values appropriate for different populations" has been stated [15]; hence there is no consensus of these values in the literature regarding hypertension in adults. Additionally, all cutoffs in the present study were adjusted according to its sensitivity and specificity to predict hypertension in a specific population. Thus, these findings contribute to the management of hypertension in the studied population.

Once office measurements of BP may not reflect the true BP levels (i.e., they do not reflect diurnal variation and nocturnal BP levels) [12], our first choice to determine hypertension was based on participant's answers to the medical history questionnaire. Consistent with previous reports [5], the prevalence of hypertension found in this investigation (24.3%, 95% CI: 20.3–28.0) is similar to that of the overall Brazilian population of big urban centers (around 24.8%) [5]. These values are higher than the prevalence found recently in Canada (19.5%), but lower when compared to other developed countries such as the United States of America (29.1%) and England (30.0%) [2]. When compared to other middle-income countries such as México (44.6%), China (42.7%), and India (37.8%), the prevalence of hypertension among the present sample was found to be lower. Some lifestyle habits may be related to this high prevalence of hypertension in developing countries. For instance, in Brazil, daily consumption of sodium is more than twice (4.7 g per 2000 kcal) the recommended levels of intake according to the World Health Organization [23]. In addition, despite the fact that around 60% of the sample of this study reported being physically active (data not shown), sedentary lifestyle in leisure-time is high (around 65% of the people) among Brazilians [5, 24]. Of note, incidence of hypertension and other cardiovascular and metabolic diseases is growing worldwide. Once hypertension is a common condition that may lead to myocardial infarction, stroke, renal failure, and death if not detected early and treated appropriately [4], public health strategies to overcome this disease are imperious.

The present study has several strengths and limitations. Representative sample and novelty of the results are strengths. We opted to evaluate body adiposity using easy-access and low-cost clinical indices in a large sample instead of gold standard that would certainly demand higher costs and lower external validity. The study is limited by its cross-sectional design, which precludes cause-effect inferences. Thus, although the present report adds information to the literature, longitudinal studies are recommended to establish the temporal influence of predicting ability of clinical adiposity indices and hypertension in adults.

5. Conclusions

Consistent with previous reports, various adiposity indices are associated with hypertension in Brazilian adults with different degrees. We observed that indices which consider abdominal adiposity such as WC, WHR, and WSR have a stronger relationship to hypertension compared to others. Of note, adiposity indices were more sensitive to predict hypertension in men and this is probably related to the differences of fat distribution between genders. Given that WC, WHR, and WSR are accurate, are simple to measure, and have minimal cost, they should be routinely employed in the assessment of Brazilian adults at high risk for hypertension.

Acknowledgments

The authors acknowledge the technicians who helped in collecting data.

References

[1] Sociedade Brasileira de Cardiologia, Sociedade Brasileira de Hipertensão, and Sociedade Brasileira de Nefrologia, "VI Diretrizes Brasileiras de Hipertensão," *Arquivos Brasileiros de Cardiologia*, vol. 95, 1, no. 1, pp. 1–51, 2010.

[2] M. Joffres, E. Falaschetti, C. Gillespie et al., "Hypertension prevalence, awareness, treatment and control in national surveys from England, the USA and Canada, and correlation with stroke and ischaemic heart disease mortality: a cross-sectional study," *BMJ Open*, vol. 3, no. 8, Article ID e003423, 2013.

[3] P. Lloyd-Sherlock, J. Beard, N. Minicuci, S. Ebrahim, and S. Chatterji, "Hypertension among older adults in low and middle-income countries: prevalence, awareness and control," *International Journal of Epidemiology*, vol. 43, no. 1, pp. 116–128, 2014.

[4] P. A. James, S. Oparil, B. L. Carter et al., "2014 Evidence-based guideline for the management of high blood pressure in adults. Report from the panel members appoints to the Eighth Joint National Commitee (JNC 8)," *Journal of the American Medical Association*, vol. 1097, pp. 1–14, 2013.

[5] Brasil. Ministério da Saúde. Secretaria de Vigilância em Saúde. Departamento de Vigilância de Doenças e Agravos não Transmissíveis e Promoção da Saúde, "Vigitel Brasil 2014: vigilância de fatores de risco e proteção para doenças crônicas por inquérito telefônico., Ministério da Saúde, Brasília, DF," 2015.

[6] B. D. Cox, M. J. Whichelow, and A. T. Prevost, "The development of cardiovascular disease in relation to anthropometric indices and hypertension in British adults," *International Journal of Obesity*, vol. 22, no. 10, pp. 966–973, 1998.

[7] M. Gus, S. C. Fuchs, L. B. Moreira et al., "Association between different measurements of obesity and the incidence of hypertension," *American Journal of Hypertension*, vol. 17, pp. 50–53, 2004.

[8] S. A. Patel, M. Deepa, R. Shivashankar et al., "Comparison of multiple obesity indices for cardiovascular disease risk classification in South Asian adults: the CARRS study," *PLoS ONE*, vol. 12, no. 4, Article ID e0174251, 2017.

[9] R. N. Bergman, D. Stefanovski, T. A. Buchanan et al., "A better index of body adiposity," *Obesity*, vol. 19, no. 5, pp. 1083–1089, 2011.

[10] S.-Y. Ho, T.-H. Lam, and E. D. Janus, "Waist to stature ratio is more strongly associated with cardiovascular risk factors than other simple anthropometric indices," *Annals of Epidemiology*, vol. 13, no. 10, pp. 683–691, 2003.

[11] Associação Brasileira para o Estudo da Obesidade e da Síndrome Metabólica (Abeso), *Diretrizes Brasileiras de Obesidade 2009-2010*, AC Farmacêutica, Itapevi, SP, Brazil, 3rd edition, 2009, http://www.abeso.org.br/pdf/diretrizes_brasileiras_obesidade_2009_2010_1.pdf.

[12] E. Grossman, "Ambulatory blood pressure monitoring in the diagnosis and management of hypertension," *Diabetes Care*, vol. 36, no. 2, pp. S307–S311, 2013.

[13] M. V. B. Malachias, W. K. S. B. Souza, F. L. Plavnik, C. I. S. Rodrigues et al., "7^a diretriz brasileira de hipertensπo arterial," *Arquivos Brasileiros de Cardiologia*, vol. 107, pp. 1–103, 2016.

[14] R. W. Taylor, I. E. Jones, S. M. Williams, and A. Goulding, "Evaluation of waist circumference, waist-to-hip ratio, and the conicity index as screening tools for high trunk fat mass, as measured by dual-energy X-ray absorptiometry, in children aged 3-19 y," *American Journal of Clinical Nutrition*, vol. 72, no. 2, pp. 490–495, 2000.

[15] C. Nishida, G. T. Ko, and S. Kumanyika, "Body fat distribution and noncommunicable diseases in populations: overview of the 2008 WHO Expert Consultation on Waist Circumference and Waist–Hip Ratio," *European Journal of Clinical Nutrition*, vol. 64, pp. 2–5, 2010.

[16] N. M. Al-Daghri, O. S. Al-Attas, K. Wani et al., "Sensitivity of various adiposity indices in identifying cardiometabolic diseases in Arab adults," *Cardiovascular Diabetology*, vol. 14, no. 1, article no. 101, 2015.

[17] S. Gupta and S. Kapoor, "Body adiposity index: its relevance and validity in assessing body fatness of adults," *ISRN Obesity*, vol. 2014, Article ID 243294, 5 pages, 2014.

[18] D. S. Freedman, J. C. Thornton, F. X. Pi-Sunyer et al., "The body adiposity index (Hip Circumference ÷ Height$^{1.5}$) is not a more accurate measure of adiposity than is BMI, waist circumference, or hip circumference," *Obesity*, vol. 20, no. 12, pp. 2438–2444, 2012.

[19] D. S. Freedman, H. M. Blanck, W. H. Dietz, P. DasMahapatra, S. R. Srinivasan, and G. S. Berenson, "Is the body adiposity index (hip circumference/height(1.5)) more strongly related to skinfold thicknesses and risk factor levels than is BMI? The bogalusa heart study," *British Journal of Nutrition*, vol. 109, no. 2, pp. 338–345, 2013.

[20] A. J. Cameron, D. J. Magliano, and S. Söderberg, "A systematic review of the impact of including both waist and hip circumference in risk models for cardiovascular diseases, diabetes and mortality," *Obesity Reviews*, vol. 14, no. 1, pp. 86–94, 2013.

[21] M. T. Dutra, A. B. Gadelha, O. T. Nóbrega, and R. M. Lima, "Body adiposity index, but not visceral adiposity index, correlates with inflammatory markers in sarcopenic obese elderly women," *Experimental Aging Research*, vol. 43, no. 3, pp. 291–304, 2017.

[22] F. D. Fuchs, M. Gus, L. B. Moreira et al., "Anthropometrie indices and the incidence of hypertension: a comparative analysis," *Obesity Research*, vol. 13, no. 9, pp. 1515–1517, 2005.

[23] F. Sarno, R. M. Claro, R. B. Levy, D. H. Bandoni, and C. A. Monteiro, "Estimated sodium intake for the Brazilian population, 2008-2009," *Revista de Saúde Pública*, vol. 47, no. 3, pp. 571–578, 2013.

[24] A. C. D. S. Andrade, S. V. Peixoto, A. A. D. L. Friche et al., "Social context of neighborhood and socioeconomic status on leisure-time physical activity in a Brazilian urban center: the BH health study," *Cadernos de Saúde Pública*, vol. 31, pp. S136–S147, 2015.

Using Anthropometric Indicator to Identify Hypertension in Adolescents: A Study in Sarawak, Malaysia

Whye Lian Cheah,[1] Ching Thon Chang,[2] Helmy Hazmi,[1] and Grace Woei Feng Kho[1]

[1] *Department of Community Medicine & Public Health, Faculty of Medicine & Health Sciences, Universiti Malaysia Sarawak, Kota Samarahan, Sarawak, Malaysia*
[2] *Department of Nursing, Faculty of Medicine & Health Sciences, Universiti Malaysia Sarawak, Kota Samarahan, Sarawak, Malaysia*

Correspondence should be addressed to Whye Lian Cheah; wlcheah@unimas.my

Academic Editor: Tomohiro Katsuya

This cross-sectional study was conducted to determine the predictive power of anthropometric indicators and recommend cutoff points to discriminate hypertension among adolescents in Sarawak, Malaysia. A total of 2461 respondents aged 12-17 years participated in this study with mean age of 14.5±1.50 years. All anthropometric indicators had significant area under the ROC curve, with body mass index (BMI) and waist circumference (WC) ranging from 0.7 to 0.8. The best anthropometric indicators for predicting hypertension for boys were WC, BMI, and waist-to-height ratio (WHtR). For girls, BMI was the best indicators followed by WHtR and WC. The recommended BMI cutoff point for boys was 20 kg/m^2 and 20.7 kg/m^2 for girls. For WC, the recommended cutoff point was 67.1 cm for boys and 68.2 cm for girls. BMI and WC indicators were recommended to be used at the school setting where the measurement can easily be conducted.

1. Introduction

Adolescent obesity has become a growing health concern, an epidemic that affects both developing and developed countries [1]. The prevalence has reached to the level that warrant an immediate attention on the primary and secondary prevention of overweight and obesity in children and adolescents. It is during the childhood and adolescents period where they develop their eating and activity pattern that can affect their lifestyle in adulthood. With the current nutritional transition that involved availability of fast foods, soft drinks, sedentary lifestyle, physical inactivity, and increase use of technology related gadgets, many adolescents aged 10-19 years were found to be less active and eat more, resulting with increase of body mass index (BMI) and fat [2]. Such unhealthy trends contributed to the increase of comorbidities such as elevated blood cholesterol, type 2 diabetes mellitus, and hypertension [3].

There were many studies that linked hypertension with overweight and obese among the adolescents. Although the evidences gathered have a mixed conclusion on the relationship between hypertension and body fat [4], measurement of body fat using anthropometric indicators had proven to be an effective approach in predicting hypertension, particularly in a large population and community-based studies [5]. Beside the use of BMI in assessing nutritional status, other indicators such as waist circumference (WC), waist-height ratio (WHtR), and conicity index (C index) were other common assessment tools where WC measures the overall body fat, WHtR assess the proportion of central fat by height, and C index measures the abdominal fat.

It is not a common practice to screen for hypertension among adolescents in the community routinely. However, detection of high blood pressure plays an important role in control and prevention of hypertension. However, young people are less likely than older adults to be aware of their risk for hypertension and screen for hypertension on their own. Perhaps one of the reasons is that they may think themselves as invincible and unlikely to be at risk for chronic diseases such as hypertension [6]. Provision of healthcare to this segment of population is often been less emphasized as compared to other age groups.

In Malaysia, the prevalence of prehypertension and hypertension among adolescents was reported to be 11.1% and 11.6%, respectively [7]. Adolescents who are hypertensive tend to be hypertensive in their adult life [3]. The Malaysia National and Health Morbidity Survey (NHMS) 2011 reported that 43.5% of the Malaysian adult population was affected by hypertension [8], an increased trend from previous years (42.6% under NHMS III 2006 and 32.9% under NMHS II 1996) [8–10]. These findings indicated the importance of controlling and preventing of hypertension at a younger age.

Using anthropometric indicators as the preliminary screening tool indirectly help to detect elevated blood pressure at the school environment. As the method does not involve the use of complicated gadget and involvement of specialized skills, the measurement can be taken routinely by the school authorities. If the anthropometric indicators show abnormality results, further assessment of blood pressure with subsequently referral for hospital management can be carried out. Thus, the aim of this study was to determine the prevalence of hypertension and predictive power of anthropometric indicators and recommend cutoff points to discriminate high blood pressure among adolescents.

2. Methods

This was a cross-sectional study assessing the blood pressure profile among adolescents in Sarawak, Malaysia. The study was funded by the Fundamental Research Grant Scheme, Ministry of Higher Education Malaysia.

Sarawak is the largest state of Malaysia, located at the Island of Borneo. Based on 2015 census, it has an estimated population of 2,636,000, with more than 40 subethnic groups, each with its own distinct language, culture, and lifestyle. The six major ethnic groups are Iban, Chinese, Malay, Bidayuh, Melanau, and Orang Ulu.

The study population comprised 186 secondary school students aged 13-17 years in Sarawak, with enrolment of 200,130 students, obtained from the Ministry of Education (February 2014). Using the sample size formula for finite populations [11] s= [X2Np(1−p)]÷[d2(N−1)+ X2p(1−p)], where s is required sample size, X is Z-score for 99% confidence interval (2.58), N is population size (200,310), p is population proportion (assumed to be 0.5 since this would provide the maximum sample size), d is degree of accuracy or margin of error (0.028), and minimum sample size needed was 2100. A quota of 18 schools were decided for each state and systematic sampling was employed in the selection of schools based on the size of enrolment as well as stratification by urban-rural location. In each selected school, one class was randomly selected for each level of schooling from secondary one to secondary six. The inclusion criteria were those respondents without physical and mentally disability, prediagnosed hypertension, or any illness that could lead to secondary hypertension.

Data collection was carried out by a team of trained field personnel. Anthropometric measurement was done using SECA body meter and portable weighing scale. Respondents were weighed with light clothing without footwear. When measuring height, the respondents were to stand upright barefooted on a flat surface with their back of the heels and occiput against the equipment. Measurement of height was to the nearest 0.1 cm. The weight was recorded to the nearest 0.1 kg. Assessment of body mass index was based on WHO 2007 reference using indicators such as thinness, normal, overweight, and obese [12].

Waist circumference (WC) was measured using a plastic nonelastic tape at the midpoint between the last rib and top of hip bone (iliac crest). The respondents were asked to relax their abdomen and stand upright. The cutoff points for abdominal obesity were based on >90 cm for men and >80cm for women [13].

The waist-to-height ratio (WHtR) was calculated based on WC (cm) by height (cm). As for conicity index (C index), the calculation was based on the following equation [14]:

$$CI = \frac{Waist\ Circumference\,(m)}{0.109 \times \sqrt{Body\ Weight\,(kg)\,/Height\,(m)}} \qquad (1)$$

Blood pressure was taken using a digital blood pressure monitor, calibrated with auscultation (a mercury sphygmomanometer) with the correct cuff size for arm circumference. Respondents were asked to rest for 5 minutes and check for no intake of caffeine or medication or no exercise before measurement. Two measurements with an interval of one minute were taken. In the case when the differences of the two readings were above 5 mm Hg or the respondent was found to be in the prehypertension or hypertension level, a third reading was taken. The final reading would be based on the average of all readings taken [15]. Classification of hypertension is based on the Fourth Report on the Diagnosis, Evaluation, and Treatment of High Blood Pressure in Children and Adolescents 2004 [16], where BP is less than the 90th percentile for age, gender, and height; it is classified as normal. BP that falls within 90th to just below 95th percentile is categorized as prehypertension or high-normal.

Statistical analyses were performed using IBM Statistical Package for Social Sciences (SPSS) version 22. Descriptive and inferential statistical analysis was performed based on confidence interval of 95% and p-value of less than 0.05 was regarded as significant. For inferential analysis, prehypertension is regrouped into hypertension, resulting in dichotomous dependent variables, normotensive and hypertensive. The predictive power of anthropometric indicators for hypertension was determined by Receiver Operating Characteristic curves (ROC). The area under ROC curve is used to determine the discriminating power of the anthropometric indicators on hypertension in adolescents. The larger the area under ROC curve, the better the discriminating power of the indicators. This study has adopted 60% as the acceptable value for sensitivity and specificity value, based on the rule of thumbs by Maroco [17] where sensitivity and specificity value between 50% and 80% are considered as acceptable. Using the Youden Index (J) method, the optimal cut point was determined based on the difference between true positive rate and false positive rate over all possible cutpoint value [18].

Ethical approval was obtained from the Medical and Ethical Committee of Universiti Malaysia Sarawak (UNIMAS/TNC (AA)-03.02/06-11 Jld.3(1) and Ministry of Education Malaysia. Informed consent was obtained from the parents/caregivers of the respondents prior to the day of data collection. A research information sheet was given to each of the respondents as well as their parents/caregivers. The respondents were also being briefed the research information on the day of the data collection. Respondents were ensured of the confidentiality of their data and they have the right to withdraw from the study at any time.

3. Results

A total of 2540 respondents have consented to participate in this study. However, 79 (3.1%) were excluded due to absent from school on the day of data collection and a number have refused despite parental consent, so the final sample size was 2461 (96.9% response rate). There were more girls than boys (58% versus 42%), mean age of 14.5±1.50 years, with majority from Iban and Malay ethnic groups. The mean weight, height, and waist circumference were higher among boys compared to girls, while BMI and WHtR were higher among girls. However, the gender differences were found significant only in weight, height, and WHtR. Both gender has similar C index. There were more boys than girls who were found to be prehypertensive and hypertensive and this difference was significant. More girls were found to be overweight than boys; however, in the obese category, the reverse was true. The detailed information is presented in Table 1.

BMI showed an increasing trend among respondents, especially age group 13 years and above. Waist circumference and systolic and diastolic blood pressure also showed similar pattern but were not consistently increased from younger to older age groups (refer Table 2).

Table 3 and Figures 1 and 2 show the final models using Stepwise logistic regression analyses and ROC analyses. All the anthropometric indicators showed significant association with hypertension for both logistic regression and ROC curve, with BMI and WC taking over larger area and fair readings (0.7-0.8). Based on cutoff point, sensitivity, and specificity results, the preferred anthropometric indicator for predicting hypertension for boys was WC and BMI, followed by WHtR. However, for girls, BMI was the best indicator followed by WHtR and WC.

4. Discussion

The prevalence of hypertension in this study was 22.5% for males and 12.9% for females. In terms of prehypertension, the prevalence was found to be slightly lower with 19.3% for males and 8.8% for females. Our results showed higher prevalence compared with other local studies [7], indicating that in a short span of five years the prevalence of prehypertension and hypertension has increased although the study location was different but it was a representative of Malaysia. Another finding of this study also indicated that the prevalence of overweight and obese is also high among males (overweight 11.7%, obese 13.7%) and females (overweight 12.7%, obese 10.7%) which might be closely related to the high prevalence of hypertension. Such observation strongly suggested an immediate attention to address this health issues which may lead to hypertension and obesity related health complication in the later life.

One of the purposes of this study was to determine the predictive power and establish the cutoff points of anthropometric indicators for the prediction of hypertension. It is hoped that with this finding a routine health checkup using anthropometric measurement at the school level can be routinely implemented to screen and detect adolescents with signs of hypertension for further investigation at the clinical setting.

Among all the anthropometric indicators, BMI and WC had the highest sensitivity and specificity value, supporting the evidence from previous study that both indicators were equally well related to hypertension regardless of age and gender [19]. However, in one study, such findings were argued where central obesity measured by WC was perceived as a stronger predictor in hypertension. This is supported by a big population study in China where the findings based on 500,000 adults reported that central obesity was the main predictor [20]. In adolescent studies, the evidences regarding anthropometric indicators with hypertension in children and adolescents are inconclusive. Some studies showed that BMI and WC were significant predictors for hypertension with OR 2.60 and 1.85, respectively [21]. While one study found that WHtR and WC are better predictors than BMI for hypertension, another study would exclude WHtR and supported BMI and WC [22, 23].

According to Sardinha et al. [24], such findings need to be interpreted with cautious. This is because the magnitude of the association between anthropometric indicators and cardiometabolic risk was stronger in overweight and obese children and adolescents compared to their counterpart. In their study, they found that being overweight was associated with more than twofold increased odd of having clustered cardiometabolic risk in adolescents while being obese was associated with more than 14 times increased risk compared to their normal weight samples. They concluded that although BMI, WC, and WHtR may not be strong predictors of cardiometabolic risk, at higher level of adiposity, the cluster of cardiovascular risk factors increases as BMI, WC, or WHtR increases.

Consistent with literatures, C index in this study presented a lower predicting power, sensitivity, and specificity as compared to other anthropometric indicators. Cutoff point for this indicator was 1.12, similar to other studies ranging from 1.13 to 1.23 [25, 26]. The sensitivity and specificity were lower as compared to literatures (ranging from 57.4 to 64.3%) [25, 26]. The evidences on C index and its relationship with hypertension was limited; however studies among risk of diabetes and hypertension in women showed that there was an association between C index with HDL cholesterol [27].

In terms of cutoff point for WC, the current study showed that girls had higher WC as compared with boys, consistent with other studies [25, 28]. The results also indicated a lower

TABLE 1: Sociodemographic and health profile among male and female respondents (N=2461).

Variables	mean±SD / n(%) Male (n=1033)	Female (n=1428)	*p* value
Age (years)	14.4 ± 1.48	14.5 ± 1.51	0.04
Weight (kg)	55.5 ± 14.78	51.0 ± 12.80	<0.001**
Height (m)	1.6 ± 0.08	1.5 ± 0.06	<0.001**
BMI (kg/m^2)	21.3 ± 4.72	21.6 ± 4.78	0.08
WC (cm)	71.3 ± 11.56	70.2 ± 18.46	0.106
WHtR	0.4 ±0.07	0.5 ± 0.11	<0.001**
C Index	1.1±0.07	1.1±0.27	0.654
Ethnicity			0.223
Iban	308 (29.8)	429 (30.0)	
Malay	301 (29.1)	380 (26.6)	
Bidayuh	116 (11.2)	140 (9.8)	
Chinese	181 (17.5)	294 (20.6)	
Others	127 (12.4)	185 (13.0)	
Blood pressure			<0.001**
Normal	602 (58.3)	1118 (78.3)	
Pre-hypertension	199 (19.3)	125 (8.8)	
Hypertension	232 (22.5)	185 (12.9)	
BMI			0.004**
Thinness	78 (7.6)	71 (5.0)	
Normal	692 (67.0)	1022 (71.6)	
Overweight	121 (11.7)	182 (12.7)	
Obese	142 (13.7)	153 (10.7)	

** Significant at p<0.001; BMI: body mass index; WC: waist circumference; WHtR: waist-to-height ratio; C Index: conicity index.

TABLE 2: Anthropometric measurement and blood pressure according to age among male and female respondents (N=2461).

	Sex	Age (year±SD) 12 years M=106; F=149	13 years M=240; F=292	14 years M=215; F=261	15 years M=180; F=281	16 years M=214; F=308	17 years M=78; F=137	*p* value
BMI	M	21.09±5.30	20.80±4.97	20.96±5.03	21.57±4.21	21.78±4.46	21.85±3.89	0.161
	F	21.38±5.62	20.55±4.27*	20.86±4.10	21.96±4.86*	22.76±5.06*	22.32±4.56*	<0.01
WC	M	70.42±13.30	69.77±12.59	70.66±12.09	71.80±10.08	72.92±10.33	72.81±10.03	0.045
	F	73.73±49.48*	67.68±9.20*	68.58±8.62	70.21±9.71	72.04±10.70	70.75±9.82	0.006
WHt	M	0.46±0.08	0.45±0.07	0.44±0.07	0.44±0.06	0.44±0.06	0.44±0.06	0.070
	F	0.49±0.31*	0.45±0.06*	0.45±0.05*	0.46±0.06	0.46±0.07	0.46±0.06	0.01
C Index	M	1.14±0.08*	1.12±0.07	1.12±0.07	1.11±0.06*	1.12±0.06*	1.11±0.06	0.006
	F	1.20±0.81*	1.12±0.06*	1.12±0.07	1.11±0.06*	1.12±0.06*	1.11±0.06	0.03
SBP	M	112.35±13.18*	116.23±13.77	118.66±14.36*	119.34±13.09*	120.59±12.96*	120.54±13.90*	<0.01
	F	112.41±14.30	109.39±11.23*	109.93±11.40	111.79±10.81	112.29±12.58*	111.69±13.11	0.013
DBP	M	63.12±10.19*	63.89±9.50*	65.15±10.23	64.73±9.27	66.92±9.58*	65.17±7.88	0.007
	F	65.66±9.90	64.62±8.61*	65.25±9.02	66.40±7.50	67.04±9.90*	66.84±8.87	0.011

M: male; F: female.
*One-way analysis of variance was applied to see the differences between age group and p<0.05 was considered as statistically significant.

WC for both boys and girls compared to literatures, where most of the WCs ranged from 70 cm or more for boys and 80 cm or more for girls. One possible explanation was the body frame size for Asians adolescents is smaller than those in the western population. Based on the Malaysian waist circumference percentile curves for children and adolescents aged 6 to 16.9 years [29], the cutoff point for boys was close to the 50th percentile and the girls was close to 75th percentile.

For WHtR, the cutoff point for boys was lower than girls with 0.42 and 0.44, respectively, consistent with others studies [25, 30]. In one study among adult females, WHtR indicator was ranked with the highest discriminatory power

TABLE 3: Age-adjusted Logistic regression model and discriminative capability for hypertension by sex (N=2461).

	Male				Female			
	BMI	WC	WHtR	C Index	BMI	WC	WHtR	C Index
Logistic Model								
Constant	-6.605	-8.670	-9.448	-15.021	-4.712	-7.288	-7.803	-10.632
Exp (B)	1.278	1.111	2.778	5.114	1.223	1.099	2.167	2.588
p value	<0.01	<0.01	<0.01	<0.01	<0.01	<0.01	<0.01	<0.01
Discriminative Capability								
Area under ROC curve	0.76 (0.73-0.79)	0.76 (0.73-0.79)	0.76 (0.73-0.79)	0.76 (0.73-0.79)	0.74 (0.70-0.77)	0.74 (0.70-0.77)	0.74 (0.70-0.77)	0.74 (0.70-0.77)
Cutoff point	20.0	67.1	0.42	1.11	20.7	68.2	0.44	1.12
Sensitivity	75.4	77.3	71.2	64.3	72.9	71.3	71.9	57.4
Specificity	60.3	61.8	60.5	60.0	60.0	61.6	60.0	60.0

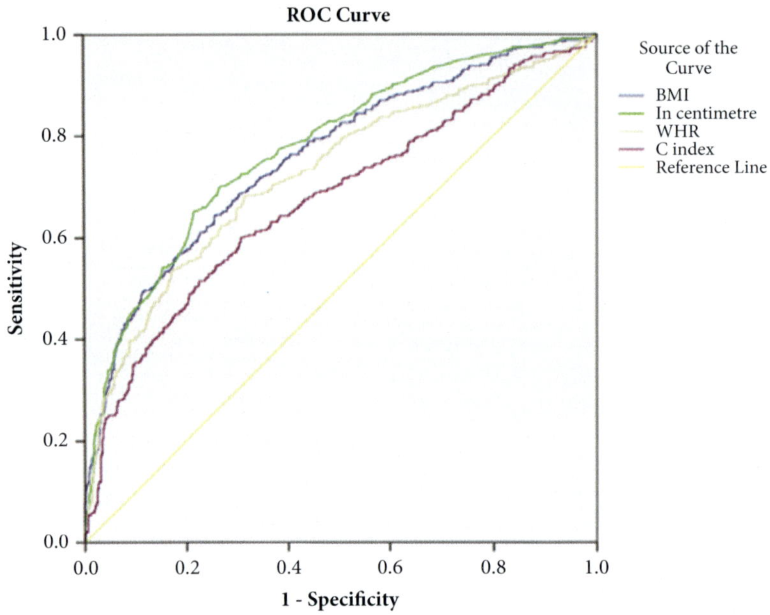

FIGURE 1: ROC curves that compare four anthropometric indicators of obesity as discriminators of hypertension (boys). BMI: body mass index, in centimeter-waist circumference; WHR: waist-height ratio; C index: conicity index.

in hypertension risk screening. It was further argued that accumulation of body fat at the abdominal part maximize the hemodynamic changes that caused endothelial dysfunction and dysregulation of hepatic metabolism that eventually promote the onset of cardiovascular disorders [31]. In additional to that, WHtR incorporated the measurement of height in its formula which proved to be more accurate in determining hypertension risk [32].

Unlike past studies on the cutoff point for BMI, this study showed higher BMI cutoff point for girls (20.7 kg/m2) as compared to boys (20.0 kg/m2). In Iran, the mean BMI for predicting hypertension among boys was higher than this study (21.9 kg/m2), but its cutoff point for girls was lower (19.1 kg/m2) [30]. Although BMI is not as accurate in differentiating distribution of fat in different body compartments as compared to WC and WHtR, it has served as the most common used anthropometric indicator in screening cardiovascular risk for children and adolescents. Perhaps a reclassification of BMI in screening for hypertension should be further explored.

Because the current study was a cross-sectional, therefore the causality association cannot be affirmed. Besides that, although the protocol of conducting the blood pressure was based on an interval of one minute [16], there might be an overestimation of the prevalence of hypertension that resulted higher sensitivity. Nevertheless, this is a common issue related to the use of screening tools at the community level.

5. Conclusion

In conclusion, based on the findings, it is recommended to use BMI and WC indicators in detecting hypertension among adolescents in Sarawak. A cutoff point of 20 kg/m^2

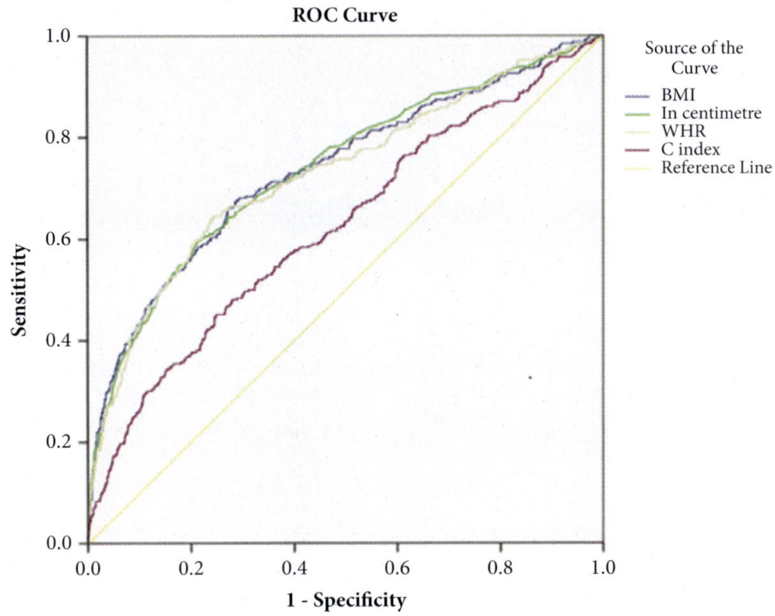

FIGURE 2: ROC curves that compare four anthropometric indicators of obesity as discriminators of hypertension (girls). BMI: body mass index, in centimeter-waist circumference; WHR: waist-height ratio; C index: conicity index.

for boys and 20.7 kg/m^2 for girls was recommended for BMI, and a cutoff point of 67.1 cm for boys and 68.2 cm for girls was recommended for WC to detect elevated blood pressure. Both indicators can be used at the school setting where scale, stadiometer, and tape measure can easily be made available. Those adolescents who are identified can be further referred for clinical investigation and subsequently go for treatment and intervention.

Acknowledgments

The authors would like to thank Ministry of Higher Education and Ministry of Education for making this study successful. This study is supported by the Fundamental Research Grant Scheme, Malaysia Ministry of Higher Education.

References

[1] N. Gupta, K. Goel, P. Shah, and A. Misra, "Childhood obesity in developing countries: epidemiology, determinants, and prevention," *Endocrine Reviews*, vol. 33, no. 1, pp. 48–70, 2012.

[2] K. Sahoo, B. Sahoo, A. K. Choudhury et al., "Childhood obesity: causes and consequences," *Journal of Family Medicine and Primary Care*, vol. 4, no. 2, pp. 187–192, 2015.

[3] A. Must and R. S. Strauss, "Risks and consequences of childhood and adolescent obesity," *International Journal of Obesity*, vol. 23, supplement 2, pp. S2–S11, 1999.

[4] C. George, J. H. Goedecke, N. J. Crowther et al., "The role of body fat and fat distribution in hypertension risk in urban Black South African women," *PLoS ONE*, vol. 11, no. 5, Article ID e0154894, 2016.

[5] D. L. Duren, R. J. Sherwood, S. A. Czerwinski et al., "Body composition methods: Comparisons and interpretation," *Journal of Diabetes Science and Technology*, vol. 2, no. 6, pp. 1139–1146, 2008.

[6] K. Bibbins-Domingo and M. Burroughs Peña, "Caring for the "young invincibles"," *Journal of General Internal Medicine*, vol. 25, no. 7, pp. 642-643, 2010.

[7] L. Rampal, K. C. Ng, I. N. Izzati et al., "Prevalence of hypertension among Malay adolescents in Putrajaya secondary schools, Malaysia, 2010," *Malaysian Journal of Medicine and Health Sciences*, vol. 7, no. 2, pp. 53–60, 2011.

[8] Institute for Public Health. and Ministry of Health Malaysia., *National Health and Morbidity Survey 2011 (NHMS 2011) vol II: Non-Communicable Diseases*, Institute for Public Health, Kuala Lumpur,Malaysia, 2011.

[9] Institute for Public Health. and Ministry of Health Malaysia., *National Health and Morbidity Survey (NHMS III) Report*, Institute for Public Health, Kuala Lumpur, Malaysia, 2006.

[10] Institute for Public Health. and Ministry of Health Malaysia., *The Second National Health and Morbidity Survey (NHMS II) Report*, Institute for Public Health, Kuala Lumpur, Malaysia, 1996.

[11] R. V. Krejcie and D. W. Morgan, "Determining Sample Size for Research Activities," *Educational and Psychological Measurement*, vol. 30, no. 3, pp. 607–610, 2016.

[12] WHO, *BMI-for-age (5-19 years)*, 2007, http://www.who.int/growthref/who2007_bmi_for_age/en/.

[13] WHO, *Waist circumference and waist–hip ratio: report of a WHO expert consultation*, Geneva, 2008, http://whqlibdoc.who.int/publications/2011/9789241501491_eng.pdf.

[14] R. Valdez, "A simple model-based index of abdominal adiposity," *Journal of Clinical Epidemiology*, vol. 44, no. 9, pp. 955-956, 1991.

[15] T. G. Pickering, J. E. Hall, L. J. Appel et al., "Recommendations for blood pressure measurement in humans and experimental animals: part 1: blood pressure measurement in humans: a statement for professionals from the Subcommittee of Professional and Public Education of the American Heart Association Council on high blood pressure research," *Circulation*, vol. 111, no. 5, pp. 697–716, 2005.

[16] National High Blood Pressure Education Program Working Group on Children and Adolescents, "The Fourth Report on the Diagnosis, Evaluation, and Treatment of High Blood Pressure in Children and Adolescents," *Pediatrics*, vol. 114, no. 2, pp. 555–567, 2004.

[17] J. Maroco, "Analise Estatistica com o SPSS Statistics," Lisboa, 2011.

[18] R. Fluss, D. Faraggi, and B. Reiser, "Estimation of the Youden index and its associated cutoff point," *Biometrical Journal*, vol. 47, no. 4, pp. 458–472, 2005.

[19] R. Nyamdorj, Q. Qiao, S. Söderberg et al., "BMI compared with central obesity indicators as a predictor of diabetes incidence in mauritius," *Obesity*, vol. 17, no. 2, pp. 342–348, 2009.

[20] Z. Chen, M. Smith, H. Du et al., "Blood pressure in relation to general and central adiposity among 500 000 adult Chinese men and women," *International Journal of Epidemiology*, vol. 44, no. 4, pp. 1305–1319, 2015.

[21] D. Gröber-Grätz, K. Widhalm, M. De Zwaan et al., "Body mass index or waist circumference: Which is the better predictor for hypertension and dyslipidemia in overweight/obese children and adolescents? association of cardiovascular risk related to body mass index or waist circumference," *Hormone Research in Paediatrics*, vol. 80, no. 3, pp. 170–178, 2013.

[22] S. C. Savva, M. Tornaritis, M. E. Savva et al., "Waist circumference and waist-to-height ratio are better predictors of cardiovascular disease risk factors in children than body mass index," *International Journal of Obesity*, vol. 24, no. 11, pp. 1453–1458, 2000.

[23] V. W. S. Ng, A. P. S. Kong, K. C. Choi KC et al., "BMI and waist circumference in predicting cardiovascular risk factors clustering in Chinese adolescents," *Obesity*, vol. 15, no. 2, pp. 494–503, 2007.

[24] L. B. Sardinha, D. A. Santos, A. M. Silva, A. Grøntved, L. B. Andersen, and U. Ekelund, "A comparison between BMI, waist circumference, and waist-to-height ratio for identifying cardiometabolic risk in children and adolescents," *PLoS ONE*, vol. 11, no. 2, Article ID e0149351, 2016.

[25] C. C. Beck, A. da Silva Lopes, and F. J. G. Pitanga, "Anthropometric indicators as predictors of high blood pressure in adolescents," *Arquivos Brasileiros de Cardiologia*, vol. 96, no. 2, pp. 126–132, 2011.

[26] S. R. Moreira, A. P. Ferreira, R. M. Lima et al., "Predicting insulin resistance in children: Anthropometric and metabolic indicators," *Jornal de Pediatria*, vol. 84, no. 1, pp. 47–52, 2008.

[27] M. D. Andrade, M. C. P. de Freitas, A. M. Sakumoto et al., "Association of the conicity index with diabetes and hypertension in Brazilian women," *Archives of Endocrinology and Metabolism*, vol. 60, no. 5, pp. 436–442, 2016.

[28] P. T. Katzmarzyk, S. R. Srinivasan, W. Chen, R. M. Malina, C. Bouchard, and G. S. Berenson, "Body mass index, waist circumference, and clustering of cardiovascular disease risk factors in a biracial sample of children and adolescents.," *Pediatrics*, vol. 114, no. 2, pp. e198–e205, 2004.

[29] B. K. Poh, A. N. Jannah, L. K. Chong, A. T. Ruzita, M. N. Ismail, and D. McCarthy, "Waist circumference percentile curves for Malaysian children and adolescents aged 6.016.9 years," *International Journal of Pediatric Obesity*, vol. 6, no. 3-4, pp. 229–235, 2011.

[30] R. Kelishadi, R. Gheiratmand, G. Ardalan et al., "Association of anthropometric indices with cardiovascular disease risk factors among children and adolescents: CASPIAN Study," *International Journal of Cardiology*, vol. 117, no. 3, pp. 340–348, 2007.

[31] J.-P. Després, S. Moorjani, P. J. Lupien, A. Tremblay, A. Nadeau, and C. Bouchard, "Regional distribution of body fat, plasma lipoproteins, and cardiovascular disease," *Arteriosclerosis, Thrombosis, and Vascular Biology*, vol. 10, no. 4, pp. 497–511, 1990.

[32] M. Ashwell, P. Gunn, and S. Gibson, "Waist-to-height ratio is a better screening tool than waist circumference and BMI for adult cardiometabolic risk factors: systematic review and meta-analysis," *Obesity Reviews*, vol. 13, no. 3, pp. 275–286, 2012.

25

Beneficial Role of Mg^{2+} in Prevention and Treatment of Hypertension

Andrea M. P. Romani

Case Western Reserve University, School of Medicine, Department Physiology and Biophysics, 10900 Euclid Avenue, Cleveland, OH 44106-4970, USA

Correspondence should be addressed to Andrea M. P. Romani; amr5@po.cwru.edu

Academic Editor: Markus P. Schlaich

Hypertension constitutes one of the most widespread pathological conditions in developed and developing countries. Currently, more than 1 billion people worldwide are affected by the condition, either as frank hypertension or as prehypertension, raising the risk for major long-term complications and life-threatening pathologies. The costs in terms of health care services, medications for the treatment of hypertension and its complications, and associated loss in productivity represent a major economic burden for the various countries. The necessity of developing treatments that are economically more sustainable and with better compliance has been increasing alongside the incidence of the pathology. Along these lines, attention has been paid to the implementation of affordable but nutritious diets that deliver appropriate levels of macro- and micronutrients as integral part of the diets themselves or as supplements. In particular, experimental and clinical evidence suggests that an appropriate intake of dietary magnesium can be beneficial in controlling blood pressure. Additional advantages of a more diffuse therapeutic and/or preventive utilization of magnesium supplements are the virtual absence of side-effects and their affordable costs. The present review will attempt to frame our knowledge of how magnesium exerts its beneficial effects on blood pressure maintenance, which may lead to the development of more effective treatments of hypertension and its main complications.

1. Introduction

Hypertension represents one of the most common human pathological conditions diagnosed. According to data published in 2013 by the World Health Organization, approximately 1.2 billion people worldwide are affected by the pathology [1], irrespective of developed or developing countries, ethnicity, gender, and age. Consistent with this trend, nearly one-third (>29% or 75 millions) of the American adult population is affected by hypertension, defined as high blood pressure [2], and another third presents with prehypertensive state [2], whereby blood pressure values are higher than normal but not yet in the high blood pressure range. More worrisome, only half of the individual with frank hypertension have their condition under medical control [2], raising the risk for the occurrence of life-threatening cardiovascular complications including stroke, myocardial infarction, and aortic aneurysm. This situation is in addition to increased risk of mortality or poor quality of life of the remaining half of the affected individuals. In terms of age and gender-related distribution, males are more affected than females as young adult [1, 2]. This gender disparity disappears during adulthood, with males and females becoming equally affected, before switching in the other direction in individuals older than 65 y.o., when females become more affected than males [1, 2]. The reasons for this gender-related change in incidence with age are not completely understood, with loss of estrogen-based cardiovascular protection in females among the proposed hypotheses [1].

The etiology of hypertension is also complex spanning from endocrinopathies with abnormally elevated levels of one of the various pressure-controlling hormones (e.g., catecholamine, renin-angiotensin II-aldosterone axis, cortisol, and growth hormone) [3], to renal pathologies (e.g., Bartter's syndrome and Gitelman's syndrome), to primary cardiac hypertrophy, to conditions in which a clear cause-effect relationship cannot be establish (idiopathic hypertension). Accordingly, the pharmacological treatment of hypertension is multifaceted and based primarily on decreasing the circulating volume through the use of diuretics (e.g., furosemide, hydrochloro-thiazide, or amiloride) that inhibit different Na^+ reabsorbing mechanisms in different portions of the nephron. Often, diuretic treatment is used in conjunction with angiotensin-converting-enzyme inhibitors (ACE inhibitors), Ca^{2+} channel blockers, or beta-blockers to regulate cardiac output, rate, and contraction and α1-adrenergic receptor blockers to control the tone of peripheral resistances, to surgical treatment to remove hormone hypersecreting adenomas, and to better address the underlying mechanism(s) responsible for the sustained increased in blood pressure [3, 4].

The complexity of hypertensive treatment and patient's compliance and responsiveness, however, result in significant costs for the health care system, without the guarantee of an effective medical control of the pathology. Consequently, the need for effective treatments that are economically more affordable and easy to comply with has increased progressively with the raising incidence of hypertension. Interest has shifted towards the implementation of diets that, while being affordable and easy to follow, do provide appropriate levels of macro- and micronutrients, and natural products (e.g., flavonoids) that can help in better controlling blood pressure and associated damaging processes such as oxidative stress.

In this regard, experimental and clinical evidence suggests that an appropriate intake of dietary magnesium can be beneficial in controlling blood pressure. Conceptually, intake of magnesium through the diet or as a supplement has the advantage of being a natural and required element for our cellular composition, of having virtual absence of side-effects, and being financially more affordable that other therapeutic agents, especially in developing countries. Practically, however, the utilization of magnesium in the contest of hypertension is still plagued by limited understanding of its true beneficial effects, limited bioavailability of some magnesium supplements, and the general misconception that because magnesium is abundantly present in our body and readily available through diet, the occurrence of magnesium deficiency is a rather rare condition.

In line with the nonpharmacological intent of this monographic issue, the present review will attempt to provide the necessary framework to understand the relevance of physiological magnesium levels for whole body well-being and for a better regulation of blood pressure.

2. Magnesium: Cellular Homeostasis and Transport

Magnesium is the fourth most abundant cation in the human body and the second most abundant intracellular cation after potassium [5]. Within the cell, magnesium ions (Mg^{2+}) are highly compartmentalized within nucleus, mitochondria, endoplasmic and sarcoplasmic reticulum, cytoplasm, and possibly other organelles, although the assessment in the latter has been hampered by technical limitations [5]. Total Mg^{2+} concentrations in excess of 16-18 mM have been measured by a variety of approaches in each of the mentioned compartments [6], with the exception of cytoplasm where 4-5 mM Mg^{2+} is present in the form of a complex with ATP and other phosphonucleotides and between 0.8 and 1 mM is in the free form [6]. Magnesium ions regulate a broad variety of physiological functions, including Ca^{2+} channels, metabolomic receptors, ATPases, cell cycle, MAPKs, IP_3 receptor, insulin signaling, and glucose transport and utilization, just to mention a few [5, 6]. At the cellular level and in the whole body, physiological Mg^{2+} contents are regulated through a series of extrusion and entry mechanisms, the operation of which is tightly controlled by a variety of hormones [5, 6]. Extrusion is mostly accomplished through a Na^+/Mg^{2+} exchanger (Slc41A1) activated via cAMP-dependent-phosphorylation, which electrogenically transports $1Na^+_{in}:1Mg^{2+}_{out}$ [5, 6]. Catecholamine, glucagon, and other cAMP-elevating hormones all promote Mg^{2+} extrusion in exchange for Na^+ [7]. Supporting the importance of the Na^+ electrochemical gradient in favoring Mg^{2+} extrusion, amiloride and other inhibitors of Na^+ transport all inhibit Mg^{2+} extrusion through this exchanger [5–7]. Under conditions in which Na^+ transport is inhibited, an alternative, less efficient, Na^+-independent Mg^{2+} extrusion pathway becomes operative. This pathway is less well characterized, and not much is known about its activation, implying the possibility that different cells utilize different Na^+-independent paths to maintain a basal level of Mg^{2+} extrusion [6, 7]. Entry of Mg^{2+} into the cell is accomplished through the operation of two distinct channels, termed TRPM6 and TRPM7 [5, 6]. While TRMP7 is ubiquitously expressed in eukaryotic cells, TRPM6 is more highly expressed in the distal convolute tubule of the nephron and in the descending colon, i.e., in locations where it can better control renal reabsorption and intestinal absorption to maintain whole body Mg^{2+} levels [5, 6]. Both these channels are maintained in the closed state by the binding of RACK1 at a specific site of the C-terminus [6]. Hormones or agents that activate protein kinase C within the cell can then scavenger RACK1 away from the channels, activating them [6]. Adding to the complexity of these channels, both TRPM6 and TRPM7 possess a α-kinase at their C-terminus, which becomes operative following Mg^{2+} entry and phosphorylates Ser and Thre residues in an alpha-helix loop [6]. Currently, only a handful of targets phosphorylated by these kinases have been identified [5, 6], *de facto* limiting our understanding of the role these kinases play in terms of whole cell function.

Because ~99% of Mg^{2+} is localized intracellularly in bones in soft tissue and ~1% is present in the circulation in both free (approximately 2/3) and bound (~1/3) form, changes in circulating Mg^{2+} levels cannot properly reflect the cellular status of the cation. Consequently, Mg^{2+} insufficiency or deficiency cannot be established using serum Mg^{2+} levels alone [5, 8], but assessment of urinary and intracellular Mg^{2+} levels should be included. Mg^{2+} deficiency, in fact, can be retrospectively identified based on the occurrence of an inverse relationship between the amount of Mg^{2+} eliminated through the urine and the amount of Mg^{2+} intake, and the variation in cellular Mg^{2+} content in more accessible pools such as red blood cells [8].

2.1. Dietary Mg^{2+} Levels and Intake. At the dietary level, Mg^{2+} is present in elevated content in green-leaf vegetables, whole grains, white potatoes, nuts, and legumes [9]. The current RDA (recommended dietary allowance) for magnesium ranges from 240 to 420 mg/day for males 31 to 70 y.o. and ~320 mg/d for females of comparable age range [10]. However, evidence is there indicating that ~60% of the US population does not consume the RDA for magnesium [11] and it is therefore considered to be magnesium insufficient if not frankly deficient. This assessment is supported by similar reports out of UK, Australia, Canada, and other industrialized countries [5], and the observation that dietary Mg^{2+} intake has declined by at least ~40% in the last 4 decades due to changes in food harvesting and processing, water purification, and overall dietary habits [12]. As a dietary supplement, magnesium is most commonly found as MgO (magnesium oxide). Other forms of mineral salts of Mg^{2+} supplements include $Mg(OH)_2$ (magnesium hydroxide), magnesium bicarbonate, carbonate, phosphate, and sulfate. Alternatively, Mg^{2+} can be provided as an organic salt (bound to aspartate, citrate, gluconate, ascorbate, etc.) or chelated with amino acids [12]. While produced at a very low cost, several of the mineral salts of Mg^{2+} have a poor bioavailability (e.g., as low as 4% for magnesium oxide) [12], which greatly limit their effectiveness.

A certain level of magnesium deficiency has been reported in several chronic diseases including hypertension, diabetes, and metabolic syndrome [5]. Yet, it is undetermined whether magnesium deficiency precedes and perhaps contributes to the onset of the disease or is instead the result of the pathology. Irrespective of the time of appearance, however, due to its involvement in a broad range of cellular and physiological functions, magnesium insufficiency or deficiency can impair to a varying extent several of these functions and aggravates the progression of the pathology and its complications.

3. Magnesium and Hypertension

Several lines of evidence suggest a role of Mg^{2+} in inversely regulating blood pressure. Studies carried out in *in vitro* and *in vivo* models in the late 1940s or early 1950s first suggested a role of circulating Mg^{2+} in inhibiting catecholamine release from both peripheral and adrenal sources [13, 14]. Later studies validated these results and showed that infusion of Mg^{2+} significantly reduces the catecholamine-induced increases in systemic vascular resistance, systolic blood pressure, and diastolic blood pressure in a dose-dependent manner and increases coronary blood flow [reviewed in [15]].

A modulating effect of Mg^{2+} on vascular tone and reactivity, and consequently on blood pressure, is in line with the clinical observation that Mg^{2+} infusion decreases peripheral vascular resistance and blood pressure and can induce hypotension through vasodilatation [16, 17]. Increasing extracellular Mg^{2+} concentration promotes vasodilation, thereby increasing blood flow systemically and attenuates agonist-induced vasoconstriction [18, 19]. Conversely, decreasing extracellular Mg^{2+} concentration increases vascular tone and agonist-induced vasoconstriction [20, 21]. The exact mechanism behind these effects is not completely clear. Because Mg^{2+} acts as a natural Ca^{2+}-channel blocker [15], it is conceivable that physiological extracellular Mg^{2+} concentrations would limit Ca^{2+} entry through the cell membrane and the increase in intracellular $[Ca^{2+}]$i necessary for smooth muscle cells contraction and endocrine-regulated increase in vascular tone. Alternatively, owing to the involvement of extra- and intracellular Mg^{2+} in modulating a variety of signaling pathways [5–8], it is possible that an increase and a decrease in cellular Mg^{2+} concentrations can have major opposite implications for smooth muscle cells contraction and relaxation, whereby influencing vascular tone and blood pressure.

The effects of Mg^{2+} are not limited to vascular tone but influence vascular endothelial functions as well [22]. The vascular endothelium regulates vessel tone by releasing nitric oxide, endothelin-1, and prostacyclin PGI_2 [22]. Magnesium ions have been reported to stimulate directly prostacyclin and nitric oxide production [23–25]. In addition, an inverse relationship between the levels of Mg^{2+} and endothelin-1 has been reported [26], further emphasizing the ability of magnesium to modulate vasodilatation through endothelium-dependent and independent mechanisms. A third possible mechanism whereby Mg^{2+} can modulate vascular tone and blood pressure is through its antioxidant and anti-inflammatory effects [27, 28]. Production of reactive oxygen species (ROS) and oxidative stress can be elevated in vascular smooth muscle cells, increasing vasoconstriction [29]. Conversely, the presence of physiological concentrations of Mg^{2+} would reduce ROS formation and antagonize the vasoconstriction effect. How exactly Mg^{2+} exerts this effect is not fully elucidated. Recently, Kolisek and collaborators [30] have hypothesized that the inverse relationship between ROS and Mg^{2+} levels is regulated through PARK7/DJ-1. This protein has antioxidant properties and tightly regulates cellular redox homeostasis. In addition, through androgen receptor activation, it would modulate the expression of SLC41A1, the main exchange mechanism responsible for Mg^{2+} extrusion in mammalian cells (see section on Magnesium: Cellular Homeostasis and Transport).

3.1. Is There a Role for Mg^{2+} in Controlling Hypertension in Human Patients? Epidemiologic studies indicate that the consumption of "hard water" with high levels of magnesium is cardioprotective whereas consumption of "soft water" (i.e., water low in minerals including magnesium) is associated with hypertension and overall higher incidence of cardiovascular diseases. This inverse association was first observed by Joffres et al. in their Honolulu Heart study [31] and subsequently confirmed by other clinical studies [32, 33]. In particular, inverse relationship between magnesium levels and systolic and diastolic pressure values [32] and risk of death from hypertension [33] have been reported, in line with a similar inverse relationship between Mg^{2+} levels and circulating renin concentrations [34] and stiffened blood vessels [35].

The presence of an inverse relationship between circulating Mg^{2+} levels and the detected concentrations of endothelin-1, PGI_2, ROS, NO, or renin, or systolic and diastolic blood pressure values, however, leaves unanswered the question as to whether magnesium supplementation can be therapeutic in restoring physiological and age-appropriate pressure values. In other words, are magnesium levels prophylactic, or they can also be therapeutic? The attempts to address this question have resulted in contradicting results, and only more recent studies appear to confirm beneficial therapeutic responses following administration of Mg^{2+} salts. The meta-analysis conducted by Dickinson and collaborators [36] assessed retrospectively 12 randomized controlled trials and indicates that diastolic pressure but not systolic pressure decreased to a significant extent as a result of magnesium supplementation [36]. Because of the limited quality of the trials included in the meta-analysis, however, the conclusion of the authors was that a causal association between magnesium supplementation and the decrease in blood pressure was weak, due to inherent bias [36]. More recently, the group of Kass has conducted a similar meta-analysis on more current studies. Twenty-two (22) trials with 23 sets of data were used, for a total of 1173 patients. While the majority of the studies assessed by Dickinson's group lasted for about 8 weeks, the studies analyzed by the group of Kass lasted anywhere from 3 to 24 weeks, with doses of Mg^{2+} ranging from 120 to ~970 mg/d [37]. The conclusion of this study was that higher doses of magnesium produced greater reduction in blood pressure, both systolic and diastolic values [37]. Similar conclusions have been attained more recently by Zhang and collaborators [38]. For their meta-analysis, this latter group assessed 34 trials involving more than 2000 participants, and magnesium supplementation (including a broad array of mineral and organic salts) ranged from 240 to 960 mg/d [38].

Based on these more recent studies [37, 38], it would appear that magnesium supplementation does achieve a statistical significant reduction in blood pressure, both systolic and diastolic values. It has to be noted that the reduction, while significant, ranges between 2 and 4 mmHg for either parameter. In clinical terms, it could be argued that such a reduction is rather small when compared to that attainable with other pharmacological treatments. Also, the presence of some variability in pressure reduction might imply that specific subgroups of patients are more (or less) magnesium-sensitive and therefore more prone to the beneficial effects of magnesium supplementation [37, 38]. At a first glance, it would appear that subgroups with higher magnesium sensitivity include patients of African descent, obese patients, patients with metabolic syndrome (see below) or preeclampsia (see also below), and patients with severe or malignant forms of hypertension [34–38]. Because our understanding of the mechanisms involved in controlling magnesium homeostasis and transport at the level of the cell and the whole body is still incomplete, it cannot be excluded that the "genetics" of magnesium homeostasis, alongside with diet composition, can be major factors in explaining this sensitivity and the effectiveness of magnesium supplementation.

3.2. Magnesium and Stroke. Cerebral insults (strokes) represent one of the most common, and feared, complications of hypertension, as they can result in paralysis, inability to speak, and difficulty in swallowing (with associated malnutrition) when they do not cause the immediate death of the patients. Strokes result from severe, not-controlled hypertension, affect ~800,000 new patients every year, and are responsible for ~140,000 deaths/year in the US alone [39]. Because of the association of this pathology with hypertension and the potential beneficial effect of magnesium supplementation in controlling hypertension, attention has been paid to the possibility that magnesium supplementation can indeed attenuate the incidence of stroke and/or their outcome. A meta-analysis study conducted by Larsson et al. [40] identified 7 prospective studies that could be used based on their criteria out of 163 articles screened. While the number of studies incorporated in the meta-analysis could be considered relatively small when compared to the starting number of articles screened, it did account for almost 6500 cases of stroke in a pool of participants of more than 240,000. The conclusion of the meta-analysis indicates once again the presence of a statistically significant inverse association between magnesium intake and risk of stroke. According to the study, an increment in magnesium intake of 100 mg/d correlates with an 8% reduction in the risk of stroke. Interestingly, this correlation applies only to ischemic strokes and not to hemorrhagic strokes [40]. While a causal relationship could not be fully validated, it is worth noting that Han and collaborators have recently reported a 5% reduction in the risk of hypertension for a similar (100mg/d) increment in magnesium intake [41].

4. Magnesium and Metabolic Syndrome

The incidence of metabolic syndrome in the human population shows a trend similar to that of hypertension, affecting more than 500 million people worldwide [42]. Haller was the first to introduce the term in 1977 to describe a pathological condition characterized by the association of obesity, diabetes mellitus, hyperlipoproteinemia, hyperuricemia, and hepatic steatosis [43]. Currently, the pathology is diagnosed based on the presence of at least 3 of the following 5 criteria: (1) central obesity (waist circumference $\geq$ 102 cm or 40 inches for males, and $\geq$ 88 cm or 35 inches for females); (2) hypertriglyceridemia (TG $\geq$ 1.7 mmol/L or 150 mg/dl); (3) dyslipidemia (HDL-C $<$ 40 mg/dL for males, and $<$ 50 mg/dL for females) with slightly or markedly elevated total cholesterol and LDL; (4) blood pressure $\geq$ 130/85 mmHg (or treated for hypertension); and (5) fasting plasma glucose $\geq$ 6.1 mmol/L (110 mg/dl) [44].

As mentioned above, an increase in systolic and diastolic blood pressure values represents one of the diagnostic criteria for this condition. Hypomagnesemia [45] and intracellular magnesium deficiency [46] are also common features of the pathology. The cause(s) for the onset of metabolic syndrome are not elucidated: for a period of time, the condition was termed Syndrome X to highlight its obscure etiology. Because of the altered triglyceride and cholesterol profiles and the presence of slightly elevated glycemia, the metabolic syndrome is currently considered the result of incipient insulin resistance [44], and progression towards type-2 diabetes mellitus is a typical complication of the syndrome [47]. Because insulin favors Mg^{2+} accumulation within cells [5, 6], reduced cellular Mg^{2+} levels in the context of insulin resistance are to be expected. According to the CARDIA study, a magnesium enriched diet or magnesium supplementation appear effective in reducing the risk of metabolic syndrome and its progression towards diabetes and cardiovascular complications [48].

5. Magnesium and Preeclampsia

The term preeclampsia refers to a clinical disorder during pregnancy characterized by hypertension after 20 weeks of gestation, with marked proteinuria [49]. The disorder affects about 5% of delivery and when left untreated it develops into eclampsia, with occurrence of tonic-clonic seizures for about 1 min, followed by a period of confusion or coma [49, 50]. Major complications of eclampsia are as follows: aspiration pneumonia, cerebral hemorrhage, kidney failure, and cardiac arrest [50]. Eclampsia affects about 1.5% or all the deliveries, with a mortality rate around 1% of all the affected women [50]. In 2015, the last year for which we have reliable collected data, eclampsia accounted to ~47,000 deaths in the world [51].

Magnesium sulfate constitutes the treatment of choice for the prevention of preeclampsia related convulsions. The first report of its effectiveness was by Pritchard in 1955 [52]. As its anticonvulsion use became more common and accepted [53], administration of magnesium sulfate has been observed to result in better outcome than other anticonvulsive (e.g., diazepam) [54]. Anticonvulsive drugs such as diazepam or phenytoin [53, 54] are still used for the treatment of eclampsia as coadjuvants of magnesium sulfate treatment. The addition of these therapeutic agents helps in maintaining magnesium dosage and circulating magnesium levels in an optimal therapeutic range, thus preventing magnesium-related toxic side-effects such as paralysis of maternal thoracic muscles and respiratory depression, which could occur at high doses of magnesium sulfate if this was the only therapeutic agent used [53]

Treatment of preeclampsia with magnesium sulfate has been reported to improve endothelial function. This improvement can be due to the previously described beneficial effects of magnesium on vascular tone (e.g., reduced stiffness and reduced Ca^{2+} entry), vascular responsiveness to endothelin-1, renin, and ROS production, and overall vascular function, including increased nitric oxide and PGI_2 production, which promote vasodilation and inhibit platelet aggregation, respectively [23–26]. Yet, it still remains controversial whether women undergoing preeclampsia have lower than normal circulating levels of Mg^{2+} and therefore are more exposed to the vascular irregularities and hypertone prevented by Mg^{2+}. Some studies have indeed reported decreased serum and intracellular Mg^{2+} levels [55, 56] whereas other studies have failed to identify similar differences between preeclamptic and healthy gravidas [57, 58]. Also in this clinical scenario, the reason(s) for such a discrepancy is/are not apparent, although patients' heterogeneity and perhaps dietary intake are possible confounders.

Despite the inconsistency in basal serum and cellular Mg^{2+} levels between healthy women and women with preeclampsia, observation by Standley and collaborators suggests that magnesium levels can still be used as a predictive/prognostic tool [59]. In studying magnesium levels at different gestational ages, this group observed that the levels of the cation decrease in both preeclamptic and healthy pregnancies, but the decrease in preeclamptic women occurs at an earlier stage as compared to the healthy counterparts and could therefore be utilized as a marker of severity of the pathology [59].

6. Conclusions and Perspectives

In this review, we have attempted to provide a general understanding of how human cells control cellular and circulating magnesium levels, the importance of these levels for wellness in general and blood pressure levels in particular, and how diet and dietary supplements can be utilized effectively to maintain physiological levels of magnesium. We have also attempted to provide an appreciation of the complexity surrounding the prophylactic and possibly therapeutic use of magnesium supplementation in hypertension, and hypertension-associated pathologies such as stroke, metabolic syndrome, and preeclampsia/eclampsia.

Despite the inherent difficulty to provide a clear cut approach and validity to the use of magnesium supplementation as a therapeutic tool, it is apparent from our reviewing of the mentioned pathologies that magnesium supplementation does have a role as a coadjuvant of more established pharmacological tools currently utilized in the various fields. The low cost of production and the virtual absence of side-effects in the normal range of doses more commonly utilized (e.g., up to 960 mg/day) add to the "appeal" of a routine use of this mineral as a dietary supplement, especially in areas where health care costs, availability of more expensive drugs, and ultimately compliance of the patients to a given therapeutic protocol represent critical factors hampering the effectiveness of medical intervention.

Acknowledgments

This study was supported by NIAAA-11593, HL 090969, and Departmental Funding to Dr. A. Romani.

References

[1] http://www.who.int/topics/hypertension/en/, May 12, 2018.

[2] R. Merai, C. Siegel, M. Rakotz et al., "CDC grand rounds: a public health approach to detect and control hypertension," *Morbidity and Mortality Weekly Report (MMWR)*, vol. 65, no. 45, pp. 1261–1264, 2016.

[3] https://www.froedtert.com/endocrinology/endocrine-hypertension, May 12, 2018.

[4] P. K. Whelton, R. M. Carey, W. S. Aronow et al., "2017 ACC/AHA/AAPA/ABC/ACPM/AGS/APhA/ASH/ASPC/NMA/PCNA guideline for the prevention, detection,

evaluation, and management of high blood pressure in adults," *Journal of the American College of Cardiology*, vol. 71, no. 19, pp. e127–e248, 2018.

[5] A. M. P. Romani, "Magnesium in health and disease," *Metal Ions in Life Sciences*, vol. 13, pp. 49–79, 2013.

[6] A. Romani and A. Scarpa, "Regulation of cell magnesium," *Archives of Biochemistry and Biophysics*, vol. 298, no. 1, pp. 1–12, 1992.

[7] A. Scarpa, "Regulation of cellular magnesium," *Frontiers in Bioscience*, vol. 5, no. 3, pp. d720–734, 2000.

[8] R. B. Costello, R. J. Elin, A. Rosanoff et al., "Perspective: the case for an evidence-based reference interval for serum magnesium: the time has come," *Advances in Nutrition*, vol. 7, no. 6, pp. 977–993, 2016.

[9] S. L. Volpe, "Magnesium in disease prevention and overall health," *Advances in Nutrition*, vol. 4, no. 3, 2013.

[10] A. C. Ross, J. E. Manson, S. A. Abrams et al., "The 2011 report on dietary reference intakes for calcium and vitamin D from the institute of medicine: what clinicians need to know," *The Journal of Clinical Endocrinology & Metabolism*, vol. 96, no. 1, pp. 53–58, 2011.

[11] F. H. Nielsen, "Magnesium, inflammation, and obesity in chronic disease," *Nutrition Reviews*, vol. 68, no. 6, pp. 333–340, 2010.

[12] https://ods.od.nih.gov/factsheets/Magnesium-HealthProfessional/, May 12, 2018.

[13] O. F. Hutter and K. Kostial, "Effect of magnesium and calcium ions on the release of acetylcholine," *The Journal of Physiology*, vol. 124, no. 2, pp. 234–241, 1954.

[14] J. B. Standbury, "The blocking action of magnesium on sympathetic ganglia," *Journal of Pharmacology and Experimental Therapeutics*, vol. 93, pp. 52–62, 1948.

[15] L. Dubé and JC. Granry, "The therapeutic use of magnesium in anesthesiology, intensive care and emergency medicine: a review," *Canadian Journal of Anesthesia*, vol. 50, no. 7, pp. 732–746, 2003.

[16] M. I. Akhtar, H. Ullah, and M. Hamid, "Magnesium a drug of diverse use," *Journal of Pakistan Medical Association*, vol. 61, no. 12, pp. 1220–1225, 2011.

[17] L. M. Resnick, R. K. Gupta, B. DiFabio et al., "Intracellular ionic consequences of dietary salt loading in essential hypertension. Relation to blood pressure and effects of calcium channel blockade," *The Journal of Clinical Investigation*, vol. 94, no. 3, pp. 1269–1276, 1994.

[18] P. Tammaro, A. L. Smith, B. L. Crowley, and S. V. Smirnov, "Modulation of the voltage-dependent K + current by intracellular Mg 2+ in rat aortic smooth muscle cells," *Cardiovascular Research*, vol. 65, no. 2, pp. 387–396, 2005.

[19] R. M. Touyz and G. Yao, "Modulation of vascular smooth muscle cell growth by magnesium-role of mitogen-activated protein kinases," *Journal of Cellular Physiology*, vol. 197, no. 3, pp. 326–335, 2003.

[20] P. Laurant, R. M. Touyz, and E. L. Schiffrin, "Effect of magnesium on vascular tone and reactivity in pressurized mesenteric resistance arteries from spontaneously hypertensive rats," *Canadian Journal of Physiology and Pharmacology*, vol. 75, no. 4, pp. 293–300, 1997.

[21] M. Yoshimura, T. Oshima, H. Matsuura, T. Ishida, M. Kambe, and G. Kajiyama, "Extracellular Mg2+ inhibits capacitative Ca2+ entry in vascular smooth muscle cells," *Circulation*, vol. 95, no. 11, pp. 2567–2572, 1997.

[22] J. A. Maier, D. Bernardini, Y. Rayssiguier, and A. Mazur, "High concentrations of magnesium modulate vascular endothelial cell behaviour in vitro," *Biochimica et Biophysica Acta (BBA)—Molecular Basis of Disease*, vol. 1689, no. 1, pp. 6–12, 2004.

[23] K. Satake, J.-D. Lee, H. Shimizu et al., "Effects of magnesium on prostacyclin synthesis and intracellular free calcium concentration in vascular cells," *Magnesium Research*, vol. 17, no. 1, pp. 20–27, 2004.

[24] N. Soltani, M. Keshavarz, H. Sohanaki, S. Z. Asl, and A. R. Dehpour, "Relaxatory effect of magnesium on mesenteric vascular beds differs from normal and streptozotocin induced diabetic rats," *European Journal of Pharmacology*, vol. 508, no. 1-3, pp. 177–181, 2005.

[25] R. Landau, J. A. Scott, and R. M. Smiley, "Magnesium-induced vasodilation in the dorsal hand vein," *BJOG: An International Journal of Obstetrics & Gynaecology*, vol. 111, no. 5, pp. 446–451, 2004.

[26] P. Laurant and A. Berthelot, "Endothelin-1-induced contraction in isolated aortae from normotensive and DOCA-salt hypertensive rats: effect of magnesium," *British Journal of Pharmacology*, vol. 119, no. 7, pp. 1367–1374, 1996.

[27] W. B. Weglicki, T. M. Phillips, A. M. Freedman, M. M. Cassidy, and B. F. Dickens, "Magnesium-deficiency elevates circulating levels of inflammatory cytokines and endothelin," *Molecular and Cellular Biochemistry*, vol. 110, no. 2, pp. 169–173, 1992.

[28] W. B. Weglicki, I. T. Mak, J. H. Kramer et al., "Role of free radicals and substance P in magnesium deficiency," *Cardiovascular Research*, vol. 31, no. 5, pp. 677–682, 1996.

[29] Y. Taniyama and K. K. Griendling, "Reactive oxygen species in the vasculature: molecular and cellular mechanisms," *Hypertension*, vol. 42, no. 6, pp. 1075–1081, 2003.

[30] M. Kolisek, A. C. Montezano, G. Sponder et al., "PARK7/DJ-1 dysregulation by oxidative stress leads to magnesium deficiency: implications in degenerative and chronic diseases," *Clinical Science*, vol. 129, no. 12, pp. 1143–1150, 2015.

[31] M. R. Joffres, D. M. Reed, and K. Yano, "Relationship of magnesium intake and other dietary factors to blood pressure: the Honolulu heart study," *American Journal of Clinical Nutrition*, vol. 45, no. 2, pp. 469–475, 1987.

[32] W. H. L. Kao, A. R. Folsom, F. J. Nieto, J.-P. Mo, R. L. Watson, and F. L. Brancati, "Serum and dietary magnesium and the risk for type 2 diabetes mellitus: the atherosclerosis risk in communities study," *JAMA Internal Medicine*, vol. 159, no. 18, pp. 2151–2159, 1999.

[33] C.-Y. Yang and H.-F. Chiu, "Calcium and magnesium in drinking water and the risk of death from hypertension," *American Journal of Hypertension*, vol. 12, no. 9 I, pp. 894–899, 1999.

[34] L. M. Resnick, J. H. Laragh, J. E. Sealey, and M. H. Alderman, "Divalent cations in essential hypertension: relations between serum ionized calcium, magnesium, and plasma renin activity," *The New England Journal of Medicine*, vol. 309, no. 15, pp. 888–891, 1983.

[35] L. M. Resnick, D. Militianu, A. J. Cunnings, J. G. Pipe, J. L. Evelhoch, and R. L. Soulen, "Direct magnetic resonance determination of aortic distensibility in essential hypertension: relation to age, abdominal visceral fat, and in situ intracellular free magnesium," *Hypertension*, vol. 30, no. 3, pp. 654–659, 1997.

[36] H. O. Dickinson, D. J. Nicolson, F. Campbell et al., "Magnesium supplements for the management of essential hypertension in adults," *Cochrane Database of Systematic Reviews*, no. 3, 2006.

[37] L. Kass, J. Weekes, and L. Carpenter, "Effect of magnesium supplementation on blood pressure: a meta-analysis," *European Journal of Clinical Nutrition*, vol. 66, no. 4, pp. 411–418, 2012.

[38] X. Zhang, Y. Li, L. C. Del Gobbo et al., "Effects of magnesium supplementation on blood pressure: a meta-analysis of randomized double-blind placebo-controlled trials," *Hypertension*, vol. 68, no. 2, pp. 324–333, 2016.

[39] https://www.cdc.gov/media/releases/2017/p0906-vs-stroke .html, January 2018.

[40] S. C. Larsson, N. Orsini, and A. Wolk, "Dietary magnesium intake and risk of stroke: a meta-analysis of prospective studies," *American Journal of Clinical Nutrition*, vol. 95, no. 2, pp. 362–366, 2012.

[41] H. Han, X. Fang, X. Wei et al., "Dose-response relationship between dietary magnesium intake, serum magnesium concentration and risk of hypertension: a systematic review and meta-analysis of prospective cohort studies," *Nutrition Journal*, vol. 16, no. 1, 2017.

[42] http://www.cdc.gov/obesity/data/adult.html, January 2018.

[43] H. Haller, "Epidermiology and associated risk factors of hyperlipoproteinemia," *Zeitschrift für die gesamte innere Medizin und ihre Grenzgebiete*, vol. 32, no. 8, pp. 124–128, 1977.

[44] S. M. Grundy, H. B. Brewer Jr., J. I. Cleeman, S. C. Smith Jr., and C. Lenfant, "Definition of metabolic syndrome report of the national heart, lung, and blood institute/american heart association conference on scientific issues related to definition," *Circulation*, vol. 109, no. 3, pp. 433–438, 2004.

[45] R. Lopez-Ridaura, W. C. Willett, E. B. Rimm et al., "Magnesium intake and risk of type 2 diabetes in men and women," *Diabetes Care*, vol. 27, no. 1, pp. 134–140, 2004.

[46] F. Guerrero-Romero and M. Rodríguez-Morán, "Low serum magnesium levels and metabolic syndrome," *Acta Diabetologica*, vol. 39, no. 4, pp. 209–213, 2002.

[47] G. M. Reaven, "The insulin resistance syndrome: definition and dietary approaches to treatment," *Annual Review of Nutrition*, vol. 25, pp. 391–406, 2005.

[48] K. He, K. Liu, M. L. Daviglus et al., "Magnesium intake and incidence of metabolic syndrome among young adults," *Circulation*, vol. 113, no. 13, pp. 1675–1682, 2006.

[49] G. Lambert, J. F. Brichant, G. Hartstein, V. Bonhomme, and P. Y. Dewandre, "Preeclampsia: an update," *Acta Anaesthesiologica Belgica*, vol. 65, no. 4, pp. 137–149, 2014.

[50] Williams, *Obstetrics*, McGraw-Hill Professional, 24th edition, 2014.

[51] GBD 2015 Mortality and Causes of Death Collaborators, "Global, regional, and national life expectancy, all-cause mortality, and cause-specific mortality for 249 causes of death, 1980-2015: a systematic analysis for the Global Burden of Disease Study," *Lancet*, vol. 388, pp. 1459–1544, 2015.

[52] J. A. Pritchard, "The use of the magnesium ion in the management of eclamptogenic toxemias," *Surgery, Gynecology & Obstetrics—Journals*, vol. 100, pp. 131–140, 1955.

[53] J. M. Smith, R. F. Lowe, J. Fullerton, S. M. Currie, L. Harris, and E. Felker-Kantor, "An integrative review of the side effects related to the use of magnesium sulfate for pre-eclampsia and eclampsia management," *BMC Pregnancy and Childbirth*, vol. 13, article 34, 2013.

[54] L. Duley, D. J. Henderson-Smart, G. J. Walker, and D. Chou, "Magnesium sulphate versus diazepam for eclampsia," *Cochrane Database of Systematic Reviews (Online)*, vol. 12, Article ID CD000127, 2010.

[55] J. Seydoux, E. Girardin, L. Paunier, and F. Béguin, "Serum and intracellular magnesium during normal pregnancy and in patients with pre-eclampsia," *BJOG: An International Journal of Obstetrics & Gynaecology*, vol. 99, no. 3, pp. 207–211, 1992.

[56] L. He, L. Lang, Y. Li, Q. Liu, and Y. Yao, "Comparison of serum zinc, calcium, and magnesium concentrations in women with pregnancy-induced hypertension and healthy pregnant women: a meta-analysis," *Hypertension in Pregnancy*, vol. 35, no. 2, pp. 202–209, 2016.

[57] R. Sanders, A. Konijnenberg, H. J. Huijgen, H. Wolf, K. Boer, and G. T. Sanders, "Intracellular and extracellular, ionized and total magnesium in pre-eclampsia and uncomplicated pregnancy," *Clinical Chemistry and Laboratory Medicine*, vol. 37, no. 1, 1999.

[58] Y. Frenkel, M. Weiss, M. Shefi, A. Lusky, S. Mashiach, and E. Dolev, "Mononuclear cell magnesium content remains unchanged in various hypertensive disorders of pregnancy," *Gynecologic and Obstetric Investigation*, vol. 38, no. 4, pp. 220–222, 1994.

[59] C. A. Standley, J. E. Whitty, B. A. Mason, and D. B. Cotton, "Serum ionized magnesium levels in normal and preeclamptic gestation," *Obstetrics & Gynecology*, vol. 89, no. 1, pp. 24–27, 1997.

Changes in Angiotensin Receptor Distribution and in Aortic Morphology Are Associated with Blood Pressure Control in Aged Metabolic Syndrome Rats

Verónica Guarner-Lans,[1] Elizabeth Soria-Castro,[2] Rocío Torrico-Lavayen,[2] Araceli Patrón-Soberano,[3] Karla G. Carvajal-Aguilera,[4] Vicente Castrejón-Tellez,[1] and María Esther Rubio-Ruiz[1]

[1] *Department of Physiology, Instituto Nacional de Cardiología "Ignacio Chávez", 14080 Mexico City, DF, Mexico*
[2] *Department of Pathology, Instituto Nacional de Cardiología "Ignacio Chávez", 14080 Mexico City, DF, Mexico*
[3] *National Laboratory of Nanoscience and Nanotechnology, Molecular Biology Division, Instituto Potosino de Investigación Científica y Tecnológica (IPICYT), 78216 San Luis Potosí, SLP, Mexico*
[4] *Laboratorio de Nutrición Experimental, Instituto Nacional de Pediatría, 04530 Mexico City, DF, Mexico*

Correspondence should be addressed to María Esther Rubio-Ruiz; esther_rubio_ruiz@yahoo.com

Academic Editor: Tomohiro Katsuya

The role of the renin-angiotensin system (RAS) in blood pressure regulation in MS during aging is unknown. It participates in metabolic syndrome (MS) and aging regulating vascular tone and remodeling. RAS might participate in a compensatory mechanism decreasing blood pressure and allowing MS rats to reach 18 months of age and it might form part of therapeutical procedures to ameliorate MS. We studied histological changes and distribution of RAS receptors in aortas of MS aged rats. Electron microscopy images showed premature aging in MS since the increased fibrosis, enlarged endothelium, and invasion of this layer by muscle cells that was present in control 18-month-old aortas were also found in 6-month-old aortas from MS rats. AT1, AT2, and Mas receptors mediate the effects of Ang II and Ang 1-7, respectively. Fluorescence from AT2 decreased with age in control and MS aortas, while fluorescence of AT1 increased in aortas from MS rats at 6 months and diminished during aging. Mas expression increased in MS rats and remained unchanged in control rats. In conclusion, there is premature aging in the aortas from MS rats and the elevated expression of Mas receptor might contribute to decrease blood pressure during aging in MS.

1. Introduction

Metabolic syndrome (MS) is a disease that accelerates aging [1]. Aging is associated with endothelial dysfunction and structural and functional vascular changes [2]. We have previously studied changes in blood pressure during aging in a MS rat model and found an increase at 6 months of age in comparison to control groups and a further decline from then onwards until 18 months of age. Rats that survive to reach 18 months are few and could be the ones that develop compensatory mechanisms to the effects of MS, the fall of arterial pressure being one of them [3, 4]. These compensatory mechanisms might be the same that underlie the condition of healthy obese or healthy MS patients and could be the basis for the development of therapeutical approaches to complications of MS. The renin angiotensin system (RAS) might participate in these mechanisms and particularly the Ang 1-7/MAS pathway.

RAS is involved in the development of MS [5] and in aging [6–8]. Moreover, long-term treatment with an angiotensin converting enzyme (ACE) inhibitor or an Ang II receptor antagonist ameliorates the MS effects [9–11]. It has long been recognized as an important regulator of systemic blood pressure and renal electrolyte homeostasis, and local RAS has also been implicated in pathological changes of organ structure and function by modulation of gene expression, growth, fibrosis, and inflammatory responses. RAS dysregulation influences the development and progression of cardiovascular disease [12].

Angiotensin II (Ang II) is a potent proinflammatory, prooxidant, and prothrombotic agent that favors endothelial dysfunction by increasing catecholamines, endothelin-1 (ET-1), and thromboxane A_2which increase blood pressure [13]. Ang II also alters the structure of vessels modifying processes such as growth, apoptosis, and cellular migration of vascular smooth muscle cells as well as changes in the components of the extracellular matrix [14]. It causes an increase in the intima-media thickness, vascular rigidity, endothelial dysfunction, and proinflammatory state [2]. Ang II binds to highly specific membrane receptors types 1 and 2 (AT1 and AT2). Increased levels of Ang II have been observed in both obese and diabetic patients.

Angiotensin 1–7 (Ang 1-7) is a heptapeptide, primarily formed from Ang II and Ang I by angiotensin converting enzyme 2 (ACE2) that has actions that oppose those of Ang II, acting through Mas. The components of RAS in white adipose tissue (WAT) are present in our rat model of MS by chronic ingestion of sucrose and WAT is an important source of Ang 1-7 [4]. Mas receptor is also expressed in the vascular endothelium which, at the same time, is an important site for Ang 1-7 generation [15]. The ACE2/Ang 1-7/Mas axis induces the release of vasodilators, including prostanoids, nitric oxide (NO), and endothelium-derived hyperpolarizing factor [16]. The vasodilator actions of Ang 1-7 depend on an intracellular signaling mechanism, as yet not fully characterized, that may be caused by secretion of prostacyclin, release of NO, amplification of the vasodilator effects of bradykinin, or vasopressin liberation alone or in combination [17].

Activation of endogenous ACE2 reduces arterial blood pressure in normal and hypertensive rats and relaxes many vascular beds [18]. Angiotensin 1-7 and its receptor Mas (Ang 1-7/Mas) were described later and antagonize the effect of AT2; therefore, they could represent a target for therapeutical strategies. The elevated expression of Mas receptor might contribute to decreases of blood pressure.

There is little information on the location AT1 and AT2 receptors in the different cell types of the vasculature and thus the identification of their function is complex. Moreover the belief that AT2 receptors are more significant during development than in adult life and so might regulate growth and development of blood vessels rather than having acute actions on the vasculature has delayed the study of their function in adult vessels [19]. During aging, Ang II, ACE, and AT1 increase in the vascular wall [20].

Therefore, the aim of the present study was to document the premature aging of the vessels in MS by comparing the structural changes in aortas from control and MS animals and to analyze the expression of AT1, AT2, and Mas receptors in these vessels as important components of RAS which might participate in the compensatory mechanisms that allow the 18-month-old MS rats to survive.

2. Materials and Methods

2.1. Animals. The experimental protocols in this study were reviewed and approved by the Laboratory Animal Care Committee of our institution and performed in accordance with the institutional guidelines for research and animal use.

Weanling male Wistar rats aged 25 days and weighing 50 ± 4 g were divided randomly into two groups: (1) control rats were given tap water for drinking and (2) MS rats received 30% sucrose in drinking water. Control and MS animals aged 6, 12, and 18 months were used. At least 6 animals were used per group. Animals were fed Purina 5001 rat chow (Richmond, IN) *ad libitum* under controlled temperature and a 12 : 12 h light/dark cycle.

Systolic arterial blood pressure was measured in conscious animals using the tail cuff method previously described [3].

2.2. Blood Samples. After overnight fasting (12 h), the animals were killed by decapitation and blood was collected. It was spun and the serum was separated by centrifugation at 600 g during 15 min at room temperature and stored at −70°C until assayed. Plasma triglycerides were measured using a commercially available kit (Randox, Laboratories LTD, Antrim, United Kingdom). Serum insulin was determined using commercial radioimmunoassay (RIA) kit specific for rat (Linco Research, Inc.; EMD Millipore, Missouri, USA). Glucose concentration was assayed using an enzymatic kit SERA-PAK^R Plus from Bayer Corporation (Bayer Corporation, Sées, France). Seric concentrations of Ang II and Ang 1-7 were evaluated by capillary zone electrophoresis as previously described [4]. Abdominal fat was dissected and weighted.

2.3. Histologic Staining, Immunohistochemistry of Angiotensin Receptors, and Image Analysis. The fixed aortic tissues were embedded in paraffin and cut into 5 μm thick sections. The sections were then stained with Masson trichrome stain to reveal histological changes. For electron microscopy, the rings of aortas were obtained and immediately fixed and embedded in Epon (Epon 812 EMS); ultrathin sections were then viewed using a Jeol 10-11.

For immunohistochemistry studies, rat aorta samples were quickly frozen in Tissue-Tek (Sakura Finetek USA, Inc., Torrance, CA). Sections were fixed with acetone and were blocked with PBS/Azide 0.02%/BSA 1% for 30 min. Subsequently, sections were incubated during 2 h at room temperature with a rabbit polyclonal antibody against AT1, AT2 (1 : 50; Santa Cruz Biotechnology, Inc., Santa Cruz, CA) and goat polyclonal antibody against Mas (1 : 50; Santa Cruz Biotechnology, Inc., Santa Cruz, CA). Antibodies were detected by using goat anti-rabbit FITC (Jackson ImmunoResearch Laboratories Inc., West Grove, PA) and rabbit anti-goat Tex Red (1 : 50; Santa Cruz Biotechnology, Inc., Santa Cruz, CA) at room temperature for 45 min. The slides were mounted with a drop of mounting medium (Dako Fluorescent mounting medium). Negative controls were prepared by substituting the primary antibody with an irrelevant antibody. Images from six different sections were collected

Table 1: Characteristics and biochemical parameters from control and MS rats during aging.

Groups and age (months)	Body weight (g)	Central adiposity (g)	Blood pressure (mm Hg)	Glucose (mM)	Triglycerides (mg/dL)	Insulin (μU/mL)	HOMA-IR
Control							
6	517.1 ± 6.7	6.2 ± 0.9	101.6 ± 0.9	5.0 ± 0.9	50.9 ± 5.2	5.9 ± 1.3	1.9 ± 0.7
12	580.2 ± 9.6	10.3 ± 1.4	100.0 ± 1.8	5.1 ± 0.4	$96.1 \pm 4.3^{\$}$	6.1 ± 2.4	2.0 ± 0.9
18	$620.9 \pm 10.4^{\ddagger}$	$14.4 \pm 3.1^{\$}$	106.1 ± 1.1	5.4 ± 0.8	$149.7 \pm 6.9^{\ddagger}$	6.4 ± 0.9	1.7 ± 0.9
MS							
6	535.7 ± 12.3	$14.7 \pm 0.8^{\dagger}$	$148.6 \pm 1.2^{\dagger}$	4.9 ± 0.9	$113.3 \pm 10.4^{\dagger}$	$22.4 \pm 5.2^{\dagger}$	$4.7 \pm 2.1^{\dagger}$
12	650.7 ± 17.4	$19.9 \pm 2.1^{\dagger}$	115.2 ± 5.6	5.9 ± 0.1	$198.6 \pm 25.7^{\dagger\$}$	19.6 ± 8.1	$4.5 \pm 1.7^{\&}$
18	$806.3 \pm 18.7^{\dagger\ddagger}$	$43.3 \pm 5.2^{\dagger\ddagger}$	$100.1 \pm 2.1^{\ddagger}$	6.1 ± 0.4	$271.3 \pm 31.4^{\dagger\$}$	$6.9 \pm 2.3^{\$}$	$1.9 \pm 0.6^{\$}$

Values are means ± SEM.; HOMA-IR: homeostatic model assessment of insulin resistance; $n = 6$; $^{\&}P < 0.05$ against C; $^{\dagger}P < 0.01$ versus C; $^{\ddagger}P < 0.05$ against other ages in corresponding group; $^{\$}P < 0.05$ against 6 months in corresponding group.

and analyzed using confocal microscopy. The samples were scanned on a confocal laser scanning microscope FV1000 (Olympus, Corporation, Tokyo, Japan) attached/interfaced to an Olympus IX81 inverted light microscope with a 20x N.A. 0.85 air objective, all times with digital zoom of 3. FITC was excited employing the 488 nm line of an Argon laser and the emitted fluorescence was detected with a 500–530 nm spectral setting. Tex Red was excited employing the 543 nm line of an Argon laser and the emitted fluorescence was detected with a 500–633 nm spectral setting. All images were obtained with the same laser power percentage and confocal aperture. The comparison of fluorescence in rat aortas between groups was done using fixed setting on the confocal microscope; confocal images were viewed, processed, and converted to TIFF format with the FV10-ASW software (Olympus Corporation, Tokyo, Japan). We used Image J software that assigned a value for green or red fluorescence intensity to every pixel and the average pixel intensity was calculated [21]. To express the intensity of fluorescence, arbitrary units were used: relative fluorescence (Mean Fluorescence Intensity (FI)) was defined as the sum of the fluorescence intensity grayscale of all pixels divided by the addition of all the image pixels. The percentage of fluorescence between comparable groups was calculated:

$$\% \text{ Relative Fluorescence} = \sum \text{FI} * \frac{100}{\sum \text{Image pixels}}. \quad (1)$$

2.4. Statistical Analysis. Results are expressed as mean ± standard errors of the mean (SEM). When applicable (comparisons between two values; MS and controls at the same age), statistical analysis was done by Student's t-test. Comparisons between groups at different ages were done by analysis of variance (ANOVA) or ANOVA on ranks followed by Student-Newman-Keuls or Dunn's tests. The accepted level of statistical significance was $p < 0.05$. Data analysis was carried out using the Sigma Stat program (Jandel Scientific).

3. Results

Table 1 shows the differences among the groups. At six months, experimental animals developed MS characterized by increased abdominal fat, hypertension, hypertriglyceridemia, hyperinsulinemia, and insulin resistance (HOMA-IR). Aging *per se* increased intra-abdominal fat and triglycerides concentrations in control rats. In 18-month-old MS rats, weight, visceral fat, and triglycerides were higher than in young MS rats. Fasting serum glucose levels were not significantly different among the groups, but there was an increase at 18 months in MS rats. In MS rats insulin level was only significantly increased at 6 months when compared to controls; then it showed a decrease during aging.

In control rats, the arterial blood pressure was not modified during aging. At 6 months of age systolic arterial pressure was significantly elevated in MS rats when compared to control rats (Table 1). MS rats showed a continuous blood pressure decrease with age.

Table 2 shows that seric Ang II concentrations were not different in C and MS rats at 6 months of age. Therefore, this peptide does not seem to participate in the development of hypertension in the MS model. In the C group, Ang II concentration remained unchanged while in MS animals it decreased significantly during aging. Ang 1-7 concentrations showed the inverse relationship, increasing significantly in MS rats at 18 months of age. In the control group, these values were unchanged. These results coincide with those previously reported by our group [4].

3.1. Morphological Study of Aging in Aortas from Control and MS Rats. When Masson staining was used, aortas from 18-month-old control rats showed characteristic changes due to aging when compared to 6-month-old aortas. These changes were apparent in the intima and media layers; endothelium showed swelling and in the media there was discontinuity of elastic fibers. When comparing 6-month-old aortas from control and MS rats, discontinuity of elastic fibers in the

TABLE 2: Seric angiotensin II and angiotensin 1-7 concentrations from control and MS rats during aging.

Groups and age (months)	Ang II (pmol/mL)	Ang 1-7 (pmol/mL)
Control		
6	0.09 ± 0.02	2.31 ± 0.17
12	0.05 ± 0.01	4.21 ± 0.41
18	0.06 ± 0.01	3.16 ± 1.29
MS		
6	0.11 ± 0.03	2.61 ± 0.36
12	0.09 ± 0.01$^{\&}$	3.97 ± 0.41
18	0.008 ± 0.0006$^{\&\ddagger}$	7.91 ± 0.46†‡

Values are means ± SEM; $n = 6$; $^{\&}P < 0.05$ against C; $^{\dagger}P < 0.01$ versus C; $^{\ddagger}P < 0.05$ against other ages in corresponding group.

media was clear even in zones close to the intima and there was hyperplasia of muscular cells in the media in aortas from MS rats at 6 months of age. Deterioration continued even further in 18-month-old MS aortas (Figure 1). Electron microscopy images showed increased fibrosis, enlarged endothelium, and invasion of this layer by muscle cells in 18-month-old control aortas and in 6-month-old aortas from MS rats when compared to 6-month-old control aortas. In 18-month-old aortas from MS rats the endothelium was enlarged and infiltrated with cells from the immune system (Figure 1).

Ultrastructure studies showed differences between control and MS aortas. Aortas from 6-month-old MS rats had endothelial damage and changes in the structure of elastic fibers when compared to aortas from control animals (Figures 2(a) and 2(b)). The aging process of control aortas is seen at 18 months in which intima swelling was accompanied by cellular infiltrate which is present together with thickening of the media layer with infiltration of muscular cells. Furthermore, there is discontinuity of elastic fibers (Figure 2(c)). In the 18-month-old aortas from MS animals the above mentioned characteristics of old control vessels were also found showing adhesion of inflammatory cells in the intima layer (Figure 2(d)).

3.2. Angiotensin Receptor Expression in Thoracic Aorta. The distribution of the fluorescence signal is different for each of the receptors studied. Fluorescence from AT1 receptors from aortas from 6-month-old rats was higher in the MS group than in controls. AT1 fluorescence did not change in control rats during aging and was located in the endothelium and adventitia. In contrast, in the arteries from the rats with MS, fluorescence diminishes significantly with age and it moved from the endothelium to the elastic fibers (Figures 3 and 6).

Fluorescence from AT2 receptors is higher in aortas from control 6-month-old rats than in aortas from the MS group and is specifically located in the elastic fibers from the media. In old control rats, intensity decreases and is located in elastic fibers and in the endothelium. Fluorescence continues to decrease and by 18 months of age it is located in the media and adventitia. In aortas from MS rats, fluorescence is less than in control rats at all ages (especially at 18 months) and decreases with aging. At 6 months of age the signal looks like spots and is located in the elastic fibers. At 12 months, the signal is even lower and located in elastic fibers and in the adventitia. By 18 months, the fluorescence looks like spots and is only located in the endothelium and the elastic fibers (Figures 4 and 6).

At 6 months of age, there is no difference in the fluorescence from the Mas receptors in control and MS aortas. During aging fluorescence intensity of the Mas receptor in control aortas does not change; however its distribution is modified. The signal is higher in the adventitia at 6 months and it diminishes by 12 months; it is located in the endothelium and adventitia. At 18 months the signal increases and is located in elastic fibers. In aortas from 6-month-old rats with MS, fluorescence is low, appears in spots, and is found in the endothelium and adventitia. At 12 months, fluorescence increases and is found in the adventitia and endothelium and finally by 18 months the signal is even higher and only located in the endothelium (Figures 5 and 6).

4. Discussion

Blood pressure is controlled by baroreflex activity that modulates sympathetic neural mechanisms and by central nervous set points that adjust its long-term level. There exist nonpathological long-term regulators that act on the central nervous set points such as aging and pathological modifiers such as obesity and heart failure. The central nervous set points receive input from volume regulatory hormones including RAS [22]. RAS constitutes a hormonal system that regulates blood pressure and its dysregulation influences the development and progression of cardiovascular disease. Although the regulation of the central nervous setpoints in our rat model might be interesting, and aging and obesity might influence their activity, in this paper we only studied the possible participation of the RAS vessel receptors during aging in control and MS rats. Ang II acts as a potent vasoconstrictor to activate AT1 receptors on vascular smooth muscle and affects cardiac and vascular remodeling, cardiac contractility, and pulse rate through increased sympathetic nervous system tone [12]. Ang 1-7 counteracts Ang II pressor and metabolic effects [16].

Our results show that rats receiving 30% sucrose in drinking water developed MS characterized by central obesity, hypertriglyceridemia, hyperinsulinemia, and moderate hypertension that are similar to those previously reported [3, 4]. Glucose was increased in MS rats at 18 months and is therefore a consequence of the aging process suggesting a prediabetic state. Aging increases the tendency to develop hyperglycemia and diabetes [23, 24].

Eighteen-month-old rats are regarded as old rats by many authors and even as senescent rats [2, 25]. Although control Wistar rats can live longer than 18 months, our model of MS rats has a significantly decreased survival rate (approximately 40%) by that age and organisms show a highly deteriorated state of health. Therefore, these rats show premature aging due to the MS. Furthermore, only rats that develop compensatory mechanisms including the capacity to restore hypertension might survive.

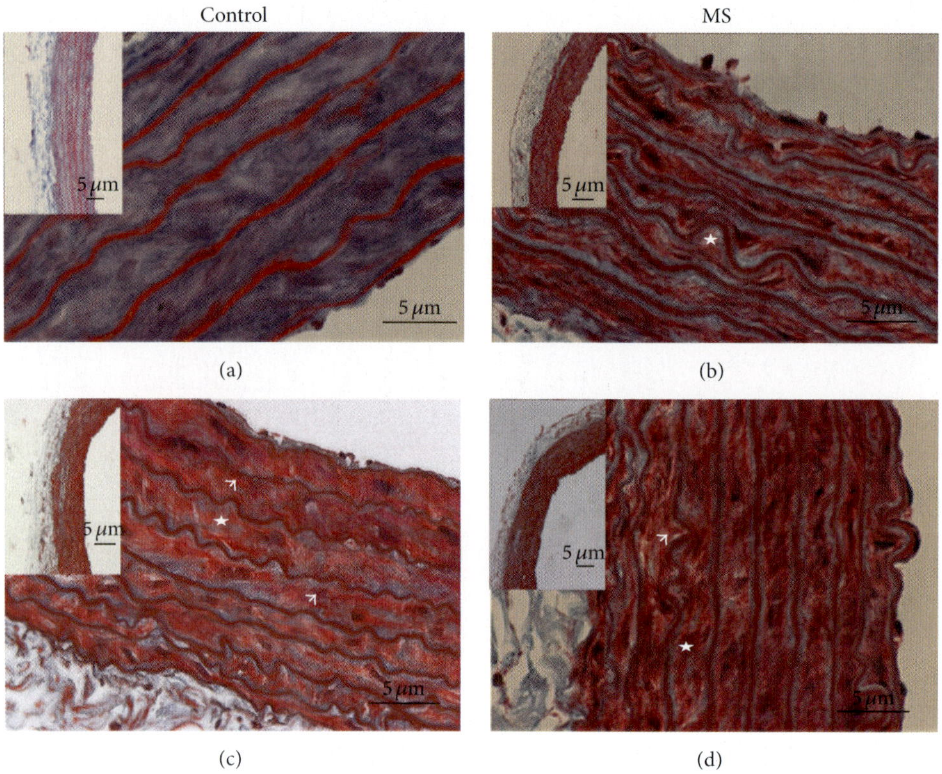

FIGURE 1: Histological images of representative rat aortas from different ages. Control ((a) 6 months and (c) 18 months) and MS ((b) 6 months and (d) 18 months) using Masson trichrome staining. The panoramic view is shown in the insert. The arrows indicate discontinuity of elastic fibers and the stars indicate hyperplasia of muscular cells.

Blood pressure in MS rats is higher than in control animals at 6 months of age and then decreases; this might be a selection of those rats with the capacity to compensate for the hypertensive state showing chronic compensatory changes in signaling molecules such as the increase in seric Ang 1-7 concentration that may restore blood pressure and a decrease in the concentration of Ang II (Table 2). This study confirms that, in control rats, the blood pressure remains constant during aging (Table 1).

Aging is associated with impaired blood vessel function, which is an early and important event leading to cardiovascular disease [26]. Aspects of vascular aging include increased arterial stiffness, dilation of central elastic arteries, and endothelial dysfunction [27]. Dysfunction is caused by the endothelium, smooth muscle, and extracellular matrix [28] and the causes of vascular dysfunction in the endothelium and in muscle have been previously described [29–36].

The aged aortic wall exhibits a proinflammatory profile that renders it a fertile substrate for the development of arterial disease. Studies in animal models demonstrate that Ang II and its downstream signaling molecules, that is, matrix metalloproteinases and monocyte chemoattractant protein-1, increase within the diffusely thickened intima of central arteries [37].

MS is a disease that accelerates aging [38], and RAS is involved in the aging process [6–8]. An increase in the intima-media thickness, vascular rigidity, endothelial dysfunction, and a proinflammatory state has been observed in MS during aging [2]. The described aging changes shown by hematoxyline-eosin staining and electron microscopy in aortas from MS agree with previous observations in pigs [39]. Premature aging in the aortas from MS rats might be the result of changes in their aortic receptors. Structural changes, inflammation, and damage have been found in vessels during aging [40].

RAS participates both in the development of MS and in aging thus rendering the evaluation of the variations in RAS receptors important in the MS aortas. During aging Ang II, ACE, and AT1 increase in the vascular wall [41]. The vascular wall is the effector organ for hormonal or plasma RAS and AT1, AT2, and Mas receptors have been identified in the vasculature. Aortas from 6-month-old MS rats showed a higher concentration of AT1 receptor than control aortas. In control rats AT1 expression did not significantly change in the vascular wall during aging. MS increases AT1 and this receptor is low during aging. Even if there is an increased expression of AT1 in 6-month-old animals, these receptors might be inactive because the cytoplasmic domain of AT1 binds to a variety of intracellular proteins involved in receptor signaling, desensitization, and endocytosis. Furthermore, alterations in homo- or heterodimerization of AT1 with other receptors may also contribute to the pathophysiological roles [42].

At 6 months of age, the aortas of the MS animals express less amount of AT2 receptors than aortas from control animals. This decrease in the expression of AT2 could be

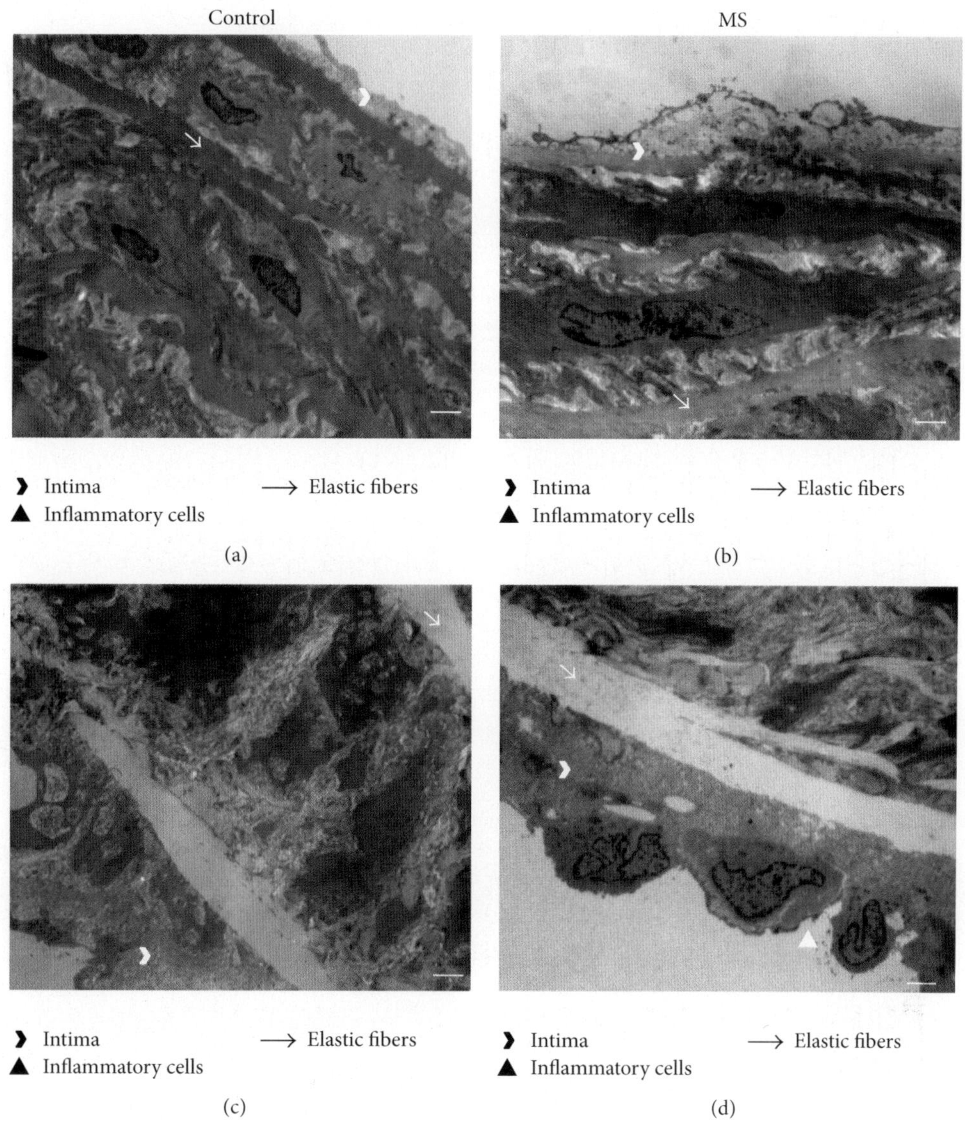

FIGURE 2: Micrographs from control 6- and 18-month-old aortas ((a) and (c), resp.) and MS 6- and 18-month-old aortas ((b) and (d), resp.). Scale bar = 2 μm.

related to the premature aging of MS animals that have a reduced vasodilator response. The distribution of the AT2 receptor in the vascular wall is nevertheless a matter of debate [43]. Advancing age is associated with arterial remodeling in diverse species. The effects of Ang II on vascular remodeling may be mediated at least in part via AT2. In this regard, AT2 may contribute to vascular adaptation and remodeling by influencing apoptosis in vascular smooth muscle cells. However, the effect of AT2 stimulation on vascular smooth muscle cells may vary between different cell phenotypes [43].

Our results show a reduction of fluorescence from AT2 in aortas from control and MS rats during aging which is consistent with the diminution found in the cardiovascular system and can be modulated in pathophysiological states associated with tissue inflammation and remodeling [44]. During aging, the fluorescence from AT2 receptor in control aortas decreases. However, we did not observe an increase in blood pressure in these animals. It is difficult to elicit a vasodilatory response directly in our aged rats; this effect may be related to AT2 receptor stimulation by Ang II. To confirm this point, we would need a more detailed description of the molecular specificity of the Ang II-AT2 pathway and to explore the possible alterations in signaling pathways in our animal model. Moreover, it has been reported that a complex interaction between Mas, AT1, and AT2 mediates the Ang 1-7 effects in blood vessels [45, 46]. The expression of Mas, which was similar in MS and controls at 6 months, increases with age only in the MS group.

Additionally, the analysis of angiotensin receptor expression by immunoblotting was done and there were no changes in AT1 and AT2 receptors in the experimental groups. Mas expression was increased in the aged MS rats (data not shown). Western blot analysis does not show the differences in the presence of the receptors in the different layers of the aortic tissue and adds little information on their location.

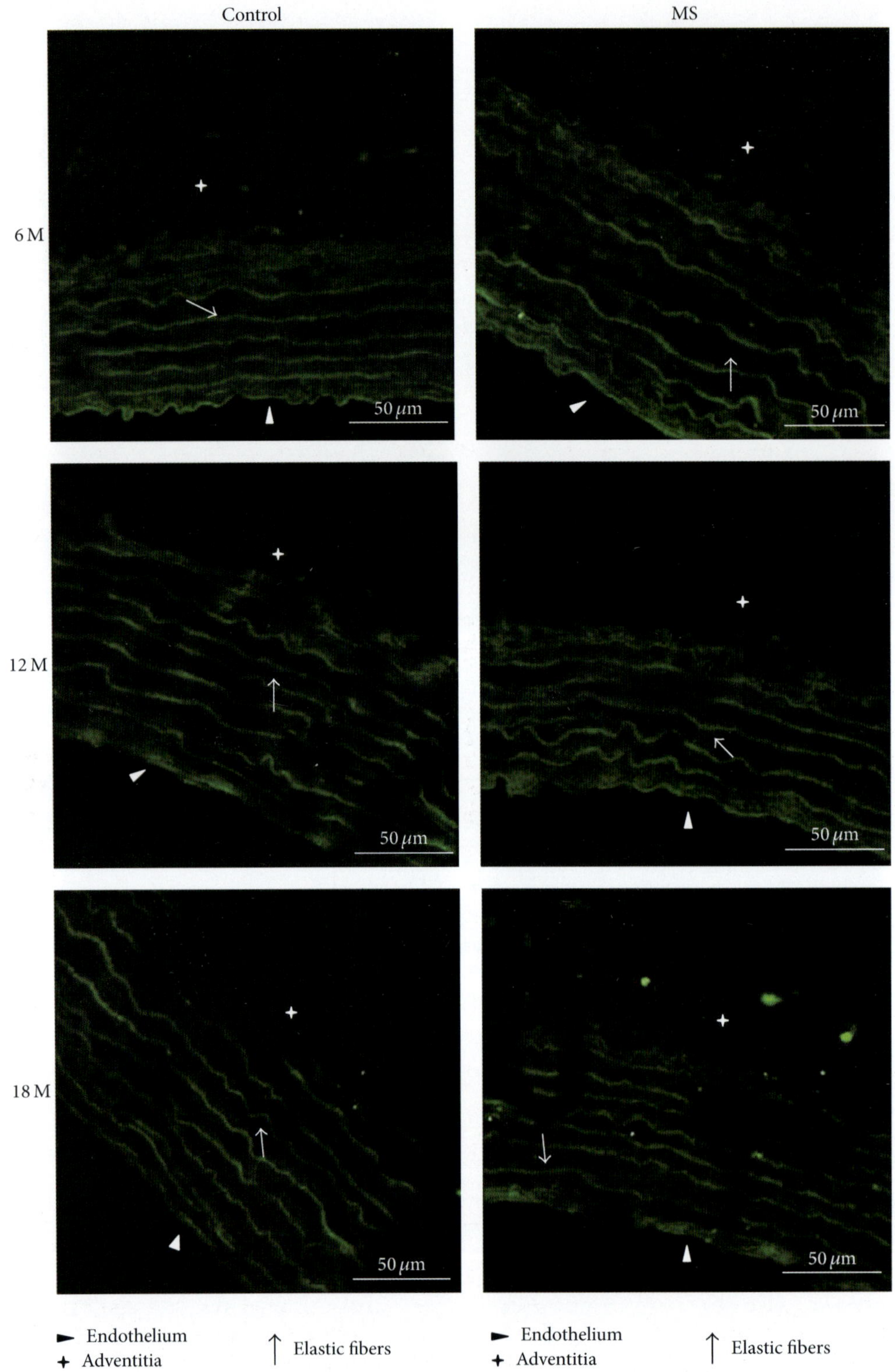

FIGURE 3: Illustrative images (×60) showing receptor AT1 immunofluorescence in aortas of control and MS rats aged 6, 12, and 18 months. Preparations were stained with FITC. Scale bar = 50 μm.

In conclusion, aging modifies body weight, abdominal fat, and triglycerides but these variables are further increased by MS. There is premature aging in this group since MS increases the progressive damage normally caused by aging. Alterations in the structure and function of the endothelium might be responsible of cardiovascular dysfunctions associated with aging in MS. The increase in Mas receptors coupled with the increased concentration of Ang 1-7 might explain, in part,

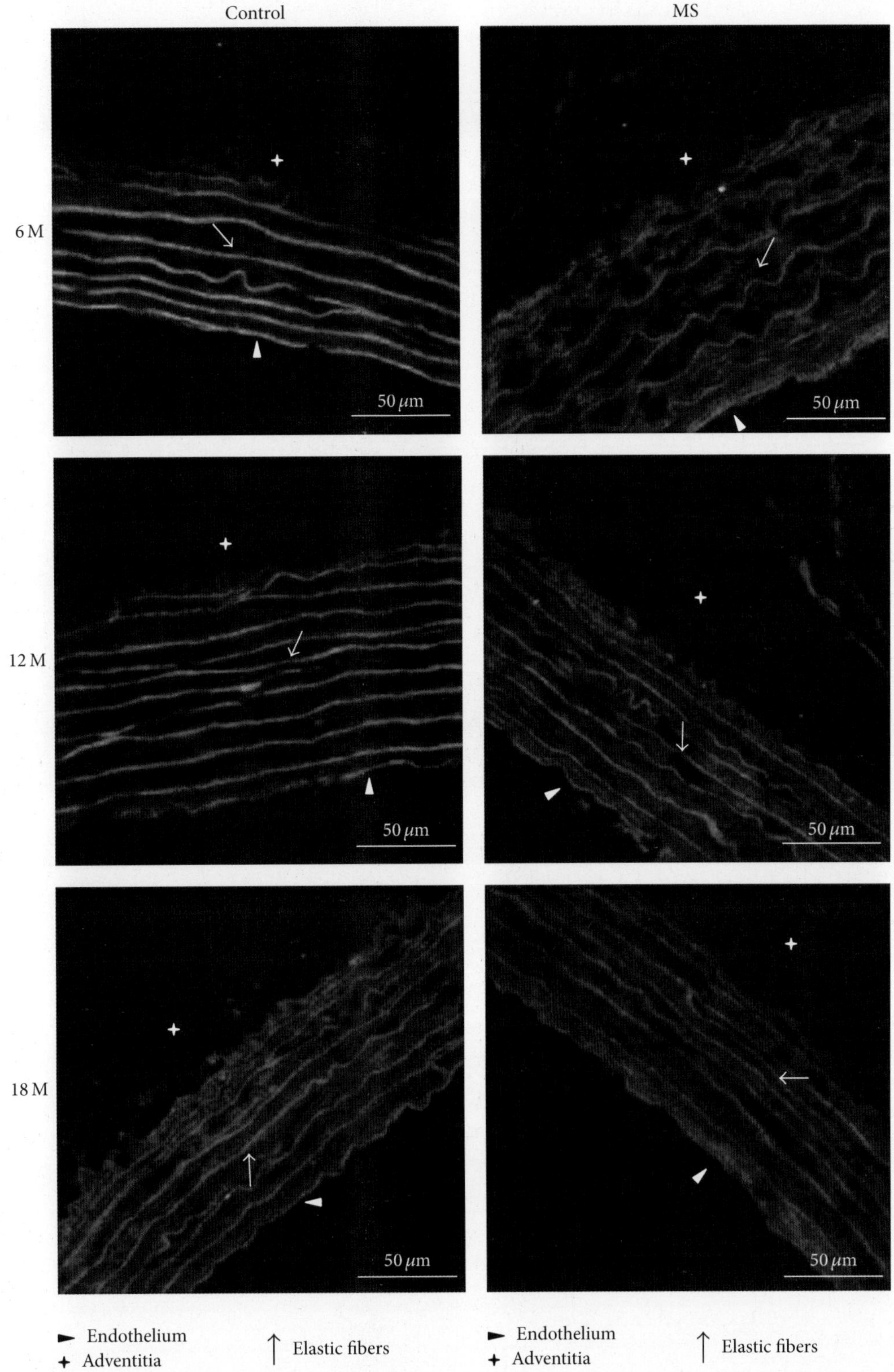

FIGURE 4: Illustrative images (×60) showing receptor AT2 immunofluorescence in aortas of control and MS rats aged 6, 12, and 18 months. Preparations were stained with FITC. Scale bar = 50 μm.

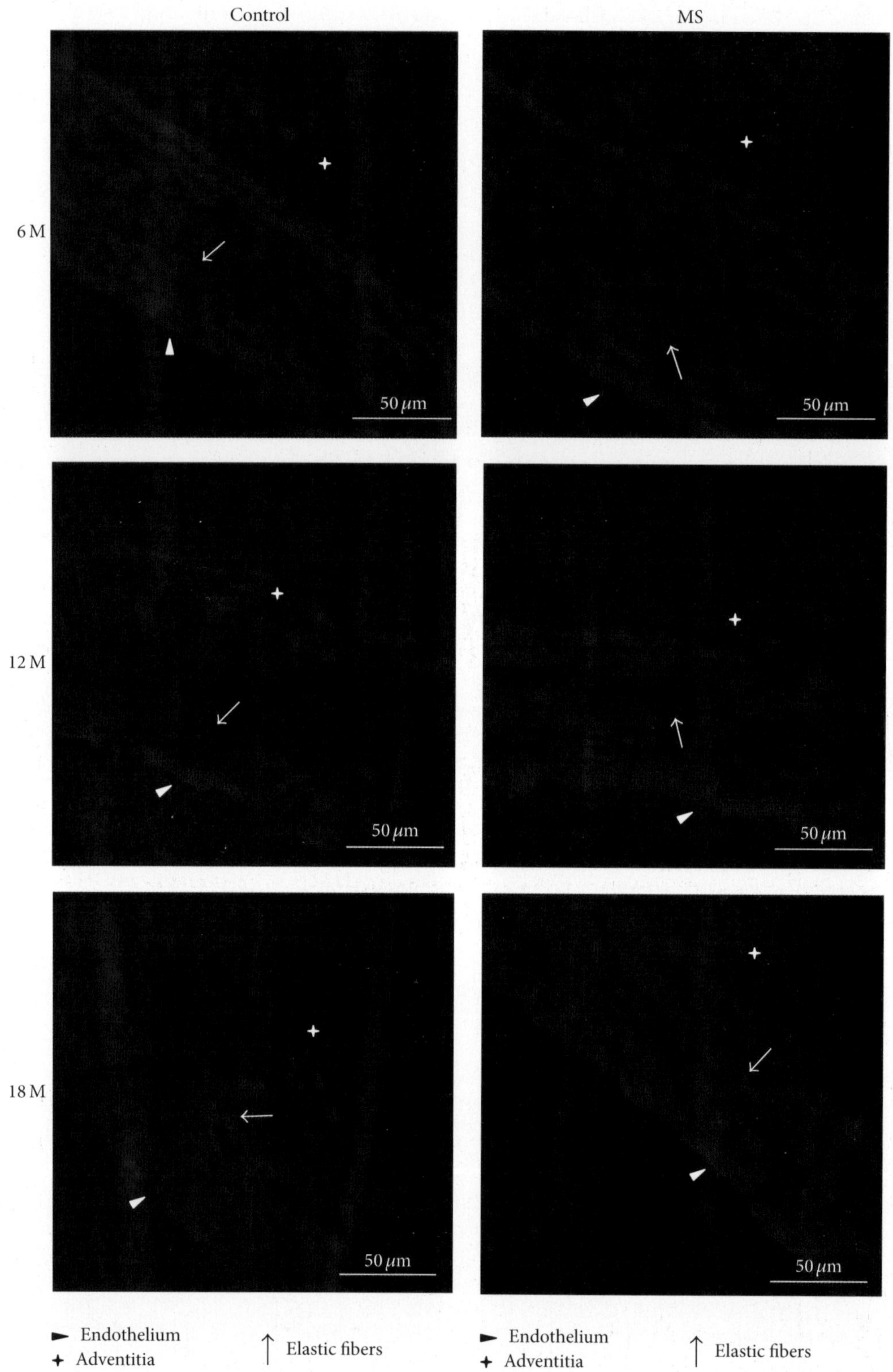

Figure 5: Illustrative images (×60) showing receptor Mas immunofluorescence in aortas of control and MS rats aged 6, 12, and 18 months. Preparations were stained with Tex Red. Scale bar = 50 μm.

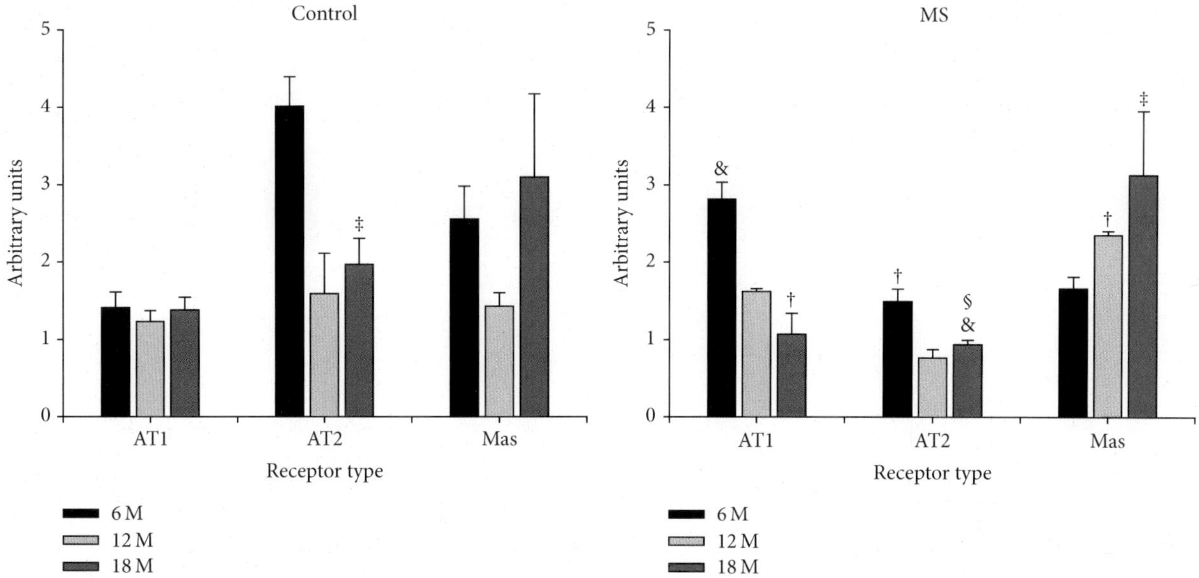

FIGURE 6: Quantitative analysis (receptor type fluorescence versus relative fluorescence) for AT1, AT2, and Mas receptors in aortas of control and MS rats during aging measured from the immunohistochemistry images in Figures 3, 4, and 5. Details of the technique are described in Section 2. Values represent mean ± SEM of six different experiments. $^{\&}P < 0.05$ against C; $^{\dagger}P < 0.01$ against C; $^{\ddagger}P < 0.05$ against other ages; $^{\S}P < 0.05$ against 6 months.

the lowering of blood pressure in the aged MS rats. The Ang 1-7/Mas axis might be an effective therapeutic target, since the surviving rats might have developed compensatory mechanisms similar to those found in healthy obese or MS patients.

Competing Interests

No competing interests exist.

Acknowledgments

The authors would like to thank Bertha Soto, Mario Pérez, Florencio Hernández, Ana B. Martínez, and Benito Chávez for technical assistance.

References

[1] J. R. Ortlepp, J. Breuer, F. Eitner et al., "Inhibition of the renin-angiotensin system ameliorates genetically determined hyperinsulinemia," *European Journal of Pharmacology*, vol. 436, no. 1-2, pp. 145–150, 2002.

[2] R. L. Matz, M. A. de Sotomayor, C. Schott, and R. Andriantsitohaina, "Preservation of vascular contraction during ageing: dual effect on calcium handling and sensitization," *British Journal of Pharmacology*, vol. 138, no. 5, pp. 745–750, 2003.

[3] M. E. Rubio, G. Baños, E. Díaz, and V. Guarner, "Effect of age on insulin-induced endothelin release and vasoreactivity in hypertriglyceridemic and hypertensive rats," *Experimental Gerontology*, vol. 41, no. 3, pp. 282–288, 2006.

[4] M. E. Rubio-Ruíz, L. Del Valle-Mondragón, V. Castrejón-Tellez, E. Carreón-Torres, E. Díaz-Díaz, and V. Guarner-Lans, "Angiotensin II and 1-7 during aging in metabolic syndrome rats. Expression of AT1, AT2 and Mas receptors in abdominal white adipose tissue," *Peptides*, vol. 57, pp. 101–108, 2014.

[5] M. Sysi-Aho, A. Ermolov, P. V. Gopalacharyulu et al., "Metabolic regulation in progression to autoimmune diabetes," *PLoS Computational Biology*, vol. 7, no. 10, article e1002257, 2011.

[6] E. L. Santos, K. de Picoli Souza, E. D. da Silva et al., "Long term treatment with ACE inhibitor enalapril decreases body weight gain and increases life span in rats," *Biochemical Pharmacology*, vol. 78, no. 8, pp. 951–958, 2009.

[7] A. Benigni, D. Corna, C. Zoja et al., "Disruption of the Ang II type 1 receptor promotes longevity in mice," *The Journal of Clinical Investigation*, vol. 119, no. 3, pp. 524–530, 2009.

[8] P. Cassis, S. Conti, G. Remuzzi, and A. Benigni, "Angiotensin receptors as determinants of life span," *Pflugers Archiv European Journal of Physiology*, vol. 459, no. 2, pp. 325–332, 2010.

[9] C. A. Aguilar-Salinas, E. García, L. Robles et al., "High adiponectin concentrations are associated with the metabolically healthy obese phenotype," *Journal of Clinical Endocrinology and Metabolism*, vol. 93, no. 10, pp. 4075–4079, 2008.

[10] S. H. S. Santos, J. F. Braga, E. G. Mario et al., "Improved lipid and glucose metabolism in transgenic rats with increased circulating angiotensin-(1-7)," *Arteriosclerosis, Thrombosis, and Vascular Biology*, vol. 30, no. 5, pp. 953–961, 2010.

[11] S. Engeli, R. Negrel, and A. M. Sharma, "Physiology and pathophysiology of the adipose tissue renin-angiotensin system," *Hypertension*, vol. 35, no. 6, pp. 1270–1277, 2000.

[12] B. Wang, Y.-H. Liao, Z. Zhou et al., "Arterial structural changes in rats immunized by AT1-receptor peptide," *Heart and Vessels*, vol. 20, no. 4, pp. 153–158, 2005.

[13] M. Barton, R. Carmona, H. Morawietz et al., "Obesity is associated with tissue-specific activation of renal angiotensin-converting enzyme in vivo: evidence for a regulatory role of endothelin," *Hypertension*, vol. 35, no. 1, pp. 329–336, 2000.

[14] Q. N. Diep, M. E. Mabrouk, J. S. Cohn et al., "Structure, endothelial function, cell growth, and inflammation in blood vessels

of angiotensin II-infused rats: role of peroxisome proliferator-activated receptor-γ," *Circulation*, vol. 105, no. 19, pp. 2296–2302, 2002.

[15] P. Xu, A. C. Costa-Goncalves, M. Todiras et al., "Endothelial dysfunction and elevated blood pressure in *Mas* gene-deleted mice," *Hypertension*, vol. 51, no. 2, pp. 574–580, 2008.

[16] R. A. S. Santos, A. J. Ferreira, T. Verano-Braga, and M. Bader, "Angiotensin-converting enzyme 2, angiotensin-(1-7) and Mas: new players of the renin-angiotensin system," *Journal of Endocrinology*, vol. 216, no. 2, pp. R1–R17, 2013.

[17] J. E. Jalil, C. Palomera, M. P. Ocaranza et al., "Levels of plasma angiotensin-(1–7) in patients with hypertension who have the angiotensin—I-converting enzyme deletion/deletion genotype," *The American Journal of Cardiology*, vol. 92, no. 6, pp. 749–751, 2003.

[18] J. A. Hernández-Prada, A. J. Ferreira, M. J. Katovich et al., "Structure-based identification of small-molecule angiotensin-converting enzyme 2 activators as novel antihypertensive agents," *Hypertension*, vol. 51, no. 5, pp. 1312–1317, 2008.

[19] M. M. Shafaroudi and C. J. Daly, "Endothelial vasodilator angiotensin receptors are changing in mice with ageing," *Research in Molecular Medicine*, vol. 2, no. 1, pp. 25–33, 2014.

[20] E. J. Henriksen, S. Jacob, T. R. Kinnick, M. K. Teachey, and M. Krekler, "Selective angiotensin II receptor antagonism reduces insulin resistance in obese Zucker rats," *Hypertension*, vol. 38, no. 4, pp. 884–890, 2001.

[21] W. S. Rasband and J. Image, U. S. National Institutes of Health, Bethesda, Md, USA, 2012, http://imagej.nih.gov/ij/.

[22] N. Charkoudian and J. A. Rabbitts, "Sympathetic neural mechanisms in human cardiovascular health and disease," *Mayo Clinic Proceedings*, vol. 84, no. 9, pp. 822–830, 2009.

[23] S. Fukuda, S. Tsuchikura, and H. Iida, "Age-related changes in blood pressure, hematological values, concentrations of serum biochemical constituents and weights of organs in the SHR/Izm, SHRSP/Izm and WKY/Izm," *Experimental Animals*, vol. 53, no. 1, pp. 67–72, 2004.

[24] R. Muzumdar, X. Ma, G. Atzmon, P. Vuguin, X. Yang, and N. Barzilai, "Decrease in glucose-stimulated insulin secretion with aging is independent of insulin action," *Diabetes*, vol. 53, no. 2, pp. 441–446, 2004.

[25] C. F. Küng and T. F. Lüscher, "Different mechanisms of endothelial dysfunction with aging and hypertension in rat aorta," *Hypertension*, vol. 25, no. 2, pp. 194–200, 1995.

[26] M. El Assar, J. Angulo, S. Vallejo, C. Peiró, C. F. Sánchez-Ferrer, and L. Rodríguez-Mañas, "Mechanisms involved in the aging-induced vascular dysfunction," *Frontiers in Physiology*, vol. 3, article 132, 2012.

[27] V. Kotsis, S. Stabouli, I. Karafillis, and P. Nilsson, "Early vascular aging and the role of central blood pressure," *Journal of Hypertension*, vol. 29, no. 10, pp. 1847–1853, 2011.

[28] R. P. Brandes, I. Fleming, and R. Busse, "Endothelial aging," *Cardiovascular Research*, vol. 66, no. 2, pp. 286–294, 2005.

[29] M. M. Bachschmid, S. Schildknecht, R. Matsui et al., "Vascular aging: chronic oxidative stress and impairment of redox signaling—consequences for vascular homeostasis and disease," *Annals of Medicine*, vol. 45, no. 1, pp. 17–36, 2013.

[30] D. A. Long, M. A. Newaz, S. S. Prabhakar et al., "Loss of nitric oxide and endothelial-derived hyperpolarizing factor-mediated responses in aging," *Kidney International*, vol. 68, no. 5, pp. 2154–2163, 2005.

[31] A. Csiszar, N. Labinskyy, K. Smith, A. Rivera, Z. Orosz, and Z. Ungvari, "Vasculoprotective effects of anti-tumor necrosis factor-α treatment in aging," *American Journal of Pathology*, vol. 170, no. 1, pp. 388–398, 2007.

[32] J. Lähteenvuo and A. Rosenzweig, "Effects of aging on angiogenesis," *Circulation Research*, vol. 110, no. 9, pp. 1252–1263, 2012.

[33] H. Matsushita, E. Chang, A. J. Glassford, J. P. Cooke, C.-P. Chiu, and P. S. Tsao, "Activity is reduced in senescent human endothelial cells: preservation by hTERT Immortalization," *Circulation Research*, vol. 89, no. 9, pp. 793–798, 2001.

[34] A. Ruiz-Torres, A. Gimeno, J. Melón, L. Mendez, F. J. Muñoz, and M. Macía, "Age-related loss of proliferative activity of human vascular smooth muscle cells in culture," *Mechanisms of Ageing and Development*, vol. 110, no. 1-2, pp. 49–55, 1999.

[35] M. S. Lundberg and M. T. Crow, "Age-related changes in the signaling and function of vascular smooth muscle cells," *Experimental Gerontology*, vol. 34, no. 4, pp. 549–557, 1999.

[36] A. Carvajal, A. Velasco, L. H. Martin Arias, and M. Maroto, "Age-related changes in contractile responses to noradrenaline in isolated blood vessels from rat and rabbit," *Journal of Autonomic Pharmacology*, vol. 15, no. 5, pp. 321–326, 1995.

[37] M. Wang, J. Zhang, L.-Q. Jiang et al., "Proinflammatory profile within the grossly normal aged human aortic wall," *Hypertension*, vol. 50, no. 1, pp. 219–227, 2007.

[38] K. Shinozaki, K. Ayajiki, Y. Nishio, T. Sugaya, A. Kashiwagi, and T. Okamura, "Evidence for a causal role of the Renin-Angiotensin System in vascular dysfunction associated with insulin resistance," *Hypertension*, vol. 43, no. 2 I, pp. 255–262, 2004.

[39] S. P. Bagby, L. S. LeBard, Z. Luo, R. C. Speth, B. E. Ogden, and C. L. Corless, "Angiotensin II type 1 and 2 receptors in conduit arteries of normal developing microswine," *Arteriosclerosis, Thrombosis, and Vascular Biology*, vol. 22, no. 7, pp. 1113–1121, 2002.

[40] M. Akishita, M. Horiuchi, H. Yamada et al., "Inflammation influences vascular remodeling through AT2 receptor expression and signaling," *Physiological Genomics*, vol. 2, no. 1, pp. 13–20, 2000.

[41] A. Csiszar, M. Wang, E. G. Lakatta, and Z. Ungvari, "Inflammation and endothelial dysfunction during aging: role of NF-κB," *Journal of Applied Physiology*, vol. 105, no. 4, pp. 1333–1341, 2008.

[42] L. Hunyady and K. J. Catt, "Pleiotropic AT1 receptor signaling pathways mediating physiological and pathogenic actions of angiotensin II," *Molecular Endocrinology*, vol. 20, no. 5, pp. 953–970, 2006.

[43] M. Paul, A. P. Mehr, and R. Kreutz, "Physiology of local renin-angiotensin systems," *Physiological Reviews*, vol. 86, no. 3, pp. 747–803, 2006.

[44] R. M. Touyz and E. L. Schiffrin, "Signal transduction mechanisms mediating the physiological and pathophysiological actions of angiotensin II in vascular smooth muscle cells," *Pharmacological Reviews*, vol. 52, no. 4, pp. 639–672, 2000.

[45] G. Gorelik, L. A. Carbini, and A. G. Scicli, "Angiotensin 1–7 induces bradykinin-mediated relaxation in porcine coronary artery," *Journal of Pharmacology and Experimental Therapeutics*, vol. 286, no. 1, pp. 403–410, 1998.

[46] R. Soares de Moura, A. C. Resende, A. F. Emiliano et al., "The role of bradykinin, AT2 and angiotensin 1-7 receptors in the EDRF-dependent vasodilator effect of angiotensin II on the isolated mesenteric vascular bed of the rat," *British Journal of Pharmacology*, vol. 141, no. 5, pp. 860–866, 2004.

27

Impaired Glucose Metabolism Is Associated with Visit-to-Visit Blood Pressure Variability in Participants without Cardiovascular Disease

Nobuo Sasaki,[1] **Ryoji Ozono**,[2] **Saeko Fujiwara**,[1] **Ryo Maeda**,[1] **and Yasuki Kihara**[3]

[1]*Health Management and Promotion Center, Hiroshima Atomic Bomb Casualty Council, Hiroshima, Japan*
[2]*Department of General Medicine, Hiroshima University Graduate School of Biomedical and Health Sciences, Hiroshima, Japan*
[3]*Department of Cardiovascular Medicine, Hiroshima University Graduate School of Biomedical and Health Sciences, Hiroshima, Japan*

Correspondence should be addressed to Nobuo Sasaki; nb7ssk7@sd6.so-net.ne.jp

Academic Editor: Christophe Tzourio

We evaluated data from 10,088 participants without cardiovascular disease (CVD) who underwent 75 g oral glucose tolerance tests and had more than four visits during the first 5 years following the test to investigate the association between impaired glucose metabolism and visit-to-visit blood pressure (BP) variability. Participants were classified into groups of normal glucose tolerance (NGT), impaired fasting glucose (IFG), impaired glucose tolerance (IGT), and diabetes. Visit-to-visit BP variability was estimated for each individual using standard deviation (SD) and coefficients of variation (CV, defined as SD/mean). SDs and CVs of systolic BP (SBP) values were divided into quartiles. The samples falling in the highest quartile were considered as having high SD/CV. The adjusted odds ratio (OR) for high SD of SBP in the IFG (OR, 1.39; $P < 0.003$), IGT (OR, 1.26; $P < 0.001$), and diabetes (OR, 1.54; $P < 0.001$) groups was significantly higher than that for high SD of SBP in the NGT group. Similarly, the OR for high CV of SBP in the IGT and diabetes groups was significantly higher than that for high CV of SBP in the NGT group. In participants without CVD, impaired glucose metabolism may modulate visit-to-visit BP variability.

1. Introduction

Visit-to-visit blood pressure (BP) variability reflects arterial stiffness and may be predictive of cardiovascular morbidity and mortality [1, 2]. Several studies in patients with diabetes have demonstrated a significant association between visit-to-visit BP variability and incident cardiovascular disease (CVD) [3–5]. Glucose fluctuation could contribute to oxidative stress, renin–angiotensin system activation, inflammation initiation, and endothelial dysfunction [6, 7], resulting in the development of atherosclerosis and increased arterial stiffness. In addition, neuropathy in diabetes could contribute to baroreflex sensitivity [8], which may modulate visit-to-visit BP variability [9]. These data suggest that visit-to-visit BP variability is a predictor of cardiovascular outcomes and may also be associated with the pathophysiology of diabetes. However, whether glucose metabolism modulates visit-to-visit BP variability remains unclear. Little is known about this BP variability particularly in participants with intermediate hyperglycemia (i.e., those with impaired fasting glucose [IFG] or impaired glucose tolerance [IGT]) [10, 11].

In the present study, we investigated the association between visit-to-visit BP variability and the status of glucose metabolism, alternating from normal glucose tolerance (NGT) to intermediate hyperglycemia including IFG, IGT, and diabetes in a large-scale population without CVD.

2. Methods

2.1. Study Participants. The present study used data collected from the Hiroshima Aging, Blood pressure, and Diabetes study (Hiroshima ABD study), a cross-sectional and longitudinal study that examined the interrelationship among aging, blood pressure, glucose metabolism, and cardiovascular outcomes. Potential participants were recruited between April

1988 and March 2012, after undergoing annual health examinations at the Health Management and Promotion Center of Hiroshima Atomic Bomb Casualty Council. Potential participants were considered eligible if they (1) were aged ≥18 years, (2) had no symptomatic heart failure, (3) had no history of treatment for diabetes, and (4) agreed to undergo the 75 g oral glucose tolerance test (OGTT). We asked all participants about their regular medications and medical histories, including treatment for hypertension, diabetes, dyslipidemia, and CVD, and information about their drinking and smoking habits. The present study reports on 10,088 participants (4,938 men and 5,150 women with mean age ± standard deviation [SD] of 65.7 ± 7.3 years and mean body mass index [BMI] ± SD of 23.2 ± 3.1 kg/m2) enrolled between April 1988 and March 2007. Included participants had no current or a prior history of CVD and had more than four visits during the first 5 years for health examinations. Among the 10,088 participants, 4,759 (47%) had hypertension (defined as taking antihypertensive medications [$n = 2{,}103$] and/or having systolic BP [SBP] ≥ 140 mmHg and/or diastolic BP [DBP] ≥ 90 mmHg); 1,072 (11%) had dyslipidemia (defined as taking antihyperlipidemic medications); 1,731 (17%) were current smokers (defined as having a current smoking habit regardless of the number of cigarettes smoked per day); and 4,388 (43%) were habitual drinkers (defined as drinking alcohol for ≥5 days per week, regardless of the amount consumed) [12]. Informed consent was obtained from all participants during their health examinations. Ethical approval for this study was obtained from the Hiroshima Atomic Bomb Casualty Council committee on the ethics of human research.

2.2. Measurements. The 75 g OGTT was conducted in the morning after an overnight fast. Blood samples were drawn just before and 30, 60, and 120 min after loading of glucose. Plasma glucose was measured using the enzymatic method. BP was measured using a standard sphygmomanometer in a seated position on a chair with back support and arm support at heart level after resting for >5 min prior to undergoing OGTT. Follow-up BP was measured under the same conditions during the annual health examinations. Mean BP was defined as the average of BP values measured on the baseline and follow-up visits. Visit-to-visit BP variability for each individual was defined by between-visit SD and coefficient of variation (CV). CV was defined as SD/mean. SDs and CVs of SBP and DBP values were divided into quartiles. The samples falling in the highest quartile were considered as having high SD/CVs and those in the remaining three quartiles as having low SD/CVs.

2.3. Participant Classification. We divided the participants into four groups according to their glycemic status as defined by the 2006 World Health Organization criteria [10] and the Japan Diabetes Society criteria [11]: (1) NGT, defined as fasting plasma glucose (FPG) < 6.1 mmol/l (110 mg/dl) and 2 h postload glucose < 7.8 mmol/l (140 mg/dl); (2) IFG, defined as FPG ≥ 6.1 and < 7.0 mmol/l (126 mg/dl) and 2 h postload glucose < 7.8 mmol/l; (3) IGT, defined as FPG < 7.0 mmol/l and 2 h postload glucose ≥ 7.8 and < 11.1 mmol/l; and (4) diabetes, defined as FPG ≥ 7.0 and/or 2 h postload glucose ≥ 11.1 mmol/l.

2.4. Statistical Analysis. Continuous variables were expressed as mean ± SD. Differences among the four groups (i.e., NGT, IFG, IGT, and diabetes) were evaluated using analysis of variance. Fisher's least-significant-difference method was used for multiple comparisons. Categorical variables were summarized as percentages and were analyzed using the chi-square test. The odds ratios (ORs) of high SD/CV of SBP and DBP were calculated using univariate and multivariate logistic regression analysis, adjusting for age, gender, BMI, habitual drinker (yes or no), current smoker (yes or no), taking antihypertensive medication (yes or no), dyslipidemia (yes or no), and number of visits. A P value < 0.05 was considered statistically significant. All statistical analyses were performed using the JMP 10 statistical software (SAS Institute, Inc., Cary, NC, USA).

3. Results

Clinical characteristics of the study population are presented in Table 1. The mean age was slightly lower in the IFG and diabetes groups and higher in the IGT group than in the NGT group. BMI was highest in the diabetes group, followed in descending order by IGT, IFG, and NGT groups. Table 1 shows the study population characteristics when participants are divided into the high and low SBP SD groups.

Table 2 shows group differences in BP measurements and BP variability. We found that SD of both SBP and DBP was significantly higher in the IFG, IGT, and diabetes groups than in the NGT group. Similarly, CV of SBP was significantly higher in both IGT and diabetes groups than in the NGT group. There was no significant difference in CV of DBP among the four groups.

Table 3 shows the results from univariate and multivariate logistic regression analyses. After adjusting for age, sex, BMI, smoking, drinking, taking antihypertensive medication, dyslipidemia, and number of visits, the OR for high SD of SBP in the IFG (OR, 1.39; 95% confidence interval [CI], 1.12–1.73; $P < 0.005$), IGT (OR, 1.26; 95% CI, 1.13–1.41; $P < 0.001$), and diabetes (OR, 1.54; 95% CI, 1.35–1.76; $P < 0.001$) groups was significantly higher than that for high SD of SBP in the NGT group. The OR for high CV of SBP in the IGT (OR, 1.15; 95% CI, 1.03–1.28; $P < 0.05$) and diabetes (OR, 1.35; 95% CI, 1.19–1.54; $P < 0.001$) groups (but not the IFG group) was significantly higher than that for high CV of SBP in the NGT group.

4. Discussion

In this study, we demonstrated higher visit-to-visit SBP variability in participants with intermediate hyperglycemia (including IFG and IGT) compared with those with NGT. The rate of high visit-to-visit SBP variability during the first 5 years gradually increased, starting with low increases in NGT cases, moderate increases in intermediate hyperglycemia cases, and highest increases in diabetes cases after the baseline

TABLE 1: Characteristics of participants with normal glucose tolerance, impaired glucose metabolism, and diabetes.

		NGT	IFG	IGT	DM	*P*
N		5235	472	2795	1586	
Mean age	(years)	65.7 ± 7.4	64.8 ±7.6[c]	66.3 ±7.2[a]	65.1 ±7.5[b]	<0.001
Female	[*n* (%)]	2887 (55)	197 (42)	1340 (48)	726 (46)	<0.001
BMI	(kg/m2)	22.6 ± 2.9	23.4 ±3.1[a]	23.7 ±3.2[a]	24.2 ±3.3[a]	<0.001
Current smoker	[*n* (%)]	838 (16)	80 (17)	486 (17)	327 (21)	<0.001
Habitual drinker	[*n* (%)]	2174 (42)	250 (53)	1263 (45)	701 (44)	<0.001
Hypertension	[*n* (%)]	2046 (39)	261 (55)	1497 (54)	955 (60)	<0.001
Antihypertensive medication	[*n* (%)]	891 (17)	110 (23)	709 (25)	393 (25)	<0.001
Dyslipidemia	[*n* (%)]	539 (10)	41 (9)	343 (12)	149 (9)	0.005
Classified by SBP SD						
High SD						
N		1150	133	754	485	
Mean age	(years)	66.7 ± 7.5	66.5 ± 7.5	67.1 ± 7.2	65.6 ±7.1[c]	0.005
Female	[*n* (%)]	624 (54)	59 (44)	396 (53)	213 (44)	<0.001
BMI	(kg/m2)	22.5 ± 2.9	23.6 ±3.4[a]	23.7 ±3.3[a]	24.0 ±3.3[a]	<0.001
Current smoker	[*n* (%)]	212 (18)	22 (17)	134 (18)	118 (24)	0.020
Habitual drinker	[*n* (%)]	490 (43)	76 (57)	314 (42)	208 (43)	0.010
Hypertension	[*n* (%)]	645 (56)	97 (73)	515 (68)	351 (72)	<0.001
Antihypertensive medication	[*n* (%)]	295 (26)	42 (32)	279 (37)	163 (34)	<0.001
Dyslipidemia	[*n* (%)]	104 (9)	11 (8)	90 (12)	37 (8)	0.059
Low SD						
N		4085	339	2041	1101	
Mean age	(years)	65.4 ± 7.3	64.1 ±7.5[b]	66.0 ±7.1[b]	64.9 ±7.7[d]	<0.001
Female	[*n* (%)]	2263 (55)	138 (41)	944 (46)	513 (47)	<0.001
BMI	(kg/m2)	22.6 ± 2.9	23.3 ±3.0[a]	23.7 ±3.1[a]	24.3 ±3.3[a]	<0.001
Current smoker	[*n* (%)]	626 (15)	58 (17)	352 (17)	209 (19)	0.020
Habitual drinker	[*n* (%)]	1684 (41)	174 (51)	949 (47)	493 (45)	<0.001
Hypertension	[*n* (%)]	1401 (34)	164 (48)	982 (48)	604 (55)	<0.001
Antihypertensive medication	[*n* (%)]	596 (15)	58 (20)	430 (21)	230 (21)	<0.001
Dyslipidemia	[*n* (%)]	435 (11)	30 (9)	253 (12)	112 (10)	0.074

Samples in the highest quartile were considered as having high SBP SDs and those in the remaining three quartiles as having low SBP SDs; BMI, body mass index; DM, diabetes; NGT, normal glucose tolerance; IFG, impaired fasting glucose; IGT, impaired glucose tolerance; SD, standard deviation; $^{a}P < 0.001$ versus NGT; $^{b}P < 0.005$ versus NGT; $^{c}P < 0.01$ versus NGT; $^{d}P < 0.05$ versus NGT.

75 g OGTT. These results suggest that, in participants without CVD, impaired glucose metabolism may modulate visit-to-visit BP variability. In particular, we found that IGT, as well as diabetes, was significantly associated with high SD and CV of SBP. Although IGT has been reported to be a significant risk factor for CVD [13], the underlying mechanisms are not fully understood. Our results indicate that visit-to-visit BP variability may be involved in adverse consequences of IGT.

Although the determinants of visit-to-visit BP variability are not completely understood, arterial stiffness is thought to be one of the key factors [14]. It is well known that arterial stiffness is prevalent in patients with diabetes [15]. Furthermore, several studies have reported that intermediate hyperglycemia, including IFG and IGT, is associated with arterial stiffness [16, 17]. Pietri et al. reported that pulse wave velocity, a marker of arterial stiffness, gradually increased with increasing degree of abnormal glucose metabolism ranging from normal to intermediate hyperglycemia and diabetes [18]. Therefore, our results may be partly explained by increased arterial stiffness that is common in patients with intermediate hyperglycemia and diabetes. Disturbances of baroreflex function also exaggerate visit-to-visit BP variability [9]. Ruiz et al. reported lower baroreflex sensitivity in patients with diabetes compared with nondiabetic participants, and the disturbance in baroreflex sensitivity does not appear to depend on carotid artery atherosclerosis [8]. In another study, Wu et al. reported that participants with IGT had impaired baroreflex sensitivity compared to NGT [19]. Thus, the disturbances in baroreflex function may partly explain the observed higher visit-to-visit BP variability in participants with IGT in this study.

In patients with diabetes, most studies reported visit-to-visit BP variability as an independent risk factor for macro- and microvascular complications [3, 5, 20, 21]. In contrast, a recent large-scale observational study revealed that higher visit-to-visit BP variability was associated with

Table 2: Blood pressure measurements of participants with normal glucose tolerance, impaired glucose metabolism, and diabetes.

		NGT	IFG	IGT	DM	P
N		5235	472	2795	1586	
Number of visits		5.5 ± 0.7	5.5 ± 0.8	5.5 ± 0.7	5.4 ± 0.8[a]	<0.001
Mean SBP	(mmHg)	129.7 ± 12.9	134.4 ± 13.0[a]	134.3 ± 12.8[a]	136.1 ± 13.3[a]	<0.001
Mean DBP	(mmHg)	75.5 ± 7.3	77.7 ± 7.2[a]	77.5 ± 7.2[a]	78.1 ± 7.4[a]	<0.001
SD SBP	(mmHg)	9.5 ± 3.8	10.1 ± 3.9[b]	10.1 ± 4.1[a]	10.3 ± 4.2[a]	<0.001
SD DBP	(mmHg)	6.3 ± 2.4	6.6 ± 2.5[b]	6.5 ± 2.5[a]	6.6 ± 2.6[a]	<0.001
CV SBP	(%)	7.4 ± 2.8	7.5 ± 2.8	7.5 ± 2.9[c]	7.6 ± 3.0[c]	0.032
CV DBP	(%)	8.4 ± 3.1	8.6 ± 3.0	8.4 ± 3.1	8.5 ± 3.3	0.565
Classified by SBP SD						
High SD						
N		1150	133	754	485	
Number of visits		5.5 ± 0.7	5.4 ± 0.8	5.5 ± 0.7	5.5 ± 0.7	0.105
Mean SBP	(mmHg)	134.6 ± 13.3	140.0 ± 12.8[a]	138.3 ± 12.6[a]	139.8 ± 13.3[a]	<0.001
SD SBP	(mmHg)	15.0 ± 2.7	14.8 ± 2.4	15.3 ± 3.0	15.3 ± 2.7	0.058
Low SD						
N		4085	339	2041	1101	
Number of visits		5.5 ± 0.7	5.5 ± 0.8	5.5 ± 0.7	5.4 ± 0.8[a]	<0.001
Mean SBP	(mmHg)	128.3 ± 12.5	132.2 ± 12.5[a]	132.8 ± 12.6[a]	134.5 ± 13.0[a]	<0.001
SD SBP	(mmHg)	8.0 ± 2.4	8.2 ± 2.5	8.2 ± 2.4[b]	8.1 ± 2.4	0.047

Samples in the highest quartile were considered as having high SBP SDs and those in the remaining three quartiles as having low SBP SDs. CV, coefficients of variation; DM, diabetes; DBP, diastolic blood pressure; NGT, normal glucose tolerance; IFG, impaired fasting glucose; IGT, impaired glucose tolerance; SBP, systolic blood pressure; SD, standard deviation; [a]$P < 0.001$ versus NGT; [b]$P < 0.01$ versus NGT; [c]$P < 0.05$ versus NGT.

Table 3: Univariate and multivariate OR for high BP variability.

	Univariate			Multivariate		
High SD of SBP	OR	95% CI	P	OR	95% CI	P
NGT	1			1		
IFG	1.39	(1.13–1.72)	0.003	1.39	(1.12–1.73)	0.003
IGT	1.31	(1.18–1.46)	<0.001	1.26	(1.13–1.41)	<0.001
DM	1.56	(1.38–1.77)	<0.001	1.54	(1.35–1.76)	<0.001
High SD of DBP	OR	95% CI	P	OR	95% CI	P
NGT	1			1		
IFG	1.13	(0.91–1.40)	0.275	1.05	(0.84–1.30)	0.655
IGT	1.12	(1.00–1.24)	0.045	1.04	(0.93–1.16)	0.477
DM	1.20	(1.05–1.36)	0.006	1.11	(0.97–1.26)	0.132
High CV of SBP	OR	95% CI	P	OR	95% CI	P
NGT	1			1		
IFG	1.09	(0.87–1.35)	0.436	1.14	(0.92–1.42)	0.226
IGT	1.12	(1.01–1.24)	0.043	1.15	(1.03–1.28)	0.015
DM	1.28	(1.13–1.45)	<0.001	1.35	(1.19–1.54)	<0.001
High CV of DBP	OR	95% CI	P	OR	95% CI	P
NGT	1			1		
IFG	1.06	(0.85–1.31)	0.588	1.07	(0.86–1.33)	0.516
IGT	1.02	(0.92–1.14)	0.694	1.02	(0.91–1.13)	0.762
DM	1.04	(0.91–1.18)	0.543	1.05	(0.92–1.20)	0.431

Multivariate model included age, gender, body mass index, smoking, drinking, taking antihypertensive medications, dyslipidemia, and number of visits; High SDs of SBP and DBP and high CVs of SBP and DBP were defined as the highest quartile; CV, coefficients of variation; DM, diabetes; DBP, diastolic blood pressure; NGT, normal glucose tolerance; IFG, impaired fasting glucose; IGT, impaired glucose tolerance; OR, odds ratio; SBP, systolic blood pressure; SD, standard deviation.

incident diabetes [22]. Although the underlying mechanisms remain unclear, these data have led to the hypothesis that visit-to-visit BP variability has an adverse effect on glucose metabolism and is associated with contributing factors for the onset of diabetes. Conversely, our study provides evidence suggesting that impaired glucose metabolism may modulate visit-to-visit BP variability. Further studies are needed to clarify the interaction between visit-to-visit BP variability and impaired glucose metabolism.

This study has some limitations. First, the types of antihypertensive agents used were not recorded for participants currently under treatment for hypertension and the effects on visit-to-visit BP variability may differ based on the use of different antihypertensive agents. Second, participants with CVD were excluded based on careful interview inquiring about regular medications, medical history, and a physical examination. Nonetheless, we cannot rule out the possibility that the present study population included participants with subclinical CVD, given that we did not assess cardiac function using more objective methods.

In conclusion, our results suggested that impaired glucose metabolism may modulate visit-to-visit BP variability. Intermediate hyperglycemia, especially IGT, was associated with visit-to-visit BP variability. This may explain the adverse cardiovascular consequences observed in patients with IGT.

Acknowledgments

The authors thank Yukari Motoyama and Naomi Yuzono for technical and secretarial assistance.

References

[1] P. M. Rothwell, S. C. Howard, E. Dolan et al., "Prognostic significance of visit-to-visit variability, maximum systolic blood pressure, and episodic hypertension," *The Lancet*, vol. 375, no. 9718, pp. 895–905, 2010.

[2] M. Nagai and K. Kario, "Visit-to-visit blood pressure variability, silent cerebral injury, and risk of stroke," *American Journal of Hypertension*, vol. 26, no. 12, pp. 1369–1376, 2013.

[3] J. Hata, H. Arima, P. M. Rothwell et al., "Effects of visit-to-visit variability in systolic blood pressure on macrovascular and microvascular complications in patients with type 2 diabetes mellitus: the advance trial," *Circulation*, vol. 128, no. 12, pp. 1325–1334, 2013.

[4] Y.-T. Hsieh, S.-T. Tu, T.-J. Cho, S.-J. Chang, J.-F. Chen, and M.-C. Hsieh, "Visit-to-visit variability in blood pressure strongly predicts all-cause mortality in patients with type 2 diabetes: A 5·5-year prospective analysis," *European Journal of Clinical Investigation*, vol. 42, no. 3, pp. 245–253, 2012.

[5] T. Takao, Y. Matsuyama, M. Suka, H. Yanagisawa, and Y. Iwamoto, "The combined effect of visit-to-visit variability in HbA1c and systolic blood pressure on the incidence of cardiovascular events in patients with type 2 diabetes," *BMJ Open Diabetes Research & Care*, vol. 3, no. 1, p. e000129, 2015.

[6] L. Monnier, E. Mas, C. Ginet et al., "Activation of oxidative stress by acute glucose fluctuations compared with sustained chronic hyperglycemia in patients with type 2 diabetes," *The Journal of the American Medical Association*, vol. 295, no. 14, pp. 1681–1687, 2006.

[7] D.-F. Su, "Treatment of hypertension based on measurement of blood pressure variability: Lessons from animal studies," *Current Opinion in Cardiology*, vol. 21, no. 5, pp. 486–491, 2006.

[8] J. Ruiz, D. Monbaron, G. Parati et al., "Diabetic neuropathy is a more important determinant of baroreflex sensitivity than carotid elasticity in type 2 diabetes," *Hypertension*, vol. 46, no. 1, pp. 162–167, 2005.

[9] J. S. Floras, M. O. Hassan, J. V. Jones, B. A. Osikowska, P. S. Sever, and P. Sleight, "Consequences of impaired arterial baroreflexes in essential hypertension: Effects on pressor responses, plasma noradrenaline and blood pressure variability," *Journal of Hypertension*, vol. 6, no. 7, pp. 525–535, 1988.

[10] World Health Organization. Definition and Diagnosis of Diabetes Mellitus and Intermediate Hyperglycemia: Report of a WHO/IDF Conclusion, World Health Org, 2006.

[11] Y. Seino, K. Nanjo, N. Tajima et al., "Report of the Committee on the classification and diagnostic criteria of diabetes mellitus: The Committee of the Japan Diabetes Society on the diagnostic criteria of diabetes mellitus," *Diabetology International*, vol. 1, no. 1, pp. 2–20, 2010.

[12] N. Sasaki, S. Fujiwara, H. Yamashita, R. Ozono, K. Teramen, and Y. Kihara, "Impact of sleep on osteoporosis: sleep quality is associated with bone stiffness index," *Sleep Medicine*, vol. 25, pp. 73–77, 2016.

[13] M. Tominaga, H. Eguchi, H. Manaka, K. Igarashi, T. Kato, and A. Sekikawa, "Impaired glucose tolerance is a risk factor for cardiovascular disease, but not impaired fasting glucose. The Funagata Diabetes Study," *Diabetes Care*, vol. 22, no. 6, pp. 920–924, 1999.

[14] Y. Imai, A. Aihara, T. Ohkubo et al., "Factors that affect blood pressure variability: A community-based study in Ohasama, Japan," *American Journal of Hypertension*, vol. 10, no. 11, pp. 1281–1289, 1997.

[15] S. B. Prenner and J. A. Chirinos, "Arterial stiffness in diabetes mellitus," *Atherosclerosis*, vol. 238, no. 2, pp. 370–379, 2015.

[16] H. Ohnishi, S. Saitoh, S. Takagi et al., "Pulse wave velocity as an indicator of atherosclerosis in impaired fasting glucose: the tanno and sobetsu study," *Diabetes Care*, vol. 26, no. 2, pp. 437–440, 2003.

[17] C.-H. Li, J.-S. Wu, Y.-C. Yang, C.-C. Shih, F.-H. Lu, and C.-J. Chang, "Increased arterial stiffness in subjects with impaired glucose tolerance and newly diagnosed diabetes but not isolated impaired fasting glucose," *The Journal of Clinical Endocrinology & Metabolism*, vol. 97, no. 4, pp. E658–E662, 2012.

[18] P. Pietri, C. Vlachopoulos, G. Vyssoulis, N. Ioakeimidis, and C. Stefanadis, "Macro- and microvascular alterations in patients with metabolic syndrome: Sugar makes the difference," *Hypertension Research*, vol. 37, no. 5, pp. 452–456, 2014.

[19] J.-S. Wu, F.-H. Lu, Y.-C. Yang et al., "Impaired baroreflex sensitivity in subjects with impaired glucose tolerance, but not isolated impaired fasting glucose," *Acta Diabetologica*, vol. 51, no. 4, pp. 535–541, 2014.

[20] E. S. Kilpatrick, A. S. Rigby, and S. L. Atkin, "The role of blood pressure variability in the development of nephropathy in type 1 diabetes," *Diabetes Care*, vol. 33, no. 11, pp. 2442–2447, 2010.

Factors Predicting Self-Care Behaviors among Low Health Literacy Hypertensive Patients Based on Health Belief Model in Bushehr District, South of Iran

Azam Larki,[1] Rahim Tahmasebi,[2] and Mahnoush Reisi[1]

[1]*Department of Health Education and Health Promotion, Bushehr University of Medical Sciences, Bushehr, Iran*
[2]*Department of Biostatistics, Bushehr University of Medical Sciences, Bushehr, Iran*

Correspondence should be addressed to Mahnoush Reisi; reisi_mr@yahoo.com

Academic Editor: Andrea M. P. Romani

The aim of this study was to determine the factors influencing adherence to self-care behaviors among low health literacy hypertensive patients based on health belief model. A cross-sectional study was conducted among 152 hypertensive patients with low health literacy. Patients with limited health literacy were identified by S-TOFHLA. The data were collected using H-scale for assessing self-care behaviors and, HK-LS for assessing knowledge of hypertension. A researcher-made questionnaire was applied for collecting data of health belief model constructs. Data were analyzed by SPSS version 22 with using multiple logistic regression analyses. Perceived self-efficacy was associated with all self-care behaviors except medication regimens. There was a significant association between perceived susceptibility and adherence to both low-salt diet (OR = 3.47) and nonsmoking behavior (OR = 1.10). Individuals who had more perceived severity (OR = 1.82) had significantly greater adherence to their medication regimens. Perceived benefits and barriers were not significantly associated with either type of hypertension self-care behaviors. It seems that designing and implementation of educational programs to increase self-efficacy of patients and promote their beliefs about perceived susceptibility and severity of complications may improve self-care behaviors among low health literacy hypertensive patients.

1. Introduction

Hypertension is an important worldwide public-health challenge, which can lead to very serious consequences such as cardiovascular and kidney disease [1]. According to reports, more than one in three adults worldwide suffer from high blood pressure, and this proportion increases with age [2]. Due to the high prevalence of hypertension and its serious complications, the World Health Organization (WHO) assigned the theme of World Health Day 2013 to hypertension as a "silent killer, global public-health crisis" [3]. Statistics showed an increase in the prevalence of hypertension. The number of patients with hypertension has increased from 600 million cases in 1980 to 1 billion in 2008; over 40 percent of adults were known to have hypertension [4]. Also, it was predicted that, by 2025, 1.56 billion adults will suffer from hypertension [5]. In this regard, it was reported to be 14 to 34 percent hypertensive patients in Iran [6].

Although this disease can lead to acute and debilitating complications and imposes many costs on the individual and the healthcare system, studies show that blood pressure control in hypertensive patients is not desirable, as the results of various studies all over the world suggest a high prevalence of uncontrolled blood pressure among people with hypertension [7, 8].

The most important strategy for controlling blood pressure and maintaining it in the optimal range is patient compliance with self-care behaviors [9]. The findings of a meta-analysis that examined the results of 87 studies indicated that optimal self-care in hypertensive patients could reduce systolic and diastolic blood pressure by 5 and 4.3 mmHg, respectively [10]. Self-care for people with high blood pressure includes compliance with a healthy diet (especially low salt), physical activity, nonsmoking, abstaining from alcohol, weight management, and following prescribed medications [11]. Despite the necessity of carrying out all self-care behaviors to succeed in the management of hypertension, globally, many patients do not follow medical or lifestyle recommendations and therefore compliance with self-care behaviors in these patients is not desirable [12].

Based on evidence, self-care behaviors and blood pressure control become worse when hypertensive patients have limited health literacy [13]. Low health literacy may impact the ability to perform tasks such as understanding basic written health information or reading a prescription correctly. Low health literacy also is associated with worse chronic disease control, increased utilization of the emergency department and hospital care, and increased mortality. Lower health literacy has been associated with worse hypertension-related knowledge, lower ability to identify hypertension medications, and reduced adherence to cardiovascular medication refills. Various studies suggest that self-care behaviors are influenced by demographic variables and modifiable psychological variables [11, 14, 15]. Information about factors that affect self-care behaviors in low health literacy hypertensive patients based on theoretical framework is scarce. In this study, the HBM (Health Belief Model) was used to explain factors related to self-care behaviors of low health literacy hypertensive patients. HBM is one of the most important theories of behavior change that has been widely considered in behavioral health sciences and successfully applied in the design of health interventions. This model has emphasized the role of moderating factors (demographic, social, and structural factors) and individual perceptions (perceived sensitivity, perceived severity, perceived benefits, perceived barriers, guidance for action, and self-efficacy) in determining the likelihood of performing a behavior [16]. According to this model, a person's decision and motivation to perform a particular behavior included items such as person's perception of being at risk (perceived susceptibility) and its seriousness (perceived severity), belief in the perceived action of usefulness to reduce the risk of disease, understanding of the health benefits (perceived benefits), person's perception of the difficulties and cost of performing behaviors (perceived barrier), and moderating factors such as demographic and psychosocial variables (awareness) and people's judgments of their capabilities to execute given level of performance (self-efficacy) [17].

Therefore, the purpose of this study was to determine the factors related to self-care behaviors among low health literacy hypertensive patients based on health belief model. The results can be used as baseline data to improve self-care behaviors and blood pressure control caused by psychological factors.

2. Material and Methods

This cross-sectional study was conducted on 152 patients with limited health literacy who had been referred to the Haft-e-Tir Comprehensive Health Service Center in Bushehr city. This study was approved by the Ethics Committee of Bushehr University of Medical Sciences (IR.BPUMS.REC.1395.128). At first, patients were identified based on initial entry criteria and entered the study by convenience sampling method. Initial entry criteria for participation in the study include having appropriate physical conditions for answering questions, age over 30 years, not having a serious complication due to hypertension (diseases such as cardiovascular disease, neuropathy, nephropathy, retinopathy, and stroke), and passing at least 6 months of definite diagnosis of the disease. The final entry criteria for the study were limited health literacy. To identify patients with limited health literacy, a Short version of Test of Functional Health Literacy in Adults (S-TOFHLA) was completed. After identifying patients with limited health literacy and before the interview, the interviewer first explained the purpose of the survey, the study participants' rights, the risk and benefit of participation, and the plan to protect the confidentiality of study participants. Further, a signed informed consent was obtained prior to the interview. Then for patients who had proclaimed their consent to participate in the study, health beliefs model and self-care behaviors questionnaire were completed. Of the 209 participants identified on the basis of initial entry criteria and convenience sampling method, 152 had limited health literacy and completed the other questionnaires.

2.1. Measurement

2.1.1. Health Literacy. Health literacy was evaluated by a shortened version of the Test of Functional Health Literacy in Adults (S-TOFHLA) that included two reading passages (36 items worth 2 points each) and 4 numeracy items (7 points each) to assess comprehension of hospital forms and labeled prescription vials that contained numerical information; this test also assesses quantitative skills and the ability to read and understand prose and documents. Possible scores on the S-TOFHLA range from 0 to 36. Based on the cut of points of the questionnaire, we categorized patients into three mutually exclusive groups: inadequate, marginal, or adequate health literacy. Scores from 0 to 55 indicate inadequate health literacy. Scores from 56 to 66 indicate marginal health literacy, and scores from 67 to 100 indicate adequate health literacy. The Persian version of the scale shows adequate internal reliability for numeracy (Cronbach's $\alpha = 0.69$) and for reading comprehension (Cronbach's $\alpha = 0.78$) [18].

2.1.2. Knowledge of Hypertension. Hypertension knowledge assessed using Hypertension Knowledge Level Scale (HK-LS). This 22-item scale prepared by Erkoc et al. [19]. HK-LS assesses respondents' knowledge in defining hypertension, lifestyle, medical treatment, drug compliance, diet, and complications of hypertension. Each item is a full sentence that is either correct or incorrect. And each item is prepared as part of a standard answer (correct, incorrect, or do not know). Zinat Motlagh et al. have validated this questionnaire in Iranian population [20]. In Persian version in the validation process, three items were excluded from the scale and the final version has 19 true/false items.

2.1.3. Health Belief Model Constructs. In order to assess the constructs of health belief model, a researcher-made questionnaire was used. Items developed for susceptibility, seriousness, benefits, barriers, and self-efficacy focused on self-care behaviors in hypertensive patients. 39 items with 5-point Likert answers was used (9 items for perceived benefits, 7 items for perceived barriers, 9 items for perceived susceptibility, 6 items for perceived severity, and 10 items for perceived self-efficacy). For determination of content validity, the list items were distributed to judges who were faculty members and Ph.D. candidates and they were quite familiar with HBM constructs. In content validity, changing the format of questions and omitting irrelevant questions were performed. Then, mean Content Validity Index (CVI) and Content Validity Rate (CVR) of the questionnaire were calculated as 0.94 and 0.91, respectively. Reliability of the scale was calculated and Cronbach's alpha values were 0.71, 0.70, 0.70, 0.82, and 0.85 for perceived susceptibility, perceived severity, perceived barriers, perceived benefits, and perceived self-efficacy, respectively.

2.1.4. Self-Care Behavior. Self-care behaviors were determined using the hypertension self-care activity level effects (H-scale). This is a 31-item scale and was prepared by Zinat Motlagh [20]. The H-scale is designed to help primary care physicians to guide hypertensive patients who are seeking to achieve blood pressure control [21]. The H-scale examines the level of self-care by asking about the number of days per week on which an individual performs a self-care behavior. The H-scale was previously validated in Persian patients with high blood pressure [20]. The Persian version consisted of 27 items that measures the hypertension self-care activities with the following domains: medication adherence (3 items), physical activity (2 items), low-salt diet (10 items), smoking (2 items), alcohol (1 item), and weight management (9 items). The Persian version of the scale shows adequate internal consistency. Cronbach alphas were as follows: medication adherence (Cronbach's $\alpha = 0.91$), low-salt diet (Cronbach's $\alpha = 0.72$), physical activity (Cronbach's $\alpha = 0.96$), smoking (Cronbach's $\alpha = 0.91$), and weight management (Cronbach's $\alpha = 0.85$).

2.1.5. Sociodemographic Characteristics. Sociodemographic attributes, including age, sex, marital status, education level, and hypertension duration, were collected. Levels of education were divided into four categories: (1) illiterate; (2) primary school (1–5 years of schooling); (3) secondary/high schooling (6–12 years of schooling); and (4) education above high school. The number of years between the diagnosis of hypertension and point of data collection were obtained as disease duration.

2.2. Data Analysis. The data obtained from the total of 152 completed questionnaires in hypertensive patients with limited health literacy. Descriptive statistics were used to examine the characteristics of the sample. Then the participants for each of self-care behaviors were divided into two groups. First group is the low literacy patients who reported to perform self-care behaviors and second group is the low literacy patients who did not perform self-care behaviors. The multiple logistic regression analyses with forward steps likelihood ratio method was used to determine of predictive HBM constructs. All statistical analyses were performed using Statistical Package for Social Sciences (SPSS) version 22.0. In all tests, the level of significance was 0.05.

Table 1: The characteristics of respondents and descriptive findings ($n = 152$).

Variables	
Age (years)	Mean age: 56.87 years (SD = 8.70)
	Range: 35–80 years
Years with hypertension	Mean: 9.46 years (SD = 5.80)
Gender	Range: 1–30 years
Male	42 (27.6%)
Female	110 (72.4%)
Marital status	
Never married	3 (2%)
Married	129 (84.9%)
Divorced	20 (13.9%)
Educational level	
Illiterate	5 (3.3%)
Primary school	61 (40.1%)
Secondary/high school	77 (48.7%)
Above high school	9 (5.9%)
Family history of hypertension	
Yes	74 (48.7%)
No	78 (51.3%)
Income	
<10000000 IR-Rial	64 (42.1%)
>10000000 IR-Rial	88 (57.9%)
Medication	
Yes	149 (98%)
No	3 (2%)

3. Results

3.1. Sample Characteristics. A total of 152 hypertensive patients with limited health literacy were studied. Their demographic features are shown in Table 1. The mean age of participants was 56.87 ± 8.70 ranging from 35 to 80 years (Table 1). Almost, 42 participants were male (27.6%) and 110 were female (72.4%). Participants had an average of 4.46 ± 5.8 years of diagnosed hypertension. Most of the subjects (84.9%) were married and had secondary/high school education (48.7%). More than half of patients (57.9%) reported earning more than 10 million IR-Rial (≥250$) a month. Most of the patients (61.8%) did not work nor were employed at the time of the study. Family history of hypertension was reported in 48.7% of patients. 34.9% of patients had their systolic hypertension above 140 and diastolic blood pressure above 90 in their last care at the health center. The most important sources for receiving health information were health professionals (42.1%) and then Internet based messaging software such as Telegram and WhatsApp (17.8).

Our results revealed that only 9.2% had a proper adherence to their medication regimen, and 5.3% avoided salt both while cooking and eating. Moreover, 19.1% had physical activity on most weekdays, and 55.9% were nonsmokers.

TABLE 2: Self-care behaviors frequencies and percentages.

Self-care behavior	Number (%)
Medication adherence	14 (9.2)
Eating a low-salt diet	8 (5.3)
Physical activity	29 (19.1)
Nonsmoking	85 (55.9)
Alcohol abstinence	120 (78.9)
Weight management	41 (27.0)

21.1% were alcohol consumers, and 27% managed their weight (Table 2).

The means and standard deviations of knowledge 7.75 (SD = 2.89) and HBM constructs related to self-care behaviors were 38.60 (SD = 7.87) for self-efficacy, 16.78 (SD = 4.01) for perceived susceptibility, 13.36 (SD = 3.35) for perceived severity, 32.90 (SD = 7.07) for perceived benefits, and 14.92 (SD = 4.70) for perceived barriers.

The multiple logistic regression analysis was used to assess the predictors of adhering self-care behaviors for HBM constructs. The results of the multiple logistic regression indicated that the knowledge about hypertension and self-care was predictor of weight management (OR = 1.247) and medication regimens (OR = 1.376), that is, the patients who had known about hypertension and self-care behaviors were one time more likely to managed their weight and more likely to adhere to their medication regimen than those who had not. Self-efficacy was predictor of all self-care behaviors except no alcohol and medication regimens. Patients with greater perceived self-efficacy were more likely to have weight management (OR = 1.174) and to be nonsmokers (OR = 1.069), physically active (OR = 1.092), and to adhere to a low-salt diet (OR = 1.259) than those with lower self-efficacy. Perceived susceptibility about hypertension complications and adherence was predictor of both low-salt diet (OR = 1.139) and non-alcohol behavior (OR = 1.562). The results also revealed that individuals who had more perceived severity (OR = 1.301) had significantly greater adherence to their medication regimens compared to those who had less perceived severity. The other components of HBM (perceived benefits and barriers) were not significantly associated with either type of hypertension self-care behaviors (Table 3) and none of the HBM components predict alcohol consumption among participants.

4. Discussion

Blood pressure control in hypertensive patients was considered as a long-standing challenge. This can be more challenging, when hypertensive patients have limited health literacy. Therefore, the aim of this study was to determine the factors related to self-care behaviors as the most important way to control high blood pressure among low health literacy hypertensive patients based on health belief model. Based on findings, low health literacy hypertensive patient's adherence to self-care tasks was low in terms of healthful diet, physical activity, weight management, and medication adherence and was moderate regarding nonsmoking and alcohol abstinence.

Based on our primary results more than 90% of the participants had not a low-salt diet and they reported that they added extra salt to their food while cooking and eating. This is while the WHO suggests that every adult should consume less than 5 grams of sodium each day [22]. However, in Iran and most countries, the daily consumption of salt per person is between 9–12 grams on average [23]. This well has been confirmed that the consumption of foods containing salt accompanied by the insufficient consumption of fruits and vegetables is an important factor that lead to high blood pressure and unsuccessful management of this disease. Thus, the implementation of health interventions to reduce the consumption of salt expenditure, as well as increasing the consumption of fruits and vegetables, is a fundamental health need.

Other results show that less than one-fourth (19.1%) of the participants took part in physical activity at least 30 minutes almost every day and only 27% of the sample managed their weight. Similar to our results the other study found that 81.2% of people with arterial hypertension did not perform any kind of physical activity [24]. This is despite the fact that the WHO has suggested 30 minutes of physical activity five days a week to prevent and control high blood pressure [25]. The amount of physical activity in the study population is much lower than what has been reported by WHO. Insufficient physical activity and lack of weight management are topics that need more attention from physicians and healthcare providers but instead seems to have been ignored by them.

The prevalence of adherence to medication as the other self-care behaviors was low in study population. The overall adherence to medication in our study was 9.2% as compared to a similar study; the adherence was 48.7% [26] and, in an Iranian study by Kamran et al., 24% of the patients were adherent [14]. Probably the reason of this difference is due to limited health literacy of this study's population. It seems that adherence to medication regimen is less important for limited health literacy patients with hypertension. Therefore, the implementation of educational interventions to inform patients with hypertension about the necessity of antihypertensive drugs are essential.

We found a moderate rate of smoking and alcohol consumption in study population. Most of patients in this study avoided tobacco use (55.9%) and did not consume alcohol (78.9%). Despite the fact that smoking and alcohol consumption in Iran are not socially and culturally accepted, and, even being illegal in case of alcohol, we still see the consumption of these substances in individuals and even in patients. Multiple factors contribute to these behaviors. It is possible that participants do not associate reducing smoking and alcohol consumption as hypertension self-care behaviors. This reasoning would suggest that health providers should intervene to increase awareness of alcohol consumption and its effects on hypertension management.

The results indicated that knowledge about hypertension and self-care was significantly associated with weight management and medication regimens. This finding declares the role of knowledge as a major source and confirm a large body of research [27] that suggests knowledge about hypertension

TABLE 3: Associations between knowledge, structures, Health Belief Model, and hypertension self-care behaviors.

	Weight management OR (95% CI)	Nonalcohol OR (95% CI)	Nonsmoking OR (95% CI)	Physical activity OR (95% CI)	Low-salt diet OR (95% CI)	Medication regimens OR (95% CI)
Knowledge	1.247 (1.064–1.461)					1.376 (1.080–1.753)
Perceived susceptibility		1.139 (1.024–1.267)			1.562 (1.031–2.366)	
Perceived severity						1.301 (1.040–1.626)
Perceived self-efficacy	1.174 (1.092–1.261)		1.069 (1.044–1.149)	1.092 (1.031–1.157)	1.259 (1.053–1.505)	

and self-care can enhance the ability to cope and comply with medical regimens and disease management.

Analyzing Health Belief Model, our study found significant associations among HBM components. The findings indicated that self-efficacy is associated with adhering to low-salt diet, engaging in physical activity, not smoking, and utilizing common weight management strategies in hypertensive patients with low literacy. Our finding supports a positive relationship between self-efficacy and self-care behaviors found in previous studies [11, 28, 29]. Self-efficacy plays a crucial role in adoption of hypertension-controlling behaviors [30] and, as mentioned in other studies [31], it seems that patients with low health literacy may feel less confident in their ability to perform self-care behaviors and may have less motivation for performing self-care tasks. Consequently, increased confidence of low health literacy patients with regard to selecting appropriate behaviors seems to improve adherence to self-care tasks. Therefore, it is useful that through educational interventions, educators promote the patient's ability to perform self-care behaviors through self-efficacy strategies.

Our results showed that perceptions of susceptibility were influential for low-salt diet and nonsmoking behavior. These self-care behaviors were worse among those who had lower perception regarding the susceptibility or vulnerability to the disease process. Perceived susceptibility is one of the most important factors affecting health behaviors. Dehghani-Tafti et al. [29] introduced perceived susceptibility as a key factor in behavioral changes among diabetic patients. For the hypertensive patients with low health literacy to adopt self-care behaviors, health providers should intervene to change their beliefs to the point that they are susceptible and at risk for the complications of the disease.

Similar to other studies, medication adherence decreased with lower perception of disease severity [14, 32]. This may be due to poor health literacy that which makes the patients to have less knowledge about hypertension and its complications among these patients. Therefore, it seems that educating patients with limited health literacy about blood pressure and its complications can be effective in creating beliefs to understand the threat of high blood pressure.

In conclusion based on findings, there was minor adherence for self-care behaviors among patients with high blood pressure and low health literacy. This is due to the inadequate knowledge, perceived susceptibility, perceived severity, and perceived self-efficacy. Therefore, it is necessary that health providers improve their actions and also their communications with the patients especially patients with low health literacy to ensure a better influence on self-care behaviors. Health education based on HBM components can be useful and educational programs for these vulnerable patients should also be expanded.

Since this study was based on a convenience sample, the findings of this study may not be generalized to all Iranian hypertensive patients with low health literacy. Self-care behaviors were evaluated with self-report, so the reliability of self-rated self-care behaviors, in particular, may be subject to recall bias or memory failure. The results reported in the study were obtained from a cross-sectional survey and no causality is established between HBM components and self-care tasks. A longitudinal study that follows the study sample and reassesses their health outcomes at a later time would help to discern the causal effects of HBM components. The S-TOFHLA, similar to other health literacy assessments, offers no indication about the respondent's communication skills, which may be equally important in determining an individual's ability to effectively navigate today's complex health care system.

References

[1] H. Chopra and N. C. Nanda, *Textbook of Cardiology (A Clinical & Historical Perspective)*, JP Medical Ltd, 2012.

[2] World Health Organization, *WHO Global Health Days*, 2009, http://www.who.int/campaigns/world-health-day/2013/event/en/.

[3] World Health Organization, *Silent Killer, Global Public Health Crisis*, 2013, http://www.who.int/campaigns/world-health-day/2013/en/.

[4] World Health Organization, *Global Health Observatory (GHO) Data*, 2017, http://www.who.int/gho/ncd/risk_factors/blood_pressure_prevalence_text/en/.

[5] P. M. Kearney, M. Whelton, K. Reynolds, P. Muntner, P. K. Whelton, and J. He, "Global burden of hypertension: analysis of worldwide data," *The Lancet*, vol. 365, no. 9455, pp. 217–223, 2005.

[6] S. F. Zinat Motlagh, R. Chaman, S. R. Ghafari et al., "Knowledge, treatment, control, and risk factors for hypertension among adults in Southern Iran," *International Journal of Hypertension*, vol. 2015, Article ID 897070, 2015.

[7] E. M. Mutua, M. M. Gitonga, B. Mbuthia, N. Muiruri, J. J. Cheptum, and T. Maingi, "Level of blood pressure control among hypertensive patients on follow-up in a Regional Referral Hospital in Central Kenya," *Pan African Medical Journal*, vol. 18, article no. 278, p. 278, 2014.

[8] R. M. Peters and T. N. Templin, "Measuring blood pressure knowledge and self-care behaviors of African Americans," *Research in Nursing & Health*, vol. 31, no. 6, pp. 543–552, 2008.

[9] S. J. Flynn, J. M. Ameling, F. Hill-Briggs et al., "Facilitators and barriers to hypertension self-management in urban African Americans: perspectives of patients and family members," *Patient Preference and Adherence*, vol. 7, pp. 741–749, 2013.

[10] J. Chodosh, S. C. Morton, W. Mojica et al., "Meta-analysis: chronic disease self-management programs for older adults," *Annals of Internal Medicine*, vol. 143, no. 6, pp. 427–132, 2005.

[11] J. Warren-Findlow, R. B. Seymour, and L. R. B. Huber, "The association between self-efficacy and hypertension self-care activities among African American adults," *Journal of Community Health*, vol. 37, no. 1, pp. 15–24, 2012.

[12] R. Shima, M. H. Farizah, and H. A. Majid, "A qualitative study on hypertensive care behavior in primary health care settings in Malaysia," *Patient Preference and Adherence*, vol. 8, pp. 1597–1609, 2014.

[13] D. E. Willens, S. Kripalani, J. S. Schildcrout et al., "Association of brief health literacy screening and blood pressure in primary

care," *Journal of Health Communication*, vol. 18, no. 1, pp. 129–142, 2013.

[14] A. Kamran, S. S. Ahari, M. Biria, A. Malpour, and H. Heydari, "Determinants of patient's adherence to hypertension medications: application of health belief model among rural patients," *Annals of Medical and Health Sciences Research*, vol. 4, no. 6, pp. 922–927, 2014.

[15] M. Reisi, F. Mostafavi, H. Javadzade, B. Mahaki, E. Tavassoli, and G. Sharifirad, "Impact of health literacy, self-efficacy, and outcome expectations on adherence to self-care behaviors in iranians with type 2 diabetes," *Oman Medical Journal*, vol. 31, no. 1, pp. 52–59, 2016.

[16] N. K. Janz and M. H. Becker, "The health belief model: a decade later," *Health Education Journal*, vol. 11, no. 1, pp. 1–47, 1984.

[17] R. Orji, J. Vassileva, and R. Mandryk, "Towards an effective health interventions design: an extension of the health belief model," *Online Journal of Public Health Informatics*, vol. 4, no. 3, 2012.

[18] H. Javadzade, G. Sharifirad, M. Reisi, E. Tavassoli, and F. Rajati, "Health literacy among adults of isfahan," *Health System Research*, vol. 9, no. 5, pp. 540–549, 2013.

[19] S. B. Erkoc, B. Isikli, S. Metintas, and C. Kalyoncu, "Hypertension knowledge-level scale (HK-LS): a study on development, validity and reliability," *International Journal of Environmental Research and Public Health*, vol. 9, no. 3, pp. 1018–1029, 2012.

[20] S. F. Zinat Motlagh, R. Chaman, E. Sadeghi, and A. Ali Eslami, "Self-care behaviors and related factors in hypertensive patients," *Iranian Red Crescent Medical Journal*, vol. 18, no. 6, Article ID e35805, 2016.

[21] J. Warren-Findlow, D. W. Basalik, M. Dulin, H. Tapp, and L. Kuhn, "Preliminary validation of the hypertension self-care activity level effects (H-SCALE) and clinical blood pressure among patients with hypertension," *The Journal of Clinical Hypertension*, vol. 15, no. 9, pp. 637–643, 2013.

[22] C. D. Domnariu, A. Cucu, and F. L. Furtunescu, "World Health Organization guidelines on salt intake in adults and children," *Acta Medica Transilvanica*, vol. 18, pp. 166–168, 2013.

[23] Organization WH, Reducing Salt Intake in Populations. Report of a WHO Forum and Technical meeting 2006, Geneva: World Health Organisation, 2014.

[24] L. C. G. Martins, N. G. Guedes, I. X. Teixeira, M. V. D. O. Lopes, and T. L. de Araujo, "Physical activity level in people with high blood pressure," *Revista Latino-Americana de Enfermagem*, vol. 17, no. 4, pp. 462–467, 2009.

[25] World Health organization, A global brief on Hypertension Silent killer, global public health crisis, 2013.

[26] S. Al-Dabbagh and S. Aswad, "Compliance of hypertensive patients to management in Duhok governorate using Morisky-green test," *Duhok Medical Journal*, vol. 4, no. 1, pp. 28–39, 2010.

[27] M. V. Williams, D. W. Baker, R. M. Parker, and J. R. Nurss, "Relationship of functional health literacy to patients' knowledge of their chronic disease: a study of patients with hypertension and diabetes," *JAMA Internal Medicine*, vol. 158, no. 2, pp. 166–172, 1998.

[28] E. Lee and E. Park, "Self-care behavior and related factors in older patients with uncontrolled hypertension," *Contemporary Nurse*, pp. 1–15, 2017.

[29] A. Dehghani-Tafti, S. S. A. Mazloomy Mahmoodabad, M. A. L. Morowatisharifabad, M. Afkhami Ardakani, H. Rezaeipandari, and M. H. A. Lotfi, "Determinants of Self-Care in Diabetic Patients Based on Health Belief Model," *Global Journal of Health Science*, vol. 7, no. 5, pp. 33–42, 2015.

[30] M. Khorsandi, Z. Fekrizadeh, and N. Roozbahani, "Investigation of the effect of education based on the health belief model on the adoption of hypertension-controlling behaviors in the elderly," *Clinical Interventions in Aging*, vol. 12, pp. 233–240, 2017.

[31] M. Reisi, F. Mostafavi, H. Javadzade, B. Mahaki, and G. Sharifirad, "Assessment of some predicting factors of self-efficacy in patients with type 2 diabetes," *Iranian Journal of Endocrinology and Metabolism*, vol. 17, no. 1, pp. 44–52, 2015.

[32] S. A. U., S. Badiger, and N. Kumar S., "Medication adherence and health belief model among hypertensive patients attending rural health centres of a tertiary care hospital in South India," *International Journal of Community Medicine and Public Health*, vol. 4, no. 4, p. 1159, 2017.

29

Characteristics of Inpatient Hypertension Cases and Factors Associated with Admission Outcomes in Ashanti Region, Ghana: An Analytic Cross-Sectional Study

Kenneth Nuamah,[1] Harriet Affran Bonful,[2] Joseph Danso Yeboah,[3] Ebenezer Antwi Amankwaah,[1] Daniel Boakye,[1] Samuel Kwame Owusu,[1] Adwoa Aduako Owusu,[4] Freddie Amponsah,[5] Fred Adomako-Boateng,[1] Alexis Nang-Beifubah,[1] Margaret Gyapong,[6,7] Anthony Ofosu,[5] Bertha Garshong,[6] and Evelyn K. Ansah[6,7]

[1]*Ashanti Regional Health Directorate, P.O. Box 1908, Kumasi, Ghana*
[2]*Department of Epidemiology and Disease Control, School of Public Health, University of Ghana, P.O. Box LG 13, Legon, Accra, Ghana*
[3]*Sekyere Central District Health Directorate, P.O. Box 36, Nsuta, Ashanti, Ghana*
[4]*Suntreso Government Hospital, P.O. Box 14775, Kumasi, Ghana*
[5]*Policy Planning Monitoring and Evaluation Division, Ghana Health Service, PMB Ministries, Accra, Ghana*
[6]*Research Development Division, Ghana Health Service, P.O. Box MB-190, Accra, Ghana*
[7]*Institute of Health Research, University of Health & Allied Science, PMB 31, Ho, Ghana*

Correspondence should be addressed to Kenneth Nuamah; kenneth.nuamah@ghsmail.org

Academic Editor: Tomohiro Katsuya

Background. Hypertension remains a cause of morbidity and mortality in the Ashanti Region of Ghana. It has been featured in the top ten causes of OPD attendance, admissions, and deaths since 2012. We investigated the sociodemographic characteristics and spatial distribution of inpatient hypertensives and factors associated with their admission outcomes. *Methods.* A 2014 line list of 1715 inpatient HPT cases aged ≥25 years was used for the cross-sectional analytic study. Accounting for clustering, all analyses were performed using the *"svy"* command in Stata. Frequencies, Chi-square test, and logistic regression analysis were used in the analysis. Arc view Geographic Information System (ArcGIS) was used to map the density of cases by place of residence and reporting hospital. *Results.* Mean age of cases was 58 (S.D 0.0068). Females constituted 67.6% of the cases. Age, gender, and NHIS status were significantly associated with admission outcomes. Cases were clustered in the regional capital and bordering districts. However, low case densities were recorded in the latter. *Conclusion.* Increasing NHIS access can potentially impact positively on hypertension admission outcomes. Health educational campaigns targeting men are recommended to address hypertension-related issues.

1. Introduction

The World Health Organization (WHO) defines hypertension as a systolic blood pressure equal to or above 140 mm Hg and/or diastolic blood pressure equal to or above 90 mm Hg [1]. Overall health and wellbeing of human rely on efficient functioning of vital organs such as the heart, brain, and kidneys [1]. This largely depends on both systolic and diastolic blood pressure being normal. If hypertension is left uncontrolled, it can lead to several cardiovascular complications including a heart attack, an enlargement of the heart, and eventually heart failure [1]. Kidney failure, blindness, rupture of blood vessels, and cognitive impairment can be attributed to hypertension [1].

The prevalence of hypertension rose from 600 million in 1980 to about 1 billion in 2013 [1]. Worldwide, there are over

17 million deaths attributed to cardiovascular diseases, which is nearly one-third of total deaths in a year [2]. Complications due to hypertension account for 9.4 million deaths every year [3]. Hypertension accounts for at least 5% of deaths from heart disease and 51% of deaths due to stroke [3].

The African region has the highest prevalence of hypertension, affecting 46% of all adult aged 25 years and above [4]. The prevalence (35%) in high-income countries is lower compared to 40% in low-income countries. The greatest health challenge facing the African region after HIV/AIDS is hypertension [4].

In sub-Saharan Africa, Noncommunicable Diseases (NCDs) have become important causes of morbidity and mortality, contributing 22% of total deaths [4]. It has been forecasted that, by 2025, the hypertensive population in developing countries will be 125.5 million people, which will correspond to an increase of 68% from 2008 to 2025 [5, 6].

Hypertension disease risk factors include age, race, family history, being overweight or obese, physical inactivity, tobacco use, high-salt diet, too little vitamin D and potassium in diet, excessive alcohol use, stress, and certain chronic conditions [3]. The prevalence of hypertension increases with increasing age. Sidhu and colleagues noted that the highest prevalence is found in ages equal to or above sixty (60 years) followed by ages between fifty and fifty-nine (50–59 years) [7] whilst Opie and Seedat also noted that, at age 65 in rural West Africa, there is a 30%–40% chance of being hypertensive as compared to 50% chance in semiurban areas in West Africa [4].

Others have identified level of education and occupation as factors associated with hypertension [8]. The risk of hypertension can vary in geographical areas depending on environmental conditions and socioeconomic position [9]

Ghana like other middle-income countries is no exception as hypertension is the number three killer today [10]. The prevalence of high blood pressure in Ghana is estimated at 12.9% and 15% for women and men, respectively [10]. The 2014 Demographic Health Survey puts the prevalence of hypertension in Ashanti at 15.3% for women and 18.1% for men, which is higher than the national average [10]. Prevalence of hypertension for Ashanti is highest among males in Ghana and second highest for females [10].

Earlier studies in the Ashanti Region have shown that there is a long-standing perception that hypertension disease is associated with affluence and that it is a disease of the rich and wealthy in society [11]. This perception has led to many people in low-income communities failing to report for medical check-ups and undertake routine exercises and not fully participate in health education programmes [11].

Over the years, some of the steps taken to control the increasing burden of hypertension in the country by the Ghana Health Service (GHS) have included the introduction of the Regenerative Health and Nutrition Program as well as the institutionalization of hypertension clinics in health facilities. In a systematic review by Tagoe and Dake in 2011, it was concluded strongly that more females exhibited healthier life style compared with males after the introduction of the Regenerative Health Policy [12]. Despite these interventions, morbidity and mortality due to hypertension continue to rise in the region. The proportion of hypertension to total OPD attendance increased from 3.8% in 2012 to 5.4% in 2014 [13]. More importantly, the proportion of admissions attributed to hypertension increased from 1.1% in 2010 to 2.4% in 2014. In 2014, hypertension was ranked sixth, third, and fifth, for top ten causes of OPD attendance, cause of admissions and deaths, respectively [13]. A review of literature suggests that there is little knowledge on the local factors driving the increasing burden of the disease and hospitalization. This study describes the characteristics of inpatient hypertension cases; establishes the factors associated with the outcomes of hypertension admissions; and also determines the geospatial distribution of these admissions in the Ashanti Region for the year 2014.

2. Materials and Methods

Data collected was used purposely for a cross-sectional analytic study. The study was conducted in Ashanti Region, which is one of the ten administrative regions of Ghana located in the middle belt of the country and covers about 10.2% of the total land surface area. It has an estimated 2014 mid-year population of 5,461,933, constituting 19.8% of the national population (projection from 2010 population and housing census, Ghana Statistical Service). The Komfo Anokye Teaching Hospital (KATH) is the teaching hospital for the region. Health services are delivered in public, private, quasi-, and mission facilities totaling 548. These facilities are comprised of 121 hospitals, 103 health centres, 282 clinics, and 133 CHPS compounds. Inpatient services are rendered in the 121 hospitals for hypertensive patients. Population to health facility ratio is 1 : 9967. Most facilities report on health indicators into the District Health Information Management System (DHIMS2) software; however, the only teaching hospital which also serves as the main referral hospital in the region does not.

This study used secondary data extracted from *DHIMS 2* for the Ashanti Region. DHIMS 2 is a developed software that operates on *DHIS2 (District Health Information Software)* application platform. DHIMS 2 is used by GHS to collect and collate data on health care service provision. DHIMS 2 helps to generate routine data, analyse reports using maps, and graphs and health profiles for indicators across facilities over a period.

The study population included records of all hypertension patients on admission aged between 25 years and above, diagnosed by clinicians within the Ashanti Region and reported in the DHIMS platform.

Diagnosis made in this study was done by prescribers in accordance with the standard Treatment Guidelines of Ghana [14]. Recruitment of study participants was based on diagnosis of hypertension by clinicians providing care in the health facility. Clinician practice is in accordance with the Standard Treatment Guidelines of Ghana and WHO. There is a system of regular supervision by different levels of health managers to ensure that the guidelines and protocols are adhered to. According to the treatment guideline, prescribers are expected to take an average of two or more properly measured blood pressure readings of a patient before diagnosing them of being hypertensive. At the point of call, the patient to be diagnosed is made to assume a relaxed and comfortable position for at least thirty (30) minutes [14]. Blood pressure (BP) of patients is checked with the use of manual mercury sphygmomanometer and a stethoscope. The arm (preferably left arm) is positioned to face the prescriber and a cuff is wrapped around the upper arm with the cuff lower edge about one inch above the antecubital fossa of the patient [14]. The average of the second and third or more outcomes of systolic blood pressure (SBP) and Diastolic Blood Pressure (DBP) within constant time intervals is recorded as the actual BP of the Patient. An adult with persistent SBP equal to or higher than 140 mm Hg and DBP equal to or higher than 90 mm Hg in nondiabetic or SBP equal to or higher than 130 mm Hg and DBP equal to or higher than 80 mm Hg in diabetics is diagnosed as being hypertensive.

Majority (>95%) of the sphygmomanometer used in the health facilities involved in this study are manufactured by Accoson from England; 3M Littmann stethoscopes from USA are also the commonly used stethoscopes in the Ashanti Region. According to the clinical engineering department, apart from the mandatory conformance to standard specifications checks made on the equipment, other factors including availability and accessibility to spare parts from manufacturers and user friendliness of the equipment, influences the choice of the equipment. Health facilities in Ghana procure clinical equipment including the manual mercury sphygmomanometer and the stethoscope with prior approval and in consultation with the clinical engineering department at the regional headquarters of the Ghana Health Service. The regional clinical engineer's approval and recommendation are paramount in the decision-making process to procure clinical equipment according to standard specifications at all levels of health care delivery (i.e., district hospitals, health centres, and polyclinics).

Hypertension-related conditions excluded in the *ICD-10-CM* (International Classification and Coding of Diseases) tabular list of diseases and injuries codes *(I10–I15)* were excluded in this study. Due to incomplete data for previous years, only data for the year 2014 was used. This study employed a cross-sectional analytic design approach.

The data was "svyset" to account for clustering in facilities and all analyses were conducted using the "svy:" command in Stata version 13 S.E (Stata Corporation, College Station, Texas). The data extracted was checked for internal consistency and completeness using simple summary statistics of the selected variables. Patient folder numbers were used as unique identifiers instead of patient names. All duplicate numbers were deleted before analysis. Frequencies were used to describe the characteristics of cases. Where there was evidence of skewness in the data, means were estimated for continuous variables after log transformation.

The independent variables were age, sex, educational level, occupation, place of residence, length of stay, facility ownership type, and District and National Health Insurance status. Educational level was recategorized from 7 levels (none, primary, JHS/middle school, SHS, technical/vocation, tertiary, and unspecified) to 4 levels (no formal education, primary, secondary, and tertiary) by merging primary and JHS, SHS, and technical vocation. Occupation was recoded from 13 to 6 groups by merging occupational status with similar characteristics as follows: *formal employment* (professional), clerical worker; *self-employed,* business person, farmer, hairdresser, and trader; *unemployed,* housewife, retiree, unemployed, and unskilled laborer; *others; student; and unspecified.* Age and length of stay were also recoded into categorical variables with uniform intervals, that is, age (5 groups with 10-year interval from 25 years to 65 and above.) and length of stay in days (5 groups from 1 day to 5 days and above).

The dependent variable, hypertension admission outcome, and a categorical ordinal variable with three categories *(died, discharged, and referred)* were used to perform Chi-square tests of associations with the independent variables. This variable was then recoded into a binary variable *(died and did not die)* by merging the referred and discharged cases. To identify the predictors of inpatient hypertension admission outcomes, univariable and multivariable logistic regression analyses were performed to determine the predictors of inpatient hypertension admission at 95% confidence level and a p value of 0.05.

2.1. Geospatial Distribution. To generate the spatial distribution of the cases, the data in Ms Excel format was imported into Arc GIS Version 10.2. The shape files for all the districts in the region adopted from the Ghana Survey Department were used to draw thematic maps for the study since the shape files for the actual communities were not available. The communities of residence (addresses) of the cases were aligned with their respective districts for the analysis of the geographical distribution. Ninety-five (95) individual records were deleted from the list because their addresses could not be linked to any district in the region.

3. Results and Discussion

The total sample size obtained after data validation was 1,715. However, there were missing data in some variables in the dataset; therefore the sample size varied for the analysis conducted on these variables. The cases reported were seen in 30 hospitals comprising 17 public (government), 10 quasi-/mission facilities, and 3 private health facilities. Majority of the cases (59.3%) were seen in public hospitals.

Females constituted 67.5%. The mean age of these patients was 58.2 (S.D 0.00685) years, ranging from 25 years to 106 years. More than half (57.7%) of the hypertensive patients on admission had no formal education with the rest having been in some form of academic training as shown in Table 1. A proportion of 85.2% (n = 1695) accessed health care with the National Health Insurance Scheme (NHIS) card. The mean length of stay on admission was 2 days, ranging from one to ninety-one (1–91) days. 90% of hypertensive patients on admission were engaged in one form of employment or the other. Less than ten percent (7.5%) were not engaged in any form of occupation.

TABLE 1: Sociodemographic characteristics of inpatient hypertension clients in Ashanti Region, 2014.

	Female		Male		Total	
	Freq	% (95% CI)	Freq	% (95% CI)	Freq	% (95% CI)
Age group				$N = 1714$		
25–34	61	35.60 (2.79–4.52)	30	1.75 (1.01–3.03)	91	5.31 (3.98–7.05)
35–44	158	9.22 (7.04–11.99)	74	4.32 (3.29–5.64)	232	13.54 (11.55–15.80)
45–54	249	14.53 (12.80–16.44)	132	22.23 (6.03–9.78)	381	22.23 (20.34–24.24)
55–64	229	13.36 (11.73–15.17)	119	6.94 (5.71–8.42)	348	20.3 (18.58–22.14)
65+	460	26.84 (24.51–29.31)	202	11.79 (8.99–15.30)	662	38.62 (36.26–41.05)
Total	1157	67.5 (61.56–72.93)	557	32.50 (27.07–38.44)	1714	100
Sex				$N = 1714$		
Female	1157	67.5 (61.56–72.93)	0	—	1157	67.5 (61.56–72.93)
Male	0	—	557	32.5 (27.07–38.44)	557	32.5 (27.07–38.44)
Total	1157	67.5 (61.56–72.93)	557	32.50 (27.07–38.44)	1714	100
Educational level				$N = 1713$		
No education	706	41.21 (31.31–51.88)	282	16.46 (12.53–21.32)	988	57.68 (45.38–69.09)
Primary	393	22.94 (16.96–30.26)	212	12.38 (8.37–17.92)	605	35.32 (25.92–46.01)
Secondary	33	1.93 (0.73–4.99)	37	2.16 (1.00–4.59)	70	4.09 (1.86–8.74)
Tertiary	24	1.4 (0.67–2.89)	26	1.52 (0.70–3.26)	50	2.92 (1.46–5.75)
Total	1156	67.48 (61.55–72.91)	557	32.52 (27.09–38.45)	1713	100
NHIS status				$N = 1694$		
Not having NHIS	148	8.74 (5.06–14.68)	103	6.08 (3.57–10.17)	251	14.82 (8.82–23.83)
Have NHIS	993	58.62 (50.21–66.55)	450	26.56 (22.69–30.83)	1443	85.18 (76.17–91.18)
Total	1141	67.36 (61.49–72.72)	553	32.64 (27.28–38.51)	1694	100
Occupation				$N = 1711$		
Unemployed	88	5.14 (1.84–13.54)	41	2.40 (12.09–5.20)	129	7.54 (3.02–17.60)
Formal employment	16	0.94 (14.38–43.87)	23	1.34 (0.66–2.73)	39	2.28 (1.23–4.18)
Self-employed	455	26.59 (14.38–43.87)	227	13.27 (7.22–23.13)	682	39.86 (20.67–62.77)
Student	1	$5.8e-02$ ($6.7e-03$–0.51)	2	0.12 ($2.5e-02$–0.54)	3	0.18 ($4.8e-02$–0.64)
Unspecified	470	27.47 (10.07–56.15)	161	9.41 (3.4–23.48)	631	36.88 (12.52–70.46)
Others	125	7.31 (3.18–15.89)	102	5.96 (2.88–11.93)	227	13.27 (6.41–25.47)
Total	1155	67.50 (61.53–72.96)	556	32.50 (27.04–38.47)	1711	100
Facility ownership				$N = 1714$		
Quasi-/mission	403	23.51 (7.12–55.23)	201	11.73 (4.97–25.22)	604	35.24 (10.8–70.97)
Public	700	40.84 (21.03–64.16)	317	18.49 (9.60–32.66)	1017	59.33 (27.20–85.07)
Private	54	3.15 (0.63–14.29)	39	2.28 (0.56–8.79)	93	5.43 (1.27–20.40)
Total	1157	67.50 (61.56–72.93)	557	32.50 (27.07–38.44)	1714	100
District status				$N = 1714$		
Rural	337	19.66 (8.29–39.84)	200	11.67 (4.87–25.43)	537	31.33 (12.48–59.34)
Urban	820	47.84 (30.18–66.06)	357	20.83 (13.86–30.08)	1177	68.67 (40.66–87.52)
Total	1157	67.5 (61.56–72.93)	557	32.50 (27.07–38.44)	1714	100

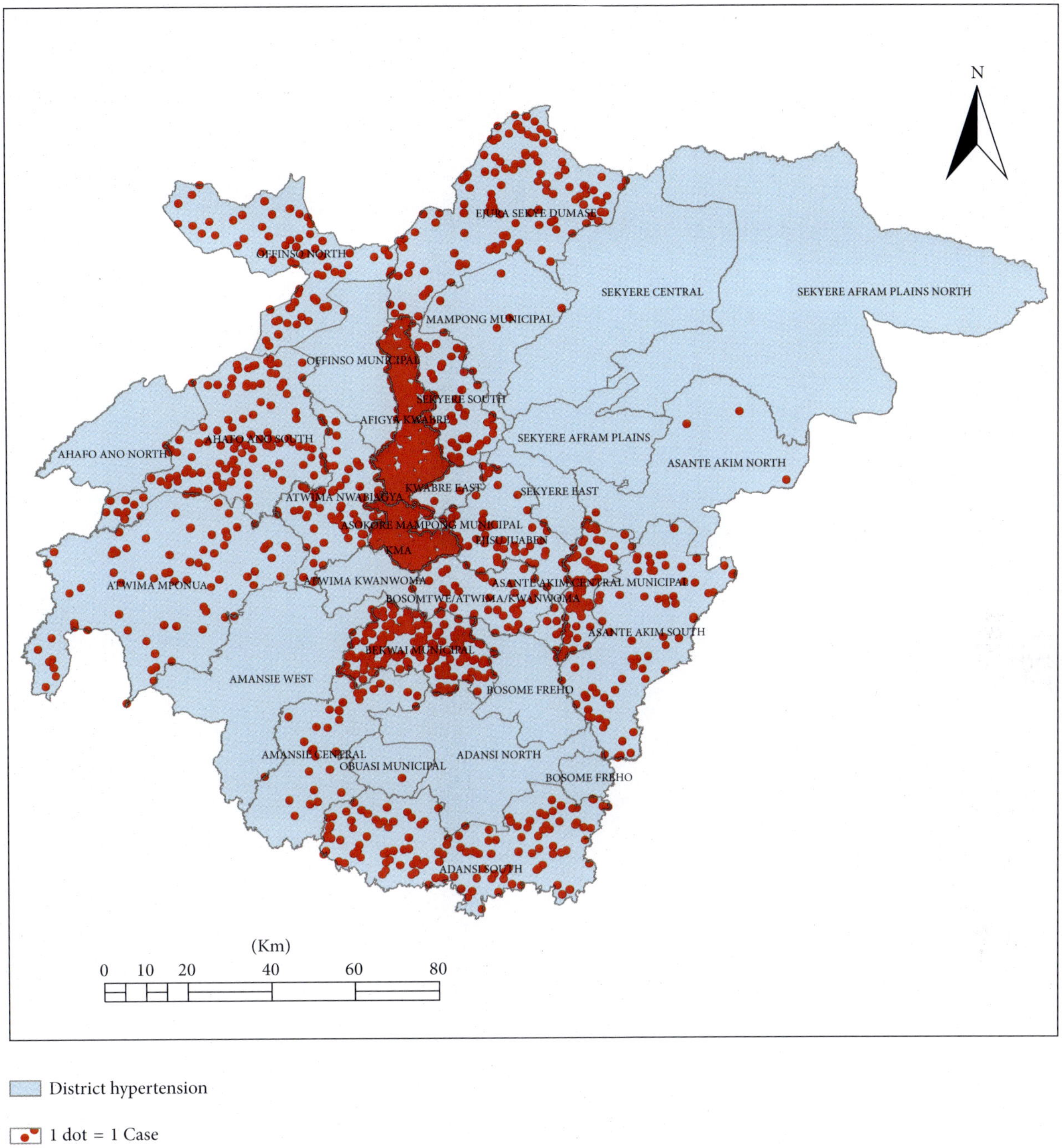

FIGURE 1: Case density of the hypertension admissions by clients place of residents, Ashanti Region, 2014.

Figure 1 shows the spatial pattern of cases by place of residence (address) across the study area. Most cases were clustered around the regional capital, Kumasi, and adjoining districts, whereas 9 districts including Sekyere Afram plains, Sekyere Central, Sekyere Kumawu, Obuasi Municipal, Ahafo Ano North, Asokore Mampong, and Sekyere East recorded admissions below 5 cases. Four out of these 9 districts do not have district hospitals.

Figure 2 is a spatial distribution of hypertension admission case density per hospital. Four (4) hospitals located in 4 districts (Ejura hospital, Nkenkaasu Hospital, Methodist Faith Healing Hospital, and Bekwai Hospital) reported hypertension admission cases constituting more than 0.1% of the district population. These 4 hospitals from 4 districts contributed 9.59% of the total admissions and 14.08% of the total deaths for 2014.

Chi-square tests of association showed no significance between the dependent variable and all independent variables except NHIS (Chi = 10.84, $p < 0.05$) as shown in Table 2.

Crude analysis of the association between the outcome of admission and predictor variables showed that gender, length of stay, and NHIS status were associated with admission

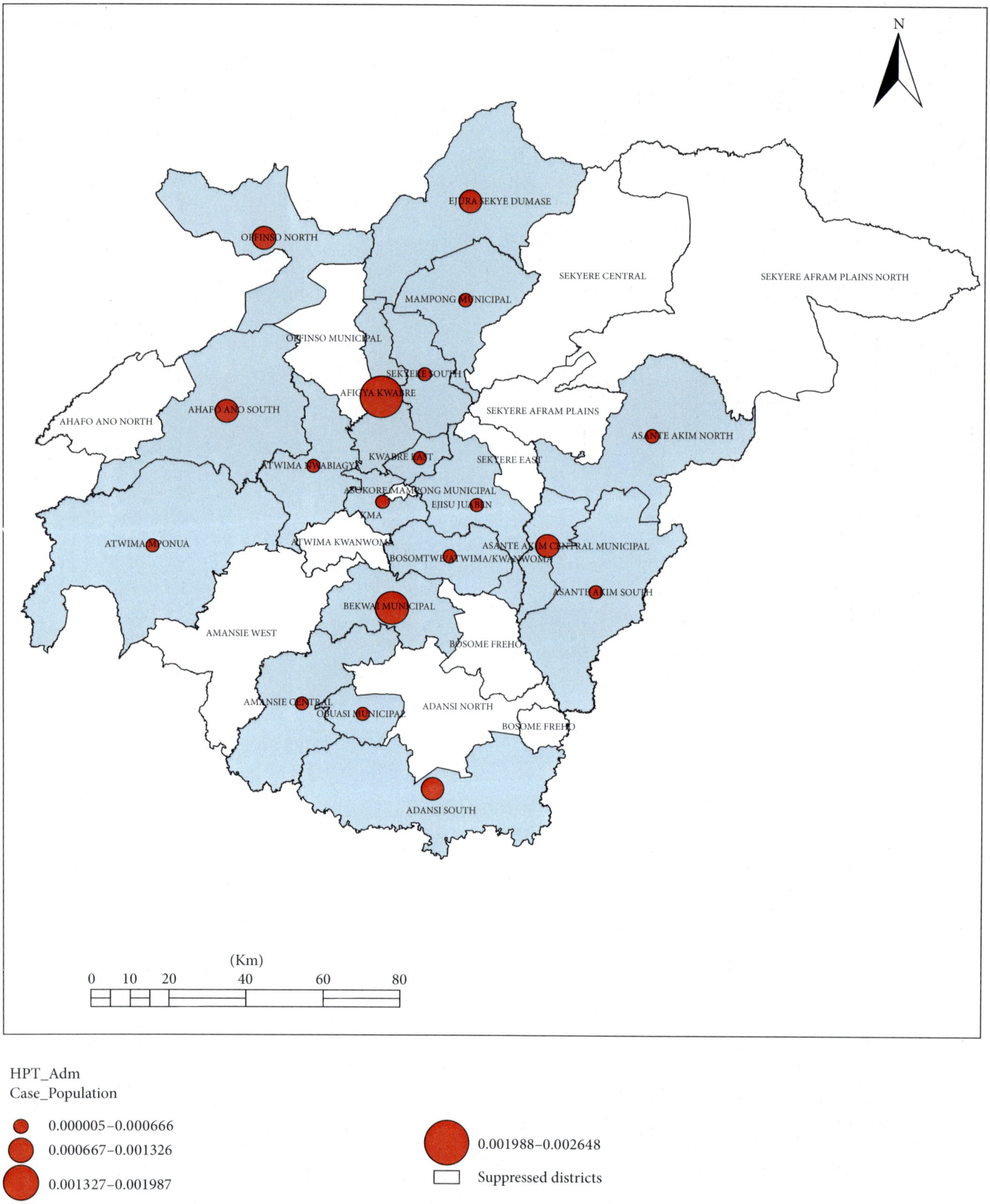

Figure 2: Case density of hypertension admission as reported by hospital, Ashanti, 2014.

TABLE 2: Chi-square test of association of sociodemographic characteristics of inpatient hypertensive clients and outcome of admission.

Variables	Hypertension outcome of admission						Total	χ^2	p – Value
	Died		Discharged		Referred				
	Frequency	%	Frequency	%	Frequency	%			
Age group									
25–34	2	3.9	86	5.39	3	4.5	91		
35–44	3	5.8	218	13.7	11	16.4	232		
45–54	10	19.2	355	22.3	17	25.4	382	8.82	0.304
55–64	8	15.4	326	20.4	14	20.9	348		
65+	29	55.8	610	38.2	22	32.8	661		
Total	*52*	*100*	*1595*	*100*	*67*	*100*	*1714*		
Sex									
Male	24	46.2	506	31.7	27	40.3	557		
Female	28	53.9	1088	68.3	40	59.7	1156	6.69	0.218
Total	*52*	*100*	*1594*	*100*	*67*	*100*	*1621*		
Educational level									
No formal education	31	59.6	921	57.8	35	52.2	987		
Primary	16	30.8	564	35.4	25	37.3	605		
Secondary	2	3.9	66	4.1	2	3.0	70	7.60	0.414
Tertiary	3	5.8	42	2.6	5	7.5	50		
Total	*52*	*100*	*1593*	*100*	*67*	*100*	*1712*		
NHIS status									
Have NHIS	36	69.2	1350	85.7	57	85.1	1443		
Not having NHIS	16	30.8	225	14.3	10	14.9	251	10.84	0.041*
Total	*52*	*32*	*1575*	*100*	*63*	*100*	*1694*		
Occupation									
Unemployed	3	5.8	113	7.1	13	19.4	129		
Formal Employment	2	3.9	33	2.1	4	6.0	39		
Self-employed	13	25.0	651	40.9	18	26.9	682		
Student	0	0.0	3	0.2	0	0.0	3	28.09	0.147
Unspecified	26	50.0	583	36.6	21	31.3	630		
Others	8	15.4	208	13.1	11	16.4	227		
Total	*52*	*100*	*1591*	*100*	*67*	*100*	*1710*		
Length of stay									
1 day	15	34.88	477	31.51	19	33.93	511		
2 days	7	16.28	473	31.24	12	21.43	492		
3 days	5	11.63	230	15.19	9	16.07	244	11.92	0.155
4 days	4	9.30	114	7.53	4	7.14	122		
5+	12	27.91	220	14.53	12	21.43	244		
Total	*43*	*100*	*1514*	*100*	*56*	*100*	*1613*		
Facility ownership									
Quasi/mission	25	48.1	556	34.9	23	34.3			
Public	27	51.9	946	59.3	43	64.2		8.41	0.706
Private	0	0	93	5.8	1	1.5			
Total	*52*	*100*	*1595*	*100*	*67*	*100*			
District status									
Rural	13	25.00	513	32.16	11	16.42	537		
Urban	39	75.00	1082	67.84	56	83.58	1177	8.41	0.221
Total	*52*	*100*	*1595*	*100*	*67*	*100*	*1714*		

*Statistically significant.

TABLE 3: Univariable and multivariable logistics regression analysis for the association between outcome of admission and sociodemographic characteristics of inpatient admissions of Ashanti.

Characteristics	Crude OR (95% CI)	p value	Adjusted OR (95% CI) $N^{*} = 1552$	p value
Age group				
25–34 (reference)	1			
35–44	0.58	0.475	0.64 (0.13–3.20)	0.573
45–54	1.19	0.836	0.74 (0.05–10.40)	0.815
55–64	1.05	0.947	0.44 (0.06–3.42)	0.420
65+	2.04	0.436	0.54 (0.02–18.13)	0.722
Age**	1.03	0.029**	1.04 (0.99–1.10)	0.087
Sex				
Male (reference)	1			
Female	0.55	0.017**	0.49 (0.29–0.82)	0.009**
Educational level				
No formal education (reference)	1			
Primary	0.84	0.581	1.43 (0.80–2.56)	0.211
Secondary	0.91	0.905	0.99 (0.13–7.86)	0.999
Tertiary	1.97	0.302	3.42 (0.38–30.49)	0.170
Occupation				
Unemployed (reference)	1			
Formal employment	2.27	0.535	Omitted	
Self employed	0.82	0.746	0.83 (0.14–4.97)	0.834
Student	Omitted		Omitted	
Unspecified	1.81	0.324	2.53 (0.49–13.11)	0.257
Others	1.53	0.533	1.15 (0.19–6.94)	0.872
NHIS status				
Not having NHIS (reference)	1			
Have NHIS	0.376	0.040**	0.22 (0.11–0.45)	0.001**
Length of stay on admission				
Length of stay	1.04	0.009**	1.05 (0.99–1.10)	0.069
Facility ownership				
Quasi/mission (reference)	1			
Public	0.632	0.260	0.69 (0.29–1.61)	0.373
Private	1 (omitted)			
District status				
Rural (reference)	1			
Urban	1.38	0.520	0.84 (0.31–2.30)	0.726

N^{*} sample size for multivariable logistic regression analysis. Age** significantly associated with the outcomes in this model when it was substituted for age category.

outcomes. After adjusting for all other variables, NHIS and sex were significant predictors of the hypertension admission outcome as shown in Table 3.

NHIS registrants were 78% less likely to die from admissions due to hypertension (AOR 0.22, 95% CI 0.11–0.45; $p = 0.001$), whilst females were 51% less likely to die from hypertension admission (AOR 0.49, 95% CI 0.29–0.82; $p = 0.009$).

In the crude analysis, for every day increase in the length of stay on admission, clients were 1.04 times more likely to die from hypertension admission. Replacing age group (categorical variable) with age (continuous variable) and using the same model, age showed a significant association with hypertension admission outcomes (OR = 1.03, 95% CI 1.00–1.05, $p = 0.029$) implying that, for every unit increase in age (years), clients were 1.04 times more likely to die from hypertension admission.

This study sought to use secondary data on hypertension admissions from the DHMIS for 2014 to determine the characteristics of inpatient hypertension cases and factors associated with admission outcomes in Ashanti Region for 2014. Females dominated the number of inpatient hypertensives in this study. This is consistent with Owusu-Sekyere and colleagues who report that there are more female hypertensives in the Kumasi metropolis than males [11]. Our finding is however not consistent with findings of Kolo and colleagues in a similar study, where females constituted 48.4% [15].

In this study, age groups were not associated with admission outcomes. However, age as a continuous variable had significant association with the outcome. Thus, for every unit increase in age (years), hypertensives on admission are 1.04 times more likely to die (OR 1.04, 95% CI 1.003–1.05 p = 0.029). This is consistent with Peck et al. study which reported in 2013 that those who die of noncommunicable diseases such as hypertension are older than those who died from communicable diseases [16].

Sex and NHIS status of clients were significantly associated with admission outcomes in this study. Contrary to popular opinions, available data showed that females were 51% less likely to die from hypertension admission. This is probably because women are more conscious of their health with a better health seeking behaviour than men [15]. It can only be inferred that men's health seeking behaviour was poor. There is the need to improve upon the health seeking behaviours of men especially through information, communication, and education programs. Earlier studies by Méndez-Chacón et al. reported that the proportion in men unaware of their hypertension status is higher than that of unaware women (32% versus 20%) [17].

Majority of the deaths recorded from HPT admissions were at the age of 65 years and above with females dominating. However, Williams et al. established the tremendous burden of hypertension-related conditions in adults in sub-Saharan Africa in a similar study which also reported that majority of hypertension-related deaths occurred in the working-age males (median age of death: 61 years) [16].

Our study reports that NHIS registrants are 78% less likely to die from admissions due to hypertension (AOR 0.22, 95% CI 0.11–0.45; p = 0.001). Others have reported that the blood pressure levels of clients who receive free medical care are lower than those who have to pay for the cost of care. Therefore, it is plausible that patients who have to pay for cost of care generally delay in seeking prompt care until their conditions are worsened [4]. Obviously, this is likely to lead to a poorer outcome when they are finally admitted. Although the proportion of patients with NHIS clients in this study was high (85.2%), the effects of lack of NHIS ownership on admission outcomes observed in this study bring to bear the need for a universal health care policy, which ensures that primary prevention and management of hypertension are included in the basic health care provided to all citizens.

Earlier reports from Nigeria indicate that case fatality for hypertension admissions is influenced by length of stay in the hospital, among others [15], and this study also answers in the affirmative regarding the crude analysis alone (OR 1.04, 95% CI, p- value = 0.009).

Our study shows that majority (59.3%) of the cases were reported by government hospitals. Out of 121 hospitals in the Ashanti Region, hospitals that reported in DHIMS by ownership were 28, 68, and 22 for mission/quasi-, private, and public facilities, respectively. However, the proportion of hospitals that reported on hypertension admission cases for the year 2014 is 35.7% of quasi-/mission, 4.4% of private, and 77.3% of public facilities. This situation contributed to the high number of cases reported by the public hospitals.

4. Conclusions

NHIS registrants and females were less likely to die on admission resulting from hypertension; therefore increasing NHIS access can potentially have an impact positively on hypertension admission outcomes. Also, IEC programs should pay more attention to men to help improve their health seeking behaviour, thereby improving hypertension admission outcomes.

Strategies must be adapted to resource quasi-/mission and private facilities in providing hypertension admission care to relieve the pressure on public hospitals.

5. Study Limitations

Due to the cross-sectional nature of this dataset, the temporal associations between NHIS status, gender, age, length of stay, and hypertension admission outcome variables may not be causal. Our study did not have any gold standard to compare the hypertension diagnosis provided in the dataset; therefore any misclassification could not have been determined. The actual cause of death could not also be validated due to the nature of the data; therefore, the death reported in this study may not be due to hypertension alone. However, generally, prescribers are all well trained and participate in compulsory continuous professional development programs coupled with regular stringent monitoring and supervisory visit from the Regional Health Administration. It could be presumed that they provide standard care to the patients. The use of routine health facility data restricted this study to the use of only variables presented in the dataset. All the public and quasi-/mission hospitals from the district levels report to the DHIMS platform, but eight out of the thirty districts in the region do not have hospitals to admit HPT cases; therefore cases from these districts could not be reported by the district. The findings of this study may not be generalizable to the whole Ashanti Region granted that even data from the only teaching hospital and biggest referral hospital (KATH) in the region was not available.

Abbreviations

AIDS: Acquired Immune Deficiency Syndrome
AOR: Adjusted odds ratio
CI: Confidence interval
DHIMS: District Health Information Management System
ERC: Ethical Review Committee
GHS: Ghana Health Service
HIV: Human Immune Deficiency Virus
HPT: Hypertension
JHS: Junior High School
KATH: Komfo Anokye Teaching Hospital
MOH: Ministry of Health
NCD: Noncommunicable diseases
NHIS: National Health Insurance Scheme
OR: Odds ratio
OPD: Out-patient department
RHMT: Regional Health Management Team
WHO: World Health Organization.

Ethical Approval

Ethical approval was obtained from the Ethics Review Committee (ERC) of the GHS (GHS-ERC: 24/09/15).

Disclosure

The Ashanti Regional Director of Health Services granted permission for the use of the retrospective health facility data, provided permission for publication, and is also a co-author of this paper. The dataset consists of routine Health Service Information obtained from the database of Ghana Health Service and as such human written informed consent was not necessary. Appropriate permission was sought from the Regional Director who had oversight over the data. There was no need for consent from study participants since we relied on retrospective health facility data. The nature of the study posed no risk to individuals whose data were used because only their unique identifiers were in the dataset. Confidentiality was maintained and only the research team had access to the data. The anonymous nature of the data used does not permit the disclosure of any individual's details since the information was not connected to individual names or identity. The Global Fund and the Ghana National Malaria Control Programme had no role in the design of the study, collection, analysis, and interpretation of data and in writing the manuscript.

Authors' Contributions

Kenneth Nuamah, Harriet Affran Bonful, Joseph Danso Yeboah, Daniel Boakye, and Ebenezer Antwi Amankwaah designed the study with inputs from Bertha Garshong, Anthony Ofosu, Margaret Gyapong, and Evelyn K. Ansah. Kenneth Nuamah, Joseph Danso Yeboah, Daniel Boakye, and Ebenezer Antwi Amankwaah extracted secondary data for analysis. Freddie Amponsah, Samuel Kwame Owusu, and Joseph Danso Yeboah generated maps for the geospatial distribution under the supervision of Anthony Ofosu. Harriet Affran Bonful, Kenneth Nuamah, Evelyn K. Ansah, Freddie Amponsah, Anthony Ofosu, Bertha Garshong, Margaret Gyapong, and Alexis Nang-Beifubah analysed and interpreted the data. Kenneth Nuamah, Harriet Affran Bonful, Joseph Danso Yeboah, Daniel Boakye, Ebenezer Antwi Amankwaah, and Evelyn K. Ansah wrote the first draft of the manuscript. Anthony Ofosu, Bertha Garshong, Margaret Gyapong, Freddie Amponsah, Adwoa Aduako Owusu, Fred Adomako-Boateng, and Alexis Nang-Beifubah contributed to the revision and finalization of the manuscript. All authors approved the final version of the manuscript. Evelyn K. Ansah and Anthony Ofosu are the guarantors.

Acknowledgments

The authors wish to acknowledge the technical support received from Dr. Abraham Hodgson, Dr. Amanua Chinbuah, and the Research Development Division of Ghana Health Service. They also wish to acknowledge the technical support from the Policy Planning Monitoring & Evaluation Division of Ghana Health Service for the extraction and use of data from the DHIMS2 database of the Ghana Health Service. The authors wish to acknowledge the organizers of the Ghana Health Service National Research Dissemination Forum where this manuscript was earlier presented as an abstract in 2016 brochure. Finally, they wish to thank the Programme Manager and staff of the National Malaria Control Programme for facilitating access to funding this study. This study received financial support from Global Fund to Fight AIDS, Tuberculosis and Malaria through the Ghana National Malaria Control Programme.

References

[1] W. H. Day, World Health Day 2013, A Glob. Br. Hypertens., p. 9, 2013.

[2] WHO, Global status report on noncommunicable diseases, 2010.

[3] S. S. Lim, T. Vos, and A. D. Flaxman, "A comparative risk assessment of burden of disease and injury attributable to 67 risk factors and risk factor clusters in 21 regions, 1990–2010: a systematic analysis for the Global Burden of Disease Study 2010," *The Lancet*, vol. 380, pp. 1990–2010, 2012.

[4] L. H. Opie and Y. K. Seedat, "Hypertension in Sub-Saharan African populations," *Circulation*, vol. 112, no. 23, pp. 3562–3568, 2005.

[5] P. M. Kearney, M. Whelton, K. Reynolds, P. Muntner, P. K. Whelton, and J. He, "Global burden of hypertension: analysis of worldwide data," *The Lancet*, vol. 365, no. 9455, pp. 217–223, 2005.

[6] O. S. Ogah, "Blood pressure, prevalence of hypertension and hypertension related complications in Nigerian Africans: A review," *World Journal of Cardiology*, vol. 4, no. 12, pp. 327–340, 2012.

[7] S. Sidhu and K. Kumari, "Socio-demographic variables of hypertension among adult punjabi females," *Journal of Human Ecology*, vol. 17, no. 3, pp. 211–215, 2005.

[8] J. Addo, C. Agyemang, L. Smeeth, A. de-Graft Aikins, A. K. Edusei, and O. Ogedegbe, "A review of population-based studies on hypertension in Ghana," *Ghana Medical Journal*, vol. 46, supplement, no. 2, pp. 4–11, 2012.

[9] Z. Wang, Q. Du, S. Liang et al., "Analysis of the spatial variation of hospitalization admissions for hypertension disease in shenzhen, China," *International Journal of Environmental Research and Public Health*, vol. 11, no. 1, pp. 713–733, 2014.

[10] H. Survey, "Ghana," 2014.

[11] E. Owusu-Sekyere, B. Ebenezer, and O. Linda, "Spatial Modeling of Hypertension Disease in the Kumasi Metropolitan Area of Ghana," *International Journal of Statistics and Applications*, vol. 3, no. 4, pp. 132–140, 2013.

[12] H. A. Tagoe and F. A. A. Dake, "Healthy lifestyle behaviour among Ghanaian adults in the phase of a health policy change," *Globalization and Health*, vol. 7, article no. 7, 2011.

[13] A. R. H. Directorate, "2014 Annual Report." 2014.

[14] G. Ministry of, Health, Standard Treatment Guidelines,.

[15] P. M. Kolo, Y. B. Jibrin, E. O. Sanya, M. Alkali, I. B. Peter Kio, and R. K. Moronkola, "Hypertension-related admissions and outcome in a tertiary hospital in northeast Nigeria," *International Journal of Hypertension*, vol. 2012, Article ID 960546, 6 pages, 2012.

[16] R. N. Peck, E. Green, J. Mtabaji et al., "Hypertension related diseases as a common cause of hospital mortality in Tanzania: a 3-year prospective study," *Global Health Action*, vol. 9, no. 1, pp. 1806–1811, 2014.

Clinical, Socioeconomic, and Psychosocial Factors Associated with Blood Pressure Control and Adherence: Results from a Multidisciplinary Cardiovascular National Program Providing Universal Coverage in a Developing Country

Daniela Sandoval,[1,2] Carolina Nazzal,[3] and Tomás Romero[4,5]

[1] *Department of Primary Care & Health Family, Faculty of Medicine, University of Chile, Santiago, Chile*
[2] *Department of Physical Therapy, Faculty of Medicine, University of Chile, Santiago, Chile*
[3] *School of Public Heath, Faculty of Medicine, University of Chile, Santiago, Chile*
[4] *School of Medicine, University of California, San Diego, CA, USA*
[5] *Institutional Review Board, Sharp Health Care, San Diego, CA, USA*

Correspondence should be addressed to Tomás Romero; tromero560@aol.com

Academic Editor: Markus P. Schlaich

Background. Limited information exists on blood pressure (BP) control factors and adherence to antihypertensive drug therapy (Rx) in developing countries. *Methods.* Cross-sectional study in randomly selected 992 hypertensive patients under a Chilean national comprehensive Cardiovascular Health Program (CVHP). Association of education, income, diabetes, obesity, physical activity, psychosocial characteristics, smoking, and alcohol abuse with BP control and adherence were evaluated by multivariate logistic regression. *Results.* BP control (<140/90 mmHg) was achieved in 63.1% of patients, with 38.4% adherent to Rx. Uncontrolled BP significantly associated with male sex (OR: 1.73 [95% CI 1.35-2.22]), low family income, high emotional-stress-depression score, body mass index, no adherence (OR: 1.83 [95% CI 1.44 - 2.32]), multiple Rx, baseline systolic BP value, and sedentary life style. Males (OR: 1.54 [95% CI 1.23 - 1.93]), low family income, high emotional stress-depression score (OR: 2.15 [95% CI 1.68 - 2.76]), low social support, and uncontrolled BP (OR: 1.52 [95% CI 1.22-1.90]) associated with no adherence. *Conclusions.* Comparable BP control (63.1%) to higher-income societies was observed. Uncontrolled BP associated significantly to no adherence and both to male sex, socioeconomic, and psychosocial factors. Global low adherence (38.4%) and improved BP control and adherence in diabetics were noted.

1. Introduction

Unsatisfactory BP control according to accepted guidelines is a persistent worldwide problem in the hypertensive population [1, 2]. In high-income countries approximately 55% of patients with access to antihypertensive drug therapy (Rx) do not reach a satisfactory BP control (<140/90 mmHg), and lack of adherence to treatment (Rx) is considered an important factor [3–5]. A World Health Organization sponsored study (SAGE) that included 47,443 adults from six middle-income countries (China, Ghana, India, Russia, Mexico, and South Africa) sampled between 2007 and 2010 documented that more than 90% of the hypertensive patients had uncontrolled BP, and insurance as well as income status emerged as significant correlates to diagnosis and treatment [6]. Unfavorable socioeconomic and psychosocial conditions have been frequently mentioned as barriers for BP control and adherence to Rx, of particular relevance in developing countries and/or social groups with limited access to health resources [6–10].

Chile is a developing country undergoing an accelerated process of socioeconomic transition and classified along with Uruguay in the high-income bracket in South America yet with one of the highest coefficients of social inequality (GINI Index 50.5) [11].

Approximately 75% of the Chilean population receives primary medical care in government sponsored primary care centers financed through FONASA (Fondo Nacional de Salud, National Health Fund) a legally mandated 7% tax on wages and from government subsidies (64% of total)[12]. Approximately 20% of the populations are affiliated to private or institutional medical services, with a different financing (private) system. FONASA guarantees coverage free of copayments for medical care at government sponsored primary care centers including approved medications for eighty medical conditions through a Health Care Policy Act approved in 2005 (Garantías Explícitas de Salud, GES, or Explicit Health Warranties) [13].

In 2002 a Cardiovascular Health Program (CVHP) (*Programa de Salud Cardiovascular*) was started in Chile implemented at the government sponsored primary care centers as part of the National Health Program aimed at reducing cardiovascular morbidity, the mayor cause of death and the third cause of disability in Chile today [10]. The increasing rates of obesity and diabetes in the Chilean hypertensive population were major determinants of this program [10, 14]. In the CVHP patients are provided access to treatment and screening for cardiovascular risk factors plus a multidisciplinary approach to modify unfavorable life style and habits free of copayments. It is estimated that approximately 500,000 hypertensive patients are followed through the CVHP in the Metropolitan region of Santiago [14]. Previous results from hypertensive patients evaluated between 2009 and 2010 enrolled in the CVHP since 2006 have been published [10]. The objective of the present study is to evaluate the association of socioeconomic and psychosocial factors, life style behavior, and adherence to Rx with BP control, not analyzed in previous studies, in 992 patients from four different primary care centers with at least one year attending the CVHP.

2. Methods

2.1. Study Population. The study was conducted in four government subsidized primary care centers in the Metropolitan region of Santiago, Chile. Patients at the primary care centers with BP ≥140/90 mmHg are referred to the CVHP and screened for associated cardiovascular risk factors (diabetes, dyslipidemias, and renal failure). Approximately every 3 months they were followed by a team of primary care physicians, dietitians, and trained medical assistants providing clinical evaluation, assessment of life style habits, and counseling for modification of unhealthy behavior.

Hypertensive patients followed in the selected centers were considered for inclusion in the study; a randomly selected sample of 992 was obtained from 14,363 patients under care in these centers. Data was collected between 2011 and 2014. The sampling size was estimated for an expected prevalence of BP < 140/90 mmHg of 50%, with 95% of confidence, estimated error of 5%, and design effect of 2.5. None of these patients have been part of a previous study completed between 2009 and 2010 in different primary care centers in the Santiago Metropolitan Region.

Inclusion criteria considered patients between 30 and 64 years of age, who had completed at least a year in the CVHP receiving antihypertensive drug therapy at the time of recruitment. Patients with significant disabilities (bedridden, mentally incompetent, and wheel chair users), pregnant women, or with frequent unjustified missed appointments were excluded (n=17). Excluded patients were replaced according to a random procedure using the EPI-Info software.

Patients were invited to participate in the study by trained medical assistants working at the primary care centers. It was explained to patients that their participation only implied an agreement to authorize the information collected to be analyzed and eventually published without compromising their privacy and ensuring confidentiality. If initial hesitation from patients to participate was encountered, follow-up of contacts was carried out to address all their concerns. Finally, all patients initially invited consented to participate (Figure 1).

Patients with documented associated cardiovascular comorbidities (coronary heart disease, valvular heart disease, and rhythm disturbances) or requiring hemodialysis were referred to secondary (specialist) level of care before randomization and therefore not included in the study (3.17% of the eligible population, 14,363 patients).

2.2. Variables. 513 patients were recruited between August 2011 and June 2012 and 479 between August 2013 and June 2014. At the time of recruitment demographic, education, income, clinical, weight, and height data was obtained and questionnaires previously validated in compatible Chilean populations regarding adherence, psychosocial variables, and life style habits (smoking, use of alcohol, and physical activity) were filled at the clinic or within a week by the patients who preferred to do it at home; assistance to clarify questions was always available as requested. The blood chemistry values used in the analysis of the study were the most recent ones available at the time of recruitment. Data analysis was completed on 07/2016.

Trained medical assistants recorded BP values at each one of the patient's visits after three successive measurements with the patient sitting at least for 5 minutes using mercury sphygmomanometers and recording the average of the two last measurements. The BP value at the time of referral to the CVHP was interpreted as the baseline BP and the average of BP measurements recorded during the last year of follow-up preceding the time of recruitment in the study was considered the final BP results. The average time of care in the CVHP was 7.5 ± 4.6 years. Presence of diabetes and other comorbidities was established by clinical diagnosis and/or therapies prescribed. Blood chemistries that included fasting blood glucose, total and HDL cholesterol, and HbA1 in diabetics were measured using standard techniques. Weight was measured using a calibrated digital scale with patients in underwear and barefoot. Body mass index (BMI) was calculated dividing the weight in kilograms by the square of height in meters. All the antihypertensive medications in use at the time of recruitment were recorded.

Family income was defined as the ratio between the total monthly family income and total number of members in the family. Low family income was defined as < than the lower quartile of monthly income for individuals (< US$ 80/per

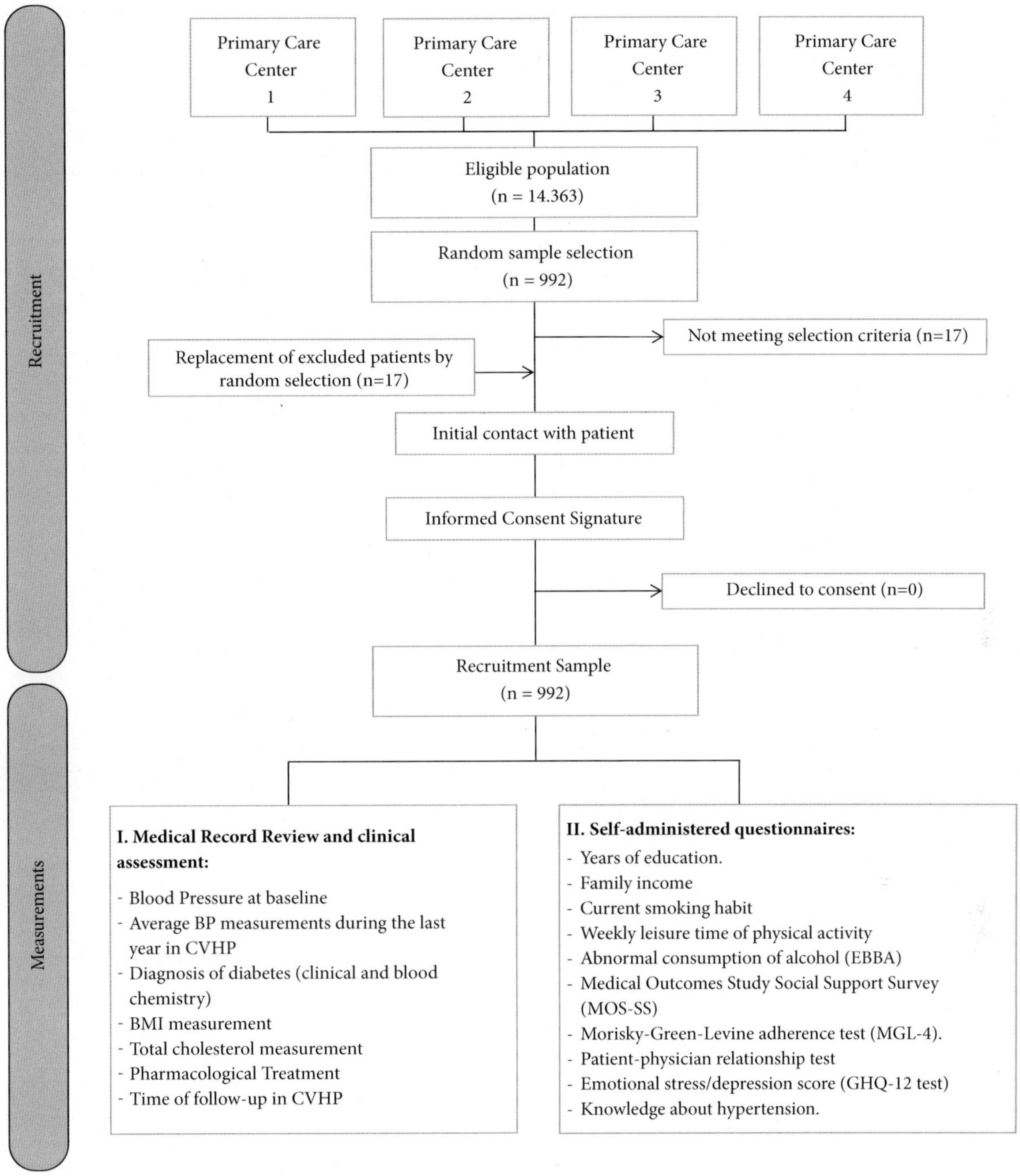

FIGURE 1: Recruitment process and procedures followed after patient's agreement to participate in the study.

person). Low education corresponded to < than 8 years of schooling.

2.3. Demographic and Psychosocial Characteristics Measurements

(1) The Morisky-Green-Levine (MGL-4) [15, 16]: a four-item questionnaire was utilized to assess adherence to Rx. A positive answer = 1 point; a negative response = 0 point. A patient is considered no adherent with a score of 1 or higher. This test has an alpha Cronbach value of 0.61 for controlled BP predictive value at 5 years [16]. A sensitivity analysis considering a score of 2 or higher for no adherence was carried out and results are included in Supplemental Table (available here) and discussed in results.

(2) MOS-SS (Medical Outcome Study Social Support Survey) [17], adapted to Spanish and validated for its use in Chilean primary care. It collects multidimensional information about the levels of support that the patient can access.

(3) Knowledge about hypertension: the following questionnaire was utilized: *Is hypertension a life-long condition? Is it possible to control it by diet and medications? Mention two or more organs that may be damaged by high BP*. An incorrect answer to any of these questions is indicative of low knowledge.

(4) Emotional Stress/ Depression score: A Chilean validated Spanish version of the GHQ-12 questionnaire was utilized [18]. This test detects and grades the levels of emotional stress and depression.

(5) Patient-physician relations: a version of a Chilean validated questionnaire by Bozzo-Martinez [19] to assess the patient satisfaction with care received at the primary care center was utilized. A score of 71 or less was considered indicative of inadequate patient-physician relation.

(6) Smoking: smokers were defined as those currently smoking at the time of the study.

(7) Use of alcohol: it was evaluated using the EBBA [20] survey (Brief Survey of Abnormal Drinking) to identify alcohol related abnormal behavior, previously validated and of common use in Chile [21].

(8) Physical activity: physically active patients were defined as those who electively exercised for at least 30 minutes three times a week [21].

Using currently accepted clinical guidelines we classified controlled BP as < 140/90 mmHg, elevated total cholesterol as ≥ 200 mg/dl, and obesity as body mass index ≥ 30 kg/m^2. Multiple antihypertensive drug therapy was defined when patients were prescribed 2 or more drugs.

The Ethic Committee of Research in Humans of the University of Chile Faculty of Medicine approved the study protocol.

2.4. Statistical Analysis. Exploratory analysis for the continuous variables was performed. Categorical variables were expressed as absolute or relative frequencies. Continuous variables were measured as medians (percentile 25 and 75). Differences according to sex, BP control, and adherence for categorical variables were analyzed using the X^2 test and Mann–Whitney test for continuous variables; p value <0.05 was considered a significant difference.

For uncontrolled BP (≥ 140/90 mmHg) odds ratio (OR) with 95% of confidence intervals was calculated. In Model 1 (unadjusted model) a univariate logistic analysis was performed in reference to uncontrolled BP, which included age (years), baseline systolic and diastolic BP (mmHg), time of care in the CVHP (years), and BMI (kg/m^2) as continuous variables and sex (male), low education (< 8 years of educations), low family income (< 80 US$ per person/month), inadequate patient-physician relation (score ≤ 71), high emotional stress-depression (score ≥7), low social support (score <57), low knowledge about hypertension (score ≥1), no adherence (score ≥ 1), multiple antihypertensive RX (≥ 2 drug antihypertensive), diabetes mellitus, elevated total cholesterol (≥ 200 mg/dL), smoking (current), alcohol related abnormal use (score ≥2), and sedentary behavior (<30 minx3/week of leisure physical activity) as dichotomous variables.

In Model 2, all variables that were statistically significant at the p<0.05 level in the unadjusted model were included in the multivariable logistic regression analysis. For no adherence a similar univariate logistic analysis was conducted (Model 1), using in the multivariable logistic regression analysis (Model 2) all the univariate variables that showed statistical significance at the p<0.05 level.

3. Results

3.1. Demographic, Socioeconomic, Clinical, and Antihypertensive Therapy and Anthropometric Characteristics. A larger number of women (n=647, 65.2%) than men (n=345, 34.8%) were part of this study. Low family income and low education level were documented in 23.0 and 33.2%, respectively. Obesity (BMI ≥ 30 kg/m^2) was found in 58.4% of patients; higher in women than men (61.1% versus 53.3%, p=0.019), and 37.8% were diabetics (42.3% men, 35.4% women, p=0.032) (Table 1).

The baseline median BP value was 146/91 mmHg. The median BP value corresponding to the last year of care in CVHP at the time of recruitment was 132/80 mmHg. BP control was achieved in 63.1% of patients (66.0% women versus 57.7% men, p=0.01). Adherence to Rx was 38.4%, greater in women (41.1% versus 33.3%, p= 0.016). Alcohol abnormal behavior was more frequent in men (25.5% versus 7.4%, p<0.001); no sex differences were observed in current smoking (25.4%) and sedentary life style prevalence (83%). Multiple drug therapy was prescribed in 46.9% (41.2% men and 49.6% women, p= 0.011).

3.2. Factors Associated with Uncontrolled Blood Pressure. Male sex (OR: 1.73 [95% CI 1.35 - 2.22]), low family income, high emotional-stress-depression score (OR: 1.32 [95% CI 1.03 - 1.70]), BMI, no adherence (OR: 1.83 [95% CI 1.44 - 2.32]), multiple antihypertensive drug therapy (OR: 1.53 [95% CI 1.21 - 1.94]), baseline systolic BP value (OR: 1.03 [95% CI 1.02 - 1.04]), and sedentary life style (OR: 1.61 [95% CI 1.15 - 2.25]) were significantly associated with uncontrolled BP in Model 2 (adjusted model). The time of care patients received in the CVHP was not predictive of uncontrolled BP in Model 2 (Table 2).

3.3. Factors Associated with No Adherence to Prescribed Antihypertensive Medications. No adherence was significantly associated with uncontrolled BP (OR: 1.52 [95% CI 1.22 - 1.90]), male sex (OR: 1.54 [95% CI 1.23 - 1.93]), low family income (OR: 1.39 [95% CI 1.11 - 1.72]), high emotional stress-depression score (OR: 2.15 [95% CI 1.68 - 2.76]), and low social support in Model 2 (adjusted). The time of care under the CVHP showed no association with no adherence in the univariate logistic analysis (Model 1). In contrast, diabetes mellitus (OR: 0.81 [95% CI 0.66 - 0.99]) was significantly associated with better adherence (in Models 1 and 2; Table 3).

It is noteworthy the associations of no adherence with uncontrolled BP, male sex, and psychosocial factors did not change after a sensitivity analysis using a no adherence MGL-4 score 2 or greater (Supplementary Table).

TABLE 1: Demographic, socioeconomic, clinical, and antihypertensive therapy and anthropometric characteristics (n=992).

Participant Characteristics	Total (n= 992)	Men (n=345)	Women (n=647)	*p-value*
Demographic and socioeconomic characteristics				
Age (years)	56.0 (50 - 61) [a]	57.0 (51 - 62) [a]	55.0 (49 - 61) [a]	<0.01
Low education (<8 years of education)	329 (33.2)	103 (29.9)	226 (34.9)	0.11
Low family income (<US$80 per person/month)	228 (23.0)	53 (15.4)	175 (27.0)	<0.001
Psychosocial variables				
Inadequate patient –physician relation[*874]	202 (23.1)	63 (21.0)	139 (24.2)	0.28
High emotional stress-depression score	258 (26.0)	59 (17.1)	199 (30.8)	<0.001
Low social support	338 (34.1)	88 (25.5)	250 (38.6)	<0.001
Low family Cohesion	366 (36.9)	95 (27.5)	271 (41.9)	<0.001
Self-perception of health (poor-very poor)	177 (17.8)	48 (13.9)	129 (19.9)	0.018
Knowledge about hypertension	542 (54.6)	190 (55.1)	352 (54.4)	0.84
Blood Pressure				
Systolic blood pressure (mmHg)	132 (123.3 – 143.2) [a]	133 (124.3 – 144.9) [a]	131 (123.0 – 142.7) [a]	0.033
Diastolic blood pressure (mmHg)	80 (75.0 – 86.7) [a]	82.0 (76.7 – 80.0) [a]	80.0 (75.0 – 86.5) [a]	0.006
Blood pressure control (BP<140/90 mmHg)	626 (63.1)	199 (57.7)	427 (66.0)	0.010
Baseline Systolic blood pressure (mmHg)	146 (140 -160) [a]	150 (140 – 160) [a]	144 (140 – 160) [a]	0.134
Baseline Diastolic blood pressure (mmHg)	91 (90 – 100) [a]	92.0 (90 – 100) [a]	90 (90.9 – 100) [a]	0.270
Time of care in CVHP (years)	7.0 (4.0 – 10.7) [a]	6.3 (3.5 – 8.9) [a]	7.5 (4.3 – 11.4) [a]	<0.001
Clinical variables				
Diabetes mellitus (clinical diagnosis)	375 (37.8)	146 (42.3)	229 (35.4)	0.032
Total Cholesterol (mg/dL)[*865]	200 (172 – 230) [a]	193.0 (166 – 227) [a]	203 (177 – 232) [a]	0.005
Elevated total cholesterol (≥ 200 mg/dL)[*865]	439 (50.8)	138 (45.7)	201 (53.5)	0.031
Antihypertensive treatment variables				
Multiple antihypertensive drug therapy (≥ 2 drugs)	463 (46.9)	142 (41.2)	321 (49.6)	0.011
Adherence to pharmacological therapy	381 (38.4)	115 (33.3)	266 (41.1)	0.016
Anthropometrics variables				
Weight (Kg)	78.0 (68.4 – 89.7) [a]	84.2 (76.0 – 96.1) [a]	75.0 (66.0 – 84.9) [a]	<0.001
Height (m)	1.57 (1.52 – 1.64) [a]	1.67 (1.63 – 1.71) [a]	1.53 (1.49 – 1.57) [a]	<0.001
Body mass index (Kg/m^2)	31.2 (28.0 – 34.9) [a]	30.6 (27.8 – 33.9) [a]	31.5 (28.2 – 35.7) [a]	0.001
Obesity (BMI ≥ 30 Kg/m^2)	579 (58.4)	184 (53.3)	395 (61.1)	0.019
Lifestyle habits				
Smoking (Current smoker)	253 (25.4)	87 (25.2)	165 (25.5)	0.88
Alcohol related abnormal behavior	136 (13.7)	88 (25.5)	48 (7.4)	<0.001
Sedentary (<30 minx3/week of leisure physical activity)	823 (83.0)	284 (82.3)	539 (83.3)	0.82

[a] Median values (percentile 25–75) or n (%); [*]number of patients in whom measurement was performed. All values included in Table 1 were determined at the time of recruitment to the study with the exception of baseline BP measurement indicative of values at the time of referral of patients to the CVHP. Systolic and diastolic BP and BP control at time of recruitment considers the average of the values in the last year at time of recruitment.

4. Discussion

The BP control (63.1%) observed in this sample of hypertensive patients enrolled in the CVHP compares favorably with results published in many high-income countries [22–25]. In addition, our results contrast with a 2004 study in a Chilean Southern region urban population that showed BP control in 30.7% of 1,838 patients under antihypertensive therapy [26], and the 2010 Chilean National Health survey that reported BP control in 45.3% of hypertensive patients who informed to be under treatment [21]. More recently, a study from a CVHP cohort showed BP control of 59.7% [10]. The adherence to antihypertensive drug therapy in our study was only 38.4%, but there is no reliable information of adherence in Chilean hypertensive patients for comparison with results prior to the CVHP. The influences of adherence in the results of our study are illustrated by the significant association found of uncontrolled hypertension to no adherence, consistent with many previous observations [3, 5, 9, 22]. Although the use of the MGL-4 questionnaire may have possibly overestimated the actual no adherence, it is also conceivable that the comprehensive multidisciplinary support provided

TABLE 2: Multivariable adjusted odds ratio for uncontrolled BP (≥140/90 mm/Hg) in hypertensive patients followed in the Cardiovascular Health Program.

	BP <140/90 mmHg n= 626 n (%)	BP ≥140/90 mmHg n= 366 n (%)	Model 1 Unadjusted Odds Ratio (CI 95%)	Model 2 Adjusted Odds Ratio* (CI 95%)
Demographic and socioeconomic characteristic				
Age (years)	56 (49 - 61)[a]	58 (50 - 63) [a]‡	**1.03 (1.01 – 1.04)**‡	1.01 (0.99 – 1.03)
Male sex	199 (31.8)	146 (39.9)‡	**1.56 (1.30 – 1.86)**‡	**1.73 (1.35 – 2.22)**‡
Low education (<8 years of education)	191 (30.5)	138 (37.7)†	**1.58 (1.31 – 1.90)**‡	1.21 (0.94 – 1.56)
Low family income (<US$80 per person/month)	189 (30.2)	124 (34.0)	1.19 (0.99 – 1.44)	**1.44 (1.13 – 1.84)**‡
Psychosocial variables				
Inadequate patient –physician relation	179 (31.1)	100 (33.4)	1.20 (0.99 – 1.47)	1.07 (0.84 – 1.37)
High emotional stress-depression score	153 (24.4)	105 (28.7)	**1.29 (1.06 – 1.57)**†	**1.32 (1.03 – 1.70)**†
Low social support	221 (33.7)	127 (34.7)	1.15 (0.96 – 1.38)	1.08 (0.85 – 1.37)
Low knowledge about hypertension	333 (53.2)	209 (57.1)	1.15 (0.97 – 1.38)	1.17 (0.93 – 1.47)
Antihypertensive treatment variables				
No adherence	360 (57.5)	251 (68.6)†	**1.67 (1.39 – 2.00)**‡	**1.83 (1.44 – 2.32)**‡
Multiple antihypertensive RX	255 (40.7)	280 (56.8)‡	**1.73 (1.45 – 2.07)**‡	**1.53 (1.21 – 1.94)**‡
Time of care in CVHP (years)	6.6 (4.0 – 9.9) [a]	7.6 (3.9 – 11.5) [a]†	**1.03 (1.01 – 1.05)**‡	1.00 (0.97 – 1.02)
Systolic blood pressure baseline in CVHP	140 (134.5 – 152) [a]	150 (140 – 164.2) [a]‡	**1.03 (1.03 – 1.04)**‡	**1.03 (1.02 – 1.04)**‡
Diastolic blood pressure baseline in CVHP	90 (90– 100) [a]	96 (90 -100) [a]‡	**1.02 (1.01 – 1.03)**‡	1.00 (0.99 – 1.01)
Anthropometrics and clinical variables				
Diabetes mellitus	248 (39.6)	127 (34.7)	0.88 (0.74 - 1.06)	0.87 (0.69 – 1.09)
Elevated total cholesterol (≥ 200 mg/dL)	289 (50.3)	150 (51.5)	1.01 (0.83 – 1.22)	1.07 (0.86 – 1.34)
BMI (Kg/m^2)	30.8 (27.8 – 34.2) [a]	32.1 (28.5 – 36.1) [a]‡	**1.05 (1.03 – 1.06)**‡	**1.04 (1.02 – 1.07)**‡
Lifestyle habits				
Smoking (current smoker)	170 (27.2)	82 (22.4)	**0.74 (0.60 – 0.90)**‡	1.00 (0.78 – 1.30)
Alcohol related abnormal behavior	69 (11.0)	67 (18.3)‡	**1.69 (1.32 – 2.15)**‡	1.23 (0.89 – 1.71)
Sedentary	505 (80.7)	318 (86.9)‡	**1.60 (1.25 – 2.05)**‡	**1.61 (1.15 – 2.25)**‡

[a] Median values (percentile 25–75); †p <0.05, ‡p <0.01. *OR adjusted for all the variables that were significant at the p<0.05 level in unadjusted model: age (years), systolic and diastolic blood pressure baseline in CVHP (mmHg), and time of follow-up in CVHP (years) and BMI (Kg/m^2) as continuous variables. Sex (male), low education (< 8 years of educations), high emotional stress-depression (score ≥7), no adherence (score≥ 1), multiple antihypertensive RX (≥ 2 drug antihypertensive), alcohol related abnormal (score ≥2), smoking (current), and sedentary (<30 minx3/week of leisure physical activity) as dichotomous variables.

the CVHP may have partially offset the negative influence of low antihypertensive drug therapy adherence in our results. The lack of association in the time patients received care in the CVHP and uncontrolled BP suggests that the beneficial influence of the program in achieving BP control may begin early and do not fade with a longer permanence of patients in it. It is of note that our findings are similar to those of the ALLHAT trial in USA that documented BP control in 56.2% of the patients after 1 year of management [25] through a similar free universal comprehensive management as in the CVHP. In this study Hispanics had 20% greater odds of achieving BP control than Non-Hispanic Whites, reversing dramatically previously documented trends between these racial/ethnic groups in USA [24].

The significant association of male sex, low family income, high emotional-stress-depression, no adherence to treatment (Rx), high BMI, multiple antihypertensive drug therapy, baseline systolic BP value, and sedentary life style with uncontrolled BP in our study is in agreement with previous studies [3, 4, 6, 7, 9]. Also we found a significant association of uncontrolled BP with low social support and male sex, factors that were also significantly predictive of no adherence. Conflictive results in the association of sex with BP control in treated hypertensive patients have been published [27, 28]. However, a study done in 5 European countries, Canada, and USA that included 73,446 patients showed that BP control in hypertensive patients was 2-fold higher in women compared with men in Spain, Italy, Canada, and the United States [29]. It is of note that none of these studies analyzed the association of BP control and adherence, or with socioeconomic and psychosocial factors. To the best of our knowledge, no previous study has documented that no adherence to Rx in men may contribute to the reported differences in BP control with women. The inferior BP control in men may be likely related to their larger no adherence, which may be also a factor partially involved in

TABLE 3: Multivariable adjusted odds ratio for no adherence risk to antihypertensive in hypertensive patients followed in the Cardiovascular Health Program.

	Adherence n= 381 n (%)	No Adherence n= 611 n (%)	Model 1 Unadjusted Odds Ratio (CI 95%)	Model 2 Adjusted Odds Ratio* (CI 95%)
Demographic and socioeconomic characteristic				
Age	56 (50 - 61)[a]	55 (49 – 61)[a]	0.99 (0.98 – 1.00)	0.99 (0.98 – 1.00)
Male sex	115 (30.2)	230 (37.6)†	**1.47 (1.22 - 1.76)‡**	**1.54 (1.23 – 1.93)‡**
Low education (<8 years of education)	119 (31.2)	210 (34.4)	1.12 (0.93 - 1.35)	1.06 (0.85 – 1.32)
Low family income (<US$80 per person month)	68 (17.8)	160 (26.2)‡	**1.66 (1.35 – 2.06)‡**	**1.39 (1.11 – 1.72)‡**
Psychosocial variables				
Inadequate patient –physician relation	95 (28.1)	184 (34.3)†	**1.33 (1.09 – 1.63)‡**	1.04 (0.84 – 1.29)
High emotional stress-depression score	76 (19.9)	182 (29.8)‡	**1.84 (1.49 – 2.26)‡**	**2.15 (1.68 – 2.76)‡**
Low social support	113 (29.7)	225 (36.8)†	**1.44 (1.19 – 1.73)‡**	**1.34 (1.08 – 1.66)‡**
Low Knowledge about hypertension	200 (52.5)	342 (56.0)	1.08 (0.91 – 1.28)	0.98 (0.81 – 1.21)
Antihypertensive treatment variables				
Uncontrolled BP (≥ 140/90 mmHg)	160 (42.0)	305 (49.9)†	**1.67 (1.39 – 2.00)‡**	**1.52 (1.22 – 1.90)‡**
Multiple antihypertensive RX	197 (51.7)	266 (43.5)†	**0.81 (0.68 – 0.96)†**	0.92 (0.75 – 1.13)
Time of care in CVHP (years)	6.9 (3.9 – 11.9) [a]	6.7 (3.9 – 10.2) [a]	0.98 (0.96 – 1.00)	0.98 (0.95 – 1.00)
Systolic blood pressure baseline in CVHP	150 (140 - 160) [a]	145 (140 - 160) [a]	1.00 (0.99 – 1.00)	1.00 (0.99 – 1.00)
Diastolic blood pressure baseline in CVHP	94 (90 - 100)	90 (90 - 100)	0.99 (0.98 – 1.00)	1.00 (0.99 – 1.00)
Anthropometrics and clinical variables				
Diabetes mellitus	156 (40.9)	219 (35.8)	**0.80 (0.67 – 0.95)†**	**0.81 (0.66 – 0.99)†**
Elevated total cholesterol (≥ 200 mg/dL)	160 (48.3)	273 (52.7)	**1.23 (1.02 – 1.48)†**	**1.26 (1.04 – 1.54)†**
BMI (Kg/m^2)	31 (28 - 35)[a]	31 (27 – 35) [a]	1.00 (0.99 – 1.02)	1.00 (0.98 – 1.02)
Lifestyle habits				
Smoking (Current smoker)	97 (25.5)	156 (25.5)	0.98 (0.81 – 1.19)	0.98 (0.78 – 1.22)
Alcohol related abnormal behavior	39 (10.2)	97 (15.9)†	**1.55 (1.19 – 2.01)‡**	1.18 (0.86 – 1.60)
Sedentary	310 (81.4)	513 (84.0)	1.16 (0.92 – 1.45)	0.98 (0.75 – 1.29)

[a]Median values (percentile 25 – 75); †p <0.05, ‡p <0.01. *OR adjusted for all the variables that were significant at the p<0.05 level in unadjusted model: sex (male), low family income <US$80 per person/month), inadequate patient-physician relation (score ≤ 71), high emotional stress-depression (score ≥7), low social support (score <57), uncontrolled BP (≥ 140/90 mmHg), multiple antihypertensive RX (≥ 2 drug antihypertensive), diabetes, elevate total cholesterol (≥ 200 mg/dL), and alcohol related abnormal (score ≥2) as dichotomous variables.

their underrepresentation in our study. It is also conceivable that the comprehensive multidisciplinary services provided by the CVHP may contribute in reducing patients negative expectations about therapies (the nocebo [30] effects that induce a reduction of their efficacy and or tolerance) and eventually lead to an improvement in compliance. In addition, conflicts with their work activities are a well-known factor limiting access of men to health care, issue that is a challenge for the Chilean health care services. Nevertheless, the proportion of men in our study (women/ men = 1.87) showed a slight increase when compared to the ratio found in a previous study (2.15) from a similar population followed in the CVHP [10], possibly reflecting a favorable trend in the recruitment of men to the program (please see Table 4).

The association of low family income, high emotional stress/depression, and low social support in our study underscored the significance of socioeconomic and psychosocial factors in BP control and adherence [6, 8, 31–34]. We also found that low income was associated with no adherence, despite patient's unrestricted free access to health care and drug therapy but consistent with previous observations and indicative of the complex causal pathways and well-documented relations of socioeconomic position and health [6, 8, 31]. Our finding that adherence to (Rx) appeared not to be hampered but favored by the association with diabetes has been noted by others in a study in hypertensive patients receiving multiple drug therapy due to comorbidities [35]. As discussed by these authors, hypertensive patients with associated comorbidities may be more aware of being at a higher risk and then more willing to follow the recommended drug therapy. It is of note that we found no differences in BP control between diabetics and nondiabetics, in contrast to a previous study from a CVHP population that showed worse BP control in diabetics [10] (Table 4). Since adherence was only measured in our current and more recent study it is uncertain if this difference also reflected adherence improvements in diabetics that plausibly may have occurred in the interim. These changes are significant achievements in

Table 4: Comparative values of BP control by sex, presence of diabetes, and adherence in the evaluation of two different groups from the CVHP.

	2009 -2010 [10] n = 1,194	*p-value*	2011-2014 n = 992	*p-value*
Sex				
Women	69.1 %	<0.01	65.2 %	<0.01
Men	31.9 %		34.8 %	
BP according to sex				
BP control in women	63.7 %	<0.01	66.0 %	0.01
BP control in men	52.4%		57.7 %	
BP control and diabetes				
BP control in diabetics	53.2 %∗	<0.01	66.1 %∗	0.12
BP control in nondiabetics	62.4 %		61.3 %	
Adherence and diabetes				
Adherence in diabetics	- -		41.6 %	0.10
Adherence in nondiabetics	- -		36.5 %	

∗ p<0.01, difference between groups.

a population with such alarming rates of obesity and diabetes (58.4 and 37.5 %, respectively).

Our study has several limitations. The underrepresentation of men as compared to women (women/men=1.87) in this cohort is a persistent problem in the CVHP, although an improvement trend may be already occurring (Table 4). As discussed, it has been attributed to conflicts with labor activities of men in Chile, but also probably reflective of the greater no adherence to therapy found in men. It is uncertain if the results of this study are applicable to patients that stayed in the program for less than 1 year or were older than 64 years of age (not included in this study). Although hypertensive patients with cardiovascular comorbidities or undergoing hemodialysis were referred to a second level of care (specialist) and not followed in the CVHP, it is unlikely that their small proportion could have influenced our results (3.17% of the eligible population). Finally, physical activity was assessed throughout a questionnaire used in the 2010 Chilean National Health Survey [21] that only counted time spend in leisure type of exercise and did not consider physical activity involved in transportation or work (bicycle, walking), common in the study population. This may explain the high number of sedentary subjects found in our study (86.9%).

5. Conclusions

Our study emphasizes the importance of socioeconomic and psychosocial factors influencing BP control and adherence in hypertensive patients in a developing society. The underrepresentation of hypertensive men enrolled in the CVHP, their worse BP control, and adherence represents an important challenge to address in this program. Nevertheless, our findings underscore an important historical improvement in BP control in Chile, a developing country in a stage of advanced socioeconomic transition, that we attribute to the implementation of a comprehensive, multidisciplinary approach in the management of hypertensive patients (CVHP) providing free of copayments medical care, and counseling in lifestyle modifying changes, with results in BP control similar to some of those reported in high-income societies [25, 35, 36]. These favorable results were highlighted by the results noted in the hypertensive diabetic group, a particularly vulnerable population, with CVHP historical improvement in BP control and similar adherence as nondiabetic hypertensive. The lack of influence of time spend by patients in the program to achieve favorable BP results provides additional support to the consideration of programs similar to the CVHP in the developing world.

Disclosure

The opinions contained in this work are exclusively from the authors and do not represent necessarily those from University of Chile School of Medicine, University of California, San Diego, California, and Institutional Review Board of Sharp Health Care, San Diego, California. A presentation of the content of this work was made at the 2017 American Heart Association QOCR meeting, April 2-3, 2017, Arlington, Virginia.

Authors' Contributions

Daniela Sandoval contributed in the study design, data collection, data analysis, and manuscript writing. Carolina Nazzal contributed in the study design, data analysis, and manuscript writing. Tomás Romero contributed in the study planning and design, data analysis, manuscript writing, and obtaining partial research funding.

Acknowledgments

This research has been partially financed by a Grant from Fundación Araucaria Foundation, San Diego, California.

References

[1] P. M. Kearney, M. Whelton, K. Reynolds, P. Muntner, P. K. Whelton, and J. He, "Global burden of hypertension: analysis of worldwide data," *The Lancet*, vol. 365, no. 9455, pp. 217–223, 2005.

[2] World Heart Federation, *Cardiovascular Disease Report*, State of the Heart, 2010, http://www.paho.org/col/index.php?option=com_docman&view=download&alias=649-state-of-the-heart-cvd-report-240910&category_slug=publicaciones-ops-oms-colombia&Itemid=688.

[3] A. V. Chobanian, G. L. Bakris, H. R. Black et al., "The seventh report of the joint national committee on prevention, detection, evaluation, and treatment of high blood pressure: the JNC 7 report," *The Journal of the American Medical Association*, vol. 289, no. 19, pp. 2560–2572, 2003.

[4] I. Hajjar and T. A. Kotchen, "Trends in prevalence, awareness, treatment, and control of hypertension in the United States, 1988–2000," *Journal of the American Medical Association*, vol. 290, no. 2, pp. 199–206, 2003.

[5] "The Task Force for the management of arterial hypertension of the European Society of Hypertension (ESH) and of the European Society of Cardiology (ESC)," in *2013 ESH/ESC Guidelines for the management of arterial hypertension*, vol. 34, pp. 2159–2219, European Heart Journal, 2013.

[6] S. Basu and C. Millet, "Determinants of Prevalence, Diagnosis, Treatment, and Control in the WHO SAGE Study," *Hypertension*, vol. 62, no. 1, pp. 18–26, 2013.

[7] D. E. Bloom, E. T. Cafiero, E. Jané-Llopis et al., *The Global Economic Burden of Noncommunicable Diseases*, World Economic Forum, 2011.

[8] M. Marmot, "Social determinants of health inequalities," *The Lancet*, vol. 365, no. 9464, pp. 1099–1104, 2005.

[9] C. Bourgault, M. Sénécal, M. Brisson, M. A. Marentette, and J.-P. Grégoire, "Persistence and discontinuation patterns of antihypertensive therapy among newly treated patients: A population-based study," *Journal of Human Hypertension*, vol. 19, no. 8, pp. 607–613, 2005.

[10] D. Sandoval, M. Bravo, E. Koch et al., "Overcoming Barriers in the Management of Hypertension: The Experience of the Cardiovascular Health Program in Chilean Primary Health Care Centers," *International Journal of Hypertension*, vol. 2012, pp. 1–8, 2012.

[11] 2016, http://www.worldbank.com.

[12] T. J. Bossert and T. Leisewitz, "Innovation and change in the chilean health system," *The New England Journal of Medicine*, vol. 374, no. 1, pp. 1–5, 2016.

[13] Ministry of Health, 2016, http://www.supersalud.gob.cl/normativa/668/articles-13722_recurso_1.pdf.

[14] Ministry of Health, *Area of Analysis*, Department of Statistics and Health Information, 2012.

[15] D. E. Morisky, L. W. Green, and D. M. Levine, "Concurrent and predictive validity of a self-reported measure of medication adherence," *Medical Care*, vol. 24, no. 1, pp. 67–74, 1986.

[16] D. E. Morisky, A. Ang, M. Krousel-Wood, and H. J. Ward, "Predictive validity of a medication adherence measure in an outpatient setting," *The Journal of Clinical Hypertension*, vol. 10, no. 5, pp. 348–354, 2008.

[17] C. D. Sherbourne and A. L. Stewart, "The MOS social support survey," *Social Science & Medicine*, vol. 32, no. 6, pp. 705–714, 1991.

[18] D. P. Golberg and V. F. Hillier, "A scale version of the General Health Questionnaire," *Psychological Medicine*, vol. 9, no. 1, pp. 139–145, 1979.

[19] G. Bozzo, B. Martínez, P. Sepúlveda et al., "Development and validation of a survey for patients satisfaction in primary care clinics," *Revista Medica De Chile*, vol. 123, pp. 1160–1164, 1995.

[20] E. Florenzano, N. Horwitz, M. Penna, and M. Valdés, "alidation of an abbreviated scale for detection of abnormal drinking behavior (E.B.B.A) (Escala Breve para la detección del Beber Anormal)," in *Mental Health and Primary Health Care subjects (Temas de Salud Mental y Atención Primaria de Salud.)*, pp. 185–193, Facultad de Medicina, Universidad de Chile, 1991.

[21] Ministry of Health (Ministerio de Salud, MINSAL), National Health Survey, Chile, Vol. 1. Santiago, 2009-2010. http://web.minsal.cl/search/node/Encuesta%20MINSAL.

[22] T. G. Pickering, "Why are we doing so badly with the control of hypertension? Poor compliance is only part of the story," *The Journal of Clinical Hypertension*, vol. 3, no. 3, pp. 179–182, 2001.

[23] A. L. Valderrama, C. Gillespie, and C. Mercado, "Racial/Ethnic Disparities in the Awareness, Treatment and Control of Hypertension- United States," in *Centers for Disease Control and Prevention*, vol. 62, 354, MMWR, 352 edition, 2013, http://www.cdc.gov/nchs/nhanes/response_rates_cps.htm.

[24] A. V. Chobanian, "The hypertension paradox - More uncontrolled disease despite improved therapy," *The New England Journal of Medicine*, vol. 361, no. 9, pp. 848–887, 2009.

[25] K. L. Margolis, L. B. Piller, C. E. Ford et al., "Blood pressure control in hispanics in the antihypertensive and lipid-lowering treatment to prevent heart attack trial," *Hypertension*, vol. 50, no. 5, pp. 854–861, 2007.

[26] E. Fasce, I. Campos, P. Ibáñez et al., "Trends in prevalence, awareness, treatment and control of hypertension in urban communities in Chile," *Journal of Hypertension*, vol. 25, no. 9, pp. 1807–1811, 2007.

[27] K. L. Ong, A. W. K. Tso, K. S. L. Lam, and B. M. Y. Cheung, "Gender difference in blood pressure control and cardiovascular risk factors in Americans with diagnosed hypertension," *Hypertension*, vol. 51, no. 4, pp. 1142–1148, 2008.

[28] S. Keyhani, J. V. Scobie, P. L. Hebert, and M. A. McLaughlin, "Gender disparities in blood pressure control and cardiovascular care in a national sample of ambulatory care visits," *Hypertension*, vol. 51, no. 4, pp. 1149–1155, 2008.

[29] K. Wolf-Maier, R. S. Cooper, H. Kramer et al., "Hypertension treatment and control in five european countries, Canada, and the United States," *Hypertension*, vol. 43, no. 1, pp. 10–17, 2004.

[30] L. Colloca and D. Finniss, "Nocebo effects, patient-clinician communication, and therapeutic outcomes," *Journal of the American Medical Association*, vol. 307, no. 6, pp. 567-568, 2012.

[31] C. M. Eze-Nliam, B. D. Thombs, B. B. Lima, C. G. Smith, and R. C. Ziegelstein, "The association of depression with adherence to antihypertensive medications: A systematic review," *Journal of Hypertension*, vol. 28, no. 9, pp. 1785–1795, 2010.

[32] A. V. Diez Roux, "Persistent social patterning of cardiovascular risk: Rethinking the familiar," *Circulation*, vol. 111, no. 23, pp. 3020-3021, 2005.

[33] C. Bane, C. M. Hughes, and J. C. McElnay, "The impact of depressive symptoms and psychosocial factors on medication adherence in cardiovascular disease," *Patient Education and Counseling*, vol. 60, no. 2, pp. 187–193, 2006.

[34] E.-L. Wu, I.-C. Chien, C.-H. Lin, Y.-J. Chou, and P. Chou, "Increased risk of hypertension in patients with major depressive disorder: A population-based study," *Journal of Psychosomatic Research*, vol. 73, no. 3, pp. 169–174, 2012.

Nebivolol Attenuates Neutrophil Lymphocyte Ratio: A Marker of Subclinical Inflammation in Hypertensive Patients

Mazhar Hussain,[1] Muhammad Saeed,[2] Muhammad Zafar Majeed Babar,[3] Moazzam Ali Atif,[1] and Lubna Akhtar[1]

[1]*Department of Pharmacology & Therapeutics, Sheikh Zayed Medical College/Hospital, Rahim Yar Khan, Punjab, Pakistan*
[2]*Department of Biochemistry, University Medical & Dental College, Faisalabad, Punjab, Pakistan*
[3]*Department of Medicine, Sheikh Zayed Medical College/Hospital, Rahim Yar Khan, Punjab, Pakistan*

Correspondence should be addressed to Mazhar Hussain; mazharhussain214@gmail.com

Academic Editor: Tomohiro Katsuya

Background. High value of neutrophil lymphocyte ratio (NLR) is a strong independent predictor and biomarker of ongoing vascular inflammation in various cardiovascular disorders. *Objective.* The main focus of the study is to investigate the effect of nebivolol on NLR in mild to moderate hypertensive patients in comparison with metoprolol. In addition, BMI, blood pressure, TLC count, blood sugar, and lipid profile were also assayed before and after treatment. *Materials and Methods.* In this 12-week prospective double-blinded randomized study, 120 patients with mild to moderate hypertension were randomly divided into two groups to prescribed daily dose of tab nebivolol 5–10 mg and metoprolol 50–100 mg, respectively, for 12 weeks. The data were analyzed using SPSS 16 software. *Results.* A total of 100 patients completed the study. Both drugs lowered blood pressure significantly, nebivolol 20.5/10.5 and metoprolol 22.5/11.2 ($p < 0.001$) from baseline. Regarding inflammation, nebivolol reduced total leukocyte count ($p = 0.005$) and neutrophil count ($p = 0.003$) and increased lymphocyte count ($p = 0.004$) as compared to metoprolol. Similarly, nebivolol but not metoprolol significantly reduced NLR ratio ($p = 0.07$). Nebivolol improved lipid profile and blood sugar compared to metoprolol, but values were nonsignificant. *Conclusion.* Nebivolol has a strong impact on reducing NLR, a marker of subclinical inflammation in hypertensive patients. Moreover NLR can be used as a disease and drug monitoring tool in these patients.

1. Introduction

Hypertension affects about one-fourth of the adult population globally and this number will increase to 29% by year 2025. The prevalence of hypertension will be much higher in developing countries in upcoming years because of strong influence of urbanization and lifestyle changes to its underlying risk factors. In addition, healthcare facilities in developing world for routine screening of hypertensive patients are grossly underutilized. Approximately one-third of deaths in the world population are mainly due to cardiovascular disease with hypertension being one of its route cause. High blood pressure itself initiates a chain of events in vessels wall in the form oxidative stress, inflammation, and endothelial dysfunction that plays a fundamental role in initiation, progression, and complication of atherosclerosis in the form of cardiovascular diseases. Therefore multifaceted and multipronged strategies are needed to handle this health issue in both developed and developing nations in order to reduce economic and social disease burden [1, 2].

The role of increased leukocytes count in the pathogenesis of atherosclerosis is well understood that initiates a cascade of inflammatory reaction in the vessel wall. Increased leukocyte counts are reliable markers of systemic inflammation in clinical practice that has very strong association with coronary heart disease, cerebrovascular disease, and vascular complications associated with diabetes [3, 4]. In recent years, there was more focus on neutrophil lymphocyte ratio (NLR), which is determined in complete blood counts by simply dividing the absolute neutrophil count to absolute lymphocyte count. NLR is reliable biomarker of low grade inflammation in various clinical conditions such as diabetes, hypertension, metabolic syndrome, obesity, and lifestyle changes [5, 6]. NLR is a reliable marker of systemic inflammation and a routinely performed test because of its easy detection, availability, and cost effectiveness. It can also be used as a drug and disease monitoring tool in various diseases. Moreover, it provides prognostic as well as diagnostic information about subclinical inflammation beyond conventional risk factors. Moreover the prognosis value of NLR is comparable to C-reactive protein, tumor necrosis factor-α, and interleukin-1 in the detection of subclinical inflammation and endothelial dysfunction in various clinical trials [7–9].

Nebivolol is a highly cardioselective 3rd-generation long acting -1 blocker which is usually prescribed once a day as monotherapy or in combination with other antihypertensive drugs. It is only beta-blocker that has vasodilating properties and is safely prescribed in diabetics patients too as it does have any adverse effect on insulin sensitivity and serum lipid profile. It also does not cause sexual dysfunction like other beta-blockers even though it improves sexual dysfunction in diabetic patients. It also inhibits platelets aggregation, improves endothelial and left ventricular systolic dysfunction, and improves arterial stiffness, coronary and peripheral blood flow in patients of angina, myocardial infarction, chronic heart failure, and various arrhythmias [10, 11].

Apart from their beneficial effects on blood pressure, nebivolol has a very strong anti-inflammatory and antioxidant potential. Nebivolol reduces the level of various oxidative and inflammatory markers like oxidized LDL, 8-isoprostanes, CRP, interleukin- (IL-) 6, adiponectin, leptin, intercellular adhesions molecule (ICAM-1), vascular cell adhesions molecule (VCAM-1), and tumor necrosis factor-α in various clinical studies [12, 13]. However lab detection of these markers is costly and usually not performed on routine clinical setting. The present study was conducted to investigate the effect of nebivolol on neutrophil lymphocyte ratio (NLR) which is easily determined from routine blood test.

2. Patients and Methods

This twelve-week prospective randomized double-blinded clinical trial was carried out at cardiology outdoor of Sheikh Zayed Medical College/Hospital, Rahim Yar Khan, from 5 November 2016 to 5 January 2017. An ethical committee permission and written informed consent was obtained from all patients before enrollment. Initially two hundred and forty patients were recruited in cardiology outdoor unit on the basis of chief complaints of headache, dyspnea, dizziness, and insomnia. Out of which 120 patients, aged 32–56 years with mild to moderate hypertensions according to World Health Organization (WHO)/International Society of Hypertension (ISH) criteria [14], who were never treated with any hypertensive drug in past, were enrolled in the study. The exclusion criteria was all conditions which affect inflammation such as smoking, alcohol, any acute or chronic inflammatory diseases, diabetes, trauma, pregnancy, secondary hypertension, dyslipidemia, liver disorders, kidney dysfunction, ischemic heart disease, and CNS disorders. In addition, detailed history was taken about drugs which affect inflammation such as statins, NSAIDS, corticosteroids, oral contraceptive, opioids, and various immunosuppressive agents.

A randomization was done by allocation of random number in ascending order in blocks to all patients generated by computed software. All patients remained unknown about the treatment plan to each other throughout the study period. After randomization patients were divided into two equal groups to prescribe daily dose of tablet nebivolol 5–10 mg and metoprolol 50–100 mg, respectively. The dose was adjusted according to their blood pressure which was kept below 140/90 mmHg. Those patients were excluded from the study if their targeted blood pressure was not achieved in spite of dose adjustment during first two weeks of therapy.

Brachial blood pressure was measured in right arm in sitting posture by auscultatory method using standard mercury sphygmomanometer apparatus as a mean of three consecutive readings at an interval of 10 minutes. BMI was calculated by standard formula weight in kg/height in m^2 without shoes and wearing light clothes. Blood sample was calculated from the median cubital vein after an overnight fasting of 12 hours. The samples were used for analyzing TLC count, blood sugar, lipid profile, serum total cholesterol (TC), HDL-cholesterol (HDL-C), serum triglycerides (TG), and LDL-cholesterol (LDL-C). Lipid profile and blood sugar were estimated by calibrated semiautomated analyzer. Total leukocyte count was analyzed by automated hematology analyzer Sysmex KX-21. Neutrophil lymphocyte ratio (NLR) was calculated by dividing the absolute neutrophil ratio to absolute lymphocyte ratio.

3. Data Analysis

All numeric data were presented as mean ± standard deviation and percentages. Continuous variables for normal distribution were assessed by using Kolmogorov-Smirnov test. With respect to these test results, we used Mann–Whitney *U* and independent *t*-test as appropriate. The comparisons between two groups in terms of statistical significance were done by chi-squared, Mann–Whitney *U* and independent *t*-test. Continuous variables were compared by two-tailed paired *t*-test by pre- and posttreatment. Data were analyzed by using SPSS 16 software. A $p < 0.05$ was considered to be statistically significant.

4. Results

A total of 120 patients were enrolled in the study, out of which, 10 patients, 4 in the nebivolol and 6 in metoprolol, cannot complete the study because they were lost of follow-up. Both groups tolerated the drug very well with no major adverse effects being reported during the study; however, two patients in nebivolol group and one patient in metoprolol group developed symptomatic bradycardia and withdrawal from the study. Three patients in nebivolol and four patients in metoprolol group were found to be nonresponders to drug regime and also withdraw from the study. A total of 100 patients completed the study, 51 in nebivolol and 49 in metoprolol group. There was no significant difference in both groups in terms of baseline demographic and clinical

TABLE 1: Comparison of baseline characteristics and inflammatory parameters between two groups.

Parameters	Nebivolol group ($n = 51$)	Metoprolol group ($n = 49$)	p value**
Age (years)	52.46 ± 8.32	54.60 ± 7.82	0.20**
Male (n = %)	35 (68.6)	32 (65.3)	0.74***
BMI (kg/m^2)			
Before	26.95 ± 4.82	27.24 ± 3.86	0.99**
After	26.25 ± 3.56	27.45 ± 4.25	0.94**
p	0.38*	0.59*	
SBP (mmHg)			
Before	149 ± 15	148 ± 14	0.36**
After	131 ± 11	136 ± 8	0.68**
p	<0.001*	<0.001*	
DBP (mmHg)			
Before	92 ± 10	93 ± 11	0.09**
After	80 ± 11	83 ± 10	0.17**
p	<0.001*	<0.001*	
WBC count × 10^9/L			
Before	9.4 ± 3.8	9.2 ± 3.6	0.66**
After	7.6 ± 3.1	9.3 ± 4.72	0.001***
p	0.005*	0.69**	
Neutrophil count × 10^9/L			
Before	7.5 ± 2.8	7.6 ± 3.2	0.26**
After	4.9 ± 3.2	7.4 ± 4.5	0.009**
p	0.003*	0.69*	
Lymphocyte count × 10^9/L			
Before	2.1 ± 0.7	2.2 ± 1.62	0.72**
After	2.4 ± 0.8	2.1 ± 1.45	0.02**
p	0.004*	0.78*	
NLR			
Before	4.4 ± 2.2	4.5 ± 3.2	0.76**
After	2.2 ± 1.5	4.4 ± 2.7	0.004***
p	0.007*	0.49*	

Values are mean ± SD; *paired t-test; **independent sample t-test; ***Mann–Whitney U test.

parameters (Table 1). Both drugs lowered blood pressure significantly, nebivolol 20.5/10.5 and metoprolol 22.5/11.2 with ($p < 0.001$) from baseline. In comparison with metoprolol, nebivolol caused a significant reduction in total leukocyte count ($p = 0.005$) and neutrophil count ($p = 0.003$) and increased lymphocyte count ($p = 0.004$). Similarly, nebivolol but not metoprolol significantly reduced NLR ratio ($p = 0.07$). Nebivolol in comparison with metoprolol also improved blood sugar and lipid profile but values were found to be nonsignificant (Table 2).

5. Discussion

The present study was conducted to investigate the effect of nebivolol on NLR, a subclinical inflammatory marker in hypertensive patients. Subclinical inflammation is a silent killer in hypertensive patients which cannot manifest clinically for years but it can cause endothelial dysfunction that predispose to atherosclerosis and its related complication in the form of various cardiovascular and cerebrovascular disorders in future [15].

NLR is a new addition in the list of inflammatory markers and has got special attention in recent years because it has strong independent diagnostic as well as prognostic value for atherosclerosis related vascular diseases and its associated risk factors such as hypertension, diabetes, metabolic syndrome, and dyslipidemia [16]. Studies have shown the important role of NLR in hypertension. Increased NLR has strong independent association with the severity of hypertension in untreated cases of essential hypertension. Similarly NLR is a strong predictor of both resistant and nondipper hypertension in various clinical studies. Similarly a large-scale epidemiological study reveals that elevated level NLR have significant correlation with an increasing risk of developing hypertension over a follow-up period of 6 years [17–20]. In addition NLR has prognostic significance in hypertension associated complications such as heart failure, coronary artery, cerebral artery, and peripheral artery

TABLE 2: Comparison of the lipid profile and blood sugar between two groups.

Parameters	Nebivolol group ($n = 51$)	Metoprolol group ($n = 49$)	p value**
Total cholesterol (mg/dl)			
Before	187.32 ± 31.22	188.82 ± 33.43	0.88
After	184.65 ± 27.35	190.68 ± 36.92	0.62
p^*	0.54	0.16	
Triglycerides (mg/dl)			
Before	130.36 ± 60.54	133.34 ± 43.86	0.73
After	126.45 ± 54.62	138 ± 52.45	0.62
p^*	0.13	0.17	
LDL-cholesterol (mg/dl)			
Before	127.42 ± 44.43	134.54 ± 42.56	0.79
After	123.65 ± 38.85	136.82 ± 36.78	0.80
p^*	0.54	0.82	
HDL-cholesterol (mg/dl)			
Before	43.85 ± 12.46	44.42 ± 8.62	0.64
After	45.32 ± 11.52	43.67 ± 11.82	0.49
p^*	0.13	0.17	
Blood sugar (mg/dl)			
Before	84.82 ± 8.82	86.42 ± 11.2	0.54
After	82.54 ± 9.89	87.56 ± 10.5	0.68
p^*	0.34	0.56	

LDL-C, low-density lipoprotein cholesterol; HDL-C, high-density lipoprotein cholesterol; values are mean ± SD; *paired t-test; **independent sample t-test.

disease. In order to detect this inflammation, neutrophil to lymphocyte ratio NLR gives valuable information about the severity of atherosclerosis in various studies. This test is simply performed by dividing the absolute neutrophil count to absolute lymphocyte count in peripheral blood sample. Moreover this test is quite inexpensive, usually not requiring a proper setup and can be used as screening and drug monitoring tool in population on large scale [16, 21].

In this study, nebivolol caused a significant reduction in NLR after 12-week treatment. Nebivolol has a strong potential to reverse hypertension associated inflammatory changes by a variety of suspected mechanisms. First nebivolol improves endothelial dysfunction that causes endothelial cells to initiate inflammation by the generation of reactive oxygen species and proinflammatory cytokines [22]. Second nebivolol increases the level of nitric oxide in vessel causing vasodilatation by interacting with L-arginine/nitric oxide pathway as inflammation blocks the ability of endothelium to generate nitric oxide and prostacyclin [23]. Finally nebivolol itself has strong antioxidant and anti-inflammatory potential by reducing the production of hs-CRP, interleukin-6 (IL-6), vascular adhesion molecule (VCAM-1), adiponectin, and leptin in hypertensive patients in various clinical studies [12–24].

Regarding antihypertensive drugs, a very limited work has been done in the past to see their effect on NLR. A study conducted by Karaman et al. [25] revealed that amlodipine (calcium channel blocker) and valsartan (angiotension receptor antagonist) improved endothelial dysfunction and vascular inflammation by decreasing the level of both Von Willebrand factor and NLR in newly diagnosed hypertensive patients, while similar type of work conducted by Fici et al. [26] demonstrated that nebivolol significantly reduced red cell distribution width (RDW), total leukocyte count, and N/L ratio as compared to metoprolol in newly diagnosed hypertensive patients over a period of 6 months. Our study showed similar results to that of Fici et al. in terms of TLC count and N/L ratio but the duration of study was 3 months.

Most of the beta-blockers have adverse effect on glucose and lipid metabolisms. In this study nebivolol did not disturb lipid and glucose metabolism. Although it improved lipid profile to some extent in comparison with metoprolol but values were found to be nonsignificant. This has additional beneficial effect as both deranged blood sugar and lipid profiles themselves initiate a process of vascular inflammation. Seeing these beneficial effects of nebivolol, it should be considered in hypertensive patients in order to prevent its future complications. Moreover, NLR, a routine test, can be used as a drug and disease monitoring tool in these patients as it has diagnostic as well as prognostic value in various cardiovascular disorders.

6. Conclusion

Nebivolol has a strong potential to decrease NLR reverse subclinical inflammation in hypertensive patients.

Additional Points

Clinical Implication. Elevated NLR is very important marker and has an important role in the detection of ongoing vascular inflammation. Treatment with nebivolol may improve cardiovascular outcome by decreasing NLR. *Limitation of Study*. The main limitation of the study was that NLR was not compared with other important inflammatory markers such as C-reactive protein which is the most studied marker to detect inflammation in various cardiovascular disorders. Further studies with large sample size should be conducted to compare the effect of nebivolol on various inflammatory markers.

Disclosure

All members hereby agree to take responsibility of the work and confirm that all questions related to the accuracy and integrity of the research have been properly and thoroughly resolved.

Authors' Contributions

Mazhar Hussain and Muhammad Saeed conceived the idea, manuscript review, and statistical analysis. Muhammad Zafar Majeed Babar and Moazzam Ali Atif designed the study and prepared the manuscript and data analysis. Lubna Akhtar searched the literature and collected the clinical data and manuscript editing.

Acknowledgments

The authors acknowledge Department of Cardiology and Pathology of Sheikh Zayed Medical College/Hospital, Rahim Yar Khan, for their cooperation during the study.

References

[1] B. V. Mittal and A. K. Singh, "Hypertension in the Developing World: Challenges and Opportunities," *American Journal of Kidney Diseases*, vol. 55, no. 3, pp. 590–598, 2010.

[2] C. Deaton, E. S. Froelicher, L. H. Wu, C. Ho, K. Shishani, and T. Jaarsma, "The Global Burden of Cardiovascular Disease," *The Journal of Cardiovascular Nursing*, vol. 10, no. 2, pp. 5–13, 2011.

[3] M. Madjid and O. Fatemi, "Components of the complete blood count as risk predictors for coronary heart disease: in-depth review and update," *Texas Heart Institute Journal*, vol. 40, no. 1, pp. 17–29, 2013.

[4] P. C. Tong, K.-F. Lee, W.-Y. So et al., "White Blood Cell Count Is Associated with Macro- and Microvascular Complications in Chinese Patients with Type 2 Diabetes," *Diabetes Care*, vol. 27, no. 1, pp. 216–222, 2004.

[5] F. Imtiaz, K. Shafique, S. Mirza, Z. Ayoob, P. Vart, and S. Rao, "Neutrophil lymphocyte ratio as a measure of systemic inflammation in prevalent chronic diseases in Asian population," *International Archives of Medicine*, vol. 5, no. 1, article 2, 2012.

[6] S. Balta, E. Kurtoglu, U. Kucuk, S. Demirkol, and C. Ozturk, "Neutrophil-lymphocyte ratio as an important assessment tool," *Expert Review of Cardiovascular Therapy*, vol. 12, no. 5, pp. 537-538, 2014.

[7] S. Balta, T. Celik, D. P. Mikhailidis et al., "The relation between atherosclerosis and the neutrophil–lymphocyte ratio," *Clinical and Applied Thrombosis/Hemostasis*, vol. 22, no. 5, pp. 405–411, 2014.

[8] C. Ozturk, S. Balta, I. Balta et al., "Neutrophil-lymphocyte ratio and carotid-intima media thickness in patients with behçet disease without cardiovascular involvement," *Angiology*, vol. 66, no. 3, pp. 291–296, 2014.

[9] K. Turkmen, I. Guney, F. H. Yerlikaya, and H. Z. Tonbul, "The relationship between neutrophil-to-lymphocyte ratio and inflammation in end-stage renal disease patients," *Renal Failure*, vol. 34, no. 2, pp. 155–159, 2012.

[10] J. Eduardo Toblli, F. Digennaro, J. Fernando Giani, and F. Pablo Dominici, "Nebivolol: Impact on cardiac and endothelial function and clinical utility," *Vascular Health and Risk Management*, vol. 8, no. 1, pp. 151–160, 2012.

[11] J. Fongemie and E. Felix-Getzik, "A Review of Nebivolol Pharmacology and Clinical Evidence," *Drugs*, vol. 75, no. 12, pp. 1349–1371, 2015.

[12] N. Merchant, S. T. Rahman, K. C. Ferdinand, T. Haque, G. E. Umpierrez, and B. V. Khan, "Effects of nebivolol in obese African Americans with hypertension (NOAAH): Markers of inflammation and obesity in response to exercise-induced stress," *Journal of Human Hypertension*, vol. 25, no. 3, pp. 196–202, 2011.

[13] M. Serg, P. Kampus, J. Kals et al., "Nebivolol and metoprolol: Long-term effects on inflammation and oxidative stress in essential hypertension," *Scandinavian Journal of Clinical and Laboratory Investigation*, vol. 72, no. 5, pp. 427–432, 2012.

[14] J. A. Whitworth, "World Health Organization (WHO)/International Society of Hypertension (ISH) statement on management of hypertension," *Journal of Hypertension*, vol. 21, no. 11, pp. 1983–1992, 2003.

[15] P. Pietri, C. Vlachopoulos, and D. Tousoulis, "Inflammation and arterial hypertension: From Pathophysiological links to risk prediction," *Current Medicinal Chemistry*, vol. 22, no. 23, pp. 2754–2761, 2015.

[16] T. Bhat, S. Teli, J. Rijal et al., "Neutrophil to lymphocyte ratio and cardiovascular diseases: a review," *Expert Review of Cardiovascular Therapy*, vol. 11, no. 1, pp. 55–59, 2013.

[17] T. Cimen, H. Sunman, T. H. Efe et al., "The relationship between 24-hour ambulatory blood pressure load and neutrophil-to-lymphocyte ratio," *Revista Portuguesa de Cardiologia*, vol. 36, no. 2, pp. 97–105, 2017.

[18] M. Sunbul, F. Gerin, E. Durmus et al., "Neutrophil to lymphocyte and platelet to lymphocyte ratio in patients with dipper versus non-dipper hypertension," *Clinical and Experimental Hypertension*, vol. 36, no. 4, pp. 217–221, 2014.

[19] N. Dagli, O. Dogdu, O. Senarslan et al., "Relation of neutrophil/lymphocyte ratio to resistant hypertension," *The European Research Journal*, vol. 2, no. 3, p. 211, 2016.

[20] X. Liu, Q. Zhang, H. Wu et al., "Blood Neutrophil to Lymphocyte Ratio as a Predictor of Hypertension," *American Journal of Hypertension*, vol. 28, no. 11, pp. 1339–1346, 2015.

[21] B. D. Horne, J. L. Anderson, J. M. John et al., "Which white blood cell subtypes predict increased cardiovascular risk?" *Journal of the American College of Cardiology*, vol. 45, no. 10, pp. 1638–1643, 2005.

[22] J. G. Howlett, "Nebivolol: Vasodilator properties and evidence for relevance in treatment of cardiovascular disease," *Canadian Journal of Cardiology*, vol. 30, no. 5 S, pp. S29–S37, 2014.

[23] M. Polakowska, J. Orzelska-Gorka, and S. Talarek, "Drugs modulating the L-arginine:NO:cGMP pathway - Current use in therapy," *Current Issues in Pharmacy and Medical Sciences*, vol. 29, no. 1, pp. 14–20, 2016.

[24] T. Celik, A. Iyisoy, H. Kursaklioglu et al., "Comparative effects of nebivolol and metoprolol on oxidative stress, insulin resistance, plasma adiponectin and soluble P-selectin levels in hypertensive patients," *Journal of Hypertension*, vol. 24, no. 3, pp. 591–596, 2006.

[25] M. Karaman, S. Balta, S. A. Ay et al., "The comparative effects of valsartan and amlodipine on vWf levels and N/L ratio in patients with newly diagnosed hypertension," *Clinical and Experimental Hypertension*, vol. 35, no. 7, pp. 516–522, 2013.

[26] F. Fici, T. Celik, S. Balta et al., "Comparative effects of nebivolol and metoprolol on red cell distribution width and neutrophil/lymphocyte ratio in patients with newly diagnosed essential hypertension," *Journal of Cardiovascular Pharmacology*, vol. 62, no. 4, pp. 388–393, 2013.

Permissions

All chapters in this book were first published in IJH, by Hindawi Publishing Corporation; hereby published with permission under the Creative Commons Attribution License or equivalent. Every chapter published in this book has been scrutinized by our experts. Their significance has been extensively debated. The topics covered herein carry significant findings which will fuel the growth of the discipline. They may even be implemented as practical applications or may be referred to as a beginning point for another development.

The contributors of this book come from diverse backgrounds, making this book a truly international effort. This book will bring forth new frontiers with its revolutionizing research information and detailed analysis of the nascent developments around the world.

We would like to thank all the contributing authors for lending their expertise to make the book truly unique. They have played a crucial role in the development of this book. Without their invaluable contributions this book wouldn't have been possible. They have made vital efforts to compile up to date information on the varied aspects of this subject to make this book a valuable addition to the collection of many professionals and students.

This book was conceptualized with the vision of imparting up-to-date information and advanced data in this field. To ensure the same, a matchless editorial board was set up. Every individual on the board went through rigorous rounds of assessment to prove their worth. After which they invested a large part of their time researching and compiling the most relevant data for our readers.

The editorial board has been involved in producing this book since its inception. They have spent rigorous hours researching and exploring the diverse topics which have resulted in the successful publishing of this book. They have passed on their knowledge of decades through this book. To expedite this challenging task, the publisher supported the team at every step. A small team of assistant editors was also appointed to further simplify the editing procedure and attain best results for the readers.

Apart from the editorial board, the designing team has also invested a significant amount of their time in understanding the subject and creating the most relevant covers. They scrutinized every image to scout for the most suitable representation of the subject and create an appropriate cover for the book.

The publishing team has been an ardent support to the editorial, designing and production team. Their endless efforts to recruit the best for this project, has resulted in the accomplishment of this book. They are a veteran in the field of academics and their pool of knowledge is as vast as their experience in printing. Their expertise and guidance has proved useful at every step. Their uncompromising quality standards have made this book an exceptional effort. Their encouragement from time to time has been an inspiration for everyone.

The publisher and the editorial board hope that this book will prove to be a valuable piece of knowledge for researchers, students, practitioners and scholars across the globe.

List of Contributors

Sudhiranjan Gupta
Division of Molecular Cardiology, Department of Medicine, Texas A and M Health Science Center College of Medicine, Temple, TX 76504, USA
Baylor Scott and White Health, Temple, TX 76508, USA
Central Texas Veterans Health Care System, Temple, TX 76504, USA

Li Li
Division of Molecular Cardiology, Department of Medicine, Texas A and M Health Science Center College of Medicine, Temple, TX 76504, USA
Department of Physiology and Pathophysiology, Peking University Health Science Center, Beijing 100191, China

Mehdi Mirsaeidi, Golnaz Ebrahimi and Micheal Campos
Division of Pulmonary, Critical Care, Sleep and Allergy, Department of Medicine, University of Miami, FL, USA

Hesham R. Omar
Internal Medicine Department, Mercy Medical Center, Clinton, IA, USA

Rafael V. Picon
Postgraduate Studies Program in Cardiology, School of Medicine, Universidade Federal do Rio Grande do Sul, R. Ramiro Barcelos 2600, 90035-003 Porto Alegre, RS, Brazil

Juvenal S. Dias-da-Costa and Maria Teresa A. Olinto
Postgraduate Program of Collective Health, Universidade do Vale do Rio dos Sinos, São Leopoldo, RS, Brazil

Flavio D. Fuchs
Division of Cardiology, Hospital de Clinicas de Porto Alegre, Universidade Federal do Rio Grande do Sul, Porto Alegre, RS, Brazil

Niteesh K. Choudhry
Division of Pharmacoepidemiology and Pharmacoeconomics, Brigham and Women's Hospital, Harvard School of Medicine, Harvard University, Boston, MA,USA

Sandra C. Fuchs
Postgraduate Studies Program in Cardiology, School of Medicine, Universidade Federal do Rio Grande do Sul, R. Ramiro Barcelos 2600, 90035-003 Porto Alegre, RS, Brazil
Postgraduate Studies Program in Epidemiology, School of Medicine, Universidade Federal do Rio Grande do Sul, R. Ramiro Barcelos 2600, 90035-003 Porto Alegre, RS, Brazil

Azin Behnood-Rod
Islamic Azad University, Tehran Medical Branch, Tehran, Iran

Omid Rabbanifar
Zanjan University of Medical Sciences, Zanjan, Iran

Pirouz Pourzargar, Zahra Saadat and Habibollah Saadat
Cardiovascular Research Center, Shahid Beheshti University of Medical Sciences, Tehran, Iran

Alireza Rai
School of Medicine, Kermanshah University of Medical Sciences, Kermanshah, Iran

Yashar Moharamzad
Cardiovascular Research Center, Shahid Beheshti University of Medical Sciences, Tehran, Iran
School of Medicine, Kermanshah University of Medical Sciences, Kermanshah, Iran

Donald E. Morisky
Department of Community Health Sciences, UCLA Fielding School of Public Health, Los Angeles, CA, USA

Christian Akem Dimala
Faculty of Epidemiology and Population Health, London School of Hygiene and Tropical Medicine, London, UK
Department of Orthopaedics, Southend University Hospital, Essex, UK
Health and Human Development (2HD) Research Network, Douala, Cameroon

Benjamin Momo Kadia
Presbyterian General Hospital Acha-Tugi, Acha-Tugi, Cameroon
Grace Community Health and Development Association (GRACHADA), Kumba, Cameroon

Ben-Lawrence Kemah
Health and Human Development (2HD) Research Network, Douala, Cameroon
Department of Vascular Surgery, Ashford and St Peter's Hospitals NHS, Surrey, UK

Maxime Tindong
Health and Human Development (2HD) Research Network, Douala, Cameroon
Department of Public Health, Université libre de Bruxelles, Brussels, Belgium

Simeon-Pierre Choukem
Health and Human Development (2HD) Research Network, Douala, Cameroon
Diabetes and Endocrinology Unit, Department of Internal Medicine, Douala General Hospital, Douala, Cameroon
Department of Internal Medicine and Paediatrics, Faculty of Health Sciences, University of Buea, Buea, Cameroon

Juan Torrado, Ignacio Farro, Yanina Zócalo, Federico Farro and Daniel Bia
Centro Universitario de Investigación, Innovación y Diagnóstico Arterial (CUiiDARTE), Physiology Department, Faculty of Medicine, Republic University, 2125 General Flores, 11800 Montevideo, Uruguay

Claudio Sosa, Santiago Scasso and Justo Alonso
Department of Obstetrics and Gynecology "C", Pereira Rossell Hospital, Faculty of Medicine, Republic University, 1550 Bulevar Artigas, 11600Montevideo, Uruguay

Tadesse Melaku Abegaz, Yonas Getaye Tefera and Tamrat Befekadu Abebe
College of Medicine and Health Sciences, School of Pharmacy, Department of Clinical Pharmacy, University of Gondar, Gondar, Ethiopia

Vaia D. Raikou
Department of Nephrology, Doctors' Hospital, Athens, Greece

Despina Kyriaki
Department of Nuclear Medicine, General Hospital "Laïko", Athens, Greece

Samuel H. Nyarko
Department of Population and Behavioural Sciences, School of Public Health, University of Health and Allied Sciences, Hohoe, Ghana

Masahiro Horiuchi
Division of Human Environmental Science, Mt. Fuji Research Institute, Japan

Arisa Ni-i-nou and Mitsuhiro Miyazaki
Faculty of Education and Human Sciences, University of Yamanashi, Japan

Daisuke Ando and Katsuhiro Koyama
Graduate School Department of Interdisciplinary Research, University of Yamanashi, Japan

Juliet Iwelunmor and Sarah Blackstone
University of Illinois, Urbana-Champaign, Champaign, IL 61872, USA

Joyce Gyamfi and Gbenga Ogedegbe
New York University, New York, NY 10016, USA

Collins Airhihenbuwa
Pennsylvania State University, State College, PA 16802, USA

Jacob Plange-Rhule and Richard Adanu
University of Ghana, Legon, Accra, Ghana

Bamidele Tayo
Loyola University Chicago, Chicago, IL 60660, USA

Girma Fikadu and Seblewengel Lemma
Addis Continental Institute of Public Health, Addis Ababa, Ethiopia

Alejandro Diaz
Instituto de Investigación en Ciencias de la Salud, UNICEN, CONICET, Tandil, Argentina

Yanina Zócalo and Daniel Bia
Physiology Department, School of Medicine, Centro Universitario de Investigación, Innovación y Diagnóstico Arterial (CUiiDARTE), Republic University, General Flores 2125, 11800 Montevideo, Uruguay

Edmundo Cabrera Fischer
Instituto de Medicina Traslacional, Trasplante y Bioingeniería (IMTTyB), Universidad Favaloro, CONICET, Buenos Aires, Argentina

Tarek M. Mousa and Olakunle O. Akinboboye
Queens Heart Institute, 234 36 Merrick Boulevard, Laurelton, NY 11422, USA

Oluwaseun A. Akinseye
Department of Medicine, Icahn School of Medicine at Mount Sinai, Queens Hospital Center, 82 68 164th Street, Jamaica, NY 11432, USA

Ketevan Berekashvili
Department of Neurology, SUNY Downstate Medical Center, 450 Clarkson Avenue, Brooklyn, NY 11203, USA

Yoshio Iwashima, Fumiki Yoshihara and Satoko Nakamura
Division of Hypertension and Nephrology, Department of Medicine, National Cardiovascular Center, Osaka, Japan

Tetsutaro Matayoshi
Division of Hypertension and Nephrology, Department of Medicine, National Cardiovascular Center, Osaka, Japan
Department of Cardiovascular Medicine, Nephrology and Neurology, University of the Ryukyus, Okinawa, Japan

Kei Kamide
Division of Hypertension and Nephrology, Department of Medicine, National Cardiovascular Center, Osaka, Japan
Division of Health Sciences, Osaka University Graduate School of Medicine, Osaka, Japan

Ryoichi Tanaka
Department of Radiology, National Cardiovascular Center, Osaka, Japan
Division of Cardiovascular Radiology, Department of Radiology, Iwate Medical University, Iwate, Japan

Tetsuya Fukuda
Department of Radiology, National Cardiovascular Center, Osaka, Japan

Takeshi Horio
Division of Hypertension and Nephrology, Department of Medicine, National Cardiovascular Center, Osaka, Japan
Department of General Internal Medicine 3, Kawasaki Medical School, Okayama, Japan

Hajime Nakahama
Division of Hypertension and Nephrology, Department of Medicine, National Cardiovascular Center, Osaka, Japan
Diage Kobe Clinic, Hyogo, Japan

Yusuke Ohya
Department of Cardiovascular Medicine, Nephrology and Neurology, University of the Ryukyus, Okinawa, Japan

Yuhei Kawano
Division of Hypertension and Nephrology, Department of Medicine, National Cardiovascular Center, Osaka, Japan
Department of Medical Technology, Teikyo University, Fukuoka Campus, Fukuoka, Japan

Takuya Kishi
Department of Advanced Therapeutics for Cardiovascular Diseases, Kyushu University Graduate School of Medical Sciences, 3-1-1 Maidashi, Higashi-ku, Fukuoka 812-8582, Japan

Yoshitaka Hirooka
Department of Advanced Cardiovascular Regulation andTherapeutics, Kyushu University Graduate School of Medical Sciences,3-1-1 Maidashi, Higashi-ku, Fukuoka 812-8582, Japan

Kenji Sunagawa
Department of Cardiovascular Medicine, Kyushu University Graduate School of Medical Sciences, 3-1-1 Maidashi, Higashi-ku, Fukuoka 812-8582, Japan

Olivier Pancha Mbouemboue and Jacques Olivier Ngoufack Tsougmo
Department of Biomedical Sciences, Faculty of Science, University of Ngaoundéré, Ngaoundéré, Cameroon
General Medicine Service, Ngaoundéré Regional Hospital, Ngaoundéré, Cameroon

Diana Derew
Department of Biomedical Sciences, Faculty of Science, University of Ngaoundéré, Ngaoundéré, Cameroon

Marcel Tangyi Tamanji
Clinical Laboratory Service, Ngaoundéré Regional Hospital, Ngaoundéré, Cameroon
Faculty of Science, University of Buea, Buea, Cameroon

Debasish Banerjee and John B. Eastwood
Department of Renal Medicine and Transplantation, St Georges, University of London, Cranmer Terrace, London SW17 0RE, UK

Jacob Plange-Rhule
Department of Renal Medicine and Transplantation, St Georges, University of London, Cranmer Terrace, London SW17 0RE, UK
Department of Medicine, Komfo Anokye Teaching Hospital, Kumasi, Ghana

Nihil Chitalia
Department of Renal Medicine and Transplantation, St Georges, University of London, Cranmer Terrace, London SW17 0RE, UK
Department of Renal Medicine, Darent Valley Hospital, Dartford, Kent DA2 8DA, UK

Kwabena Kumi and Frank B. Micah
Department of Renal Medicine, Darent Valley Hospital, Dartford, Kent DA2 8DA, UK

Francesco P. Cappuccio
Division of Mental Health and Wellbeing, University of Warwick, Warwick Medical School, Gibbet Hill Road, Coventry CV4 7AL, UK

Anthony Liwa
Department of Clinical Pharmacology, Weill Bugando School of Medicine, Catholic University of Health and Allied Sciences, Mwanza, Tanzania

Rebecca Roediger
Department of Internal Medicine, Mount Sinai Hospital, 17 East 102nd St, 7th Floor, New York, NY 10029, USA

Hyasinta Jaka
Department of Internal Medicine, Weill Bugando School of Medicine, Catholic University of Health and Allied Sciences, Mwanza, Tanzania

Amina Bougaila
Weill Cornell Medical College in Qatar, Doha, Qatar

Luke Smart
Department of Internal Medicine, Weill Bugando School of Medicine, Catholic University of Health and Allied Sciences, Mwanza, Tanzania
Center for Global Health, Department of Medicine, Weill Cornell Medical College, New York, NY, USA

Stacey Langwick
Department of Anthropology, Cornell University, 261McGrawHall, Ithaca, NY, USA

Robert Peck
Department of Internal Medicine, Weill Bugando School of Medicine, Catholic University of Health and Allied Sciences, Mwanza, Tanzania
Center for Global Health, Department of Medicine, Weill Cornell Medical College, New York, NY, USA

Christiana Aryee
Department of Molecular Medicine, School of Medical Sciences, Kwame Nkrumah University of Science and Technology, Kumasi, Ghana
Becton Dickinson Biosciences Technical Services, West Africa, Accra, Ghana

William K. B. A. Owiredu and Edwin F. Laing
Department of Molecular Medicine, School of Medical Sciences, Kwame Nkrumah University of Science and Technology, Kumasi, Ghana
Department of Clinical Biochemistry, Diagnostic Directorate, Komfo Anokye Teaching Hospital, Kumasi, Ghana

James Osei-Yeboah
Department of Molecular Medicine, School of Medical Sciences, Kwame Nkrumah University of Science and Technology, Kumasi, Ghana
Department of Medical Laboratory Sciences, School of Allied Health Sciences, University of Health and Allied Sciences, Ho, Ghana

Ellis Owusu-Dabo
School of Public Health, Kwame Nkrumah University of Science and Technology, Kumasi, Ghana
Kumasi Centre for Collaborative Research in Tropical Medicine, Kwame Nkrumah University of Science and Technology, Kumasi, Ghana

Isaac K. Owusu
Department of Medicine, School of Medical Sciences, Kwame Nkrumah University of Science and Technology and Komfo Anokye Teaching Hospital, Kumasi, Ghana

Kathy D. Wright
College of Nursing, Discovery Themes-Chronic Brain Injury, The Ohio State University, Columbus, OH 43210, USA

Carolyn H. Still and Karen O. Moss
Frances Payne Bolton School of Nursing, Case Western Reserve University, Cleveland, OH 44106-4904, USA

Lenette M. Jones
School of Nursing, University of Michigan, Ann Arbor, MI 48109, USA

Karl Peltzer
HIV/AIDS/STIs and TB (HAST), Human Sciences Research Council, Pretoria 0001, South Africa
Department of Research and Innovation, University of Limpopo, Sovenga 0727, South Africa

Supa Pengpid
Department of Research and Innovation, University of Limpopo, Sovenga 0727, South Africa
ASEAN Institute for Health Development, Mahidol University, Salaya, Thailand

Maurílio T. Dutra
Technical School of Health, State Department of Education of the Federal District, Brasília, Brazil
Federal Institute of Education, Science and Technology of Brasília, Brasília, Brazil

Diego B. V. Reis and Karla G. Martins
Technical School of Health, State Department of Education of the Federal District, Brasília, Brazil

André B. Gadelha
Mauá Institute of Research and Education, Vicente Pires, Federal District, Brazil

Whye Lian Cheah, Helmy Hazmi and Grace Woei Feng Kho
Department of Community Medicine and Public Health, Faculty of Medicine and Health Sciences, Universiti Malaysia Sarawak, Kota Samarahan, Sarawak, Malaysia

Ching Thon Chang
Department of Nursing, Faculty of Medicine and Health Sciences, Universiti Malaysia Sarawak, Kota Samarahan, Sarawak, Malaysia

Andrea M. P. Romani
Case Western Reserve University, School of Medicine, Department Physiology and Biophysics, 10900 Euclid Avenue, Cleveland, OH 44106-4970, USA

Verónica Guarner-Lans, Vicente Castrejón-Tellez and María Esther Rubio-Ruiz
Department of Physiology, Instituto Nacional de Cardiología "Ignacio Chávez", 14080 Mexico City, DF, Mexico

Elizabeth Soria-Castro and Rocío Torrico-Lavayen
Department of Pathology, Instituto Nacional de Cardiología "Ignacio Chávez", 14080 Mexico City, DF, Mexico

Araceli Patrón-Soberano
National Laboratory of Nanoscience and Nanotechnology, Molecular Biology Division, Instituto Potosino de Investigación Científica y Tecnológica (IPICYT), 78216 San Luis Potosí, SLP, Mexico

Karla G. Carvajal-Aguilera
Laboratorio de Nutrición Experimental, Instituto Nacional de Pediatría, 04530 Mexico City, DF, Mexico

Nobuo Sasaki, Saeko Fujiwara and Ryo Maeda
Health Management and Promotion Center, Hiroshima Atomic Bomb Casualty Council, Hiroshima, Japan

Ryoji Ozono
Department of General Medicine, Hiroshima University Graduate School of Biomedical and Health Sciences, Hiroshima, Japan

Yasuki Kihara
Department of Cardiovascular Medicine, Hiroshima University Graduate School of Biomedical and Health Sciences, Hiroshima, Japan

Azam Larki and Mahnoush Reisi
Department of Health Education and Health Promotion, Bushehr University of Medical Sciences, Bushehr, Iran

Rahim Tahmasebi
Department of Biostatistics, Bushehr University of Medical Sciences, Bushehr, Iran

Kenneth Nuamah, Ebenezer Antwi Amankwaah, Daniel Boakye, Samuel Kwame Owusu, Fred Adomako-Boateng and Alexis Nang-Beifubah
Ashanti Regional Health Directorate, Kumasi, Ghana

Harriet Affran Bonful
Department of Epidemiology and Disease Control, School of Public Health, University of Ghana, Legon, Accra, Ghana

Joseph Danso Yeboah
Sekyere Central District Health Directorate, Nsuta, Ashanti, Ghana

Adwoa Aduako Owusu
Suntreso Government Hospital, Kumasi, Ghana

Freddie Amponsah and Anthony Ofosu
Policy Planning Monitoring and Evaluation Division, Ghana Health Service, PMB Ministries, Accra, Ghana

Margaret Gyapong and Evelyn K. Ansah
Research Development Division, Ghana Health Service, Accra, Ghana
Institute of Health Research, University of Health and Allied Science, PMB 31, Ho, Ghana

Bertha Garshong
Research Development Division, Ghana Health Service, Accra, Ghana

Daniela Sandoval
Department of Primary Care and Health Family, Faculty of Medicine, University of Chile, Santiago, Chile
Department of Physical Therapy, Faculty of Medicine, University of Chile, Santiago, Chile

Carolina Nazzal
School of Public Heath, Faculty of Medicine, University of Chile, Santiago, Chile

Tomás Romero
School of Medicine, University of California, San Diego, CA, USA
Institutional Review Board, Sharp Health Care, San Diego, CA, USA

Mazhar Hussain, Moazzam Ali Atif and Lubna Akhtar
Department of Pharmacology and Therapeutics, Sheikh Zayed Medical College/Hospital, Rahim Yar Khan, Punjab, Pakistan

Muhammad Saeed
Department of Biochemistry, University Medical and Dental College, Faisalabad, Punjab, Pakistan

Muhammad Zafar Majeed Babar
Department of Medicine, Sheikh Zayed Medical College/Hospital, Rahim Yar Khan, Punjab, Pakistan

Index

R

S

T

V

W